You and Your Health
Volume 2
Dealing With Disease

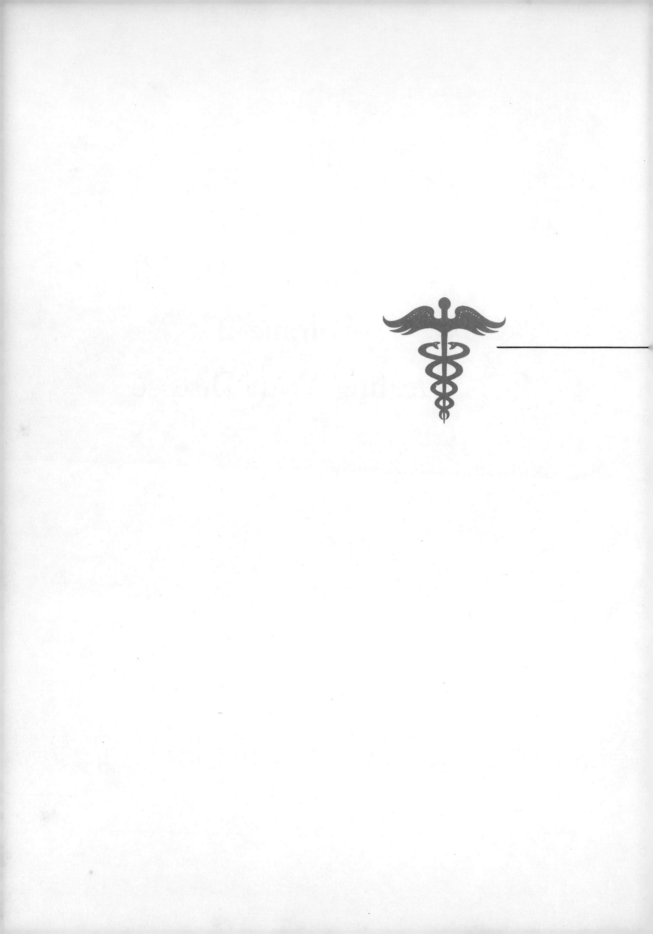

VOLUME 2

You and Your Health

In three volumes
Illustrated
Revised Edition

Dealing With Disease

Harold Shryock, M.D.

**In Collaboration With 38
Leading Medical Specialists**

Southern
Publishing
Association,
Nashville,
Tennessee

Pacific Press Publishing Association,
Mountain View, California
Omaha, Nebraska   Oshawa, Ontario

Review and
Herald
Publishing
Association,
Washington, DC

CONTENTS

Volume 1—More Abundant Living

Volume 2—Dealing With Disease

Volume 3–The Human Body, Emergencies, Signs and Symptoms

SECTION I — Marvels of the Human Body

The Whole Man - The Body a Living Machine - The Body's Framework - The Body's Motive Power - The Body's Covering - The Body's Transportation System - A Filtering System for the Tissues - The Organs for Breathing and Speaking - The Mouth and Teeth - How the Body Is Nourished - The Body's Waste Disposal System - The Glands - The Nervous System - Sensation - The Reproductive Organs - The Body's Defenses

SECTION II — Emergencies, First Aid, Home Treatments

First-aid Kits and Home Medicine Chests - Handling Emergencies - Home Care for the Sick - Simple Home Treatments

SECTION III — Signs and Symptoms

Detecting Signs of Disease - List of Signs and Symptoms

FAMILY MEDICAL RECORDS

GENERAL INDEX

INTRODUCTION

Volume 1 of this set provides instruction on how to live healthfully, successfully, and happily. It deals with family life, care and training of children, and relationships between husband and wife. It goes into the development of a well-rounded personality and the means of preserving good health and maintaining physical fitness. Its message is optimistic in tone and forward-looking in perspective.

This volume serves a different purpose. It is built on the recognition that sickness and suffering do exist, whether we like it or not. Much of the illness that prevails could have been prevented had such instruction as that contained in volume 1 been heeded. But mere regrets do not restore health. So the present volume is intended for the person who, finding himself sick, asks, Now what do I do?

Volume 2 is also intended to reinforce the message of volume 1, not only by saying, "This is what may happen if you fail to take good care of your body," but also by providing scientific information for the health-conscious.

By its very nature, the realistic message of *Dealing With Disease* is not as cheerful as that of volume 1. But it needs to be given and heard, for it can be lifesaving to those who, even though stricken with illness, will employ right means of aiding the body's capabilities for healing.

SECTION I

Combating Disease

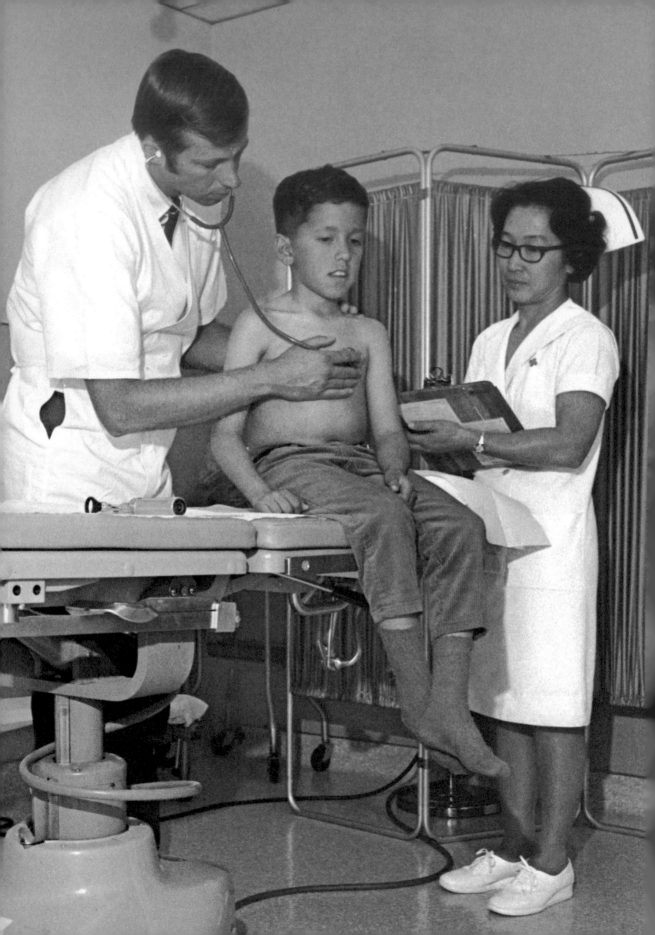

Why Disease?

Medicine's remarkable progress today in combating disease is largely traceable to one outstanding development—a growing understanding of the causes of disease. In fact, medicine's entire system of prevention and treatment is based on this understanding.

Every disease has its cause. The words of Scripture are just as true here as in other phases of life: "The curse causeless shall not come." Proverbs 26:2. Only as we understand what causes disease can we intelligently prevent it. And also only then can we prescribe a rational and effective program of treatment.

Admittedly, a patient who consults a doctor is not as much concerned over the cause of his disease as over how to obtain relief from his symptoms. He suffers because of a headache or a bad cough, or he feels weak and dizzy. To him the important problem is to find a quick remedy. But the doctor, in order to do the best by his patient, must look beyond the symptoms to the cause.

A national health survey conducted by the United States Bureau of Census indicates that 17 million Americans are limited in various degrees in their ability to work, keep house, or conduct routine activities. Five million cannot move about without help, and about one million are unable to leave their homes.

This same national health survey reveals that the average American becomes ill or suffers an injury about two and a half times a year. Upper respiratory disease accounts for 31.1 percent of all acute illnesses, with other respiratory ailments bringing the total for acute respiratory afflictions to 65 percent. Injuries account for 10.9 percent of acute illnesses, infections and parasitic diseases for 8.8 percent, and acute conditions of the digestive organs for 5.5 percent. Miscellaneous acute conditions make up the remaining 9.8 percent of the total.

Germs

Ask any high school student what causes infectious disease, and he will doubtless answer, "Germs." But this answer represents a comparatively modern concept. Only during the latter part of the nineteenth century did medical scientists first recognize the important part germs play in infectious diseases.

Germs are living organisms, many of them belonging to the vegetable kingdom (these are also called bacteria), so small that they can be seen only through the microscope. It would take 2,000, even of the largest ones, placed end to end to make a line an inch long.

Within recent years viruses, which

1

are much smaller, have also been found to cause disease. One must use an electron microscope, with its tremendous magnifying power, to see them.

About the turn of the century scientists began to catalog germs and the respective diseases caused by them. They learned that when a certain kind of germ invades the body's tissues, a definite disease results. This observation led them to assume that to prevent disease one had only to keep germs from entering the human body. This concept is good as far as it goes.

Some disease-producing germs are breathed into the body—for instance, those carried by the spray of tiny droplets thrown into the air by a cough or sneeze. Also some are carried by dust particles in the air, even house dust. But street dust understandably carries many more kinds of germs.

Then there are the germs injected into the blood by mosquitoes or other blood-sucking insects. Malaria, yellow fever, and dengue are transmitted in this way. The germs which cause bubonic plague are carried from rat to man by the bite of fleas. The germs of African sleeping sickness are carried by the tsetse fly. The germs of typhus fever are carried by body lice or fleas, and those of relapsing fever and Rocky Mountain spotted fever, by ticks.

Other common germs are carried by contaminated ice and water and by foods such as salads and milk. The greatest source of danger here is from domestic water supplies contaminated by human excreta. Flies, rats, mice, or unclean hands may carry disease-producing germs and deposit them where they contaminate milk or other food materials. By this means typhoid fever, dysentery, and other gastrointestinal infections are often spread.

The modern science of sanitation is built around a knowledge of the role germs play in producing disease. This science consists essentially of controlling the growth and transmission of

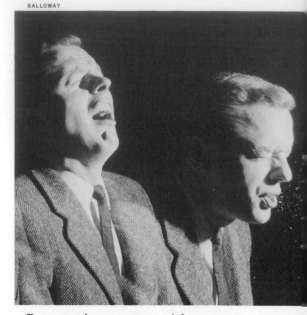

By a cough or sneeze a sick person discharges disease-producing germs into the air around him.

germs and of guarding against invasion.

Conditions Under Which Germs Thrive. All germs must have moisture in order to live and multiply. Most of them need air also, but a few can grow without it. The germ which causes tetanus (lockjaw), for example, grows only in the absence of air.

Most germs which produce disease in human beings thrive best in about the same temperature as that of the human body (98.6° F. or 37° C.). Very few germs grow at temperatures below 50° F. (10° C.). This fact makes refrigeration of food an effective means of preventing disease. As long as food is kept at low temperatures, any germs it may contain cannot multiply. But some germs remain alive for long periods of time even below the freezing point of water.

On the other end of the scale, the growth of germs is hindered by temperatures above about 115° F. (46° C.). Most germs are killed above 145° F. (63° C.) when these temperatures are maintained for as long as half an hour.

This is the basis on which surgical dressings and other such materials are made "sterile" (free from germs) by the use of heat.

Most germs thrive better in darkness than in light. Sunlight is particularly effective in destroying germs.

Certain germs can stop growing and remain dormant for long periods of time, even in spite of dryness and unfavorable temperatures. Then when conditions become favorable again, such germs are revitalized. These dormant forms are called spores.

Chemical Means of Controlling Germs. A great deal of progress has been made in the control of disease-producing germs by the use of chemical disinfectants. Time-honored disinfectants include iodine, phenol solution, potassium permanganate, silver nitrate, and chlorine; but newer and more practical ones are constantly being made available. Care must be exercised in using disinfectants, for almost all are poisonous when taken into the body.

Spores (the dormant form of germs) are difficult to kill. For them it is necessary to use strong disinfectants or high temperatures.

How Germs Harm the Body. Disease-producing germs harm the body in more than one way. Some kinds, such as the one that causes tuberculosis, actually destroy certain body tissues. Others produce toxins (poisons) that circulate in the blood and damage organs or tissues apart from those where the germs originate. The diphtheria germ, for example, multiplies best in the tissues of the pharynx (throat), but its toxin tends to damage the heart and nerves.

The control of germs, important as it is, does not constitute the only means of preventing disease. The human body has ways of altering its resistance to the invasion of germs. There-

Vaccinia virus particles, or cowpox (here magnified 70,000 times by electron microscope) are used in vaccinations against smallpox.

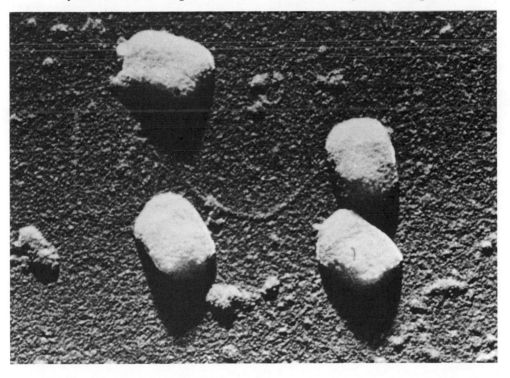

fore it is important to approach the matter from two directions—(1) to protect the body, as far as possible, from invasion by germs, and (2) to maintain such a high level of general health that the body will be able to combat the germs that may enter.

Some germs are so powerful in their ability to cause disease that once they gain entrance into the body they will produce serious illness in spite of the body's usual defense mechanisms. On this account special procedures of immunization must be used to combat them. Diseases such as diphtheria and smallpox fall in this class.

Heredity

In a few diseases, heredity plays a part.

Long before men knew the relationship between germs and disease, they observed that certain maladies tend to run in families. Examples would be diabetes and certain forms of anemia.

The fact that a certain disease may be more common among members of a given family does not prove that faulty heredity is the sole cause of the disease. The habits of the family may have something to do with it too. Faulty diet, indifference to the principles of sanitation, and emotional tensions which lower the body's vitality—any of these, if part of a family's pattern of living, may render the members more susceptible to illness.

Sex difference also constitutes a factor in the incidence of certain diseases. Men more commonly than women are victims of coronary heart disease, of diseases of the lungs, of liver disease, and of tuberculosis. Women, on the other hand, suffer more frequently from diseases of the thyroid. Even after allowing for the influence of a man's way of life in contrast with a woman's we must still recognize that a man's body is peculiarly more susceptible to certain diseases.

Some persons are inherently more resistant to disease because of factors transmitted from parent to child. It is

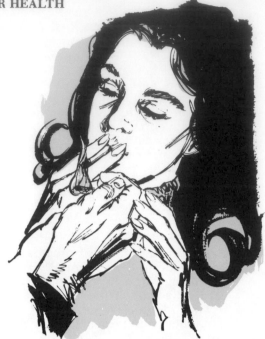

Irritation produced by the use of cigarettes plays a causative role in the development of lung cancer.

now established that irritation produced by the smoking of cigarettes is an important factor in lung cancer. A heavy smoker runs a much greater risk of contracting this ailment than a non-smoker. Even so, certain individuals, in spite of having smoked, do not contract lung cancer. They doubtless inherited such vitality of tissue that they can tolerate the irritating effects of tobacco smoke. Of course, even a person with such natural resistance to certain diseases may still suffer in other ways because of intemperance or indulgence.

In recognizing that heredity plays an important part in determining the individual's susceptibility or resistance to disease, we still cannot order a person's heredity. Everyone must be reconciled to whatever handicaps or assets he may inherit. Especially encouraging then is the fact that heredity is only one of several factors affecting health. Even the person with poor heredity may, by following a plan of healthful living, rise above his inherited tendencies to disease. Contrariwise, the person with a favorable hereditary background may lower his resistance through careless habits and become an easy victim of disease.

Most Diseases Have Multiple Causes

When disease-producing germs were still being discovered and classified, it was easy to assume that a given disease was the direct result of a particular kind of germ. It was then supposed that if a person could remain free from contact with disease-producing germs, he would remain healthy. But if he encountered the germs that produce a given disease, he would fall victim to that disease.

It is now understood, however, that the mere presence of germs in the human body does not always produce disease. Consider tuberculosis for example. The germ *Mycobacterium tuberculosis* is the active agent in causing this illness. This germ is quite widely distributed, however, and even healthy individuals have had many exposures to it. Admittedly, without exposure to the germ, one would not contract tuberculosis. But even when exposed, many people do not contract the disease because of the inhibiting factors of inherent vitality and tissue resistance.

Present evidence indicates that many children, before they reach adulthood, have had contact with *Mycobacterium tuberculosis*. But only a few, proportionately, contract the disease. The factors of personal vitality and tissue resistance figure more prominently in determining whether a person will become ill with tuberculosis than does the factor of exposure to the germ.

Take pneumonia as another example. Any one of several germs may be involved in causing this disease. The most common is *Diplococcus pneumoniae*. But simple contact with this germ does not determine that a person will inevitably become sick with pneumonia. This germ is present in the mouth cavities of many healthy individuals. The factors that tend to prevent the development of pneumonia may vary, but in one way or another they make the individual's tissues less vulnerable to the germ or germs which cause pneumonia.

On the other hand, weakening factors contributing to pneumonia could be loss of sleep, fatigue from overwork, or undue exposure to cold. In addition, possibly a background of unfavorable experiences such as anxiety and worry may have depleted the individual's nervous reserves, thus weakening the brain's usual influence over the body tissues and lessening their ability to function efficiently.

Even in the case of a broken leg a combination of factors may be the cause. It is proverbial among skiers that broken legs occur near the end of the day or, at least, when the persons involved have become weary and careless. Skiers go so far as to predict that a person who says, "I am going down the hill just this once more," is the one most likely to have an accident. Weariness, then, shows up as an important contributing factor to misfortune.

Accidents on the highways typically occur when the drivers concerned are overweary, emotionally upset, or mentally beclouded by the use of alcohol or drugs.

Illnesses occur in "clusters" during a person's lifetime. Extensive studies have been made on the relationship of environmental factors to the incidence of disease, and it has been demonstrated that even unrelated illnesses tend to group themselves in various periods of life. A person may be susceptible to several kinds of illness for a period of several months or years. Then a period of relative freedom from illness can follow, only to be succeeded by another "cluster." On closer study, it may become apparent that these periods of illness came at times when the person was making a poor sociologic adjustment to life. Perhaps he was uncertain over

5

the outcome of a financial undertaking. Maybe tensions within the home robbed him of the vital force necessary to maintain his resistance to disease. Perhaps he was insecure during a period of education or training for future responsibilities. As Lord Lytton once remarked, "Half our diseases come from neglect of the body in overwork of the brain."

Habits of Life

Nutrition. The body tissues are built of the food elements in the diet. If these elements are adequate both in quality and variety, then the body tissues will be able to carry on their functions properly. But if some of the necessary nutritional elements are lacking in the diet, the body tissues suffer accordingly.

One's ability to resist disease-producing germs depends in part upon the adequacy of the diet. Carefully controlled animal experiments have demonstrated that the outcome of a given infection depends not only upon the nature of the germs but also upon the quality of the diet—whether or not it promotes the development of tissue resistance to infection. More is said elsewhere in this set about the means of ensuring an adequate diet.

Excessive intake of food has as detrimental an effect on the state of health as does an inadequate diet. Too great an intake promotes excess body weight; and this, in turn, lays the foundation for diseases of the heart and blood vessels—diseases which favor chronic illness and short life.

Nutritional research indicates that a diet which includes too great a proportion of foods with a high percentage of fats (particularly saturated fats) lays the foundation for degenerative diseases. More is said in volume 1, chapter 50, on the proper selection of foods.

Living Conditions. Climate, of course, has its influence on health. Tropical climates pose their particular health hazards, which include problems of sanitation. Colder climates

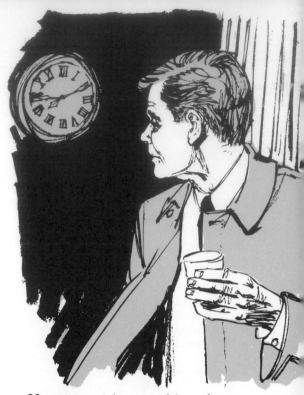

Nervous tension resulting from late hours and overwork weaken vitality and contribute to disease.

introduce elements of fatigue and exposure.

Living conditions in the home also have a definite influence on health. The ideal home provides adequate protection from extremes of temperature and also is designed for cleanliness and sanitation. A cheerful atmosphere promotes contentment and optimism, both favorable to good health.

Personal Habits. The laws of health, like the laws of moral conduct, imply a promise for obedience as well as a penalty for disobedience. An individual may choose whether he will live in harmony with the principles which favor good health or whether he will disregard them and pay the penalty in the form of increased susceptibility to disease. Even a person handicapped by inherited susceptibility to disease may, by compliance with the laws of healthful living, improve his general resistance and enjoy as great a degree of health as the more fortunate person endowed with a rich heritage of vitality.

Two kinds of personal habits influence health: (1) positive habits which are health-promoting, and (2) negative habits which are health-destroying.

Adequate physical exercise, adequate sleep, recreation in the out-of-doors, regular meals with nothing between, an attitude of optimism—all of these habits tend to conserve vitality and to improve resistance to disease.

Personal habits which deplete one's store of vitality and increase the risk of disease include excesses in eating, irregular hours of sleeping, the use of tobacco and alcohol, unnecessary recourse to drugs, and the use of such stimulants as coffee, tea, and cola drinks.

Popular customs do not provide a reliable guide for health habits. It is easy for a person to become the victim of his habits without realizing that his way of life is making him a candidate for invalidism. No personal sacrifice is involved in avoiding health-destroying habits. Quite the contrary, a person lives even more happily.

The Wear-out Diseases

Before we conclude this chapter on the causes of disease we must mention that certain illnesses result from a deterioration of the body's tissues. Aging is a progressive process by which, throughout life, the tissues become less efficient in performing their functions.

The tissues of a certain organ, such as the heart or the kidneys, may wear out before those of other organs. Thus, the final illness may be described as "heart trouble" or "kidney disease" just because these organs have failed first in performing their vital functions.

Inheritance plays a part in determining how fast a person's tissues will deteriorate. So also does one's way of life—a factor of even greater importance to the individual. One who lives conservatively and with due consideration to the laws of health, will live longer than another person who, with

a comparable heredity, dissipates his vital forces by careless living and personal indulgence.

What It Means

Sickness, then, is not something that arbitrarily overtakes a person, descending "out of a clear sky" to bring invalidism here and sudden death there. True, some of the causes of disease, such as heredity, are beyond the individual's control. But many illnesses can be prevented—an obvious fact, now that we understand better the causes of disease.

The primary benefit, therefore, of this discussion on the causes of disease is to encourage you, the reader, to follow such a way of life that will enable you to avoid as many of the causes as possible and thus to prolong your health and usefulness.

The second value is to impress the truth that in order to treat a disease intelligently and effectively, attention

Sleep promotes health, thus increasing resistance to disease.

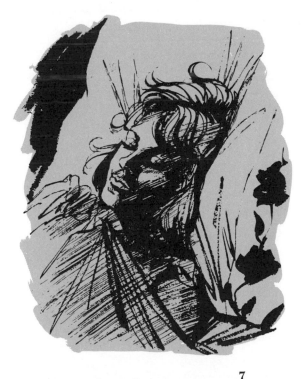

must be focused on its fundamental cause. When a person suffers from a disease caused by a dietary deficiency, he accomplishes nothing worthwhile by taking pain relievers or sedative pills. He must discover and correct the cause. And this is where a physician comes into the picture. Any drugstore salesman can suggest medicines that will relieve a person's pain or otherwise make him less aware of his suffering. But only a physician trained in discovering the actual causes of illness can devise and direct a treatment program that will cure by removing the cause.

Periodic Physical Checkups

For centuries it was assumed that the job of physicians is to *treat* disease. To this extent, physicians were cast in the role of repairmen trained to patch up the human organism, as best they could, once it was injured by disease or accident. It was considered foolish to consult a doctor unless a person was actually sick.

But with the advance of medical science has come an increasing understanding of the causes of disease. Knowing the cause, the next logical step is to remove it and thus prevent the disease. Preventing a disease is better in every way than treating it after it has developed. Suffering is avoided. Complications and resulting handicaps are bypassed. The life-shortening influence of illness is prevented.

With a knowledge of how to prevent disease as well as how to treat it has come a relatively new branch of medical science called "preventive medicine."

Witness the strides that have been made in improving the health of the nation and of the world since the advent of preventive medicine. Contagious diseases are now largely under control. Deaths from typhoid fever, poliomyelitis, smallpox, and diphtheria, to name a few, are almost unheard-of now.

People laughed at physicians and medical research workers when they first began placing emphasis on preventing disease. They said, "You doctors are about to run yourselves out of business." But physicians are happy for the change in the picture of disease as we now see it.

Even though the average person lives much longer now than he did a few decades ago, people still fall and get hurt and therefore still need the care of physicians. But physicians are now able to give more attention to the relief of suffering, to making their patients' lives more enjoyable, and to preventing many of the ordinary illnesses. This type of medical practice brings greater rewards to the physician in terms of human satisfaction than the strictly conventional type generally considered merely curative.

Disease Prevention Requires Cooperation

In order to help his patients stay well, a physician must have their cooperation. A doctor can try to educate people in disease prevention. But unless they take it upon themselves to use the methods taught, they will not be able to rise above the usual dangers of illness.

Modern medical training makes of the physician a specialist in health and the means of keeping people healthy. True, a doctor knows how to treat disease when it occurs, but he prefers to place the emphasis on *keeping* people well rather than on *making* them well. The wise person, then, will consult a doctor and learn from him how to prolong health—that greatest of all human assets.

Imagine a person who has just inherited a large fortune. This newly rich person is not trained in business methods. He realizes the danger, however, of losing his fortune if he does not handle it properly. But he knows also that his wealth can be increased if invested wisely.

If this person is wise, he will seek out an investment counselor—a person trained in business methods and up-to-date on the relative values and reliability of investment opportunities. By soliciting such help the newly rich person, even though not trained in business, can invest his inheritance wisely and can expect to receive satisfactory returns.

Similarly, every normal human being is "wealthy" by having inherited a healthy body. If he uses this body wisely, he will be rewarded by years of good health and resulting happiness. If he is careless and fails to take precautions for the prevention of disease, he runs the risk of shortening life and of forfeiting happiness because of suffering and illness.

In order to handle his health investment wisely, a man or a woman should follow the same pattern as would the wise newly rich person—he finds a counselor trained in matters of health and capable of advising him on how most effectively to promote and maintain his health. This health counselor is none other than the family physician.

The Personal Physician

A personal physician is one to whom a person or a family goes first for matters of sickness or for counsel in ways to prevent illness. This type of physician is interested in the person's or the family's total well-being. It matters not what a person's ailment may be, the personal physician either treats the specific illness or helps his patient to arrange an appointment with a physician who specializes in the treatment of just such problems.

We have been accustomed to speaking of personal physicians as "general practitioners." But recently it has become customary to call them "family physicians." However, personal physicians may include not only the typical family physicians but also the pediatricians who specialize in the health problems of children, as well as specialists in internal medicine who have been trained beyond their regular medical course in handling the diseases which affect the heart, the lungs, the endocrine organs, and the organs of digestion.

It used to be customary to think of the general practitioner as a doctor who had not chosen to specialize in any particular branch of the practice of medicine. Beginning in 1969, however, family medicine was established by the American Medical Association as a specialty in its own right. A young physician who wishes to specialize in family medicine receives training beyond the regular medical course just as does a physician who wishes to specialize in urology or any other specialty. Each receives supervised training in the field of his choice. At the end of such a period of training the specialist in family medicine must pass an examination in order to be certified in this specialty.

The training of the modern family physician includes training in the handling of emergencies, training in hospital procedures, and training in the behavioral sciences as these relate to the health problems of the various members of a family. Such training enables him to evaluate the stresses under which persons in our modern society find themselves. He is qualified to give counsel on the problems of human relations. He evaluates illnesses, treats those that come within his range of experience, and refers others to the proper specialists.

Every married couple and every family should select a family physician to become their personal doctor. This selection should not be delayed until illness occurs. Just as the head of a family does not wait until his house catches on fire to arrange for fire insurance, so there should be an ongoing relationship with the family physician. This enables the physician to guide the family members in their health habits, in their needs for immunizations, in their major decisions that relate to the state of health, and in their illnesses when these occur. By making periodic checkups he can even detect and correct tendencies to illness before the person becomes sick.

Selecting a Family Physician

Certain reliable evidences help a layman to determine whether a particular physician is thorough and dependable in the care of his patients. One, he takes a careful medical history upon the patient's first visit. He goes back to the time of the patient's birth, checking every event that might pertain to his state of health. He keeps this record on file along with the records of the various visits.

Two, he performs a complete physical examination when a patient visits him for the first time and at any time thereafter when such a checkup seems desirable. A complete physical examination means one in which all parts of the body are examined and which includes pertinent laboratory tests.

A competent physician is not content to base his plan of treatment simply on the list of symptoms which the patient recites to him. Rather, he first makes a diagnosis of the patient's basic difficulty and then plans his treatment around the actual cause of this difficulty. This means that an accurate diagnosis must be made before the treatment program is outlined.

You may be new in your community

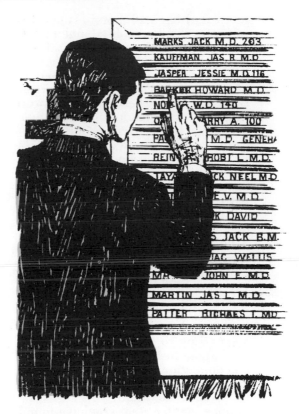

and therefore may not feel well enough acquainted to select one physician from among the several available. The following suggestions should be helpful to you, then, as a means of checking on a physician's reputation and professional qualifications.

1. Write to the national headquarters of the American Academy of Family Physicians in Kansas City, Missouri, requesting a list of the certified family physicians in your area.

2. Call the office of the county medical society and ask for a list of the family physicians in your county.

3. Talk to the administrator or the chief of the medical staff of your local hospital and ask for the names of qualified family physicians. If there are several hospitals in your area, make sure that the hospital where you make inquiry is an accredited institution. If the physician in whom you are

11

interested has staff membership, this indicates that his professional qualifications meet the standards of the hospital.

4. In all medical libraries and in most hospitals, *The American Medical Directory*, published by the American Medical Association, is available. This book lists the names and qualifications of all licensed physicians in the United States. For each physician it gives his age, the types of training he has received, his qualifications for a particular type of practice, and his affiliation with recognized medical organizations.

Before making your final selection, arrange for interviews with physicians you consider likely prospects. Talk to each one frankly about your desire to select a physician who will carry the responsibility for maintaining your health. Ask him about his policy for responding to night calls, about his fees, about his training and his hospital connections. Tell him that you are more interested in keeping well than in being treated after you are sick.

Once you feel that you have found the physician properly qualified to take care of your personal needs, trust him, rely upon him, and follow his suggestions.

Who Needs Checkups?

It is easy to assume that young people are naturally healthy and that, therefore, only older people need the advantage of health consultations. Many of the serious diseases do become manifest in later life. But even these may have had their beginnings years before they caused symptoms. Just as the wise investment of money is a long-range enterprise, so the maintenance of health should begin in childhood and continue throughout life.

Periodic checkups at the doctor's office begin at birth and continue with the preschool child. On starting to school a child is subjected to new demands for adjustment and to new circumstances which may undermine

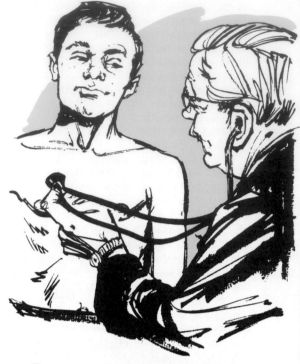

Do young people need checkups?

his health. The preschool child deserves the advantage of being prepared well for his first major venture in life—attending school.

In one carefully recorded study of preschool children, the surprising fact was uncovered that 55 percent of five- and six-year-old children presented at least one health problem. Once the health handicap of a child this age is discovered and properly handled, the prospect for future good health increases. In many five- and six-year-olds who appear healthy, the health problems are not serious. But in others there are such difficulties as orthopedic problems; defects of the heart; allergies; problems of nutrition; problems involving the genito-urinary organs; nervous disorders; diseases of the ear, nose, and throat; and emotional problems.

Still another important factor in the checkup of a preschool child is to make sure he has been immunized against the various contagious diseases. On entering school, a child associates with many others his own age, and the danger of contracting diseases carried from child to child is greatly increased. The preschool checkup, therefore, provides an opportunity to protect the child against illness, loss of school days, and lowered general resistance.

Another era of life when the checkup becomes important is at the beginning of adolescence. At this time, when a child is becoming a man or a woman, he may have fears and anxieties that ordinarily he is too timid to express. If accustomed, however, to having a checkup at the doctor's office each year, he will have learned to respect and trust the doctor and will be able to seek his advice on matters of concern. The girl just coming into womanhood needs professional advice on the meaning of menstruation and on the proper care of her body. The boy becoming a man can benefit by advice from his doctor regarding his newly acquired capacities.

Teen-agers have some special health problems. It is during the teens that problems of nutrition often become acute. It is during these years that growth is most rapid and the demands greatest for adequate vitamins and minerals in the diet. It is during these years that girls sometimes develop the false notion that they should avoid even slight gains in weight. There is danger that with the limited diet sometimes used to keep the weight down, anemia and even tuberculosis may result and handicap the teen-ager.

At the time of courtship and marriage, the family doctor's services are again very important. The adjustment to marriage, the prospect of parenthood, the anxieties that come from trying to make a living while finishing college—all of these have their effect on a person's general health and point up the need for expert advice from the family's health counselor.

Beyond the time of marriage and on through middle age, the advantages of periodic checkups increase progressively, as pointed out in the paragraphs which follow.

What Facts Are Discovered

The average person, even though not trained in medical matters, feels that he is able to detect whether he is in good health. He may feel that it is unnecessary to consult a doctor unless he has symptoms that suggest his need of medical service. In this connection, an interesting study was made at the Tulane University School of Medicine. More than 10,000 apparently healthy persons were given careful examinations to determine how many had health problems of which they were not aware. These 10,000 persons were in the age bracket of thirty to forty-nine years—a time of life when they felt that they were in their prime and not in need of medical service. Very surprisingly, 92 percent of this group of apparently healthy persons had findings of one kind or another that deserved medical attention. It is true that fewer than 1 percent had cancer or other serious disease. However, the minor illnesses which were discovered were such that the health and happiness of the individuals could be improved by receiving the needed attention.

Many physicians who specialize in diseases of women encourage their patients to come to the office each year for an examination and reevaluation of their health status. During the childbearing period and thereafter, cancer is the dread of womankind. Modern medicine provides means of detecting cancer at such an early stage that the physician speaks of it as "precancerous." For example, in one series of cases in which 137,000 women were given the cytologic test for cancer of the uterus and related organs, 659 cases of early cancer were discovered. The cytologic study is made by examining with a microscope the cells contained in a sample of mucus taken from the lining of the vagina. This is a simple procedure

13

which causes no pain or discomfort, yet it provides an accurate means of discovering cancer at the early stage in which it can be treated successfully.

As indicated in the accompanying charts, cancer is only one of many important diseases that can be discovered by periodic examinations at an early stage before symptoms develop. More on what a doctor looks for in making a physical examination is outlined in chapter 21 of volume 3.

Women do not have a monopoly on the advantages to be derived from periodic checkups. Another study was recorded in the city of Philadelphia in which business executives were given routine examinations. In a group of more than 1,500 men, 40 percent were found to have disease of one kind or another which had not been previously recognized. Dealing with these newly discovered diseases in the early stages of their development prevented many months of invalidism as well as many premature deaths.

A wise businessman recognizes that his health constitutes his most valuable asset. He may carry what he considers to be adequate life insurance. But insurance payments give meager consolation when declining health deprives a man of his opportunities to pursue success in business or to continue as the stabilizing influence in his family.

Why Do People Hesitate?

In the face of the obvious advantages resulting from the periodic physical checkup, it seems strange that more people do not accept their doctor's suggestion to come to his office on each birthday. Some people are just naturally fatalistic and think that what is going to be will be. They are aware that many persons are stricken by poor health even in the prime of life. They read about persons who have had to give up important

CAREFUL EXAMINATION CAN DETECT THESE AND OTHER DISEASES BEFORE THEY PRODUCE SYMPTOMS

*Heart disease—various kinds
*High blood pressure and hardening of the arteries
*Cancer of the breast
      lung
      stomach
      colon
      rectum
      uterus
      skin
Lesions of the rectum and lower bowel
Anemia
Kidney disease
Diabetes
Tuberculosis
Glaucoma

*The first three on this list are today's "major killers." Valuable time can be gained and lives can be saved by discovering and treating them early.

careers because of premature illness. But they still cling to the belief, "It can't happen to me."

Ask any surgeon, "What is the best method of preventing death from cancer?" and he will doubtless reply, "Early detection and early treatment."

The performing of a complete physical examination, plus reporting the results to the person being examined and advising him on how to take better care of his health, takes two hours or more of the physician's time in his office. The doctor usually charges $45 or more for the time he spends. In addition there are laboratory procedures and screening tests that provide tangible evidence of the person's present condition of health. These cost an additional $25 or more.

Many persons have complained, after receiving a clear bill of health, "All I received in return for my money was the assurance that I am disgustingly healthy." But such a person will not hesitate to take his car to an automotive service center for its 5000-mile service and pay up to $60. Probably the car runs very little better after the service than it did before. But its period of usefulness will be prolonged by the care which the periodic service provides. From a business standpoint, this is money well spent. Why should there be any difference, then, in spending money for a checkup of one's most valuable asset—his health?

Some people complain that they have to wait too long when an appointment is requested before they get to see the doctor. He may be booked up for several weeks in advance. But consider this: The time of waiting for a routine checkup does not put the person in jeopardy. But when a person waits for symptoms to develop before he requests an appointment with his doctor, every day of continued waiting allows his disease to progress just that much farther and makes the treatment more difficult.

Why the Emphasis on Cancer?

Perhaps it seems that too much emphasis has been placed on cancer in our discussion of the periodic checkup. The shocking fact remains, however, that at present rates, one out of every four persons in the United States will develop cancer of some sort during his lifetime. Because of the inherently treacherous nature of cancer, the outcome of this development in the individual case will depend upon how early and how adequately the cancer is treated. In order for a cancer to be treated early, it must first be discovered. So it is that even for the sake of detecting and treating cancer, the periodic checkup is well worth while.

Physicians are training their women patients to make their own examination of their breasts for the detection of beginning cancer. For the technique of self-examination of the breasts see the discussion of breast cancer in

One in four of the nation's population will have cancer at some time.

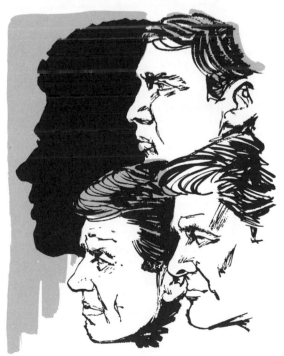

chapter 11 of this volume. Once a woman discovers a small lump in her breast, she is instructed to report at once to her physician, who will determine whether this lump is of a serious nature or whether it is harmless. If there is the possibility of its being serious, the physician will arrange for it to be examined microscopically and will plan his treatment in harmony with the results of this examination.

In men, lung cancer causes more deaths than any other form of cancer. Unfortunately, the symptoms which attract attention to lung cancer develop gradually and too late to be of much help in the treatment of the dread disease. The persistent cough which usually takes a lung cancer victim to the doctor's office comes after the cancer has grown to the extent that it interferes with the passage of air into the involved portion of the lung. The five-year survival rate for persons with the common type of lung cancer, including those who have had surgical treatment, is only about 10 percent. So high is the mortality rate from lung cancer that physicians now advise heavy smokers to come in for an X-ray examination of the chest at least every six months.

Incidental Benefits

The periodic physical checkup is usually not accomplished at a single appointment. It takes a little time for the laboratory tests to be completed and the results reported to your physician. When you return, the doctor explains his observations and the laboratory findings. He is then able to function truly as a health educator. Then he can point out trends, either good or bad. Then he

can give counsel on habits and customs that need to be changed in order to promote your good health.

Your family physician is well acquainted with life as it is lived. He has personal insight into the problems of many persons who live in his community. He is not only trained in the techniques of preventing, detecting, and treating disease, but he has experience in the best methods of dealing with people. He has proved himself to be trustworthy, otherwise he would not be successful as a physician.

Your physician is a person in whom you can safely confide your problems of a personal nature. You can tell him about tensions that may have developed between you and other members of your family. You can seek his advice regarding plans for education, problems relating to your children, prospects for changing employment, and other matters that give you concern. When your doctor sits down to tell you the results of your physical checkup, you have an ideal opportunity to seek his counsel regarding these other problems that affect your life as it is lived.

If you have questions as to what manner of living will contribute most to your prospects of continued health, ask your doctor. Question him regarding the kinds of food that are best for you to eat. Ask him about the number of hours of sleep you need. Seek his guidance on the kind of recreation best suited to your needs. Your doctor is pleased to have you take him into your confidence regarding the matters that mean most to you. If you do your part by calling on him regularly, he will give you the kind of counsel that will help you to live both healthfully and happily.

Immunizations

Immunization provides protection within a person's body, rendering it less susceptible to contagion. But this protection is generally specific for each disease. That is, immunization against smallpox, for example, protects only against smallpox, not against diphtheria, whooping cough, or tetanus. Each disease usually requires a separate defense mechanism. So, in considering the advantages of immunization, we must consider the ways by which a person can be protected against each of the common communicable diseases.

But first a word about immunization in general and the great advantage it offers mankind.

Immunization is something like insurance—it removes the element of risk. But immunization is better than insurance, for insurance only compensates for loss or tragedy, while immunization prevents the tragedy in the first place.

From a business standpoint insurance is a necessity. Without coverage for his home, his car, or his crops a person could suffer disastrous loss. Many also carry accident and hospital insurance. Even out of meager earnings a family, if wise, will pay the cost of this justifiable protection against disaster. It provides financial assistance in case of a major loss or major illness.

Perhaps the public is not as well informed on the equally great need for immunization "insurance." Every person runs the risk of contracting contagious diseases. Epidemics in the past have caused millions of deaths. Now, thanks to medical science, many such diseases can be prevented. But prevention in each case is an individual matter, each person having to take advantage of the immunization procedure effective against a particular disease.

Protection against disease is more important than protection against financial loss. Disease can deprive a person of life itself. But even though the patient survives, he will likely be left with depleted vitality. Furthermore, many contagious diseases leave complications, impairing body organs and thus shortening life expectancy.

Perhaps businessmen exercise more foresight in protecting their assets by insurance than people in general manifest in protecting their bodies against the risk of disease. Also in the matter of immunization itself, certain businessmen have set an example worthy of emulation. Cattlemen, poultrymen, and others concerned with animal husbandry make sure that the animals which represent their financial assets are protected by immunization against disease. But how much more important that the average citi-

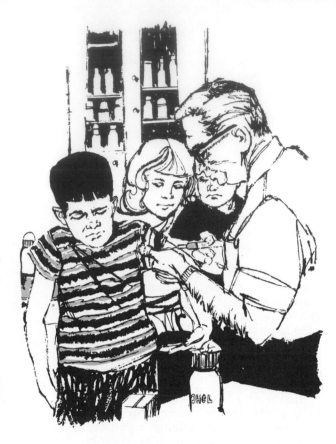

It was in the latter part of the eighteenth century that Dr. Edward Jenner, a young physician in England, became interested in verifying the rumor that milkmaids seldom contracted smallpox. In those days cows were always milked by hand. In England this work was generally done by milkmaids.

Dr. Jenner was aware of a disease called cowpox, prevalent among cows. Perhaps because of handling cows, milkmaids often contracted this disease, but generally only once. It was a mild disease, but was sometimes accompanied by a slight rash from which the milkmaid soon recovered, hardly feeling ill in the meantime.

Dr. Jenner began to wonder whether cowpox and the more severe disease, smallpox, were related. He knew that a person who had had smallpox was also not susceptible to a second attack. He wondered, therefore, whether an attack of cowpox might not cause the same defensive reaction within the body as the more severe disease.

It took many years of convincing and persuading before Dr. Jenner's method of preventing smallpox was generally accepted and before his theory of the relationship between cowpox and smallpox was admitted to be correct.

Dr. Jenner's method of immunizing against smallpox was to transmit cowpox deliberately to a person who had never had smallpox. This would make the person slightly ill, but for a period of a few years thereafter the person thus treated would remain immune to the more severe disease, smallpox.

It is now understood that both smallpox and cowpox are caused by a virus—a disease-producing organism much smaller than ordinary bacteria.

Vaccination for smallpox has of course been greatly refined since Dr. Jenner's day. The doctor now places a small amount of purified vaccine on the skin, usually on the left upper arm. Then with a needle he makes re-

zen should protect life's most valuable possession—the health and physical welfare of himself and the members of his family! He should be consistent in taking advantage of available protection against contagious diseases.

The Story of Smallpox

Smallpox was the first of the contagious diseases to be conquered. The story of how this came about provides good insight into the modern system of immunization for protection from the other contagious diseases.

Smallpox is a distressing disease which may be fatal, which sometimes causes blindness, which usually causes disfigurement, and which in previous centuries has been a scourge to the entire world. This is the disease which first lent itself to the benefits of immunization. So we will relate here the story of smallpox vaccination.

peated pressure on the skin through the droplet of vaccine. This introduces a small amount of the vaccine into the skin. In a person not previously immunized against smallpox, a reddening of skin at the vaccination site will occur a few days later and a slight feeling of illness may persist for two or three days. The reddened area on the arm should be kept dry until it has healed completely. A light gauze dressing may be strapped loosely over the area while it is healing.

Thanks to the active program of vaccination for smallpox carried on throughout the world, smallpox as a disease has been almost eradicated. Occasional cases do still occur in some places; however, in the United States it is a conquered disease. In 1971 the U.S. Public Health Service advised that it is no longer necessary to vaccinate for smallpox except in cases such as of travelers to and from countries where smallpox possibly still exists. Should it happen that smallpox is again introduced into the United States and threatens to become epidemic, there would be time enough to heed the warning of our Public Health Service and arrange for vaccination.

(For a discussion of this disease and proper treatment see *Smallpox* in chapter 28 of this volume.)

A Program for Immunization

Seven additional contagious diseases, which were formerly very common, can now be prevented by immunization. We will consider them one at a time, mentioning the methods by which they can now be prevented. Then, after considering them, we will summarize our discussion by offering an immunization schedule which if followed can give a child maximum protection.

1. *Whooping Cough (Pertussis)*. Whooping cough used to be considered a harmless disease, just a little more severe than an ordinary cold. Many persons—except the person involved—made fun of the severe

coughing, followed by near choking and finally by the characteristic "whoop."

The disease is now recognized as serious. For babies under three months of age whooping cough carries a 25 percent mortality rate. In children under four years of age the fatality rate for whooping cough is 5 percent. Deaths from this disease usually result from one or more of the serious complications such as pneumonia, damage to the lung on account of the severe coughing, or hemorrhage into various organs, including the brain. Sometimes hernia results from the severe coughing episodes.

Fortunately an effective agent is now available for immunizing against whooping cough—a vaccine administered by injection. The immunity conferred is not as long-lasting as some others. Doctors therefore recommend repeated doses during the child's first six years as recommended in this chapter.

2. *Diphtheria*. Diphtheria is another communicable disease now under good control, thanks to widespread immunization. But this comforting knowledge carries with it the danger that persons may become complacent, willingly taking a chance rather than carrying through the proper procedure for immunization.

This disease involves the tissues of the pharynx and larynx and those of the air passages into the lungs. It is characterized by the development of a thick membrane covering the tissues involved. The disease is serious because this membrane sometimes obstructs the air passages and also because the germs causing diphtheria produce a toxin very damaging to the heart. In the days before immunization, diphtheria caused the death and invalidism of many children.

Immunization for diphtheria should be begun early in an infant's life and should be renewed at intervals thereafter as specified in the recommended schedule in this chapter.

(For a discussion of this disease and

proper treatment see *Diphtheria* in chapter 28 of this volume.)

3. *Polio (Poliomyelitis).* Many adult readers of this book will recall the days before the conquest of polio when this disease was a terror to every family and every community. Children were more susceptible, but many young adults were also affected. The principal manifestation of the disease was paralysis, and this accounts for the name by which it was often called—"infantile paralysis." Just which muscles would be involved could not be predicted. The seemingly most tragic cases were those in which the breathing muscles were paralyzed so that the patient had to be given artificial respiration by means of an iron lung. When muscles of the arms, legs, or back were involved, crippling deformities resulted which often persisted throughout life. Entire hospitals were filled with those who barely survived the acute attack of the disease only to

remain invalids because of extensive paralysis. Many cases of "bulbar polio," which affected the brainstem, ended fatally.

No wonder then that people everywhere rejoiced when polio was brought under control by immunization. In 1954 there were an estimated 38,000 cases in the United States. Vaccination for polio began in 1955, and that year there were about 29,000 cases. Then the number of cases began to drop off rapidly. In 1973 there were 14 cases with three deaths. In 1974, only four cases with no deaths. A marvelous conquest of a terrible disease!

But the danger still lurks. The polio virus is still around. And because people tend to forget the tragedies of the past, they are not as insistent on vaccination for polio as they were when the children of neighbors and friends—as well as many adults— were being paralyzed by this disease.

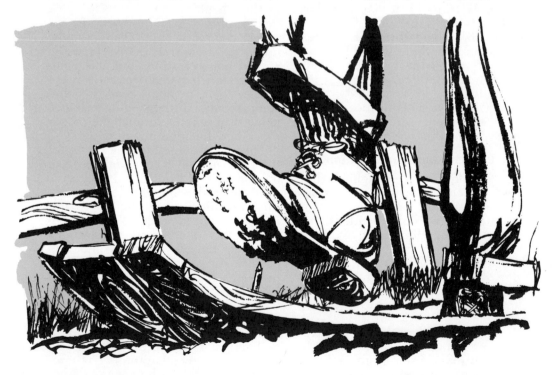

Tetanus germs, commonly present in barnyards, may be introduced into the body by a puncture wound such as caused by a nail.

A small epidemic of polio occurred among unvaccinated children in Houston, Texas, in 1968. In 1972 eleven students in a private school in Greenwich, Connecticut, contracted polio within a period of eighteen days. Paralysis developed in nine of these. None of the students or teachers in this school had been immunized!

The sensible way to keep polio under control is to take full advantage of the provision for immunization. The immunization is easily administered and causes practically no inconvenience.

The first immunization for polio should be given to the infant at two months of age. Repeat immunizations should be carried out thereafter to age six as indicated in the recommended schedule in this chapter.

(For a discussion of this disease and proper treatment see *Poliomyelitis* in chapter 28 of this volume.)

4. *Tetanus.* Tetanus, commonly called lockjaw, is a dread disease in which the toxin produced by the tetanus germs affects the nervous system, causing painful spasms of certain muscles, often those that close the jaw and that move the neck. This toxin is highly poisonous, relatively small amounts being capable of causing death.

The germs of tetanus or their spores occur commonly about barnyards, in manure, and in garden mold. Penetrating wounds, such as those caused by a nail or a splinter, may introduce the germs or spores into the deeper tissues, where they multiply most readily in locations not exposed to air.

Special care should be taken of any wound involving the deeper tissues, particularly if it has possibly been contaminated by street or barnyard dirt. Compound fractures in which the broken bones pierce the skin can easily provide entrance for tetanus germs.

The body's resistance to tetanus is not long-lasting. Even an attack of the disease, if survived, does not confer permanent immunity; but with the present good methods of immunization, the body's resistance lasts more than five years. Because immunity to tetanus wanes as time passes, physicians recommend extra protection whenever they deal with a serious penetrating wound, even though the patient may have been previously immunized. With children, the possibility of penetrating injuries is so great that it is best to maintain an active immunity to tetanus throughout the years of childhood. Then later, administer a booster injection periodically as per following schedule, or whenever a serious injury occurs.

The effectiveness of immunization against tetanus is attested by the experience of the United States Armed Forces during World War II. All service personnel were required to be immunized against this disease. As a result, only fifteen cases of tetanus occurred among two thirds of a million wounded men—a phenomenal improvement compared with previous wars, before availability of immunization.

(For a discussion of this disease and proper treatment see *Tetanus* in chapter 28 of this volume.)

5. *Measles (Rubeola).* Measles was common in the U.S. before vaccination. It is a contagious disease more prevalent among children than among adults. Ordinarily the illness is mild, and many persons feel that it is best for a child to have the disease in routine fashion whenever he happens to be exposed. Thus the child builds his own immunity and will be protected from this illness for life.

Measles carries the risk of serious complications, however, and for a frail child particularly, to have him immunized is better than to run the risk of such complications as pneumonia or encephalitis.

(For a discussion of this disease see *Measles* in chapter 28 of this volume.)

6. *German Measles (Rubella).* German measles is a comparatively mild contagious disease as far as the immediate illness is concerned. But

21

when an expectant mother becomes ill during the first three months of her pregnancy, there is grave danger that her unborn child will be so affected by the virus of this disease that it will not develop normally. Many congenital deformities of infants are traceable to such damage by German measles.

A preventive vaccine for German measles (rubella) became available in 1969.

(For a discussion of this disease and proper treatment see *German Measles* in chapter 28 of this volume.)

7. *Mumps.* For children, mumps is a relatively harmless disease. In adulthood, however, serious complications often occur. These may involve the sex organs, either the ovaries or the testes, and may occasionally produce sterility. Other complications of mumps include pancreatitis and encephalitis.

(For a discussion of this disease and proper treatment see *Mumps* in chapter 28 of this volume.)

A Model Plan for Immunization

After reading the preceding section you know that the time to provide protection from the common contagious diseases is during infancy and early childhood. The accompanying recommended schedule for immunizations is proposed by the American Academy of Pediatrics and is sanctioned by the Center for Disease Control of the U.S. Public Health Service. When followed, it provides protection against diphtheria, tetanus, whooping cough (pertussis), polio (poliomyelitis), measles (rubeola), German measles (rubella), and mumps. Your family doctor probably has a copy of this same schedule, for it is the official pattern that most physicians follow in caring for their young patients. By consulting the schedule you will know when to take your child to the doctor's office for his next immunizations.

Disease incidence and severity vary in different parts of the world. Im-

---

RECOMMENDED SCHEDULE FOR IMMUNIZATION OF INFANTS AND CHILDREN

2 months	DTP* and TOPV†
4 months	DTP and TOPV
6 months	DTP and TOPV
1 year	Measles, rubella, mumps‡
1½ years	DTP and TOPV
4-6 years	DTP and TOPV
14-16 years	Td§ and thereafter every ten years

*Diphtheria and tetanus toxoids with pertussis vaccine.
†Trivalent oral polio vaccine.
‡Combined vaccines.
§Combined tetanus and diphtheria toxoids, adult type.

From an article entitled "Current Status of Vaccine-Preventable Diseases" by John J. Witte, M.D., director, immunization division, Center for Disease Control, USPHS, Atlanta. *Postgraduate Medicine,* October 1974.

---

munization schedules as well as the list of diseases for which immunization is recommended also vary from country to country. For example, some countries use B.C.G. vaccine to protect against tuberculosis, while others do not.

Immunizations for Other Diseases

1. *Rabies.* This is a tragic disease which, once it develops in a human being, is invariably fatal. It is caused by a virus transmitted to human beings by the bite of an infected animal, the typical situation being the bite of a "mad dog." It is known that many animals besides dogs, such as bats and skunks, are susceptible to this disease and can transmit it to humans through their saliva when they bite.

Rabies does not occur commonly in

human beings; therefore it is not recommended that immunization be carried out generally. There is a period of at least two weeks after a person has been bitten by a rabid animal before the disease becomes established. During this time it is possible for the individual to be immunized and thus be saved from the tragic development of the actual disease. This requires the so-called "Pasteur treatment."

The procedure for immunizing against rabies is complicated, and it is usually undertaken only when there is evidence that the animal which bit the individual carried this disease; but to be safe, the doctor may advise injections at once. The animal at fault should be kept confined and under observation for ten days after the incident to see whether it remains well or dies because of its illness. If the animal dies, examination is then made to determine whether or not it had rabies. If so, the Pasteur treatment for the human victim must begin at once and be carried forward with thoroughness.

(For a discussion of this disease and proper treatment see *Rabies* in chapter 28 of this volume.)

2. *Influenza.* Influenza is perhaps our most prevalent contagious disease. There are several viruses that may cause it, and the particular virus or combination of viruses that causes one epidemic may differ from that which causes another. Vaccines have been developed to protect against each of the viruses that can cause influenza; but, unfortunately, the vaccine which protects against one virus does not protect against the others.

It is customary, in immunizing against influenza, to use a "polyvalent" vaccine which consists of a mixture of vaccines for the various viruses which commonly cause this disease. Even so, unusual combinations of causative viruses are often present in a new epidemic of influenza. Manufacturers of vaccines are constantly on the alert to provide vaccines that will protect against the influenza viruses currently prevalent.

Another complication in the immunization against influenza is that the immunity is not of long duration. When a person depends upon the immunity which an influenza vaccine provides, he should have the immunization procedure repeated each year. Those who need this protection most, either for their own safety or for the protection of those closely associated with them, are doctors, nurses, teachers of elementary school children, elderly people and those caring for them, and those who are caring for babies and preschool children. Also patients with respiratory or cardiac conditions should have this protection. The usual immunization procedure requires two injections, administered about two weeks apart. The preferred time of year for obtaining this immunization is early autumn.

(For a discussion of this disease see *Influenza* in chapter 28 of this volume.)

3. *Rocky Mountain Spotted Fever.* This disease occurs in several countries. In the United States it is most prevalent in the Rocky Mountain area. The disease is transmitted by the bite of an infected tick. A suitable vaccine is available to protect against this disease, and its use is recommended for those who live or vacation in areas where the disease occurs, particularly those who have unusual opportunities for exposure to the infection.

(For a discussion of this disease see *Rocky Mountain Spotted Fever* in chapter 28 of this volume.)

4. *Q Fever.* This disease somewhat resembles pneumonia and occurs commonly among persons who have close contact with domestic animals or their carcasses. It is relatively common in the southwestern part of the United States.

(For a discussion of this disease see *Q Fever* in chapter 28 of this volume.)

5. *Scarlet Fever.* This disease is caused by an infection with streptococci. These germs can cause sev-

eral serious diseases, of which scarlet fever is one. There is no satisfactory plan for long-range immunization to protect against scarlet fever. For persons who have been in close contact with a scarlet fever patient (particularly when these are young children or persons in delicate health) temporary protection can be afforded by the administration of an appropriate antibiotic drug such as that used in the treatment of the disease.

(For a discussion of this disease see *Scarlet Fever* in chapter 28 of this volume.)

When You Travel

There are several serious contagious diseases prevalent in certain parts of the world but not in others. These include cholera, epidemic typhus, yellow fever, typhoid fever, and plague. When a person travels to areas where these diseases occur, it is imperative, of course, that he be protected in advance. Travel agents and public-health officials can give advice on the particular immunization procedures to be followed and for what countries.

Conclusion

There are still some contagious diseases for which no effective immunization is available. Medical scientists are continuing their efforts along the line of developing proper protective measures for these. In the meantime we can be very grateful for the marvelous developments of the past that now provide protection from most of the diseases which in previous years killed large numbers of people.

Gradually the population has become convinced of the value of immunizations. But there is a wide gap between being convinced and the carrying out of the immunization procedures in individual cases. Among the many people who still need to be immunized, some are adults, people old enough to be responsible for their own decisions. Large numbers of children, however, are in even greater need of protection against contagious diseases, and for them parents must decide. This throws a great responsibility on parents, for the child's future health and welfare depend upon whether or not the parent is consistent in providing the protection available for the child.

If you are a parent and thus responsible for the welfare of your children, we urge you to ponder the words of Solomon as recorded twice in the book of Proverbs: "A prudent man foreseeth the evil, and hideth himself: but the simple pass on, and are punished." Proverbs 22:3; 27:12.

Protecting Community Health

Medical science has now made it possible for a much larger proportion of men and women to live out a normal lifetime than was true a hundred or even fifty years ago. The resulting increase in the average length of life has been due primarily to the control of infectious and contagious diseases, especially those common in childhood.

In this chapter we shift our attention from medical practice to the community's defenses against disease. Immunization may protect against contracting disease even in the face of exposure. The community's defenses are designed to reduce the chances of the individual's being exposed in the first place.

Modern health departments are responsible for keeping communities free from the hazards of preventable diseases, especially from communicable ones. The United States Government has several public-health agencies, the one probably most well-known to the average citizen being the Food and Drug Administration. State laws govern, for the greater part, the work done in local health departments; but any public-health problem large enough to involve more than one state or an outside country is the primary concern of the Federal Government. This being true, the general public-health program is in many respects the same throughout the country, but it varies somewhat from state to state. Additional variation exists from community to community, because local health officers must also be governed or guided by the orders and ordinances of local governing bodies—city councils or county boards of supervisors, for instance. Many of the variations exist also because of the need to fit laws and regulations to differing conditions.

Several of the most important means by which a community's health is protected are often grouped together under the heading of sanitation. By sanitation is meant care of food and drink, disposal of excreta, and regulation of environment—all focused on preservation of health and prevention of disease. We often think of the science of sanitation as a recent development, but the principles of clean living are old. They were even well documented in the first five books of the Bible. These books, written by Moses more than three thousand years ago, contain a simple code of sanitary living which enabled the Israelites to continue as a relatively healthy nation for centuries.

After the time of Christ and the downfall of Rome men seemed to forget or neglect the principles of clean living. During the Dark Ages sanitary conditions became so bad that the moats around castles were often little better than pools of sewage. Scraps of food were thrown on the floors in eating places. People seldom took baths and knew nothing about how disease is spread from person to person. They feared disease but often thought it to be an act of God and did not know how to prevent it.

During the fourteenth century a terrible epidemic of the Black Death (a good deal of it bubonic plague) swept across Europe. It killed millions of people—perhaps a third of the population of that continent. This disease thrives among rats, and the germs are readily carried to humans by rat fleas. One of the first signs that it may be threatening a community is an unusual number of dead rats lying around. The control of bubonic plague, then, centers around the control of rats—a sanitation problem.

Control of rats, a sanitation problem, aids in prevention of disease.

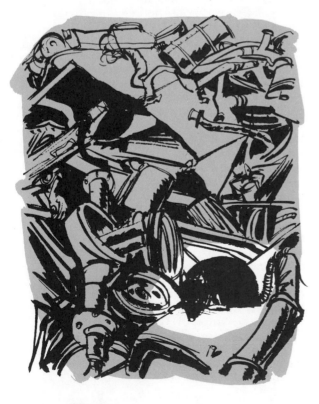

Another disease that thrives amid unsanitary conditions is typhoid fever. It is usually transmitted by contaminated food, milk, or water; and flies can spread the germs that cause it.

Diseases prevalent under poor sanitary conditions have been greatly reduced in recent decades, but they are not yet entirely controlled. Typhoid fever still occurs commonly in many parts of the world and occasionally even in the United States. Plague could still be a terrible scourge were it not for the constant vigilance of health departments and other health-guarding agencies.

The effective protection of individual health, as well as of community health, calls for the active cooperation of each citizen in obeying the rules of sanitary living. It is not enough that we pay taxes and expect the health departments to do the complete job of preventing infectious diseases. Each family needs to keep its own home and surroundings clean. Each person must be alert to the need for keeping food, milk, water, and air as free as possible from disease-producing agents.

Food Sanitation

Food sanitation includes care in producing, marketing, preparing, and serving food. For the purpose of our present discussion, vegetable and animal foods will be considered separately.

Vegetable foods are easily contaminated by contact with soil fertilizer, especially animal or human excreta of recent origin. This kind of contamination carries germs that can cause serious bowel infections and diarrhea. All vegetables to be cooked should of course be clean, but if they are to be eaten raw, they must be more than merely clean. They must also have been produced and handled with proper sanitary safeguards.

A comparatively recent new hazard in eating fruits and vegetables has come from the use of poisonous sprays

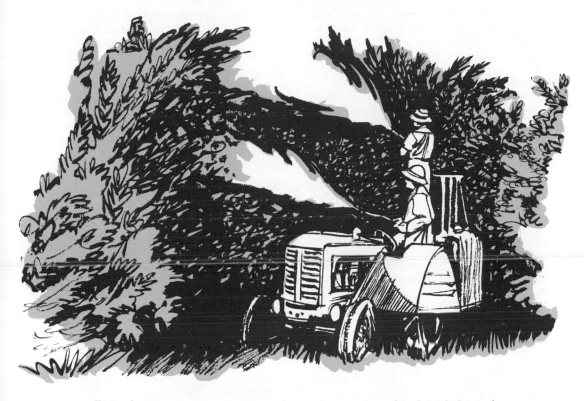

Fruit from trees recently sprayed constitutes a possible health hazard.

to kill pests. When crops are marketed too soon after the last spraying, they may carry a sufficient amount of poison from the spray to affect the health of consumers. Health officers try to avert this danger by enforcing regulations requiring that fruits or vegetables that have been sprayed be washed before being marketed. Some contaminants can be removed by washing with plain water. Others require the use of a mild acid solution or some other chemical.

Fruits and vegetables should be carefully handled while being harvested, transported, or marketed. Bruised spots on fruits cause them to decay rapidly. Fruits and vegetables are easily contaminated by germs carried by flies. Unpackaged foods, therefore, should be protected against flies while being transported and marketed.

Cooked foods should be served promptly, before there is any possibility of contamination. If such foods must be kept over from one meal to another, they should be kept in a refrigerator. Foods allowed to remain at room temperature can serve as a breeding medium for germs. The kitchen and dining room should be kept clean and free from dust. All flies and other insects should be kept out of rooms where food is handled. This is best done by screening windows and installing self-closing screen doors.

Public eating places are required to comply with state laws and regulations and with the local ordinances of the city or county. Health department inspectors visit such places as frequently as time will permit, but not on a regular schedule. Thus proprietors do not know when to expect their visits. Even so, unsanitary conditions sometimes develop in such places. If you notice what seem to be unsanitary

27

conditions in any restaurant, you will be doing your community a favor by reporting the matter to the proprietor or to the health officer. It is your health which is at stake, and the health of others in your community.

Animal foods include milk and eggs as well as all kinds of flesh foods. Milk will be discussed by itself a bit later in this chapter.

The proper production and handling of flesh foods pose many more sanitation problems than the handling of vegetable foods. It is much easier, therefore, for vegetarians to avoid diseases carried by food than for nonvegetarians. We recommend a diet largely vegetarian, but inasmuch as many of the readers of this book will be using flesh foods in their diets, a discussion of the production, handling, and preparation of these foods follows.

No diseased animal should be slaughtered for food. But even meat derived from healthy animals can easily become contaminated and then be a medium in which germs multiply rapidly, unless it is quickly cooled and kept under adequate refrigeration. Many packing companies now freeze meat promptly after slaughtering and keep it frozen until it is sold.

Unfortunately some meat inspectors and meat handlers do not adhere faithfully to the regulations designed to ensure the quality and safety of meats. But even if they did, it is not always possible to determine by ordinary inspection whether or not meat is free from disease. So it is urged that all flesh foods be thoroughly cooked before serving. Tapeworm and trichina infestations come from eating raw or partially cooked flesh foods. Thorough cooking minimizes this danger and kills whatever disease germs happen to be present in the

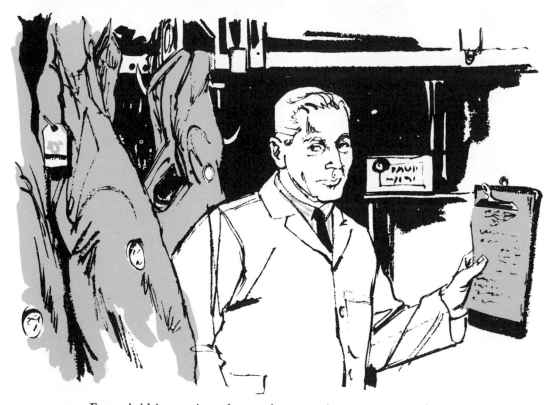

Even rigid inspection of meat does not always prove it safe to eat.

meat. The red interior of "rare" steaks or roasts cannot be considered as safely cooked.

Most of what was noted above about the handling, preparing, and serving of vegetable foods also applies in a general way to animal foods. The usual precautions are even more important in the case of animal foods, however, because of the greater ease with which germs multiply in them.

Milk

Milk is a very important food. It contains generous amounts of carbohydrate, protein, and fat. It also contains an adequate supply of calcium and phosphorus, necessary constituents for bones and teeth. It is not only the best food for babies and small children but also a good food for teenagers and adults. Nutritionists generally recommend that each child and teen-ager drink about a quart (liter) of milk a day. Adults will do well to take at least half as much, either as a beverage or in combination with other foods.

Some people argue that milk is suitable only for babies and very young children. They point out that very little milk has been or is being used in certain very populous parts of the earth, notably China. They also argue that the young of lower orders of mammals thrive without milk after the first few weeks or months of life. It would no doubt be possible for humans to do likewise if we had some practical way to supply them with the amount of calcium and phosphorus which carnivorous animals get from bones, and which herbivorous animals get from herbage and whole grains. But milk is a much more convenient source and has been widely used throughout the course of human history.

Unfortunately, milk serves as a ready medium for the multiplication of germs. Germs of diarrhea, tuberculosis, food infection, scarlet fever, septic sore throat, undulant fever, diphtheria, and other diseases are easily carried in milk. In the days before modern public-health departments controlled the handling of milk, many epidemics were traced directly to the distribution of contaminated milk.

The production of safe and wholesome milk requires careful cooperation between the dairy and the health department. The first step in producing good milk is to make sure that all cows in the dairy herd are healthy. State and local health officials cooperate in making periodic tests on each cow, eliminating diseased animals.

The second step in producing good milk is to make sure that the dairy is kept clean. In most places adequate laws regulate this matter. Floors must be smooth and easily cleaned. There must be enough windows to provide abundant light and ventilation. The cows should be given only pure water to drink, and they should be washed with pure water before being milked. Flies must be kept away from the

Cleanliness of modern dairies aids in prevention of disease.

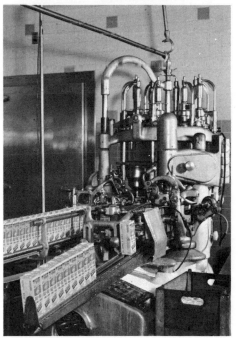

29

milk during all stages of its processing.

Prior to the days when the handling of milk was so carefully guarded, many epidemics were spread by diseased dairy workers. Now dairies are required to keep a careful health check on each employee. Dairy workers must have frequent physical examinations. One who becomes sick is not allowed to work until well again. Those who work in dairies are carefully instructed on keeping their bodies and clothes clean, thus reducing the danger of germs in the milk.

As soon as milk is taken from the cow, it should be removed to a separate milk room, a screened area kept spotlessly clean. As the milk arrives in the milk room, it should be chilled and kept cold from then on except while it is being pasteurized. Keeping milk at a low temperature prevents germs, if any, from multiplying rapidly.

More than 90 percent of the milk now marketed in the United States has been pasteurized. In some areas it is close to 100 percent. Pasteurization can be accomplished in either one of two ways: (1) heating the milk to a temperature of 145° F. (63° C.) for thirty minutes, or (2) heating it to 161° F. (72° C.) for fifteen seconds. Most germs are killed by this amount of heat, and the kinds not thus killed seldom cause disease. After being pasteurized, milk should again be quickly cooled and kept cold until it is delivered to the customer.

Some families still keep one or more cows for their own milk supply. It is not safe to continue using such milk raw. Boiling it would make it free from living disease germs, but boiling it or even heating it nearly to the boiling point spoils its taste for most people. A good method of home pasteurization is as follows: Get an accurate thermometer of the sort used to test the temperature of hot liquids. Use a heavy kettle preferably of stainless steel. Heat the milk *slowly* over low heat. It is best to put a thin asbestos pad between the kettle and the heat.

While the milk is heating, *stir it constantly*. Bring the milk to 165° F. (74° C.), and be sure it holds that temperature for about five minutes, still stirring constantly. (Extra temperature and extra time compensate for open-kettle method.) Then take the kettle from the stove and cover it. Cool the milk quickly by setting the kettle in a large pan of cold water, preferably with ice in the water. Then put it in the refrigerator until time to serve it, keeping it covered. This procedure will make the milk as safe as pasteurized market milk, and it is not likely to give it an objectionable taste.

Questions are often asked about the effect of pasteurization on the nutritional qualities of milk. Only two constituents of milk are adversely affected by pasteurization—vitamin B$_1$ and vitamin C. The loss of these vitamins is of little consequence because milk does not contain much of either one, and other foods can easily supply all that is needed. Only in cases where milk is used as the main food, as in infant feeding, does a deficiency of vitamin C constitute a problem. The lack is then made up easily by giving the baby a supplemental food rich in vitamin C, orange juice or tomato juice most often being used.

Most market milk is now homogenized. Homogenization does not take the place of pasteurization. It does not kill germs. Rather it breaks up the globules of fat into much smaller globules so that no cream line forms in the bottle or carton. It is easier to use such milk in cooking or infant feeding, since all parts of it contain the same percentage of milk fat. As a matter of fact, most market milk is both homogenized and pasteurized, as the wording printed on the containers will show.

Local health inspectors take frequent samples of milk at dairies, at processing plants, and at markets where milk is offered for sale. Laboratory tests are run on the samples to determine whether or not they show evidences of contamination by disease germs. If such evidences are seen, the milk is condemned until the cause of the trouble is located and corrected.

Water

Strangely, in the United States, generally considered to be a land of plenty, fresh water is becoming a major problem. Of the 12,000 billion gallons of water per day which flow toward the ocean through our rivers, we are now salvaging only about 325 billion gallons for domestic and commercial uses. At first this may seem like an abundant supply; but changing conditions have resulted in a continually increasing per capita demand for water.

Individual homes supplied with running water require from sixty to a hundred gallons (225 to 375 liters) per day per person. This need represents only a small part of the overall demand. Consider irrigation. We are using nearly half of our fresh-water supply to grow crops. Almost as much is required for industrial purposes. Three basic reasons for our growing need for water are: (1) the rapid increase in population, (2) the shift of population to urban areas where homes have modern plumbing, and (3) greatly increased industrialization.

When we speak of pure water, we do not mean water free from all extraneous chemical substances. Acceptable water may contain enough minerals to make it "hard." Even "soft" water may contain certain impurities. Water free from disease-producing germs and from chemical substances harmful to the body is considered "pure" from the point of view of health.

Now that the volume of sewage discharged into streams or lakes has so greatly increased, the problem of obtaining pure water for domestic use has become more complicated. However, most modern communities use sewage disposal plants to purify sewage before it goes into streams or

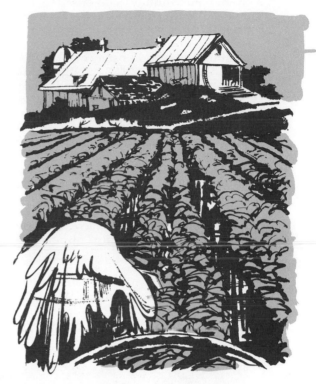

lakes. Also, water purification plants are used to make sure that domestic water supplies are free from disease-producing germs.

But a further complication is that many streams are now polluted by chemical substances discharged from industrial plants. Many of these substances stay in solution and are carried along by the water for many miles. Some are actually poisonous. In the notable example of the Animas River, a tributary of the Colorado River, the water became temporarily polluted by radioactive substances originating in a uranium mill.

Another source of chemical pollution of water is the increasing amount of pesticides now used for the control of insects, as in crop dusting. These include poisonous chemicals, sometimes carried away from cultivated areas by runoff from rainfall. To date, the amount of these pesticides entering the usual sources of water supply

31

is not measurably dangerous to humans, but this may not always remain true.

Some commercial fertilizers also contain soluble substances that can pollute ground-water supplies and eventually become a health hazard. This is especially true of the nitrogen-containing compounds in the fertilizers. If these are not already present in the form of nitrates, they are likely to be more or less slowly converted into nitrates by oxidation; and all nitrates are soluble and remain in the water as it percolates downward through the soil and deeper strata. In a few cases ground-water sources have already been found to contain nitrates in sufficient concentrations to be harmful, especially to babies.

Detergents sometimes find their way into water supplies. With the widespread use of automatic clothes washers and dishwashing appliances, the amount of detergents introduced into sewage has become enormous. The usual treatment of sewage in purification plants does not remove detergents from the water, and this water may eventually be discharged into streams or lakes which supply water for domestic use. In rural areas where cesspools or septic tanks are used for sewage disposal, the detergent chemicals seep slowly into the subsoil and eventually into the underground water reservoirs. When water is obtained from these reservoirs by the drilling of wells, traces of detergent chemicals appear in the water. Contamination with detergents may cause domestic water to produce suds when drawn from the faucet.

When detergents were first marketed they contained considerable quantities of compounds of phosphorus. The phosphorus in such detergents, when it found its way into the soil, promoted the growth of algae. More recently the amount of the

HAROLD M. LAMBERT

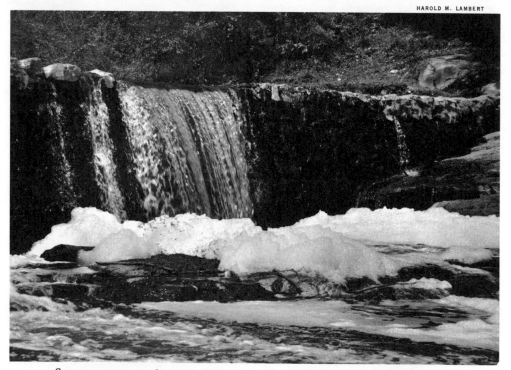

Streams apparently clear and pure may be polluted by detergents, which are not removed by the usual treatment of sewage.

compounds of phosphorus in detergents has been reduced and it may now be said that the amounts of detergent in domestic water are relatively harmless either to individuals or to the soil that absorbs such water.

In most water purification plants, the incoming water is first allowed to settle in large tanks or reservoirs, and then it is run through a sand filter. Filtering the water through sand takes out most of the foreign matter, as well as most of the germs. In some plants, chemicals are added to the water to aid the settling process or for other reasons. No chemicals harmful to human health are used which cannot be removed from the water before it is distributed into the mains. To ensure that the germs are killed, a small amount of chlorine is usually added to domestic water as it leaves the purification plant. It takes only one part of chlorine to a million parts of water to kill disease-producing germs. This amount of chlorine does not injure those who drink the water.

We cannot tell whether or not water is pure simply by looking at it. Some people consider all clear running water safe to drink. This is not always true, for disease-producing germs may be found in swiftly running water as well as in stagnant pools. The water in a beautiful mountain stream may be clear and colorless and yet carry the germs of typhoid fever or dysentery, especially if people are free to roam about in the vicinity.

People living or traveling in an area where the source of the water is unknown or unprotected should employ a means of purifying their drinking water. Also, there are times following disasters, such as earthquakes or tidal waves, when a city's water supply may be contaminated by broken water mains or overflowing sewers. The usual and safest way to make questionable water safe to drink is to boil it vigorously for at least a full minute. Then it should be kept in a covered utensil while it is cooling and until it is used. Other methods ap-

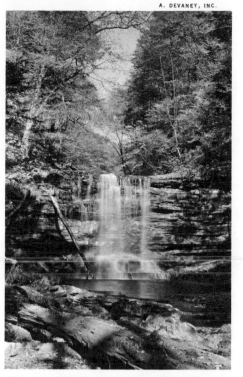

Even mountain water may be impure.

proved by the United States Public Health Service for making water reasonably safe for drinking are as follows:

1. Iodine or chlorine tablets, designed for the purification of water, are available in most drugstores. When using them, follow the directions printed on the packages.

2. Tincture of iodine from the medicine chest may be used to purify water. After adding three drops of the standard tincture to a quart (liter) of water and mixing well, allow to stand for half an hour before using.

3. Chlorine bleach solution from the home laundry may also be used to purify water. After reading the label to determine the percentage of chlorine in the bleach solution, add it to the water as follows:

Chlorine	Drops per Quart (Liter) of Water
1%	10
4-6%	2
7-10%	1

After being mixed well, the water must stand at least half an hour before it can safely be used. For purifying muddy or turbid water, twice the amount of the chemicals listed above should be used.

Fluoridation of Domestic Water

Within recent years accumulated scientific evidence seems to indicate that a small amount of the element fluorine (the active form of fluorine called fluoride ion) is necessary in the body's tissues in order to ensure proper development and health of the teeth. The United States Public Health Service has made comparative studies of communities where the water supply naturally contains an adequate amount of fluorine and those where fluorine is wholly or nearly absent. In the communities where an adequate amount of fluorine is present, children are remarkably free from dental caries (cavities in the teeth), in contrast to the high incidence of caries in communities where fluorine is deficient. Furthermore, careful investigation has shown that when fluorine is naturally present in much more than the desirable amount, no damage to the health of the water users is detected aside from the somewhat unsightly mottled appearance of the enamel of the teeth.

These findings have prompted the practice of adding fluoride to the domestic water (one part of fluoride to one million parts of water) in areas where fluoride is naturally deficient. Some oppose the practice, fearing possible poisoning by fluorine gas and some of its compounds. But there is no more danger in this procedure than in adding iodine to salt in areas where iodine is deficient. In both cases the compounds used are not those which are poisonous in ordinary amounts, and the amounts used are always very small.

As a result of continued studies made by national health organizations, two conclusions may now reliably be drawn with respect to the use of fluoride in domestic water: (1) The presence of fluorine as fluoride ion in domestic water in concentrations of approximately one part per million is effective in reducing the incidence of dental caries as much as 60 to 70 percent; and (2) the addition of fluorine to domestic water has produced no harmful results in the general health of those using such water.

Sewage Disposal

The disposal of human excreta is a most important problem in sanitation. Water and sewer systems in modern cities take care of this problem for individual households. There was a time when such sewer systems discharged their waste directly into nearby rivers or lakes; but now most municipalities operate disposal plants where sewage is treated and made safe before being discharged into a body of water used for domestic or irrigation purposes.

When a house has a supply of running water piped into it, but no city sewer available, a flush toilet with a septic tank can be installed. Local building codes and health department regulations must be consulted in this case.

Swimming Pools

The water in swimming pools may become a health hazard, entirely apart from the danger of drowning. It not only comes in contact with the swimmer's skin but also gets into his eyes and ears and some of it may accidentally be swallowed. As a general rule, civic regulations govern the sanitation of public swimming pools; and inspectors make frequent checks on cleanliness and possible disease germs, taking water samples for laboratory examination. But private pools, the number of which is rapidly growing, are usually less carefully supervised, perhaps receiving no attention at all except that which the owners may give them spasmodically or on rare occasions.

34

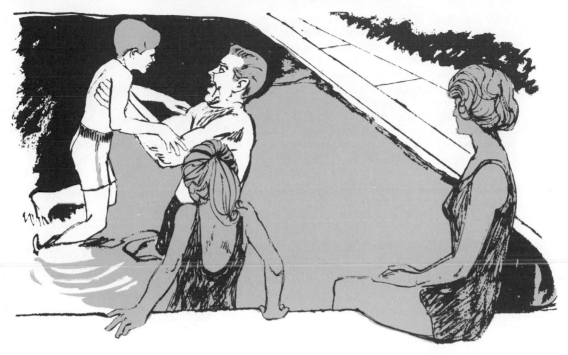

Care must be taken that the water in private swimming pools
does not become a health hazard.

Defenses Against Insects and Vermin

A hundred years ago, cities throughout the world were dirty. Garbage was not carried away quickly. Rats thrived in the litter scattered in alleys and backyards. Flies swarmed over exposed refuse and then flew into people's houses, carrying disease-producing germs. Now most modern cities provide for frequent collection of garbage and rubbish. Officers from health departments inspect streets and alleys and require that they be kept clean. This policy goes far in controlling flies, mice, rats, and the fleas carried by rats.

Flies, fleas, and mosquitoes are the worst insects for carrying disease germs. Ticks, not true insects, are also dangerous carriers. In controlling these pests, it is important to kill those that already exist; but it is even more important to prevent the propagation of the young.

Ticks are more difficult to combat than flies, fleas, or mosquitoes. The most dangerous ones are found in the wilds or out-of-the-way places, where they live on wild animals. Clearing and burning brush at certain seasons of the year, destroying wild rodents, and the periodic spraying of sheep and cattle will help to reduce the number of ticks.

Flies will breed in filth of almost any kind, but the ordinary housefly prefers the filth of an ill-kept stable or barnyard. The control of flies, therefore, consists essentially of maintaining sanitary conditions where animals are kept and where refuse of any kind is deposited. All refuse, as well as fertilizer, should be kept in tightly covered containers. Make sure that flies have no access to the interior of buildings. Careful screening and the use of traps and sticky paper will help in this objective.

The control of disease-carrying

35

fleas consists in large part in exterminating rats. As long as food is available to them, rats will breed freely. Even methods of trapping and poisoning them only partially succeed as long as the rats can obtain food. Rats thrive on most kinds of human food and on feed for poultry and domestic animals. All buildings should be carefully ratproofed. When in doubt as to the best means of doing this, consult building inspectors for the techniques of ratproofing, and health department representatives for methods of controlling rat breeding grounds. Piles of lumber, plywood, or rubbish often serve as living quarters for rats.

Mosquitoes can be most easily destroyed in the larval or pupal stage. Periodic oiling of standing water will suffocate the larvae. Dusting the surface of standing water with DDT will poison the immature mosquitoes, but may also poison any fish in the water. Certain varieties of small fish feed on the larval or pupal forms of mosquitoes. Stocking ponds with such fish is often effective in checking the propagation of mosquitoes. Vegetation growing in the water of such ponds should be cleared away so the fish can find the mosquito larvae. Stagnant ponds and marshes should be drained if possible. Some species of mosquitoes breed in very small amounts of water, such as in empty cans, broken dishes, flowerpots, roof gutters, and even in knotholes in trees.

In controlling mosquitoes, both individual effort and community cooperation are necessary. Such measures as the draining or filling of swamps and ponds are of permanent value. Other measures may have to be repeated year after year, and sometimes several times a year.

When people find it necessary to live in an area where community-wide control of mosquitoes has not been accomplished, they will have to combat mosquitoes the best they can on their own premises. Having a house on a breezy elevation, well

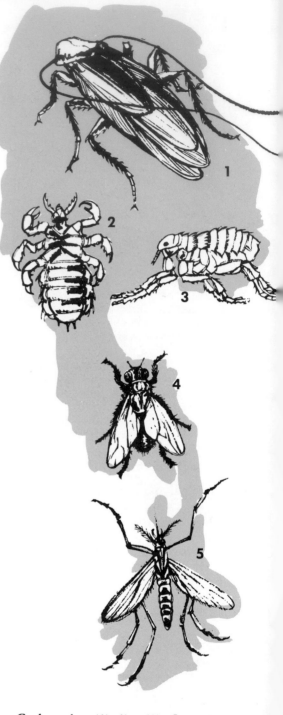

Cockroaches (1), lice (2), fleas (3), flies (4), and mosquitoes (5) carry germs, thus constituting a serious public-health problem.

away from known breeding places, will help. Vines and bushes should not be planted in the immediate vicinity of a house. Adequate screens on windows and doors, as well as the use of bed nets, will protect against mosquitoes. Remaining indoors after sunset is also a help in preventing mosquito bites.

The Problem of Air Pollution

Current population growth everywhere, with accompanying shift of population to urban areas, has in recent years increased the problem of air pollution. Industries, for the most part, have cooperated in trying to prevent pollution of the atmosphere. But some, by their very nature, continue to discharge smoke and chemical fumes into the air in spite of the most modern means of prevention. Also the exhaust fumes from an ever-increasing number of cars and trucks pollute the air and irritate eyes and air passages.

Air may be polluted by soot, smoke, gases, dust, finely divided chemical particles, and offensive odors. For this reason some large cities prohibit the use of incinerators and other air-polluting equipment. Also in some areas smog-control devices are required on automobiles and trucks.

Heavily polluted air impairs health. Evidence for this generally accepted opinion comes partly from known interference of polluted air with the growth of plants and partly from statistics indicating that certain diseases are more prevalent, and death rates from them higher, in urban areas than in rural areas, especially in urban areas where the air is frequently heavily polluted. Several cases are on record where air pollution became both extreme and persistent, and a sharp increase in deaths from respiratory ailments resulted.

Inasmuch as the factors which contribute to air pollution are not easy to control, the prospect for complete release from this health hazard is doubtful, except as scientists may

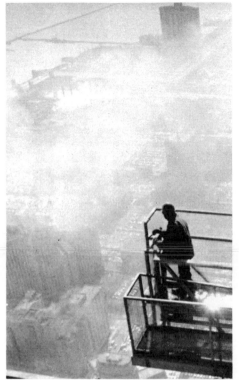

UNITED PRESS INTERNATIONAL

devise means of control at present unknown. But in any case the cooperation of all citizens will be required. Every person living in areas where the air is easily polluted should do his best to promote health by curtailing those activities that pollute the atmosphere.

Your Health Department

It is easy to take for granted the many services of city, county, and state health departments. We reap the benefits of modern medical and scientific achievements without realizing how much governmental agencies do to secure our relative freedom from disease.

Earlier in this chapter the work of various inspectors, especially in the field of sanitation, was mentioned. These officers maintian general sanitary conditions. Some keep constant vigil to make sure that rubbish and

37

garbage are removed and that vermin are not allowed to multiply. Others guard the purity of water supplies and see that sewage is disposed of safely. Still others are concerned with dairies and the milk supply. Then there are inspectors who specialize in the supervision of food handling and public eating places. These men often work in cooperation with representatives of the Federal Food and Drug Administration and with state health departments.

Because health departments have the control of communicable diseases as one of their primary concerns, and because prevention is the most effective method of control, these agencies maintain clinics and conduct programs of immunization against contagious diseases. And, while these immunizations may, from one point of view, be considered a medical service to the individuals receiving them, from the public-health point of view

the chief aim is protection of the public. Studies have indicated that when 75 percent or more of the individuals in a community have been immunized against a contagious disease, an epidemic of that disease is highly unlikely.

Another important function of local health department service in most parts of the United States concerns maternal and child health. This is carried on by means of clinics, conferences, and home visits. In the prenatal clinics prospective mothers not under the care of private physicians can be given periodic examinations and advice aimed at protecting and promoting their own health and that of their babies. In the child-health conferences babies and young children who for financial or other reasons are not being taken to the offices of private physicians can be weighed, measured, physically examined, and given immunization treatments. The

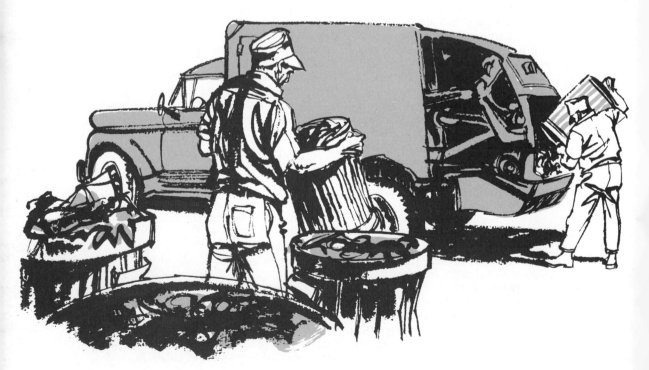

mothers can be advised about feeding and other child-care problems. When what is seen or learned in the clinics or conferences indicates that home visits might be helpful, such visits can be arranged.

A modern health department includes nurses on its staff. Public-health nurses assist in clinic and conference work and in the control of communicable diseases. They make home visits and conduct health classes to inform people about their health needs and to instruct them as to the best ways to maintain good health. In some places the law makes it automatically the duty of public-health nurses to visit schools periodically, with a view to promoting the health of students. In other places such service can be made available to the schools through agreements or contracts between school authorities and local governing bodies. In the course of such visits the nurses confer with school administrators and teachers on health problems of individual students, of special groups of students, or of the whole student body. They also give health talks to teachers or students and assist in periodic physical examinations.

Laboratory tests have been mentioned in connection with the work of sanitary inspectors. Such tests are also needed to aid public-health physicians in the detection of communicable diseases. A laboratory, therefore, is an essential part of a modern health department. The work of such laboratories consists chiefly of testing milk and water samples and examining specimens of body fluids or discharges for evidence of communicable disease. Most of this work is done on samples or specimens brought in by health department personnel. But private physicians who may suspect patients of having communicable diseases are also permitted to send in specimens.

Another activity of local health departments is the keeping of records, not only birth and death certificates

but also statistics of diseases legally reportable in the areas concerned. By studying such records, much valuable information can be obtained as to the changing incidence of diseases, the prospects of epidemics, the proper methods of preventing diseases, and the causes of death. Also, legal copies of birth or death certificates can be obtained when necessary.

A growing number of local health departments are adding mental health clinics to their list of services. A common argument justifying this step is that mental diseases are to a great degree preventable, and the primary concern of public health is disease prevention. On the other hand, many people experienced in the field of public health do not consider mental health clinics effective in preventing mental disease. They have observed that whenever a mental health clinic is set up, it is almost sure to become

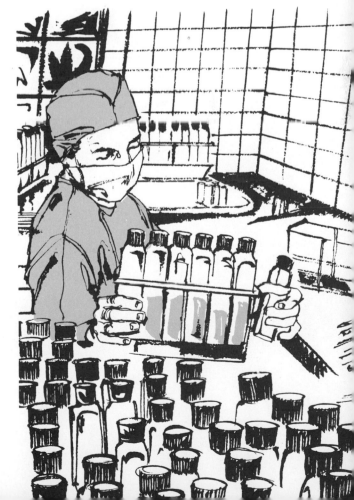

bogged down in the treatment of mental disease that already exists, with little or no time left for preventive work.

It seems logical that in the mental health field prevention should in most cases begin very early in life. More effective mental disease prevention could probably be done by enlarging the scope of prenatal clinics and child health conferences in health departments than by setting up separate mental health clinics and opening them to people of all ages. But in one way or another, health departments seem destined to become more and more concerned with mental health, and people with mental health problems can increasingly look to health departments for counsel.

We are fortunate to be living at a time when problems of health are given such high priority by scientists, newspapers and journals, community leaders, and governing bodies. This is true in most modern nations. Let us each cooperate fully with those measures and practices which will continue to promote the health of the nation and of its individual citizens.

Wonder Drugs

For centuries man has sought cures for disease. Before the recent scientific understanding of the causes of disease, remedies used were generally chosen either because of supposed mystical properties in them or because of an observed association between them and improvement in a particular disease condition.

With the discovery of germs and the recognition, late in the nineteenth century, that many a disease is caused by a specific germ, there developed a general impression that the eventual conquering of germ-produced diseases would consist of discovering the means for killing the responsible germs.

This hope of conquering disease by killing germs began to be realized first in the field of preventive medicine. People correctly reasoned that by keeping germs from entering the body they could largely prevent the diseases which these germs produced. Here we have the basic concept of our present methods of sanitation and hygiene, discussed in detail in the previous chapter.

The use of disinfectants for decontaminating surgical instruments and high heat for sterilizing surgical dressings also constitutes part of the program to prevent disease by destroying germs before they gain access to the human body. These methods of preventing surgical infections have been so effective as to prove beyond a doubt that germs can be killed and that many diseases can be prevented by taking precautions against the entry of germs into the body.

The next logical step in applying the growing knowledge of the relationship between germs and disease was to try to treat diseases by killing the offending germs after they had already invaded human tissues. Thus the emphasis shifted from prevention to cure. We have already dealt with immunization's role in this endeavor, a procedure which prevents contraction of disease after exposure. But what if invading germs have already made the patient ill—then what can be done to kill the germs? Such questions impelled medical scientists, beginning several decades ago, to search for drugs which would be effective in controlling infections once they had become established.

Chemical disinfectants were introduced for use in cleansing open wounds. Tincture of iodine became popular as a local application to kill germs when the skin was broken and even in cleansing the torn tissues of a deep wound. Other disinfectant solutions have now come into greater favor than tincture of iodine, but the attempt to kill germs that may enter the tissues through a damaging wound remains standard medical practice.

The real need in trying to cure disease caused by germs was to find a chemical agent which would destroy the germs without damaging the body tissues. Thus the chemical or drug, carried by blood circulation and other body fluids, would kill the germs inside the body without killing the person who harbored the germs. Many substances were known to kill germs and could thus be classed as disinfectants. But most disinfectants when taken into the body were damaging to the tissues as well as to the germs.

In the early decades of the twentieth century several poisonous drugs became popular in the treatment of germ-produced diseases. Quinine was one, a drug known to be poison-

Local application of disinfectant kills germs and controls infection.

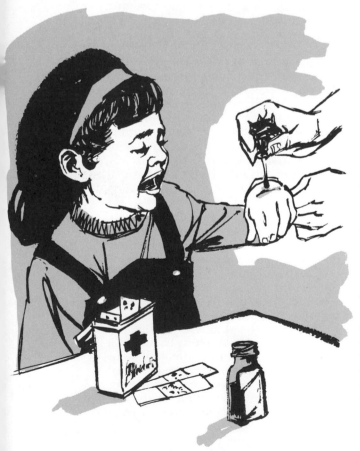

ous and to produce such symptoms as ringing in the ears, loss of hearing, impairment of vision, convulsions, irregularities of the heart, and even collapse and death. But even though poisonous when taken in sizable doses and thus dangerous, quinine was able to kill the parasites which cause malaria. Thus, physicians used quinine for the prevention and cure of malaria even though they realized the damage it could cause within the human body. Their attempt was to give just enough of the drug to kill the malarial parasite but not quite enough to kill the malaria patient.

A similar approach was made to the treatment of patients with intestinal parasites. The drugs used in such cases, though highly poisonous, were administered in carefully graduated doses within the level of human tolerance but fatal to the organisms lodged within the intestine.

The most effective drugs in the early part of the century for the treatment of syphilis contained either arsenic or bismuth. Both of these metals are highly poisonous and, even when used in the concentrations necessary to kill the spirochetes which cause syphilis, produced symptoms of mild poisoning. Justification for the use of such preparations was simply that the patient would die prematurely if the syphilitic infection was allowed to go untreated. Even though his life might be shortened somewhat by the use of such powerful drugs, this loss was considered better than allowing the syphilis to run its course.

The Sulfonamides

It was in the early 1930s that rumors began making their rounds in medical circles that a "wonder drug" was in the offing. Of course medical scientists can't believe rumors. They deal with matters of life and death. They must possess verified facts before they dare alter their method of treating disease in human subjects.

But in 1936 the rumors were backed

up by scientific reports emanating from Germany and France. The reason for the delay in making final announcement was that it took time to check results. A new drug must be tried out first in the laboratory. If it passes scrutiny, then, cautiously, it can be tried on humans.

As the exciting story unfolded, it indicated that "prontosil," as used by certain medical scientists in Germany, had prevented the death of laboratory animals infected with streptococci—the germs responsible for many severe infections, including many of the skin, one form of meningitis, and the infection accountable for the death of mothers following childbirth.

Prontosil is a member of a chemical family of substances developed for use in the dye industry. Sulfanilamide, the original member of this group, had been developed in 1908. A few scattered observations indicated that certain members of this group of dye substances had the effect of killing bacteria; but, strangely, no research had been done to determine how toxic they might be to living tissues. Now, in the middle 1930s, it was demonstrated that their toxicity was low, meaning that living tissues tolerated these chemicals well, whereas germs were apparently brought under control by their action.

A great deal of professional enthusiasm developed in both the United States and Britain over the hope of curing infections by the use of sulfonamides. In Britain the early successes attended treatment of infections following childbirth. In the United States sulfonamides were administered to laboratory animals to discover possible dangers in their use. Then they were given cautiously to human patients suffering from various kinds of infection.

In this early use of the sulfonamides enthusiasm ran high. Medical scientists hoped they had found the miracle drug which would prove harmless to the human body but destructive to all

or nearly all germs that invade it. There were mixed emotions, then, as the results began to be tabulated and reported in medical literature. Cures wrought in certain infections were truly remarkable. Patients with infections caused by the streptococcus germ began to show improvement within a matter of hours, and many cases were practically rid of infection within two or three days. At the same time similar cases without such treatment ended fatally or had to suffer through many days, even weeks, of serious illness.

But it was soon apparent that not all infections responded as dramatically as did those caused by the streptococcus germ. Infections caused by the staphylococcus germ were usually reduced by sulfanilamide, but the improvement was not so dramatic as in those caused by the streptococcus.

Pneumonia can be caused by more than one kind of germ, one common type being pneumococcus. Inasmuch as pneumonia was at that time one of the major killers, it had been sincerely hoped that the new drugs would be as helpful in controlling infections by this germ as they had been with others. Gradually the truth dawned, however, that sulfanilamide rendered practically no benefit in the treatment of infections caused by the pneumococcus. It did provide some benefit, however, in the treatment of infections caused by the germ which commonly produced meningitis (the meningococcus). It also relieved infections caused by gonococcus, the bacterium responsible for many cases of venereal disease and other serious infections such as those of the eyes.

Disappointment over sulfanilamide's failure to help in the conquest of pneumococcic pneumonia did not last long. While physicians were gathering data on the advantages and limitations of sulfanilamide, chemists were busy in the laboratory developing chemical modifications of this same preparation. Presently sulfapyridine, another sulfonamide developed in England, proved effective in the control of pneumococcic pneumonia. With the use of this new drug, the mortality rate of this type of pneumonia dropped suddenly from more than 25 percent to a little less than 10 percent. This type of pneumonia was so common that this sharp decline in mortality represented a saving of thousands of lives per year.

Collaboration between physicians and chemists continued, with the result that other sulfonamides soon came into general use, each with its particular advantages and limitations. In addition to sulfapyridine, the list soon included sulfathiazole, sulfadiazine, sulfamerazine, sulfaguanidine, and sulfasuxidine. All these various sulfonamides closely resemble each other in chemical structure but differ just enough so that some are adapted to the treatment of one infection and others to another.

Following the realization that the sulfonamides really were effective agents in the control of infections, medical scientists began to concern themselves with the question of how the sulfonamides produced their marvelous results. Previously physicians had been so concerned with finding out what the drugs would do in the control of infections that they had hardly taken time to ask the question, How do they accomplish what they do?

Even to the present time, the exact means by which the sulfonamides inhibit germs that cause infection is not known. It seems certain, however, that they bring about conditions within the tissues that retard the growth and reproduction of germs that may be present. Under favorable circumstances germs within the tissues multiply very rapidly. But under the influence of the sulfonamides this rapid multiplication is prevented.

Sulfonamides can safely be used only under a doctor's supervision.

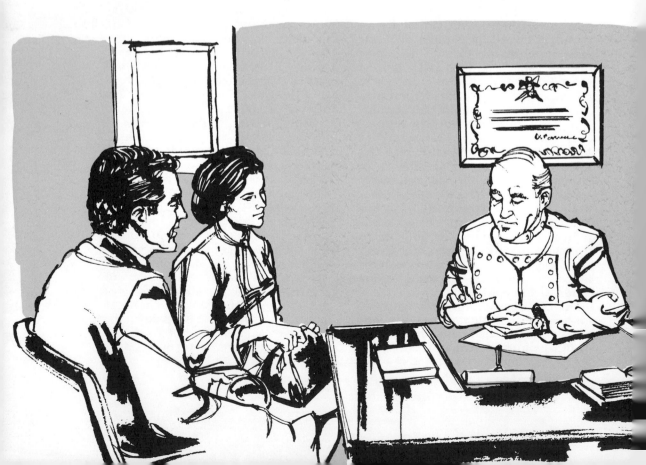

Fortunately, however, the body can and does still produce antibodies to resist the invasion of germs just as well as usual.

Thus far in our story of wonder drugs it probably seems that the sulfonamides provided a nearly perfect answer to the problems of the control of infection. And as yet we have not come to the part of the story relating to the antibiotics. At this point the reader might even ask, Why was it necessary to have any other drugs in addition to the sulfonamides?

No drug is perfect, and the longer the sulfonamides have been used, the more apparent it has become that they have limitations. When used in doses too large for the individual's tolerance, they produce signs of intoxication, meaning that a person can tolerate only so much of the sulfonamides within his body fluids. The limit of tolerance varies from one person to another.

The commonest signs of intolerance of the sulfonamides or of an overdose are nausea, vomiting, and mental confusion. These signs usually disappear quickly when the drug is reduced or discontinued. Prolonged use of the sulfonamides may interfere with the production of blood cells. Another possible complication is an irritation of the tissues of the kidneys, resulting in a reduced production of urine. It was soon learned that this effect on the kidneys can be largely prevented by requiring the patient to drink a larger than usual volume of fluid during the time the sulfonamides are being taken and by using some chemical substance to keep the urine's reaction from becoming acid.

The sulfonamides continue to be valuable drugs even though, in the meantime, antibiotics have been developed. The antibiotics did not replace the sulfonamides in the treatment of disease but only served as a supplement, so that the physician now has more than one effective treatment as he deals with serious infections that affect the human body.

The Antibiotics

Research developments were taking place, even while the sulfonamides were being acclaimed, which soon produced an entirely separate group of wonder drugs—the antibiotics. The story starts in 1928 with an accidental observation made by Sir Alexander Fleming. After serving as a medical officer in World War I, Fleming devoted himself to research in bacteriology at St. Mary's Hospital Medical School in London. One day when examining a culture plate of the staphylococcus germ which had become contaminated by the growth of mold, he suddenly became fascinated as he observed that surrounding the area of the mold was a zone in which no germs were growing.

This caused Fleming to speculate on whether the mold was capable of producing a substance that was deadly for staphylococcus germs. His sub-

Dr. Alexander Fleming, 1881-1955

THREE LIONS, INC.

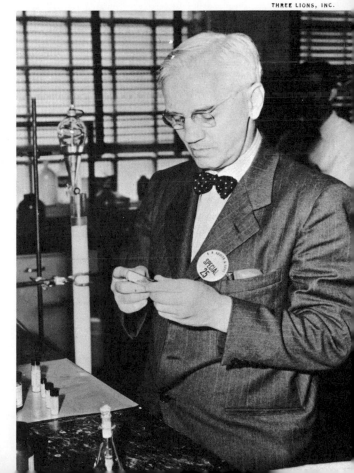

sequent experiments indicated that this was indeed true. Thus Alexander Fleming became famous as the discoverer of the mold culture which he named penicillin. For this and his continuing research in the field, he was awarded the Nobel Prize in 1945.

As far as its application in the treatment of germ-produced diseases is concerned, Fleming's discovery lay dormant for eleven years. Then it was, in 1939, that a group of research workers at Oxford University, as they searched for drugs that would supplement the sulfonamides, decided to make a trial run with penicillin. In their experiments on laboratory mice, it proved surprisingly effective in controlling infections caused by the staphylococcus as well as by some other germs. Then, cautiously, they tried it on human beings and were highly gratified to find it effective in controlling certain infections and also remarkably low in toxicity for human cells.

Next came the problem of developing ways to produce penicillin in large enough quantities to make it available wherever needed as a medicinal agent. Cooperation between pharmaceutical manufacturers in England and the United States soon resulted in methods of mass production. Its manufacture still uses the processes of mold fermentation, just as in Fleming's laboratory.

In the intervening years, scientists have developed several hundred antibiotic compounds, all of them related, as far as the structure of their molecules is concerned, to the original penicillin. Most of these have limited uses because they are toxic or because of side effects when used medicinally. Of these, about a score have found important places in the treatment of infections.

Antibiotics are particularly effective in the treatment of infections caused by the staphylococcus germ. They are also useful in combating the pneumococcus and the germs of the common venereal diseases.

Antibiotic drugs can be administered by mouth and also by either intramuscular or intravenous hypodermic injection. They are used not only in the treatment of infections, but also, very importantly, in the prevention of certain infections. One member of the group (streptomycin) is important in the treatment of tuberculosis.

During the years since antibiotics have come into use, many varieties of germs have become resistant to these drugs. This is one of the facts that has urged medical scientists to develop other forms of antibiotics. When a certain germ becomes resistant to one member of the antibiotic group, another member which differs slightly in its chemical structure may still be effective.

Another complication seriously af-

A technician examines microorganisms of penicillium.

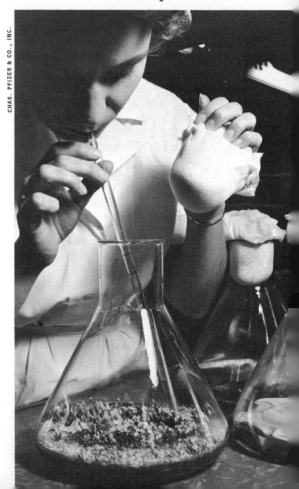

CHAS. PFIZER & CO., INC.

fecting the usefulness of antibiotics is that a small percentage of persons develop an allergic reaction by which, after they have received some such drug on a previous occasion, they manifest a dangerous sensitivity to its subsequent use. Physicians now test a patient for sensitivity before administering certain antibiotics.

Cancer Chemotherapy

Another frontier along which medical science is making progress is the development of chemical substances helpful in the control of some types of cancer. Popular reports on these chemicals have sometimes given the false impression that they are "cancer cures." But when we understand the means by which these anticancer agents act, we recognize that they are only adjuncts in the treatment of cancer.

There are now three general methods used in the treatment of cancers: (1) removal of the affected tissue by surgery, (2) radiation of the cancerous tissue by X ray (radiation therapy), and (3) the administering of chemical substances which have the effect of inhibiting the growth and reproduction of the cells composing the cancer (cancer chemotherapy). A fourth method—still essentially in the experimental stage—is immunotherapy in which attempt is made to immunize the patient against the virus supposed to be responsible for the development of the cancer.

Each of these general methods of treatment has its limitations. That is, no one method is a cure-all. Some types of cancer are best treated by one method and some by another. The treatment of a given case must therefore be individualized. In many cases, particularly in the most malignant types of cancer, best results are obtained by using a combination of the available methods. Our modern clinics for the treatment of cancer are equipped to do this and have staff members who are trained and experienced in such matters.

Cancer chemotherapy is especially helpful in the treatment of cancers that are widely distributed in the body's tissues as in the leukemias, the lymphomas, and many solid cancers that have spread (by metastasis) to several sites in the body. However, a chemical substance which is powerful enough to affect the cells of cancer may also have detrimental effects on normal cells. The normal tissues which are in greatest danger of being harmed by chemotherapy are those which produce blood cells. Thus, anemia may develop as an unwelcome complication.

Drugs Which Influence the Brain

Two other groups of drugs which deserve mention in this chapter are the tranquilizers and the antidepressants — those that relax mental processes and those that stimulate them. The development of these drugs has greatly influenced the methods of treating persons with mental disorders. Depressed cases often benefit by the proper use of antidepressant drugs—those that whip up the mental processes. In similar fashion, patients who develop panic, fear, hostility, and delusions may be helped by the appropriate use of tranquilizers.

Many persons with mental illness can now be treated without having to go to a mental hospital. Other cases still have to be admitted, but the time spent in the hospital is greatly reduced. It must be emphasized, however, that the particular effect of any one of these drugs on a certain individual is difficult to predict. Possible side effects may be undesirable. Use of some drugs of this group may develop pathological dependence in the patient. Some may cause harmful effects on the liver, on the blood-forming organs, or in the brain itself. Some have the effect of raising the blood pressure.

Important as these drugs are, then, in the treatment of mental illness, they must be used only under the supervision of a physician skilled in this area of medical practice.

Conclusion

Treatment of disease by the use of drugs has undergone a remarkable revolution. At the beginning of the present century medicines used for treating disease were chosen empirically. In most cases the exact effect of the drug on the human body was not known, the medicine being used only because of its supposed beneficial influence or because of its relief of symptoms.

Now that medical science has advanced to the place that cause-and-effect relationships serve as the basis for the treatment for illness, the use of drugs is based on combating the cause rather than on merely relieving symptoms. Most drugs in use today are those of known effect on the body's tissues and fluids. This does not mean, however, that modern drugs are always safe. Many have marked effects on the functions of the tissues and organs of the body. In many cases a delicate balance exists between beneficial effects and harmful side effects. Reactions differ from person to person.

The wonder drugs have prolonged millions of lives, certainly a cause for gratitude. But the same drugs which, when used appropriately, may be lifesaving can, on the other hand, if used indiscriminately, produce great harm and even death. Physicians trained in chemistry, pharmacology, and modern methods of therapeutics are the only ones in a position to make available to a patient the benefits of the wonder drugs. For the layman, therefore, the only safe policy to follow is to avoid self-medication.

SECTION II

Functional Diseases

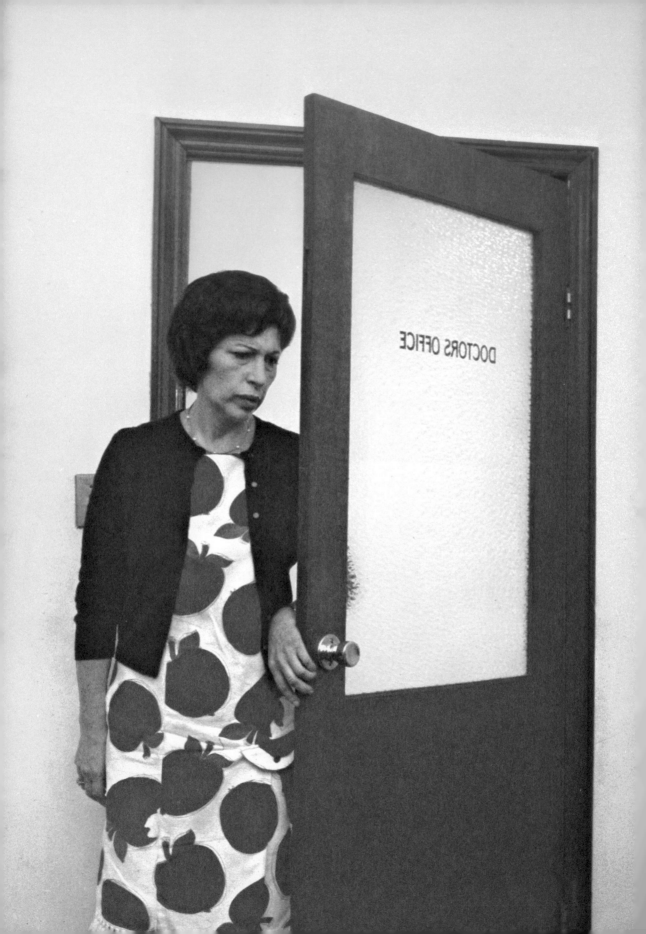

What Is Functional Disease?

"I'm sorry to hear that your husband is sick," I remarked to a neighbor lady.

"Yes, he hasn't been to work for three days now, and I am becoming concerned," she replied. "He doesn't have a cold, and I don't think he has a fever. He says he just feels miserable all over. I tell him it's all in his head, but he thinks I should be more sympathetic."

Here was a case in which the real cause of illness hadn't been determined. Maybe Mr. Jones had been working too hard. Perhaps things hadn't been going well where he worked, with resulting anxiety robbing him of his usual drive. Or possibly he was in the first stages of some serious illness such as diabetes or kidney disease. And Mrs. Jones was concerned because she didn't know how serious or how prolonged the illness might be.

Of course illnesses vary. Some, like pneumonia, we recognize as "serious." But even then we take comfort in the thought that modern methods of treatment can save most patients. We consider a person with cancer to be seriously ill because some kinds of cancer carry a high mortality rate. But we minimize the seriousness of indigestion because it usually runs a short course and few ever die from it.

A given attack of indigestion, however, could be more serious than supposed. Indigestion may result from carelessness in eating. It can also be caused by emotional factors that disturb the normal functioning of the digestive organs. A single attack of indigestion may be quite harmless, but recurring bouts associated with emotional unrest may become serious.

Thus we see the need for a discussion of diseases which result from emotional tensions and conflict—the so-called functional or nonorganic diseases.

The term "functional diseases" refers primarily to illnesses involving no structural change in the tissues of the body. The symptoms of functional diseases result from changes in the nervous control of certain organs.

Functional diseases may develop into organic diseases, depending upon factors relating to emotions. When the causative emotional upset is short-lived, the illness will be relatively harmless and short-lived; but when repeated or continuous, the patient will be susceptible to repeated occurrences of the functional disorder. If the disturbance is so deep-rooted as to persist for days, weeks, and months, the resulting illness will probably progress until what began as a simple functional illness develops into an organic disease.

Emotional disturbances often affect

the organs of breathing. A person so affected may feel that he is about to suffocate. He rushes to an open window, turns on a fan, or by other means attempts to increase the amount of available air, not realizing that the difficulty stems from his own emotional state.

This problem should not be confused with the shortness of breath produced by organic heart disease. In heart trouble the shortness of breath is most troublesome when the patient climbs stairs or runs to catch a bus or otherwise overexerts.

The type of difficult breathing associated with functional disease is not related to physical exertion nor is it associated with other evidences of heart trouble. It is sometimes observed as "sighing respiration" and is often accompanied by a feeling of constriction of the chest with an awareness of palpitation of the heart and even with a feeling of weakness or dizziness.

Take Mr. Harnek's case as an interesting example. Suddenly, while eating, Mr. Harnek put down his fork, pushed himself back from the table, and began to sigh and breathe in a peculiar, rapid manner. He appeared pale and anxious.

Of course everyone thought of heart attack, and while the others helped him to the sofa, Mrs. Harnek phoned Dr. Scott.

Then a frightening thing happened. The muscles all over Mr. Harnek's body began to twitch. Gradually his arms and legs drew up so that by the time the doctor arrived the patient's knees were almost under his chin.

"What is it, doctor?" Mrs. Harnek asked as Dr. Scott made a hurried examination.

"It is too early to say yet, but I don't think it is a heart attack. Just to play safe we will call an ambulance and take him to the hospital where I can make a more careful examination. By the way, has he ever had attacks like this before?"

"Yes, several," Mrs. Harnek re-

called, "the last one about three months ago when he was watching a boxing match on television."

At the hospital Dr. Scott, among other things, ordered an electrocardiogram.

The next morning Mr. Harnek was much better. He had had a good rest and said he felt like getting up and going home.

"But before I sign you out, I want to talk to you a bit," Dr. Scott explained. "I understand that you have had some previous attacks like this one. Tell me about them."

"Well, doc, I have had three or four, and it seems that they have always occurred when something happened to make me nervous."

"Like what?" the doctor encouraged.

"The first attack I had was when a friend of mine died of a heart attack. He died right there in the office while I was bending over him. It was too much for me. That night the thought of

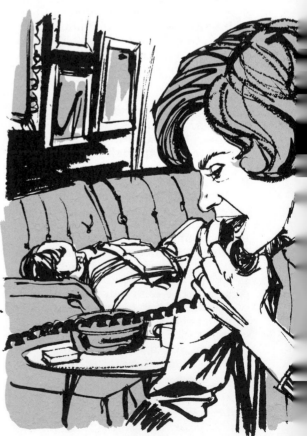

it all seemed to hit my nerves. All of a sudden I began to feel dizzy, and the skin around my mouth began to tingle. I felt a lump come into my throat. And then my chest seemed to get tight, and I felt pain in my heart. I was afraid I was having a heart attack, and for about half an hour it seemed that I couldn't get my breath. Yes, I have had three or four attacks since then, but always when I was alarmed or nervous about something. Do you think it may be my heart?"

"Before I answer that, I want you to do something for me. I want you to breathe real deeply and real quickly for about two minutes. Don't stop breathing even if you feel light-headed."

"All right, doc," Mr. Harnek responded. "Here goes."

After he had been breathing rapidly for almost a minute, he began to move his lips as though the skin around his mouth were tingling.

"Keep on breathing," the doctor encouraged.

Then Mr. Harnek put his hand to his heart. By this time his face bore an anxious expression. Then his muscles began to twitch and his legs to draw up just as they had on the previous day.

At this point Dr. Scott held an open paper sack over the patient's mouth and pressed it tightly against his face as he breathed into the sack. As if by magic, the symptoms began to disappear. Within two or three minutes Mr. Harnek was feeling all right again except that he was weary from the ordeal. Then Dr. Scott began to explain.

"You see, we have produced another attack just by having you breathe too actively. This confirms my opinion that nothing is basically wrong with your heart. Your symptoms are the result of breathing too fast—hyperventilation, we call it."

"But, doc, I didn't try to breathe that way yesterday. The symptoms came out of a clear sky."

"I know you didn't try to do it. But there was something that made you alarmed or uneasy or anxious. And it is quite normal for a scared person to breathe more energetically as though he were getting ready to run or fight or do something about whatever makes him alarmed. That is nature's normal response to fright. But you didn't use up the extra oxygen you were breathing. What was more important, by breathing so rapidly you exhaled a lot of carbon dioxide. This sudden loss of carbon dioxide from your body made your blood more alkaline, and that, in turn, caused your symptoms. Of course, being already frightened, your imagination provided some of the symptoms and thus you became more frightened because of your symptoms and the symptoms continued because you were frightened."

"Is this hyperventilation, as you call it, a common disease?"

"It isn't a disease in the true sense of the word. It is just a group of symptoms which sometimes occur in nervous persons who have become ill at ease. But I would like to know what caused you to be anxious and fearful yesterday when you had that attack."

"I might as well admit, doc, that my wife and I haven't been getting along too well of late. It isn't anything serious, I hope, but we have been having our differences. And here we were at my wife's sister's house with all the relatives gathered round. I knew that some of them had heard of the differences Suzan and I were having. This made me feel out of place and mad at the same time. In fact, I thought Suzan was probably laughing up her sleeve because she had me where she wanted me for once. I tried to act unconcerned, but then my brother-in-law made a sly remark, and the next thing I knew I was on the sofa all drawn up like a monkey."

"Now you see that your real trouble is with your personal problems and your emotions. I don't know how you and your wife are going to settle your differences, but I can tell you that you are not suffering from heart trouble."

"But how did you get me out of this

attack this morning, doc? I'd like to know how to do it so that if I have another attack I can cure it myself."

"Whenever you get to feeling so nervous that you think another attack is coming on," Dr. Scott replied, "just take a paper sack as I did, hold it tightly over your face, and breathe into it for a few minutes. What it does is to save the carbon dioxide that you would otherwise be breathing out into the atmosphere. By breathing it over and over again, as you breathe in and out of the paper sack, you do not lose it from your body, and therefore the symptoms are alleviated."

Another common manifestation of functional disease is nausea and vomiting, a result which often follows a sudden emotional shock.

In a case reported by Drs. Hubert Smith and Stanley Cobb, of the Harvard Medical School, a practical joker telephoned a lady that her husband had been involved in an accident in which both his legs had been broken. Supposing the report to be true, the wife experienced a violent type of nervous shock associated with intense vomiting. Although she was soon informed that her husband was all right, her functional illness lasted several weeks.

Tiredness is another symptom of functional disease which may appear as the result of protracted emotional tension. For example, a healthy-appearing man, thirty-two years of age, had complained of this symptom for at least eight months. The tiredness had been getting worse for the previous three or four months.

This patient had been an only child, and his mother had always dominated him. Following his discharge from the Army, he had married and settled in his parents' home. The patient's wife, quite like his mother, tried to run his affairs. A baby was born slightly less than a year after their marriage; but the couple resented its arrival, feeling that they were not ready for the responsibility of parenthood. Also the patient's father openly disapproved of

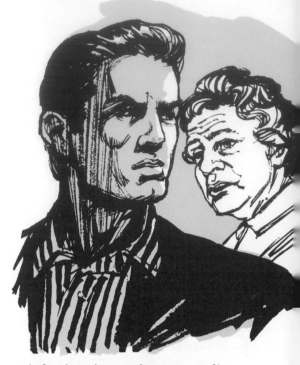

A domineering mother may predispose a child to functional disease.

the methods used by the patient's wife in caring for the baby.

Here we find a group of circumstances that produced serious emotional tension. The patient had resented his mother's domination and had supposed that he would be free from this once he was married. Upon marriage, he found that his wife manifested similar characteristics of dominance. Then he developed a troubled conscience because of his uncordial feelings toward the baby. Finally came the difficulties which resulted from living with his parents.

Another common symptom of functional disorder is the sensation of a "lump in the throat." A thirty-eight-year-old woman who complained of this symptom admitted undue inclination to worry about her health. She said, "Probably the lump in my throat is not serious, but I came for an examination to determine whether it is only nerves or something that really deserves treatment." When she was asked what she feared the lump in her throat might be, she said, "I'm afraid it might be cancer."

The doctor made a thorough examination, on the strength of which he assured the patient that she did not have cancer. As a result of this assurance, the symptom quickly disappeared.

Another patient who complained of a lump in the throat was a twenty-eight-year-old man who operated a hoist for a steel construction company. In this case, also, there was no evidence of actual disease. Inquiry revealed misunderstandings between him and his wife. His work throughout the day was lonely in nature. He simply stood at the controls of his machine and watched for the signals which the other workmen gave. Thus he had ample opportunity to brood over his marital disagreements. This buildup of emotional tension formed the background of the functional disorder of which he complained.

Dr. Canby Robinson of Johns Hopkins University School of Medicine tells of a twenty-one-year-old baker who became almost incapacitated by certain vague symptoms. Shortly after his marriage, seventeen months before he came to see the doctor, he had begun to experience attacks characterized by a choking sensation. They usually occurred at mealtime and were so severe as to force him to leave the table. Also they were accompanied by the apprehension that he was about to die.

A complete examination disclosed no organic disease. Dr. Robinson then tried to become better acquainted with the young man, in the hope of discovering a reason for his anxiety. The patient finally confided that he was afraid he might get tuberculosis. A boyhood friend of his had died of this disease.

Now his own marriage and eventually the knowledge that his wife was pregnant intensified his fear of tuberculosis. He remembered that his friend had passed away shortly after his first child had been born.

Once the doctor explained to the young man that a thorough examination offered positive proof against his having tuberculosis, he immediately felt much better.

Any childhood circumstance leading to persistent feelings of insecurity or apprehension can cause troublesome anxiety and functional disorders in years to come. When faulty relations between a child and his parents stifle the child's normal tendencies to self-assertion, he becomes chronically fearful of any circumstances which require self-assertion. This may so mold his personality that even in adult life, conditions demanding personal initiative and agression provoke anxiety. Anxiety, being emotionally charged, brings about an overflow of emotional energy into that portion of the nervous system which regulates the function of the various organs. This is the mechanism by which tension-producing circumstances produce the symptoms of functional disease.

Not all anxiety states have their background in childhood. The ambitious schoolteacher, desirous of advancement and success, may find herself hopelessly torn between her desire to maintain high professional standards on one hand and the unreasonable demands of parents on the other. The salesman, in his effort to increase his commissions, may find it difficult to reconcile the desires of his customers with the policies of his company. Such circumstances may produce anxieties and tensions that upset the delicate balance of the nervous system and initiate functional disease.

A woman in her middle forties was troubled with "nervousness" and with numbness in her fingertips. As a child she had known unpleasantness between her parents, who finally separated when she was sixteen. Thereafter she lived with her mother, but had to discontinue school in order

55

to earn money. At eighteen she was married to a man ten years her senior. This marriage also ended in separation, when she was twenty-four.

Later she married again, the second marriage being a happy one. She continued her employment for several years, until shortly before she consulted the doctor. Her husband had upheld her in the decision to discontinue employment; but her employer, for whom she had worked for many years, objected.

It was the adjustment to spending her entire time at home, in the face of her employer's displeasure, that seemed to provoke her symptoms. Now that she no longer had to work, her emotions provided the excuse by which she could say to the employer, "My poor health makes it impossible for me to work."

In one group of functional diseases either an imitation, or else an actual development, of organic disease occurs. In these cases, illness begins as a simple disturbance of the function of certain organs. As it progresses, definite tissue changes finally occur. These diseases produce suffering even early in their courses. As they bring about actual changes in the tissues, they endanger the future health and even the lives of their victims.

A forty-three-year-old man complained of sleeplessness, loss of appetite, loss of weight, occasional diarrhea, and intermittent pain in the pit of his stomach. These symptoms had become more severe during the past year and a half. The patient thought he was suffering from ulcer of the stomach and feared cancer.

The doctor made a thorough examination, including X-ray studies and laboratory tests. The evidence was conclusive against both ulcer and cancer. The doctor therefore talked with the man about the circumstances surrounding the onset of his symptoms.

The patient's wife had died suddenly about the time his symptoms first appeared. Her chief complaint had been pain in the pit of her stomach. About six months prior to the wife's death, a seven-year-old girl whom they had reared from infancy was taken from their home and returned to the custody of her own mother. The patient and his wife were greatly disappointed, for they had loved the girl as if she were their own.

When the patient understood that he had neither an ulcer nor a cancer, and that his symptoms were the result of his emotional tensions during the previous two years, he began to feel better.

Another case which illustrates the relation between emotional tensions and illness is that of a middle-aged woman who complained of sleeplessness, headaches, spots before her eyes, irritability, and extreme nervousness. Physical examination revealed a small goiter. Also, her blood pressure was high. The physician reasoned that some factor must have stimulated this woman's thyroid gland to function beyond its usual limits, thus giving rise to goiter. Increased activity of the thyroid gland could then account for the increased blood pressure. On careful inquiry he found the suspected factor to be the patient's anxiety over the infidelity of her husband.

Functional disease is not limited to adults. Drs. Hamilton Ford and Lamar Ross cite the case of a nine-year-old girl. This little patient had attacks in which the rate of her heartbeat ran as high as 130 per minute, and her blood pressure rose to high levels. During each of these attacks she was afraid she might die.

The girl's parents had indulged in frequent quarrels. These quarrels centered around a domineering mother-in-law who lived in the home and was said to be suffering from heart disease. She used to attempt to control her granddaughter's behavior by threatening, "Grandma may die of heart trouble if you aren't a good girl."

Examination showed the child's

heart and blood vessels to be fundamentally normal. Their function had been altered because of the unfortunate emotional experience. But had this little patient continued in her unfavorable situation, she doubtless would have developed permanent high blood pressure.

In some cases functional disease takes the form of hysterical ailments. These manifestations do not pose the serious health threat offered by the group just considered, but they do incapacitate the patient.

In hysteria the emotional difficulty is often deep-seated. Patients become victims of their imaginations, to the extent even of believing their illnesses to be genuine.

Sometimes hysterical manifestations take the form of paralysis of one or more of the extremities. Such paralysis incapacitates the patient for performing regular work. Thus handicapped, he hides behind the excuse of illness. In this way hysterical paralysis serves its mischievous func-

Emotional problems in children often stem from quarreling parents.

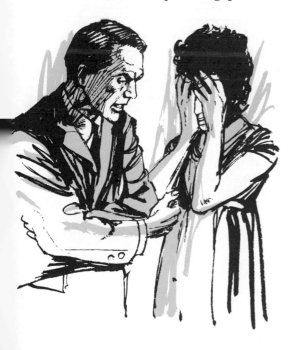

tion of relieving the patient's emotional tension. He unwittingly takes recourse to the supposed illness, rather than work out a satisfactory adjustment to the situation which has provoked his emotional unrest.

There are many forms of hysteria. But all have one feature in common—they enable the patient to sidestep the real factor in his environment which he considers intolerable.

Dr. E. D. Edie cites the case of a seventeen-year-old girl who complained of blurred vision in one eye. The blurring occurred after reading for a few minutes.

The girl had previously consulted an eye specialist who, after a thorough examination, found nothing abnormal. On questioning the parents about the girl's childhood and record in school, the doctor learned that she had always had difficulty in school. She was older than the other pupils in her class.

In view of there being nothing actually wrong with the eye, it became apparent that this girl had unconsciously resorted to a hysterical maneuver to enable her to say, "The reason I cannot do well in school is that I cannot see well enough to read my assignments." Had she been able to progress normally in school and to obtain the usual satisfactions that come from success, her eyes would not have bothered her.

Doctors today know that certain illnesses are closely related to emotional tensions and anxieties. Pychosomatic illnesses, they call them. It is as though emotional energy, once accumulated, must find an outlet. If circumstances make it difficult for the individual to control the situation that produces emotional tension or anxiety, this pent-up energy will find its own outlet through the portion of the nervous system which controls the organs. In so doing, it disturbs the normal delicate controls, thus producing symptoms.

Background of Functional Disease

Emotional tensions and emotional conflicts are listed along with germs, injuries, dietary deficiencies, and tissue degenerations as causes of disease. The importance of distraught emotions as a disease-producing factor is often overlooked; but more Americans suffer from physical and mental disorders resulting from emotional problems than from those resulting from all other causes combined.

A classic example from medical literature is the forty-nine-year-old stockbroker who consulted Dr. Fremont-Smith in 1929. The man had been ill, off and on, for about twenty years. After a checkup, the doctor arrived at a diagnosis of duodenal ulcer (ulcer in the first portion of the intestine).

The patient, placed on a treatment program, was getting along well when, on October 29, the evening newspapers described the great stock-market crash. Within minutes the typical symptoms of ulcer reappeared.

Dr. Fremont-Smith, noting that the symptoms recurred soon after the patient had read the bad news, inquired and obtained an admission from the patient that on several former occasions symptoms had appeared in direct relation to emotional upsets.

In angina pectoris—a form of heart disease—a patient can usually tolerate moderate exercise better than emotional stress. In cases of peptic ulcer, as mentioned above, the patient's condition is often more affected by his emotional experiences than by the type of food he eats.

What are these emotions that work so much mischief with a person's health, and how do they operate?

Emotions are complex feeling states which include all the variations from pleasant to unpleasant. One type represents a stirred-up state with accompanying preparation throughout the body, to respond to whatever stimulus has provoked the emotion. For example, with the unpleasant emotion of fear the individual is automatically prepared by his bodily responses to flee from the object which provokes the fear.

Suppose a child, walking alone in the woods, hears a rustling of leaves. His childish imagination pictures some wild animal about to pounce upon him. This produces the emotion of fear. His body responds, enabling him to run faster and longer than he otherwise could.

The nervous connections between the brain and various organs of the body are such that the emotion of fear automatically stimulates the adrenal gland to produce extra quantities of its hormone. This circulates in the blood, stepping up the rate of the heartbeat, contracting the blood vessels, and increasing the blood pressure. It stimulates the liver to pour increased amounts of blood sugar into the blood. It increases the rate of breathing and temporarily paralyzes the stomach and intestinal tract.

These combined responses provide a large volume of blood, carrying a high concentration of energy food, to all muscles of the body. Furthermore, the rapid rate of blood circulation, together with increased breathing, provides a larger amount of oxygen so the muscles can use to advantage the extra energy food now available. For this reason a frightened person can perform feats otherwise impossible.

Though not a part of conscious thought, one's emotions provide a background of consciousness—a stage setting for conscious thought.

Emotions depend upon the thoughts, and thoughts upon the emotions. The frightened child in the woods would have had no fear had not his conscious thoughts first provided the subject matter for fear. An emotion, then, is a sort of undercurrent of mental experience which induces the whole body to respond to some unusual situation.

Similar is the case of a man sitting at his desk and opening a letter containing bad news—perhaps about danger of losing a large sum of money. Even though he sits quietly at his desk, he will experience an emotion of fear as definite as that experienced by the boy in the woods. This fear will have the same effect on the organs of his body as it did on those of the child—it will prepare him for sudden and intense physical activity.

Running pell-mell would not solve the man's financial problem. Even so, his heart speeds up, his blood pressure rises, his breathing becomes rapid, his blood carries more energy

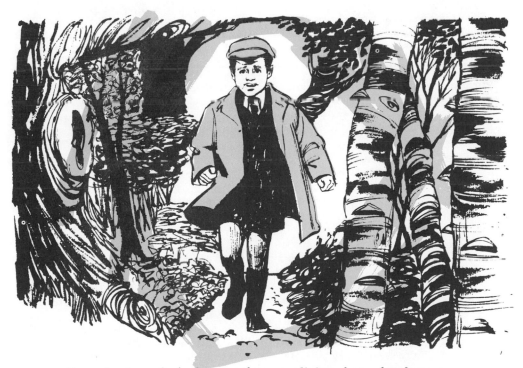

Fear stimulates the body to perform prodigious feats of endurance.

food, and he is as ready to go as though he were on a sprinting course.

Not being in a position to respond physically, the man is worse off for having experienced the emotion of fear. The increased blood pressure, the increased amount of energy food in the blood, and the various other effects serve no useful purpose. The organs of his body are thereby placed under undue strain. They now have to dispose of the excess substances liberated into his blood. His final condition is worse than if he had actually used his muscles in response to his fear.

Persistent emotional states, such as commonly brought about by modern high-pressure ways of living, keep the organs of the body on an emergency footing much of the time. No wonder health suffers as the result!

But fear is not the only emotion. Anger, for instance, produces about the same effects on the body as fear.

Often opportunity for physical response—the natural outlet for pent-up feelings—does not exist, or is inappropriate. As a student nurse once wrote on her examination paper, "The worst thing about emotional excitement is that the organs of the body get ready, set, but there is no go."

Warning should be given, however, against the opposite viewpoint that every emotion should find prompt outlet in activity. This doctrine carried to its ultimate always makes the individual the loser. When he gets angry, he strikes. When he hates, he may kill. When afraid, he becomes dejected. When in love, he seeks access to the object of his affection without consideration to propriety or moral issues. The unrealistic doctrine that permits emotions to dictate unrestrained action must be condemned.

Emotions must not be allowed free rein. Their overstimulation must be the exception rather than the rule. They can thus serve their true purpose of preparing for an emergency, rather than being perverted by constant stimulation through artificial, un-

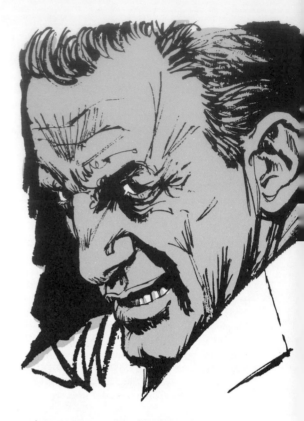

Anger gets a man's adrenaline up.

healthy patterns of living.

It must not be assumed that all emotions produce unfavorable effects. We are mostly concerned here with the unpleasant emotions, those that tend to deplete the mental and physical forces. But the pleasant emotions, such as happiness and joy, have a favorable influence. In this discussion of emotions as causes of illness, we mention the favorable emotions only to commend them as important adjuncts to healthful living. More is said about them in section IX of volume 1.

Emotional responses are automatic, controlled by certain of the deeper brain centers. Though they do not involve a strictly conscious process, they are touched off by conscious thoughts.

When a person experiences the emotion of love, his love is directed toward another person. He is in love with *someone*, so his love depends upon his conscious thoughts about that person.

Similarly, the emotion of fear involves an automatic emotional response. In order to be afraid, the individual must be afraid of something or of someone. Even in fear, the circumstances that touch off the emotion are determined by the conscious thoughts.

Emotions can be increasingly provoked by circumstances which do not ordinarily produce strong feelings, an effect resulting from a process called "conditioning."

For example, consider the case of Mildred. She had two brothers and one sister. Her parents had adopted the unfortunate custom of using mealtime for free discussion of family problems. Often conversational topics produced definite emotional responses. For instance, thorough review of the injustices perpetrated by the next-door neighbor stirred Mildred, as well as her brothers and sister, to anger. At other times one of Mildred's parents would take advantage of the presence of the whole family to point out the faults of one of the children. This child would be humiliated and would attempt to retaliate. On some occasions the father would berate the mother, or vice versa. Thus mealtime became an occasion when emotions ran riot.

As pointed out already, the effect of an emotional buildup is to prepare the organs of the body for an emergency. Anger, for example, not only increases the amount of available energy food, quickens the heart, and speeds the respiration, but also paralyzes the digestive organs. So in Mildred's case, when a heated discussion took place at the table, her organs of digestion ceased to function. Naturally this interfered with her general health. But what was more, nature's trick of conditioning gradually became effective.

In the process of conditioning, there develops a substitute stimulus which touches off the emotional responses.

In Mildred's case this substitute stimulus became the dining room. She became so conditioned that the mere sight of the dining room provoked the emotional responses ordinarily awakened by quarreling and sharp criticism.

How unfortunate! This meant that every time Mildred came to the dining room for a meal, her organs of digestion became paralyzed. She responded as unfavorably to the sight of knives, forks, and dishes as she used to respond to the active contention and debate. Her indigestion became chronic, so that by the time she reached adulthood she was the victim of poor appetite and of constant digestive disorders.

Another example is the conditioning by which an individual experiences intense grief every time he visits a relative's grave. Actually nothing inherent in a gravestone or a mound of sod-covered earth should produce grief. This response to a grave site dates back to the time when bereavement provoked its normal emotional response. At that time a conditioning occurred. Ever since, just the sight of the grave brings back the grief and anguish of the original bereavement.

How clear, then, looms the importance of a child's background in determining the course of its later life. Many adults with functional illnesses are suffering the consequences of unfortunate childhood situations. This is why the physician speaks in terms of the "longitudinal perspective." He recognizes that, in order to get a complete understanding of his patient's present difficulty, he must go into the background for insights concerning various contributing factors.

Take the case of the man in his late thirties who consulted the doctor because of complaints referable to his digestive organs. The physician's examination uncovered no serious disease. Had he been content with a superficial inquiry, the doctor would not have helped his patient much.

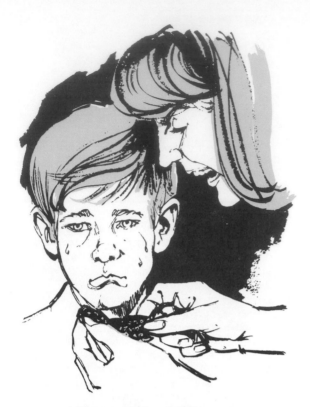

Unreasonable scolding may cause future maladjustment in children.

But by emphasizing the "longitudinal perspective" and inquiring into the patient's background, the doctor discovered an interesting sequence of events. The patient, when young, had married against his father's will. This caused an estrangement. Not long after the marriage the father had died of cancer of the stomach. This circumstance, with its deep-seated emotional implications, left the patient with the haunting suspicion that his own course of action had had something to do with precipitating his father's death. His emotions played a trick on him to the extent that, almost as a gesture of penance, his own digestive organs began to function poorly.

Had the doctor been hasty, he might simply have attributed the patient's stomach trouble to poor heredity. But when the full "longitudinal perspective" became known, it was apparent that the man's emotional responses, rather than a hereditary factor, had caused his illness.

The problem is not always this simple. Sometimes antagonistic emotional reactions bring about a state of frustration, causing the patient to develop a sense of inadequacy. Not being able to find his way out of a difficult situation, he takes recourse, more or less subconsciously, to a condition of ill health.

A fifty-year-old man sought medical aid for a supposed ulcer of the stomach. His symptoms suggested ulcer, but thorough examination and laboratory tests did not confirm the suspicion.

The patient for most of his life had taught school but had discontinued teaching about a year before he consulted the doctor. He said that he had enjoyed teaching, but that year by year disciplinary problems were becoming more difficult. He had developed the conviction that students were becoming progressively more unruly. Thus his natural fondness for teaching was offset by his feeling of inadequacy.

On being asked about his family life, he confided certain intimate problems that had diminished his affection for his wife. They had always been true to each other, but certain traits in her personality had caused him to love her less than he should.

After the patient had discontinued teaching, he had established a real-estate business, doing well for a time. Not long before he came to see the doctor, another real-estate man had taken an unfair advantage and had cheated him out of the sale of a house.

The patient now had several emotional conflicts: his fondness for teaching versus his disdain for disciplinary problems, the deep-seated emotional tension between himself and his wife, and now hatred for the other real-estate man plus a feeling of helplessness as he realized his inability to secure justice. These conflicts formed the basis on which his acute illness had developed.

As the physician gave counsel and guidance, this patient's symptoms cleared. Consequent recovery offered tangible evidence that his illness had resulted from his unhealthy emotional state.

Another case in which the emotional background played an obvious part was that of a forty-eight-year-old woman who appeared to have had a heart attack. As the husband answered the doctor's questions about the patient's history, he told of an operation, about a year before, for bowel obstruction. Following her recovery from surgery, she had developed the unwarranted fear that she had cancer. It was this combination of circumstances that seemed to have precipitated the supposed heart attack.

A checkback over the hospital records as well as a complete physical examination enabled the doctor to dispel her fear of cancer. But this simple assurance did not suffice to relieve her anxiety.

In a subsequent conversation the patient revealed a fear that her husband was untrue to her. She did not recognize, until the doctor pointed it out, that this was the real background of her illness. Subconsciously she had supposed that her invalidism would require her husband to remain at home, or that the grief which her illness might bring to her husband would be the equivalent of punishment for his supposed lack of social rectitude.

It was finally possible for this patient to accept the doctor's reasoning that the best way for her to inspire and retain the affections of her husband was to shake off the shackles of ill health. As she did so, her companionship with her husband would become so pleasant that there would be little danger of his becoming untrue to her.

We typically think of the things that a person can *do* or keep from *doing* in order to maintain good health. But there is another important factor in this matter of keeping well. *Thinking* is as important as *doing*.

The Bible says, "As he thinketh in his heart so is he." Proverbs 23:7. Although the text refers especially to the relationship between thoughts and character, the principle applies also to the relationship between thoughts and health. The person who pictures himself as being frail and delicate is the person who will have more than the average amount of sick leave. But the person whose thoughts are centered on what makes life worthwhile will experience both a mental and a physical stimulation by which he can rise above much of the tendency to illness. Attitudes of optimism and courage have a vitalizing influence on the human body.

We do not want to give the impression that a person's determination to keep well will enable him to escape illness in spite of his own disregard for the rules of healthful living. We are not advocating a brand of magic by which a person can "kid himself" into thinking that he is well even when he is sick. But we contend that the person with a wholesome outlook will find life so interesting and challenging that he will automatically want to keep well in order to pursue the activities he enjoys. And by wanting to keep well, he does two things: (1) He gladly follows a health-promoting pattern of living; and (2) he refuses to indulge in self-pity. It is this refusal to pity himself that can tip the balance in favor of health.

The human body is constituted so that its organs and tissues modify their functions to harmonize with mental attitudes. Unhappiness, grief, anxiety, and guilt all have their influence in producing an unfavorable effect. When these unfavorable mental attitudes persist for long, the body's tissues actually suffer from the continued handicap under which they are placed. Unfavorable mental attitudes, then, lay the foundation for actual illness.

Common Functional Manifestations

There are many kinds of functional illness—so many, in fact, that functional disease is sometimes said to imitate all forms of organic disease plus a few others. This problem makes the work of a physician all the more difficult because he has to sort the symptoms caused by emotional tensions from those caused by germs or by actual organic disturbances often confusingly the same. Treatment in a given case must be directed at the cause of the illness, and so treatments for functional illnesses differ markedly from those for organic illnesses. To diagnose properly and then treat a case in which the symptoms might be caused by either functional or organic disease challenges a doctor to exercise keen discernment. We will now consider some of the common outcroppings of functional illness, a few of the hundreds of such symptoms that might occur.

Headache

Headache is perhaps the commonest symptom of which patients complain. Probably half the persons who consult a doctor mention headache among the things that bother them. An estimated one fourth of the absences among industrial workers are caused by or related to headache. Some headaches come and go rather quickly, while others persist or recur. It is stated that 12 percent of the urban population of the United States suffer from chronic headaches of one kind or another. Headache occurs as a symptom of many diseases, some of them serious. So when a patient complains of headache, the doctor must make a thorough examination for a possible background disease needing specific treatment. Laymen often fear brain tumor. They have heard of someone with a brain tumor who suffered from headache, so it is easy for them to assume that a pain in the head indicates something wrong inside the brain. As headaches go, however, very few are caused by brain tumors; for brain tumors, fortunately, are rare. The usual pain in the head (headache) is caused by a stretching of the blood vessels and their related tissues inside the skull. The tissues which compose the blood vessels contain many sensitive nerve endings, and when these are stimulated, as by stretching, they initiate the sensation of pain. When the stretching of the vessels occurs with each pulsation of the bloodstream (with each heartbeat), the pain is throbbing in nature.

High blood pressure can stretch the cranial blood vessels and thus cause headache. So can a reflex constriction (tightening) of the veins that carry blood away from the brain. So can the wearing of a tight collar which compresses the veins of the neck and interferes with the return of blood from the head. A brain tumor, in the rare cases in which it does occur, can stretch the blood vessels in its vicinity and thus cause headache.

Not all headaches result from the stretching of vessels and tissues inside the skull. A major source of head pain is muscular tension on the attachments about the back of the neck and head. The head is encased in muscles, and tension can cause a bandlike headache. An inflammation of the sinuses related to the nasal cavities can cause severe pain which the patient may interpret as coming from inside his skull. Sometimes this pain of sinusitis is reflexly projected to some distant part of the head.

Many systemic diseases associated with fever and toxemia cause headache. The exact means by which they cause the tissues inside the skull to be stretched is hard to understand. This kind of headache will be considered more specifically in the following sections.

"Eyestrain" is acknowledged to be a common cause of headache, and here again the exact mechanism by which the pain is produced is hard to determine.

In our present discussion we are primarily interested in headaches which come from nervous and emotional excesses—the so-called "tension headaches." Consider the case of John Jones as an illustration.

After the doctor had taken John's blood pressure and temperature, examined his heart, and checked his eyes for evidences of pressure within the skull, he remarked, "I don't find anything organically wrong. More often than not, persons who complain of headache are responding unfavorably to some of life's everyday problems."

"You mean it is all in my head?" John interrupted.

"That's where a headache usually is," the doctor chuckled. "Seriously,

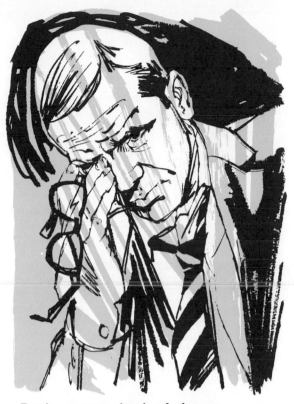

Persistent, recurring headache may be a symptom of functional illness.

though, I am not accusing you of imagining that you have headaches. I know that the pain is very real. But I do think that some unsolved problem or some source of tension in your life may be setting the stage for the symptom of headache. Please tell me more about yourself."

"Perhaps I should report," John began, "that the only problem that I have at home centers around my wife's mother. She's a headache!"

"What's that you say?" the doctor broke in. "Do you mean to admit that she is the cause of your symptom?"

"Well, I hadn't suspected any cause-and-effect relationship here," John remarked, "because she and I don't have much in common, and usually she comes to see my wife while I am at work. She lives across town from us, you see. What I wish is that my wife had enough spunk to do things her own way without doing what her mother tells her to do all the

65

time. As far as my nervous tensions are concerned, she is only one of several. Most of my tensions come from my work at the office."

"Perhaps your antagonism toward your mother-in-law is just a 'last straw' type of thing," the doctor suggested. "But when it is added to the tensions you experience all day at the office, it tips the balance of your nervous equilibrium unfavorably. Tension headaches are often triggered by some inner personal conflict which involves hostility or resentment. Usually such a factor operates unconsciously without the affected person's realizing such a relationship.

"Everyone has problems to solve," the doctor continued. "Everyone operates under a certain amount of nervous tension. Persons who get along without having symptoms of tension are those who learn to live within their personal limitations, keeping their expenditures of nervous energy at a lower level than the point at which a headache can develop.

"Now for the remedy. Let me suggest a four-point program:

"1. Get at least eight hours of sleep each night.

"2. Eat a well-balanced diet, and eat your meals regularly.

"3. Take some pleasant physical exercise each day, preferably out of doors.

"4. Every hour of the day during working hours, knock off for ten minutes and do nothing but relax. You may spend this ten minutes in lounging, in listening to relaxing music, or in sitting with your eyes closed."

"Must be you never ran a business of your own, doc," John objected. "This item about working fifty minutes and resting ten minutes all day

long just doesn't fit in with my program."

"I know that's the hard part, all right," the doctor sympathized. "But I think you can find a way. A doctor in Boston recently tried this same program with a group of fifty patients who had tension headaches. Some of his patients were college students and some were employees. The employees had to make special arrangements with their employers. After six weeks of this program thirty-three out of the fifty had complete or almost complete relief from headaches. And the seventeen who didn't have such good results were the ones who had not followed the program consistently."

Dizziness

Dizziness is not a disease; it is a symptom. It consists of a false sense of movement. The patient *feels* that he is moving or that his surroundings are moving when, actually, he *knows* that neither is the case.

Dizziness may herald the onset of various diseases, or, strangely, it may not indicate any disease at all. But, in any event, dizziness is unpleasant.

Before we discuss the causes of the symptom of dizziness, we need to consider the means by which a normal person can detect movement. First, vision helps a person to tell whether he is stationary or moving. Second, a person detects motion by sensations which come to his brain from the various muscles and joints of his body. A third means is by sensations from the semicircular canals located in connection with the organs of hearing inside his skull. These tiny canals are filled with fluid which moves slightly with every change in the position of the head.

Of these three systems, we are here primarily concerned with the semicircular canals. When they do not function normally, the individual experiences dizziness.

A normal person sitting quietly receives equal nervous impulses from the two sets of semicircular canals in

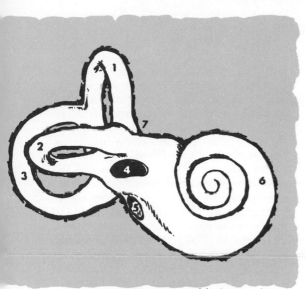

Inner ear, the organ of balance: (1, 2, 3) semicircular canals; (4) vestibular window; (5) round window; and (6) cochlea.

each side of his head. When he moves in any direction except straight ahead, the canals on one side will be stimulated somewhat differently from those of the other side. Thus he detects movement by the fact that he receives differing impulses from the right and from the left.

Now, back to the symptom of dizziness. When, because of an abnormal situation, a person sitting quietly receives differing impulses from the right and the left, he will naturally *feel* that he is in motion even though he *knows* better. This is the basis for dizziness. This difference in the sensations coming from the two sides of his head can be produced by an irritation of the semicircular canals on one side or by a loss of function (complete or partial) from one side. To produce dizziness it is necessary only to have an abnormal *difference* in the sensations from the two sides.

The underlying cause of dizziness may be some serious disease, it may be an injury, it may be a minor disturbance of function, or it may be some emotional disturbance. For this reason, a person who experiences dizziness is entitled to a thorough examination.

A serious head injury which damages the semicircular canals can produce dizziness. So also can a brain tumor which either interferes with the nerves which carry impulses from the semicircular canals or interrupts the connections of these nerves within the brain. Diseases of the blood vessels such as occur in hardening of the arteries may have the effect of disturbing the normal function of the semicircular canals. If the blood supply to the semicircular canals on one side of the head is reduced more than that on the other side, the patient will experience dizziness. Some diseases, such as mumps and encephalitis, irritate or damage the semicircular canals enough to produce the symptom of dizziness. Drugs taken to excess may do the same. Even the poisons which some infections set free in the blood may affect the semicircular canals and cause dizziness.

One young secretary complained of dizzy spells which occurred every day she was at work. Finally she was found to be allergic to one of the ingredients of the mucilage used on postage stamps. When she began to use a sponge to moisten the stamps, her dizziness promptly disappeared.

In many instances, dizziness is caused by psychic factors of nervousness, emotional tension, or anxiety. Concern over a financial problem may cause dizziness. Prolonged tension between relatives can do the same. Some attacks of dizziness follow climaxes in personal experience. One woman had her first attack of severe dizziness as she left the courtroom where her husband had been declared bankrupt. A man experienced a sudden bout of dizziness soon after his wife had committed suicide. Another person complained of dizziness after reading some old letters which brought back vivid memories of previous family troubles.

Probably the development of dizziness caused by tensions and anxieties is due to reflex changes in the flow of blood through the semicircular canals, and occasionally from spasm of the neck muscles.

Heart Symptoms

It is estimated that 10 million people in the United States are afflicted with some form of organic heart disease. Probably another 15 million have normal hearts but think they have heart trouble. Many of these have symptoms which they interpret to be serious.

Of all the organs of the body, the heart is the most symbolic of one's personal and emotional welfare. Who ever clutches his liver, as he does his heart, when seized with mortal fear? One doesn't say, "My kidneys are sick," when stricken with anguish. Instead, he says, "I am sick at heart."

The symptoms of real heart disease and of pseudo heart disease are so much alike that it is proper to ask, How can a person know when he has real heart disease? Admittedly, when one is in doubt over the meaning of his palpitation or his chest pain, he suffers the same amount of concern as he would in the face of proven organic disease—perhaps even more.

So let us consider the common symptoms which attract a person's attention to his heart, symptoms which may or may not be caused by genuine heart disease.

Palpitation. When a person complains of palpitation, he means that he has become aware of the action of his heart and that he notices that it seems to be beating too forcefully, too fast, or with irregular rhythm.

The heart is under precise nervous control, and its rate and forcefulness change in response to the body's momentary needs. During vigorous exercise the heart can perform several times as much work as during rest. A

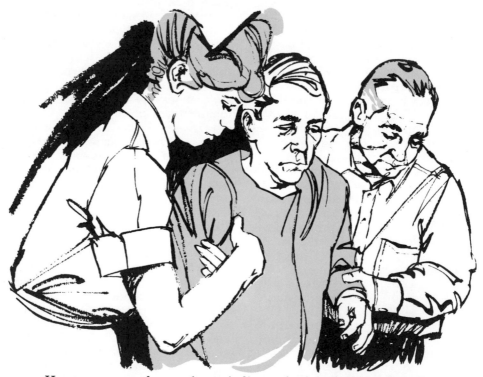

Heart symptoms do not always indicate physiological impairment.

person is not surprised, after exercising vigorously, to feel his heart pumping fast and vigorously within his chest, or possibly even to hear its pulsations. It is when he has not been exercising and feels or hears his heart action that he becomes alarmed.

The normal heart responds not only to exercise but also to the body's demand to be ready for an emergency. The body knows only one response to fear, and that is to prepare for activity. The person who is fearful or anxious places a strain upon his heart just as though he were actually passing through the experience of which he is afraid.

As for the irregular beats which attract a person's attention to his heart, these may be caused either by disease or by variations in the nervous control of the heart's action. Feeling the pulse or listening to the heart does not reveal the cause of the irregular beats. An electrocardiographic tracing, interpreted by a competent physician in the light of the patient's clinical history, will answer the question for or against organic disease of the heart.

Pain. Not all pain that originates in the vicinity of the heart comes from the heart proper. The reason a person is so fearful of pain in his chest is that he knows that such pain is often associated with the dreaded "heart attack." But other disorders also cause pain in the region of the heart. The pain of pleurisy, of spasm in the muscles between the ribs caused by neuralgia, of muscle spasm at the opening into the stomach—these may cause discomfort in the chest which, to the uninformed, is similar to that of actual heart disease. Excessive use of tobacco may cause terrorizing pain in the chest. Pains are sometimes transmitted to the chest from organs in other parts of the body as in gallbladder disease and stomach ulcer.

Here again, the person whose symptoms make him fearful of heart disease should trust his case to a competent physician and accept the physician's findings.

Difficult Breathing. There are many causes of shortness of breath, some from heart disease and some not. When, as in serious heart disease, the heart is not able to pump a sufficient quantity of blood to satisfy the body's needs for oxygen, the organs of breathing are reflexly stimulated, and breathing becomes labored. Other circumstances which also deprive the body of the amount of oxygen it needs will similarly stimulate the organs of respiration. Certain lung diseases make breathing difficult. In anemia, in which the oxygen-carrying capacity of the blood is reduced, the patient may exhibit a similar symptom of difficult breathing. In obesity, breathing is commonly handicapped.

Heart Murmur. A heart murmur is an unusual blowing sound which the physician hears through the stethoscope when the flow of blood through the heart or the large blood vessels causes eddy currents in the bloodstream. With modern, refined methods of studying the heart and its action, doctors now understand that about half the persons with heart murmurs have no disease of the heart. Innocent heart murmurs occur very commonly in children. A heart murmur may come and go with the onset and cure of a fever. Sometimes it is related to exercise.

Heart murmurs are not properly classed as "symptoms." The patient does not know whether he has a heart murmur unless his examining physician tells him. Modern physicians recognize that they must double-check heart murmurs by other means of diagnosis before suspecting heart disease.

Now to the important question— What should you do if you have symptoms that make you fear heart disease? Should you take things easy "just in case"? Should you be fatalistic? Should you try to stifle your fears by a "work till I drop" attitude?

Logically, the first thing to do is to seek out a physician and learn from him the exact cause of your symptoms.

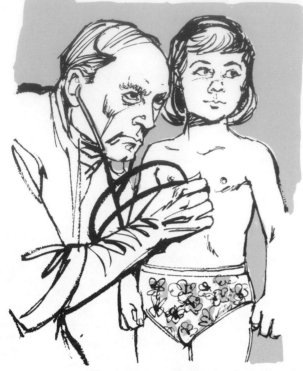

For a correct diagnosis of suspected heart trouble see a doctor.

If careful examination and study of your case indicate a diseased heart, then follow the doctor's advice on how to get along best with your limitation. If the symptoms are caused by some other disease, then that disease should be treated. If they are caused by anxiety, nervous tension, and fear, then the best approach is to learn to carry on normally in spite of the symptoms, of course at the same time trying to ease the stresses and anxieties. Thus, with assurance that your heart is healthy and with a determination to live normally, you should be able gradually to eliminate your symptoms.

Constipation

When a person complains of constipation on Monday through Friday but not on weekends, there must be something about his work program that predisposes to this ailment.

Definitions of constipation vary.

One person claims to be constipated just because he does not have a bowel movement every day. Another states that he is constipated whenever he must tarry too long at the toilet. Some people are perfectly healthy and still have a bowel movement only every three or four days. On the other extreme are those who feel uncomfortable or even ill if they do not have a bowel movement after every meal. Someone else uses the word constipation when a bowel movement is painful. As we try to harmonize these various ideas, the best definition we can arrive at is that constipation involves a delay in bowel action, and this delay causes the individual discomfort or anxiety or both.

The intestine, along with the other organs of digestion, is regulated quite precisely by delicate nerve filaments of the autonomic nervous system. When a person is alarmed, fearful, anxious, angry, or otherwise nervously tense, the usual contractions in the wall of his intestine are altered. Nervous tenseness causes a tightening of the muscle in the wall of the large intestine, retarding the passage of intestinal contents. Let us notice the case history of a thirty-four-year-old woman who complained of constipation.

This woman was the youngest of her parents' four children. When she was a child, her family had lived in a rural area in which modern plumbing facilities were not available. As a small child she had dreaded the long trip to the outdoor toilet. Her mother therefore gave instructions that one of the older children accompany her whenever she needed to go to the toilet. In typical childlike fashion, these older children resented having to take care of their baby sister in this manner and used to tease her by saying, "The boogeyman will get you if you don't hurry up." Thus, each trip to the privy became associated with unpleasant emotions. Resulting tenseness had its effect on the action of the muscle in her intestine and made it almost impossible for her to accomplish a normal bowel movement. Chronic constipation became so firmly established that it persisted into her adult years.

Many a person becomes constipated for no other reason than that he follows a strenuous pattern of living. The office worker who grabs a bite of breakfast, hurries to catch his bus, and rushes into the office in fear of a reprimand from the boss is a ready candidate for constipation. He does not allow opportunity for the natural contraction wave of his intestine, which should follow the eating of breakfast, to culminate in a normal bowel movement. If stress and strain continue throughout his day, the muscle in the wall of his intestine remains spastic, unable to carry forward its usual rhythmic contractions. As the contents of his large intestine remain for a longer than normal period, more and more water is absorbed, thus making the fecal mass hard and more difficult of evacuation.

On weekends or during vacation periods such a person has relief from his constipation for the simple reason that a more relaxed way of life frees him from the nervous tenseness which accompanies his work at the office. If only he could learn to live at ease with the regular routines of his work, he could be free from constipation even during weekdays.

The only rational remedy for any complaint is to discover and remove the cause. In the type of constipation which results from nervous tenseness, the victim should deliberately alter his way of life. Three considerations in this connection deserve special attention: mealtimes, pleasant physical activity, and the development of attitudes of faith and confidence.

Grabbing a snack, eating hurriedly at the lunch counter, and eating during a business conference should give way to making mealtime pleasant and leisurely. This will allow the digestive organs to carry on their functions normally. Spasticity of the muscle in the wall of the digestive organs will be replaced then by normal, rhythmic contractions which promote the mixture of digestive juices with food and which move the intestinal contents progressively to the large bowel.

Physical exercise favors the normal digestive and eliminative processes. Exercise in pleasant surroundings should become part of one's program of recreation. Thus it provides proper release from the day's tension.

Finally, the cultivation of calm attitudes of faith and confidence allows the autonomic nervous system to carry on its control of the body's organs in a normally balanced fashion. The person who makes such attitudes habitual increases his enjoyment of life both on account of improved health and because of the accompanying feelings of cheerfulness and optimism.

Diarrhea and Colitis

Most of the body's organs have a dual control provided by the nerves which regulate their functions, one set of nerves accelerating the organ's activities and the other inhibiting them. As already pointed out, the nerves that supply the organs are readily influenced by emotions. It is often said that the nervous energy concerned with emotions "spills over" into the nerves that control the organs. Thus when the emotions are extreme, the influence on the organs will be greater than when the individual is calm.

Just which set of nerves—those that activate an organ or those that inhibit it—will receive the greatest influence from excessive emotions is hard to predict. In one person the accelerator nerves seem most reponsive, and in another the inhibitor. And even this may vary from one organ to another in the same person.

In the case of the large intestine, some persons respond to emotional states by becoming constipated, as mentioned under the previous head-

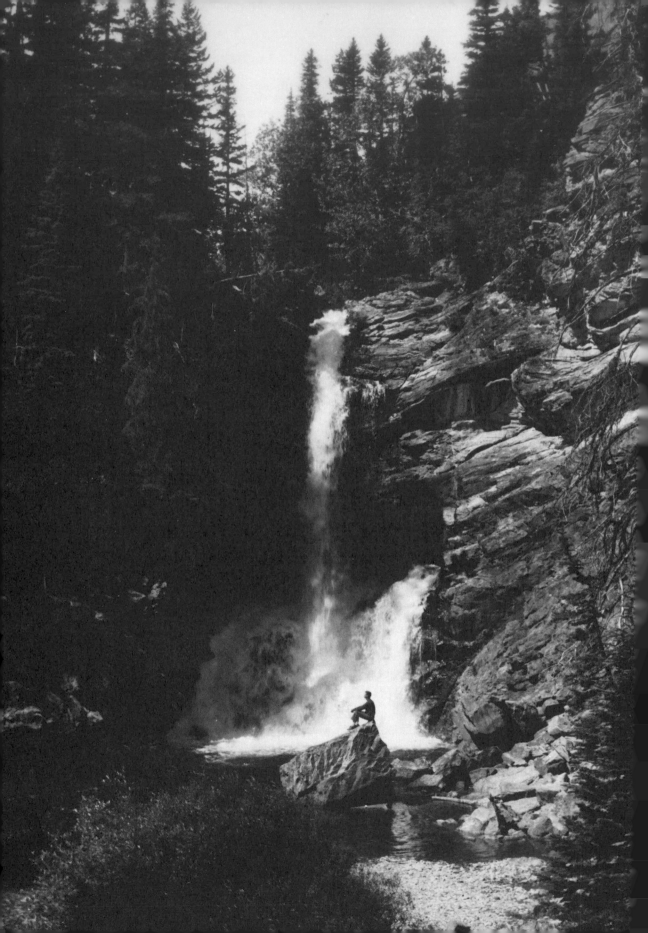

ing. Others react by having diarrhea.

Right here it should be admitted that other factors besides emotional stresses and tensions can also cause diarrhea. Actual diseases of the tissues of the large intestine will, of course, cause this. But about 90 percent of all instances of diarrhea are caused by some kind of nervousness.

The young physician, taking his state board examination, is naturally concerned over the outcome. Even though he has prepared well, he is distressed by knowing that in the past there have been failures in state board examinations. Should he fail, his plans for the future would be delayed, he would be humiliated, he would feel defeated in his chosen enterprise. With all of this hanging over him, his emotional tensions become strong. His autonomic nervous system responds by stimulating his colon to such activity that the intestinal contents are hurried on their way. Diarrhea results.

Many a public speaker has experienced a comparable reaction when scheduled to deliver an important address. He has staked his reputation on this particular talk. He has prepared his remarks systematically and well. Even so, his apprehension over the outcome generates so much nervous energy that the excess overflows into the nerves that regulate the action of his organs. Temporary diarrhea commonly occurs under these conditions.

Sometimes the symptom of diarrhea extends over such a long period of time that the tissues of the bowel become irritated. This condition is called colitis (inflammation of the colon).

A twenty-five-year-old male patient had been troubled with abdominal pain and attacks of diarrhea for several

Cultivation of calm attitudes of faith and confidence contributes to a normally balanced autonomic nervous system.

months. Careful examination indicated no organic disease of his colon or of his other organs. Interviews with the man about his emotional responses, however, revealed that he was at a critical period in relation to his chances for long-range success. He had undertaken a vocation which demanded his entire attention and challenged his abilities to the limit. Fear of failure made him ill at ease. Emotional tensions centering around this fear accounted for his attacks of diarrhea. Once this relationship was made clear to him, he determined to live more deliberately and calmly. Even so, he reported later that at times his apprehensions still manifested themselves by brief attacks of diarrhea.

Another man experienced attacks of diarrhea during a time when his brother (a politician) was involved in a scandal. The patient, who had a sensitive nervous system, felt that he shared his brother's humiliation.

A state of indecision sometimes creates emotional turmoil. One woman patient in her early thirties had been accepting the attentions of a man considerably older than she. There were reasons, she admitted, why she felt she should not marry this man. Not having other suitors at the time, however, she became emotionally tense as she tried to decide between marriage to a man who did not measure up to her ideal and the prospect of remaining single. Her symptoms during this period of indecision consisted of loss of appetite, nausea, vomiting, and diarrhea.

A young mother whose first child was one year old had complained of diarrhea for a period of nine months. The usual physical examinations revealed no organic disease. Finally the patient confided that soon after her child had been born, her husband had frightened her with stories of small children being kidnapped. She had come to live in constant fear of such a tragedy.

Self-reproach or a sense of guilt

commonly produces emotional tensions, and these in turn may alter the functions of the autonomic nervous system and produce such symptoms as diarrhea. A forty-year-old widow became overly concerned about the social welfare of her sixteen-year-old daughter. Her emotional reactions were prompted by a combination of guilt over her own previous indiscretions and a fear that her daughter might learn of the mother's past and be tempted to follow her example. With this background, the bouts of diarrhea of which the patient complained were not surprising.

Even though emotional disturbances of one kind or another constitute the commonest cause of diarrhea, a person with this symptom should not draw his own conclusion on the cause of his trouble. There are other important causes, any one of which deserves proper diagnosis and treatment. These vary all the way from a virus infection to cancer.

A person with persistent diarrhea should arrange for his physician to make a careful study of his case. If in the course of the examination an organic disease is found, the handling of the case from then on will depend upon the physician's recommendations. But if the diarrhea is the result of emotional stress, the patient should alter his way of life so that he can overcome or learn to live above the conditions that produce his tensions and conflicts. Without this willingness to get to the bottom of the emotional problem and correct the basic causes, the symptom of diarrhea tends to persist for as long as the unhappy emotional state continues. In protracted cases the tissues of the colon may even become so damaged that the patient cannot again enjoy perfect health.

The successful handling of a case of persistent diarrhea resulting from emotional tensions requires provision for adequate rest, periods of pleasant relaxation, a wholesome, balanced diet, and, most important, release from disquieting fears and anxieties. The person with emotional diarrhea must learn to follow a new way of life. Even though convinced of the need for living differently, it will take more than a few weeks to become accustomed to the new program. Such a patient cannot expect to be *cured* to the extent that he can go back to his former, tense way of living. He must learn to live within the limits of his own tolerance for emotional stresses. An occasional recurrence of symptoms should serve as a warning to the patient that he is again exceeding his tolerance. His continued good health depends upon his willingness to follow the simpler way of life and upon his learning to accept life's uncertainties with confidence.

Inability to Become Parents

About one out of ten couples (an estimated 5 million couples in the United States) do not become parents even though they want children. This inability to conceive is commonly called *sterility* or *infertility*.

The ability to have children is greatest among those couples in which the wife was less than twenty-five years old at the time of marriage. In those married at older ages, the ability to become parents declines progressively as the age of the wife at marriage increases.

Until recent years it was commonly assumed that "barrenness" was usually the fault of the wife. But with modern scientific insight and with present methods of studying childless couples, it becomes clear that the husband is about as often responsible for the inability to conceive as is the wife.

In the marvelous process of becoming parents, husband and wife each contribute a "germ cell." These two cells unite to form a single cell which, by one of the most remarkable sequences known to biologists, develops into a complete human organism. For further details on the subject of conception and human fertilization, the reader should consult relevant sections in volume 1.

The causes of sterility can be listed under five general headings: (1) failure in production of germ cells, (2) inadequate vitality of germ cells, (3) hindrances to the transmission of germ cells to that part of the uterine tube where ovum and spermatozoon may unite, (4) interference with the nourishment of the new life after the germ cells have united, and (5) the occurrence of emotional factors which alter the normal functioning of the sex organs.

1. *Failure in production of germ cells.* The wife's ability to produce an ovum every month depends upon the normal functioning of the ovaries and their proper control by such endocrine organs as the pituitary. In men, the production of spermatozoa may be reduced or prevented by certain diseases that affect the testes. The testes may be permanently damaged as one of the complications of mumps. Exposure to X rays or other forms of radiation may damage the sex organs of either men or women so as to prevent normal production of germ cells. (The usual X-ray examinations ordered by a physician do not thus affect the sex organs. The danger attends those employed around X-ray equipment or working with other forms of radiation.)

2. *Inadequate vitality of germ cells.* This factor is particularly important in the spermatozoa—germ cells produced by the husband.

3. *Hindrances to the transmission of germ cells* to that part of the uterine tube where ovum and spermatozoon may unite. These hindrances usually occur in the organs of the wife and may interfere either with the transmission of the ovum or with the transmission of the spermatozoa.

4. *Interference with the nourishment of the new life* after the germ cells have united. If there is any serious interference with the complicated process by which the new cells receive their nourishment, the new

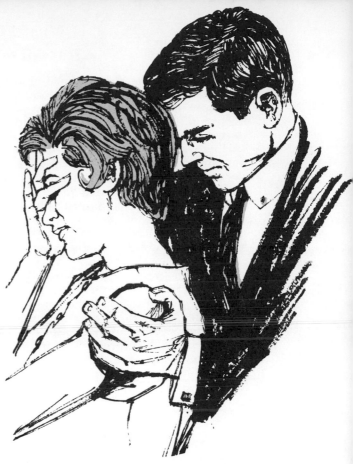

life will necessarily perish. Many cases of sterility or of premature termination of pregnancy result from a defect in the supply of nutrition to the developing embryo.

5. *The occurrence of emotional factors* which alter the normal functioning of the sex organs. Many a woman has observed that following some emotional shock the usual monthly cycle of her menstruation is interrupted. Thus, it becomes apparent that the sex organs, along with other organs of the body, are susceptible to the stresses and strains of one's emotional experiences. Time and again an interesting circumstance has developed by which a couple, previously childless, has been "blessed" with a pregnancy right after having completed the arrangements for the adoption of a child. Careful studies of many cases indicate that personal problems and emotional conflicts can actually prevent conception. Such circumstances as sharing an apart-

ment with parents, worry over financial matters, the thwarting experience of enforced military service—any of these can interfere with the ability to become parents.

How can emotional states change the functions of the reproductive organs? In some cases emotional tensions alter the usual cycle of menstruation and thus interfere with the production of an ovum each month. Obviously, unless an ovum becomes available, pregnancy cannot occur. In other cases, emotional tensions cause reflex spasms of the uterine tubes so that germ cells cannot normally unite. In still other cases, the body's response to emotional situations changes the normal tissue activities within the uterus, either interfering with the transport of sper-matozoa through the uterus or making it impossible for the newly formed cells, following a union of the ovum and spermatozoon, to obtain an adequate supply of nourishment.

Once the cause of sterility in a given case has been determined, the plan of treatment must be directed toward the removal of the specific cause. The family physician will gladly help a childless couple to find a qualified consultant who specializes in the study and treatment of cases of sterility. Endocrine therapy, general health-building programs, and proper attention to the removal of emotional stresses all have their beneficial effects in selected cases. Thanks to medical science, many childless couples can yet experience the joys and satisfactions of parenthood.

SECTION **III**

The
Treacherous
Trio

The Treacherous Trio

Interesting things have happened during the present century in the kinds of disease from which people die. In 1900 it was influenza and pneumonia that caused the greatest number of deaths. Then came tuberculosis in second place. Infectious diarrhea and other forms of gastroenteritis were in third place. Diseases of the heart and the various kinds of stroke came in fourth and fifth places, respectively. Cancer was in eighth place in 1900 as a cause of death.

Notice what has happened in the meantime. Modern antibiotics now do very well in controlling pneumonia and the complications of influenza. These diseases, although still serious when they occur, have dropped into fifth place among the causes of death. And tuberculosis, which used to be in second place, does not even appear anymore among the first ten of the major causes of death. In fact, at the mention of tuberculosis, many a modern school child would probably ask, "What is that?" Also gastroenteritis, which used to be in third place, very seldom causes death anymore.

Those diseases which were major killers at the beginning of the century have been brought under reasonably good control by the improved methods of prevention and cure which the advance of medical science has made possible. And with this near-conquest of the infectious diseases there has come a very great increase in life expectancy in America from about forty-five years in 1900 to about seventy years at the present time. But people still die eventually. And the diseases which now top the list of the causes of death are those which typically occur in older people—diseases of the heart, cancer, and stroke. These three cause well over half of all the deaths in the United States today. President Johnson, recognizing this, established a commission in 1964 to reduce the incidence of heart disease, cancer, and stroke. We respect a statesman who is thus concerned with the health of his nation.

Dr. Michael D. DeBakey, eminent heart surgeon, was appointed chairman of the President's commission. In December of 1964 he submitted his report to the President, and the commission's findings shocked the nation. They had determined that the three diseases— heart disease, cancer, and stroke—"account for more than 70 percent of the deaths in this country." Fortunately, a concerted attack on these diseases by health agencies has caused a slight roll-back, but the three still exact a staggering toll of two thirds of all deaths.

THE TREACHEROUS TRIO

It is fitting that we devote the next three chapters, placed in a section by themselves, to a consideration of this "Treacherous Trio." The very fact that these three diseases are now the major killers is, in one sense, a triumph for medical research. The diseases they superseded now have rare incidence. And even today's major killers are responding to progress in the relief of suffering and the postponement of their fatal outcome.

The three chapters which follow include not only a description of the various forms which these high-mortality diseases manifest, but also an emphasis on how a health-conscious person may avoid these diseases as far as possible and may detect them early enough to institute appropriate treatment.

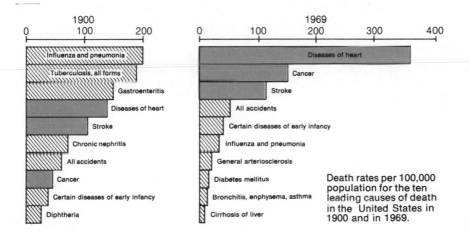

Death rates per 100,000 population for the ten leading causes of death in the United States in 1900 and in 1969.

Diseases of the "Treacherous Trio" now account for 66% of all deaths.

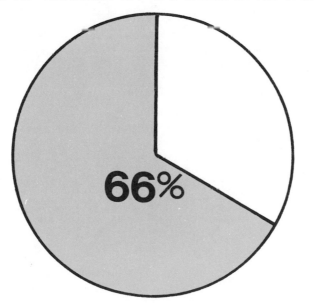

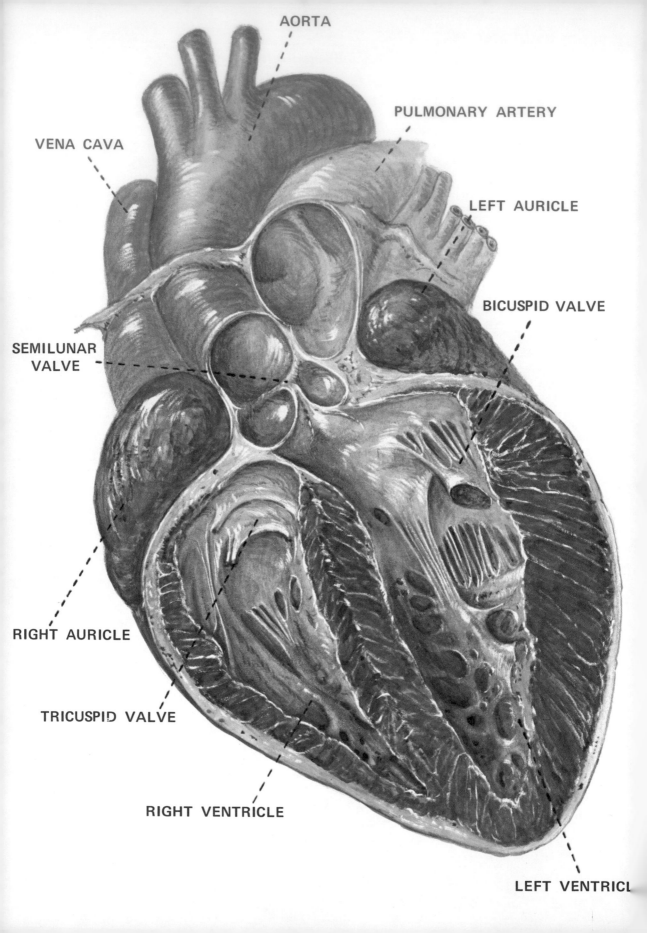

AORTA

PULMONARY ARTERY

VENA CAVA

LEFT AURICLE

BICUSPID VALVE

SEMILUNAR VALVE

RIGHT AURICLE

TRICUSPID VALVE

RIGHT VENTRICLE

LEFT VENTRICL

Heart Disease

The heart is one of the vital organs —vital because all other tissues and organs of the body depend on the heart's action to provide them with blood. If the heart stops functioning for only a few minutes, changes take place, some of which cannot be repaired. Cells within the brain are the first to suffer such damage.

For a discussion of the structure and function of the normal heart, see chapter six of volume 3.

More people suffer and die from heart disease than from any other ailment. Heart disease is at the top of the list, even among the three major killers that constitute the "Treacherous Trio." One out of every eight adults in the United States has some form of heart ailment. Probably there are many others who have minor degrees of heart disease without realizing it.

Of the several forms of heart disease, some are more serious than others. Some strike suddenly, causing premature death or invalidism. Others allow their victims to linger for years with reduced vitality.

It is coronary heart disease—the one that causes the typical "heart attack"—that has increased so tragically in recent years and that accounts for the greatest number of deaths by far. We will give it the greatest emphasis and allow it the most space in the present chapter.

The two principal reasons why the frequency of heart disease has increased so dramatically during the present century are these:

First, people live longer now than they did at the beginning of the century. The infectious diseases that caused so many deaths a few decades ago are now under virtual control. The resulting longer life expectancy allows time for the tissues of the body, including those of the heart and the blood vessels, to deteriorate. Thus, many of the current cases of heart disease belong to the group of "wear-out diseases."

The second reason why heart disease has become more common is that the life-style of the average American includes several practices that are health-destroying and that set the stage for the occurrence of the wear-out diseases, especially diseases of the heart.

Emphasis on Prevention

The body contains only one heart— not a pair of organs like the lungs or the kidneys or certain of the body's glands. And when one's heart is damaged by disease, the damage is often irreparable. Heart disease, being our number one killer, should therefore be prevented, as far as possible, rather than being treated after disease has occurred.

Medical scientists are understanding more and more about the factors that permit the various forms of heart disease to develop. Prevention in preference to treatment is by far the best method of reducing the high death rate for which heart disease is responsible.

Heart Transplantation

In December, 1967, Dr. Christiaan Barnard, a surgeon in South Africa, performed the first successful replacement of a human heart. At once hope developed throughout the medical world that damaged hearts could now be replaced by healthy ones. In the following year 101 transplants were performed in various parts of the world. The surgical procedure consisted of removing the patient's damaged heart and inserting in its place a healthy heart taken from a person who had just died from some unrelated cause. Enthusiasm ran high, and it was predicted that soon heart transplantation in selected cases would become almost a routine procedure.

But these hopes soon faded. Even though most of these patients survived the surgical procedure and even though the transplanted hearts functioned well at first, the patients died within a few days or weeks either from their body's rejection reaction or because of an uncontrollable infection.

The human body contains a built-in mechanism by which it tends to reject implanted tissues derived from any other person's body. This rejection reaction is part of what scientists call the immune mechanism, by which the body protects itself from various "foreign" agents, including germs.

In order to improve the prospect for a transplanted organ to be retained by the recipient, the physicians in charge of a transplantation procedure must stifle, for the time being, the patient's immune mechanism. In doing so they reduce the patient's ability to fight infection. Thus tissue rejection and

Heart transplant operation in progress. Patient's own heart is held by surgeon as it is lifted from the chest cavity.

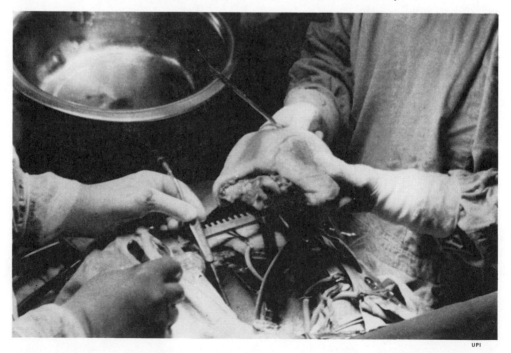

UPI

uncontrollable infection are the two unsolved problems that, at least for the present, have caused surgeons virtually to abandon heart transplantation.

It should be explained that these problems relating to heart transplantation do not apply with equal significance to the surgical transplantation of kidneys, an operation that has met with a greater rate of success.

Progress in Treatment

Although the transplantation of a normal heart to replace a diseased one has not yet become practical, great progress has been made in other forms of treating heart disease.

The development of the heart-lung machine has made it possible for specialists in chest surgery to perform surgical procedures on the heart while the circulation and oxygenation of the patient's blood are performed mechanically. Thus it has become possible for the heart to be opened for repairs as in cases in which the heart of a child developed abnormally. Also, open heart surgery makes possible the replacement of valves of the heart when these have become diseased.

Another surgical procedure which is proving to be the means of prolonging many lives is the so-called "bypass operation" in which a section of the patient's vein, taken from another part of his body, is inserted into the vessels supplying the heart so as to convey blood around an area in which the coronary arteries which supply the heart itself have become narrowed to the extent that they do not permit a sufficient volume of blood to flow through them.

High blood pressure is another one of the causes of heart disease. Progress in medical science now makes it possible for high bood pressure to be lowered by the administration of certain drugs. Thus the heart is spared the damage that would otherwise result from the extra work of maintaining the circulation of blood under high pressure.

An ingenious and life-saving device for those whose hearts have lost their ability to maintain a normal rhythm is the electronic pacemaker. One of these tiny instruments is implanted (through a small incision) beneath the skin of the patient's chest. There it remains permanently and emits a continuous series of signals which stimulate the muscle of the heart to contract at the usual, normal rate. The pacemaker supplies the lack of the heart's normal automatic control.

Congenital Heart Disease

The heart is a complicated organ. It is really two pumps in one. One pump, the so-called right side of the heart, receives blood that is returned from all parts of the body and pumps it through the lungs and back again to the other side of the heart. The other pump, the left side of the heart, receives blood that has just acquired its new load of oxygen as it passed through the lungs and then pumps it under pressure through the system of arteries to all parts of the body. Each of these two pumps that constitute the heart consists of two chambers, an atrium and a ventricle. Thus there is a right atrium and a left atrium and a right ventricle and a left ventricle— four chambers in all. They are separated from each other by partitions, and the two on each side are connected to each other by openings which are guarded by valves.

In its earliest life history the heart was not so complex. The heart begins to function about three weeks after conception, pumping blood through the developing tissues of the embryo. At this early time the heart consists of a single tube which pulsates.

It is during the next five weeks of development (weeks three to eight, following conception) that the heart becomes a four-chambered organ. The marvel of it is that it is able to continue pumping blood while it is undergoing the marvelous transformation from a simple tube to a four-chambered organ.

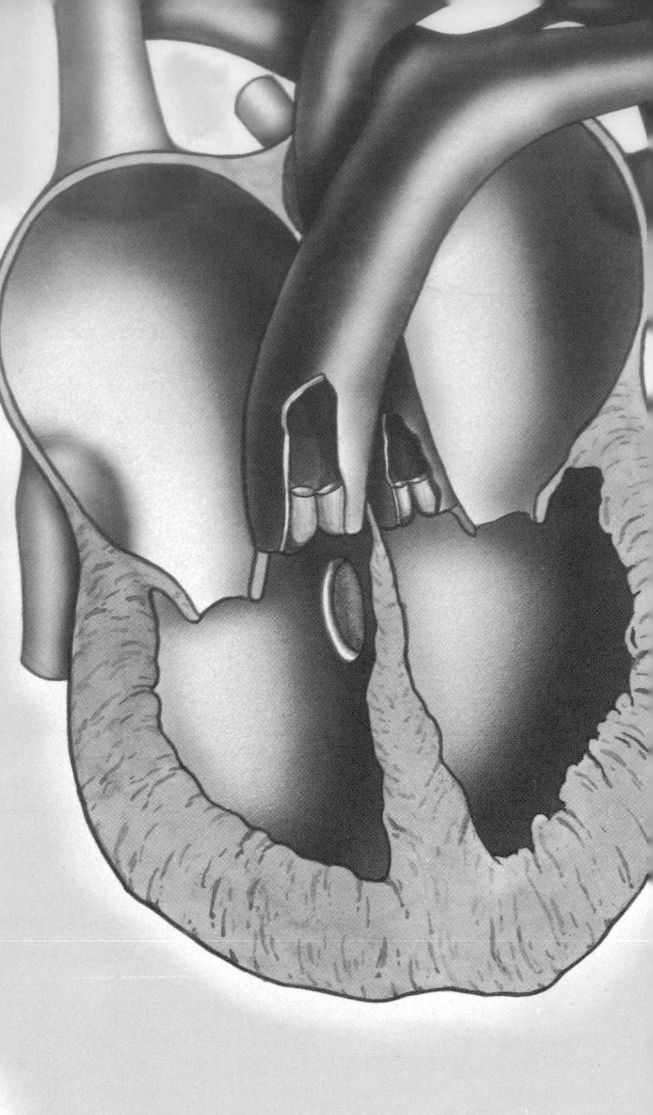

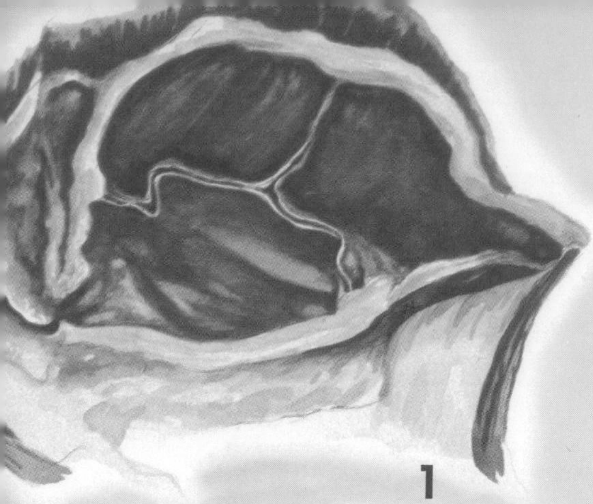

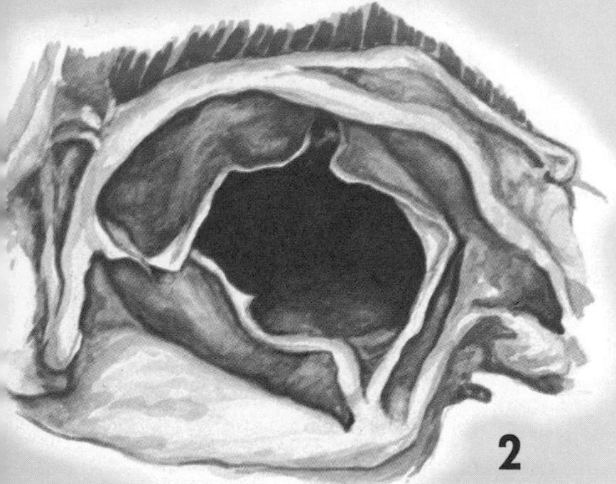

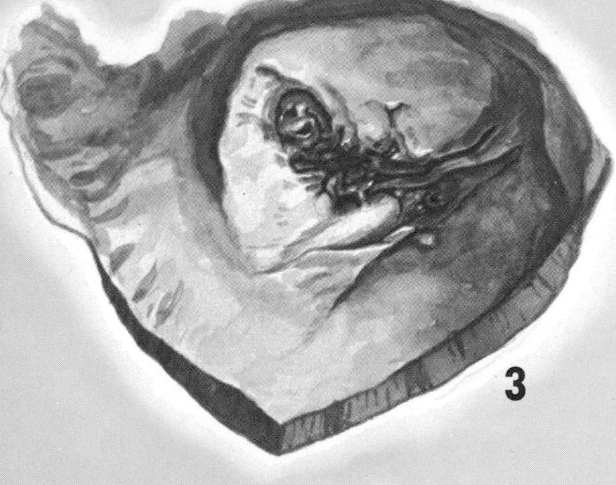

1

2

3

4

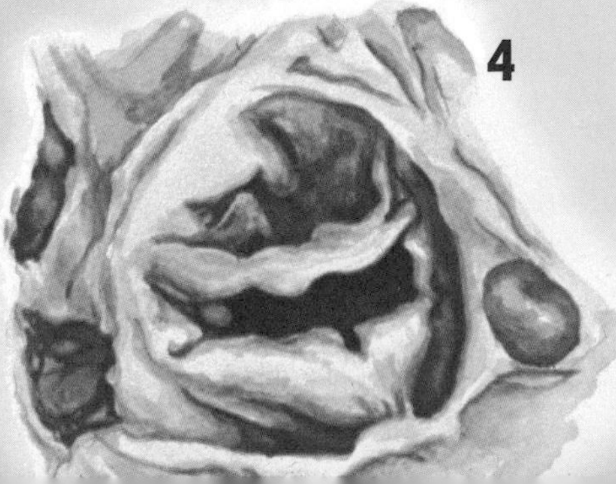

Left: Inflammation in connection with rheumatic fever may damage the heart valves. (1) Normal aortic valve closed. (2) Normal aortic valve partially open. (3) The mitral valve, showing narrowing of valve opening (stenosis) caused by scar formation. (4) Damaged aortic valve.

Above: Congenital heart defect, showing abnormal opening in the wall between the right and left sides of the heart.

The process of development is so complicated that if the circumstances in the tissues of the unborn child are not entirely favorable, there may result certain defects of structure.

Defects of the heart and its vessels account for about half the deaths caused by all types of congenital deformities. Some form of structural defect is present in about three out of every 1000 live-born babies. And because the heart's function is so important to the well-being of the entire body, the more serious defects actually threaten the life of the child.

The advent of heart surgery has made it possible to save or prolong the lives of many children who have congenital defects of the heart. It is necessary, of course, to determine the nature of the defect before a decision can be reached as to whether heart surgery might help the patient. Medical centers now have adequate facilities for determining the nature of a heart defect and thus providing information on which a judgment can be made on the proper type of treatment.

One of the procedures on which such an evaluation depends is that of cardiac catheterization. In this procedure, a small tube (catheter) is slipped through one of the patient's veins or arteries (depending on what part of the heart is to be explored) right into the interior of the heart. Its progress and position can be followed under the X-ray fluoroscope. Samples of blood are removed through the tube as it moves into the various parts of the heart. By testing these samples to determine how much oxygen and how much carbon dioxide they contain, the examining physician can know how much mixing of blood has occurred from the two sides of the heart and how serious is the defect. If it is decided that the patient would benefit by heart surgery, the usual method of using a heart-lung machine while the heart is opened and repaired makes it possible for the defect to be corrected or at least made less serious. Thus life

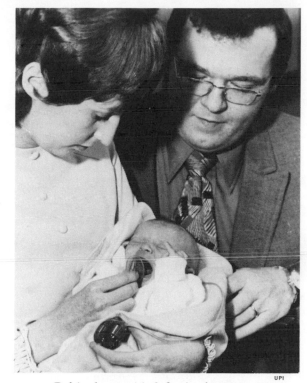

UPI

Babies born with defective hearts can often be helped by pacemaker transplants.

may be saved and health improved for a child whose prospect of long life was otherwise restricted.

The signs of congenital heart disease vary from case to case depending on the exact nature of the defect and the effect it has on the circulation of the blood. A dusky (cyanotic) color of the skin sometimes gives a clue. The term "blue baby" is often used to describe babies with defective hearts. Delayed growth and development in infants and children is obvious in many cases of congenital heart disease. Shortness of breath when the child exercises is a very frequent sign. This is related to a reduced capacity for exercise. The child with a faulty heart will often be observed to rest frequently when at play.

The severe degrees of congenital heart disease in babies are usually discovered by the doctor who attends the delivery. In less severe cases the discovery may be made by the family doctor or school nurse in making routine health checks of the child. Occasionally a person with congenital heart disease reaches adulthood before the cause of his frail health is discovered.

What to Do

Congenital heart disease is a condition that must be evaluated and treated by a specialist. For a child, it is the pediatrician who is trained to give professional guidance in such cases. Otherwise it is a specialist in internal medicine or in cardiology (diseases of the heart) who is qualified to handle such a case. For the surgical correction of such a problem, the doctor in charge will refer the case to a chest surgeon or to a medical center where a chest surgeon is available.

CORONARY HEART DISEASE.

It has already been emphasized that heart disease in its various forms stands at the top of the list of diseases that cause death and invalidism. And of the various forms of heart disease, it is coronary heart disease that largely accounts for this high figure.

An average healthy man living in the United States has about one chance in five of developing coronary heart disease before he reaches the age of 65. Notice that we mentioned the average *man*. Coronary heart disease is more common among men than among women.

It is coronary heart disease that accounts for practically all the instances of "heart attack" that strike suddenly and end, so many times, in sudden death. About 25 percent of persons who have a first heart attack die within three hours of the onset of the attack. Another 10 percent of this group of first-heart-attack victims die within the next four weeks. This leaves 65 percent who survive their first heart attack, only to live with the knowledge that they are quite vulnerable to another heart attack and that, at best, their life expectancy is reduced.

Another way of emphasizing the importance of coronary heart disease is to observe that about half of all the deaths in middle-aged men are caused by this form of heart disease. Each year, in the United States, about one out of every 100 men between the ages of 35 and 64 will experience a first heart attack.

Major Risk Factors

Most of the heart attacks resulting from coronary heart disease come unexpectedly. The victim may have seemed perfectly well and may have carried on his usual activities right up to the moment of the heart attack. The attack may occur while he is driving his car, sitting at his desk, or eating his dinner. It may strike while he is asleep.

Emergency treatment, if given promptly, reduces the prospect of death during this first attack. Even so, damage has already occurred to the tissues of the heart.

With these facts in mind, medical scientists have made careful studies of the circumstances and conditions that serve to identify persons who are susceptible to heart attack. These investigations have resulted in the listing of certain "risk factors"—three major and several minor ones. With a knowledge of the risk factors, the person who finds himself at risk should take precautions in advance.

Interestingly and significantly, the method of favorably modifying the risk factors is about the same as the program for the treatment and rehabilitation of a person who has already suffered a heart attack. In other words, the person at risk should take the treatment first and thus, hopefully, avoid the actual heart attack.

The three major risk factors are these: (1) an increase in the amount of cholesterol in the blood (hypercholesterolemia) which is associated with developing arteriosclerosis, (2) uncontrolled high blood pressure (hypertension), and (3) the use of cigarettes.

The influence of these three major risk factors becomes compounded when more than one of them is present in a given case. That is, when two risk factors are present, the prospect of a heart attack is more than twice as great as the prospect when only one risk factor is present. And when all three risk factors are present in a given case, the probability of a heart attack is more than three times as great as when only one factor is present.

Each of these primary risk factors is considered in greater detail elsewhere. The abnormal increase in cholesterol as this is related to arteriosclerosis is considered in the next chapter (chapter 10) under the heading of *Arteriosclerosis*. High blood pressure, its significance and treatment, is also considered in chapter 10 under the heading of *High Blood Pressure*. The use of cigarettes as this relates to coronary heart disease is treated in chapter 53 of volume 1.

Additional factors, the secondary risk factors, which also have their influence in determining a person's susceptibility to coronary heart disease, include these: (1) lack of sufficient physical exercise, (2) the personality type in which the person finds himself under continual emotional stress, (3) a metabolic predisposition in which there is a low tolerance for glucose (sugar), (4) obesity, and (5) a family record in which relatives have had a tendency to coronary heart disease.

Prevention

The prevention of coronary heart disease consists essentially of avoiding or correcting the risk factors mentioned above. Some of the secondary risk factors, admittedly, cannot be changed. But the primary risk factors and several of the secondary ones can be eliminated by the person who really chooses to do so.

Consider the first one of the major risk factors—increase in cholesterol in a person's blood. Medical scientists do not yet understand completely the manner in which an increase in cholesterol within the body's tissues and blood signals the development of arteriosclerosis. Cholesterol is a normal constituent of the body's tissues and blood. So cholesterol itself is not necessarily "bad." The body manufactures some of its cholesterol. The rest comes from the diet.

What is significant is an *increase* in the amount of cholesterol above normal limits. And this is usually related to the kinds of food a person eats. It has been noted that the people living in countries where the diets are high in saturated fats and in sugar have higher average values of cholesterol in their blood and a greater incidence of arteriosclerosis than those living in countries where the diets are low in saturated fats and sugar.

What are saturated fats? Chemically they are those fatty substances in which there is a high ratio of hydrogen to carbon within the molecules. From a practical standpoint, the saturated fats are those, for the most part, that are derived from animal sources such as the fatty cuts of meat, dairy butter, cream, and hard cheeses.

The average American diet contains too great a component of these foods which bring about an increase of cholesterol in the body's tissues and blood. This is indicated by the remarkably early age at which the first evidences of excess cholesterol appear in people living in our Western countries. The beginnings of arteriosclerosis occur commonly as early as the teens and early twenties. This fact was verified by a study of the tissues of American soldiers who met death in South Vietnam. These young men had not yet reached the age when coronary heart disease develops. However, the arteries throughout their bodies already contained evidence that arteriosclerosis was in progress.

The prevention of arteriosclerosis,

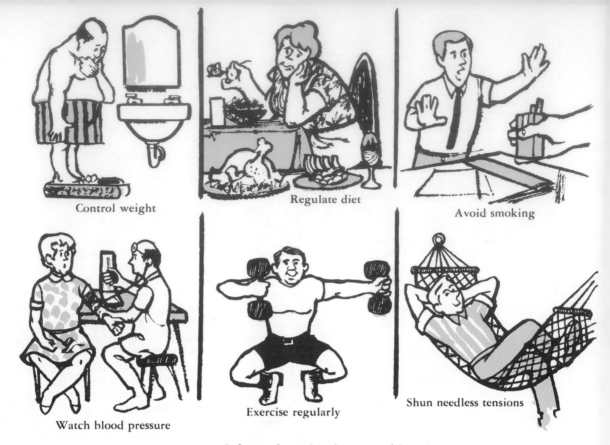

Control weight

Regulate diet

Avoid smoking

Watch blood pressure

Exercise regularly

Shun needless tensions

Safeguards against heart trouble.

then, should really begin during childhood, for it is the result of a lifetime pattern of unwholesome eating. (See under *Arteriosclerosis* in chapter 10 of this volume.)

Consider next the second of the primary risk factors—high blood pressure. This is often a concomitant of arteriosclerosis. As the name implies, it is a condition in which the blood which leaves the heart is under greater pressure than normal. This means that the heart must maintain a greater work load in order to sustain this high pressure.

An important aggravating factor in high blood pressure is emotional tension. Persons who live under unusual emotional stress or who are otherwise distraught and under competitive pressures sometimes develop high blood pressure. The prevention of this second primary risk factor may therefore require a person to modify his way of life. (See under *High Blood Pressure* in chapter 10 of this volume.)

Even in a perfectly healthy person blood pressure rises from time to time to surprisingly high levels, as when a person is greatly frightened or otherwise faces a serious emergency. But normally the blood pressure returns to its normal level as soon as the critical situation is over. Some people have a natural predisposition to high blood pressure. Aggravating factors keep the blood pressure at high levels for long periods of time and may promote the tendency for it to remain high. It is this sustained high blood pressure that causes damage to the body's tissues and sets the stage for unfavorable complications. Physicians have learned that even in these established cases of high blood pressure, the complications can often be avoided by artificially reducing the blood pressure. Certain chemical substances are now available that have the effect of reducing blood pressure. Even though these chemicals sometimes produce side effects, the prospects of continued health and longer life are improved by keeping the blood pressure at near normal levels. It is better, then, to have the doctor control high blood pressure by prescribing appropriate medicines than it is to allow the high blood pressure to run its unfavorable course.

The third primary risk factor—the use of cigarettes—seems to operate by favoring the development of arteriosclerosis. As detailed in chapter 53 of volume 1, those who smoke are much more susceptible to coronary heart disease than are nonsmokers. Furthermore, the risk of developing coronary heart disease is proportionately higher among those who smoke the greater number of cigarettes.

Finally, while we are speaking of the ways to prevent coronary heart disease, we should mention the importance of physical exercise. A program for using the large muscles of the body systematically each day in maintaining physical fitness is very important in arresting or delaying the progress of arteriosclerosis which, after all, is the basic cause of coronary heart disease. A well regulated program of exercise is an important part of the rehabilitation of the patient who has survived a heart attack. The fact that it is beneficial at such a time is sufficient evidence that it would be beneficial earlier in life as a means of keeping the heart attack from occurring at all.

What Happens in a Heart Attack?

We have said that arteriosclerosis is the basic cause of coronary heart disease and that the risk factors in this disease are those conditions that favor the development of arteriosclerosis.

The heart is a very active organ, functioning as it does twenty-four hours every day. Being thus active, its tissues require an abundant supply of oxygen and energy food. These are not derived from the blood as it flows through the chambers of the heart. Instead, the heart has its own system of blood vessels which provide the muscle in its wall with a continuous flow of freshly oxygenated blood. These arteries are called the coronary arteries. They branch off the aorta just as it leaves the left ventricle of the heart. Therefore the blood conveyed by the coronary arteries is the best blood, in terms of its oxygen content, of any blood within the body.

The coronary arteries are just as susceptible as any other arteries in the body to the development of arteriosclerosis. In arteriosclerosis, the walls of the arteries deteriorate. An abnormal amount of fibrous tissue develops in the walls, along with deposits of calcium and cholesterol. With the weakening of the arterial wall there comes also a thickening. Thus the lumen of the artery becomes smaller.

It is the narrowing of the coronary arteries, as part of the process of arteriosclerosis, that accounts for the usual case of coronary heart disease. There comes a time when some part of the coronary artery system becomes suddenly closed so that it no longer carries blood to that portion of the heart which it serves. It is this sudden plugging of a coronary blood vessel that brings on the typical heart attack.

Every branch of the coronary artery system has its own area of the heart to supply with blood. When any part of the system becomes unable to convey blood, the corresponding area of the heart begins to die.

The shock produced by the chemical changes in this area of dying tissue causes the immediate symptoms of a heart attack. The sudden death of the patient that so often occurs early in the course of the attack comes as a part of this shock reaction.

But this is not all. The area of the heart which is now deprived of its blood begins to soften and with this comes the danger that it may even rupture under the stress of continued heart action. This accounts, in part, for the deaths that occur a few hours or even a few days after the heart attack begins. Half of the deaths due to heart

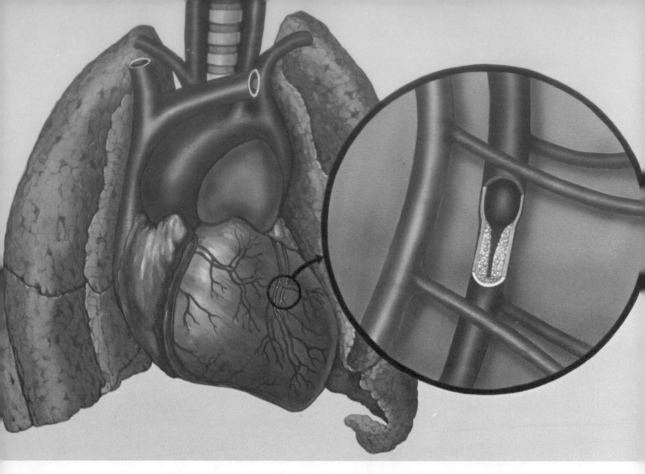

Obstruction in a major branch of the coronary system (shown in circle), as by a coronary thrombosis, deprives a certain area of the heart wall of its blood supply, bringing on myocardial infarction.

attacks are caused by uncontrolled irregularity of the heart rhythm.

For those who survive a coronary heart attack, the healing process involves replacing the muscle of the affected part of the heart with scar tissue. The scar, of course, does not have the ability to contract; therefore it is unable to do its share of the work of the heart. The healed heart is never as efficient as it was before the heart attack. What is more, the person who has survived one heart attack is still a prospect for another heart attack because the fundamental condition of arteriosclerosis still exists, and other parts of the coronary artery system may yet become obstructed.

Angina Pectoris

In some cases of coronary heart disease the symptoms result from a gradual reduction in the blood supply rather than from a sudden incident as in a typical heart attack. In these cases of gradual reduction of blood flow there often occurs a series of painful episodes to which we apply the term angina pectoris.

The attack of pain in angina pectoris usually occurs after the person has engaged in some strenuous exertion such as running to catch the bus. Such extra exertion makes additional demands on the functioning heart. If the heart were normal, it could rise to the occasion by beating faster and more forcefully, thus sending out a greater volume of blood. In the case, however, in which the coronary blood flow is reduced, the heart soon exceeds its limit of tolerance. With a limited supply of oxygen and energy food, it can perform only so much work and no

90

more. When its tolerance is exceeded there develops reflex pain which usually centers just beneath the breast bone. The pain is described as "pressing," "boring," or "gripping." Its intensity varies a great deal from case to case. Often the pain radiates to the left shoulder and down the left arm. The episode of pain usually lasts only a few minutes, typically not more than five minutes. It subsides as the person rests, because the rest reduces the demand for extra work by the heart.

The symptoms of angina pectoris may be brought on by emotional shock or even by a bad dream in which the person's body reacts as to some sudden emergency. Often the painful episode occurs during or just after a heavy meal.

Angina pectoris may be mistaken for a genuine heart attack. However, the pain due to a heart attack usually lasts longer. In both conditions the pain may be intense, originating beneath the sternum (breast bone), and often radiating to the left shoulder and down the left arm. When in doubt as to which condition is causing the pain, the safe procedure is to assume that the situation is the more serious of the two possibilities—the heart attack of coronary occlusion. This deserves immediate attention as specified a few paragraphs later under *What to Do*.

The person who has had previous episodes of angina pectoris has usually been instructed by his doctor to carry with him a small supply of nitroglycerine tablets. One or two of these tablets placed under the tongue at the time of an attack will cause the tiny muscles in the walls of the coronary arteries to relax and thus relieve the pain. In the meantine the person should be kept quietly at rest, lying on his back with his head and shoulders elevated slightly.

The Actual Heart Attack

When the stoppage (occlusion) of one of the coronary arteries occurs suddenly, we then have an actual heart attack—an emergency situation

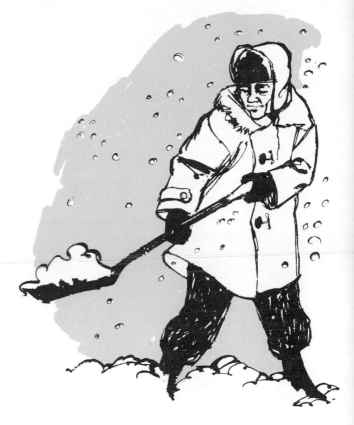

Overexertion or vigorous exercise may precipitate heart attack.

in which the patient's life hangs in the balance. This is the condition that the physician calls a "coronary occlusion." It results in myocardial infarction—dead heart muscle.

The symptoms strike suddenly. One minute the victim is carrying on his usual activities; the next minute he is incapacitated with intense pain which originates in the chest, or even in the region of the upper part of the stomach, and radiates to the left shoulder and left arm. The patient often feels that his chest is being squeezed, pressured, or constricted. The attack may begin under almost any circumstances: while the person is resting, while he is driving his car, while he is working, or even while he is sleeping. Often the pain is so intense that there is difficulty in breathing. The person becomes weak. He may be nauseated and may even vomit. He often perspires freely. His skin may be moist and cold. The skin may appear pale or dusky. He often expresses fear of impending death. The pain usually persists for half an hour or more.

The above description applies to the usual case of heart attack. But the symptoms may vary a great deal from case to case, both in the intensity of the pain and in its duration. Also, some of the associated symptoms may be absent in any particular case.

The location and nature of the pain in heart attack resembles that of an episode of angina pectoris. This is reasonable, for in both situations there is a reduction in blood supply to the heart. The symptoms of heart attack may also be confused with those of indigestion, especially when the pain of a heart attack begins in "the pit of the stomach" and is accompanied by nausea.

Doubt as to what is causing the symptoms, plus the natural desire to believe the best rather than the worst, explains why so many cases of heart attack are not given the prompt care they so urgently deserve.

Actually, the care the victim receives during these first few minutes of his attack may make the difference between life and death.

The American Heart Association puts it this way: "Don't you wait. If you think someone is having a heart attack, call the fire department rescue squad immediately. Seconds count. Don't wait for severe pain, dizziness, fainting, sweating, or shortness of breath. . . . Don't let fear of embarrassment delay your call. If you're wrong about the existence of a heart attack, it doesn't matter. If you're right, nothing could matter more."

You may not live near a fire department that has a rescue squad. But call whatever help is available: a doctor, an ambulance. Many ambulances are now operated by trained paramedics and are equipped so that they can give necessary emergency care to a patient with heart attack even while he is being transported to the hospital emergency room.

What to Do

1. Call for the doctor, the fire department rescue squad, or an ambulance. Make the message urgent, stating that a person is having a heart attack. Give your name, address, and telephone number.

2. Place the victim in a half reclining position with his head and shoulders elevated slightly. Keep him in this position until seen by the doctor or until trained help arrives.

3. Insist that the victim remain absolutely at rest, not even moving a finger.

4. Loosen the victim's clothing where it might constrict his neck or waist.

5. Allow him to breathe fresh air. If a tank of oxygen is available, play a gentle stream of the oxygen over the victim's face thus allowing him to breathe the oxygen.

6. If tablets of nitroglycerine are available, place one of these under the victim's tongue, allowing it to be dissolved there.

7. When trained help arrives, follow instructions.

8. Allow the patient to be transferred to the emergency room of the hospital or, if available, to a hospital coronary care unit.

Treating the Heart Attack Patient

The proper care for a person who has just suffered a coronary heart attack requires professional expertise and a great deal of technical skill. It is best accomplished in the coronary care unit of a hospital. Here the necessary equipment is available for monitoring the heart's action continuously through 24 hours each day. The personnel of a coronary care unit are trained to deal with each complication that may develop.

The principle of caring for a recent

case of heart attack requires that the work load of the heart be reduced as much as possible during the time the damaged portion of the muscle is being healed. Therefore during this early period the patient must be kept at rest so as to reduce the work of his heart to the minimum. Sometimes medicines are necessary to relieve pain. In some cases oxygen is administered to make the patient's breathing easier.

Depending on what part of the heart was damaged by being deprived of its blood supply, many different problems can develop. The modern methods of monitoring the heart's action will indicate these complications, if and when they develop, so that they can be treated appropriately.

Rehabilitation After Heart Attack

The patient who is recovering from a heart attack should have a bland diet which is low in calories—so low that he loses some weight. As he continues to improve, the number of calories in his daily diet can be raised to about 1500 which is still on the low side compared with the average diet for an adult.

Such a person should live at a slower pace than he is accustomed to until his heart has completely healed. If he has been a smoker, he should permanently discontinue the use of cigarettes.

Physicians have learned in recent years that the person who has had a heart attack benefits greatly thereafter by following a systematic program of graduated physical exercise. The exact amount of exercise that a given patient can tolerate can be determined by measuring the response of his heart to the added work load as exercise is increased. A simple way to determine how much exercise such a patient can tolerate is to keep a record of his heart rate. The patient will usually tolerate the amount of exercise necessary to increase his heart rate to 120 beats per minute. Where sophisticated equipment is available, the prescription for the proper amount of exercise can be determined by the amount of oxygen the patient uses during a period of monitored physical activity.

Angiocardiography

Many patients who have a high risk of heart attack or who are candidates for a subsequent heart attack after having survived a previous one, are benefited by the modern surgical procedure known as coronary bypass. This was described earlier in the chapter. Whether a patient will benefit by this has to be determined by making a careful examination of his heart's coronary arteries. This requires the use of the special technique known as angiocardiography. This involves an X-ray study of the heart, using rapid motion picture methods while a dye is injected into the bloodstream. The dye can be seen as it moves through the coronary arteries and it can be thus determined what particular sites in the arteries have been narrowed by the process of arteriosclerosis. If the narrowing of these vessels is limited to one or two sites, the surgical procedure of coronary bypass may serve to carry the blood through a newly established detour route past these locations where the arteries have become narrow.

Men vs. Women

It is a remarkable observation that during middle life a much higher percentage of men than of women suffer from coronary heart disease. Between the ages of 30 and 59, more than four times as many men as women die from heart attack. After age 60, the incidence of heart attack among women begins to approach that of men. The reason for this difference in the susceptibility of men and women to heart attack probably centers around the biologic advantage that women have in their resistance to illness during the child-bearing period. Also the female hormone protects against atherosclerosis.

DISTURBED FUNCTIONS OF THE HEART.

The most common disturbance of the heart's function is *palpitation,* a condition characterized by awareness of a rapid, forcible or irregular action of the heart and noticeable to the person concerned. It may cause anxiety, difficulty in breathing, and, at times, distress around the heart.

Palpitation may be caused by emotional stress, such as fear, anger, joy, grief, or anxiety; by certain drugs or poisons, such as may be found in tea, coffee, tobacco, or alcoholic drinks; or by reflex impulses from disease in some other part of the body. The attacks may last from a few seconds to several hours; and the victim may become very nervous and mentally distressed, though there is seldom any real danger to life.

Sinus tachycardia is an abnormally rapid rate of otherwise normal heartbeats, the rate being a hundred or more per minute. It may or may not be a sign of actual heart damage. Sinus tachycardia may occur in response to exercise or excitement even in a person whose heart is healthy. The symptom may call for an examination by a physician.

Paroxysmal tachycardia consists of spells, usually brief, of very rapid but regular beating of the heart, the rate often being 150 or more per minute. It may have several different causes, which often require careful study by a physician to detect; and it may or may not be serious.

Atrial fibrillation is a very rapid but irregular beating of the atria; but, since the beating of the atria does not create the pulse, this condition cannot be directly detected by feeling and counting the pulse or by any ordinary examination. A physician can detect it by using special instruments or equipment. It should be strongly suspected whenever the pulse is somewhat rapid and shows irregularity both in rate and force. It is often a sign of serious heart impairment.

Atrial flutter is a very rapid but

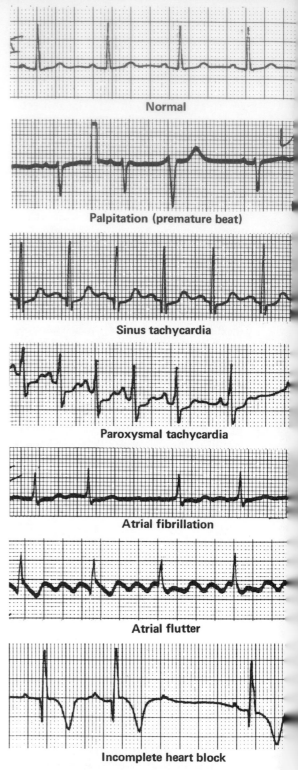

Normal

Palpitation (premature beat)

Sinus tachycardia

Paroxysmal tachycardia

Atrial fibrillation

Atrial flutter

Incomplete heart block

Typical electrocardiogram (EKG) tracings, made by an electrocardiograph and used in diagnosing irregularities of heart action.

94

regular beating of the atria. It should be suspected if the pulse continues to be as rapid as 140 or more per minute, but regular, for a considerable period of time. It fairly often indicates the presence of heart damage.

Heart block is a term applied to a condition in which the contraction impulses are delayed or fail to get through from their source in the right atrium to the ventricles. In such a case the ventricles may keep on beating because of a natural rhythm in their own muscles, but the rate, while regular, is very slow—perhaps forty or less per minute. The block may be partial, resulting in delayed or dropped beats. Heart block, especially complete block, usually indicates the presence of serious heart damage.

Pulsus alternans or alternating pulse, consists of alternate strong and weak heartbeats with a regular rhythm. It usually indicates an impaired heart muscle and is an omen of future trouble. This is a rare condition.

There is a very common group of symptoms—some of them heart symptoms—called by many names, among which are soldier's heart, effort syndrome, and neurocirculatory asthenia. The prominent symptoms are palpitation, shortness of breath, pain in the heart region, and exhaustion on moderate exertion. A person with this condition rarely if ever dies of it; but it is distressing, disabling, and difficult to cure. The cure depends largely upon the victim's being brought to understand the true nature of his ailment and his being willing to undertake the changes in his living program that his physician is likely to recommend.

It is a remarkable fact that many of the disturbances that a person himself may observe about his heart are symptoms of trouble that have no real relation to heart muscle, heart valves, or the blood vessels of the organ; and their true nature cannot be determined without careful study by a physician. Consequently, one who fears that he has heart disease should seek medical counsel. If his heart is found to be healthy in spite of possibly alarming symptoms, which may well be the case, his mind can the sooner be set at rest. If he really has a diseased heart, the sooner he begins the proper treatment the better.

HEART FAILURE.

Acute dilatation of the heart is a phrase that explains itself. If a diseased heart is suddenly forced to work beyond its strength, it may dilate markedly and become filled with blood, but be unable to pump this blood out into the arteries. This condition is a serious menace to life. If the left side of the heart is chiefly affected, the victim will develop cyanosis, weakness, breathlessness, and a cough with much sputum. More rarely, when the right side of the heart is chiefly affected, there will be pain and pulsation in the liver, pulsation in the large veins, and other symptoms that may lead to a suspicion that appendicitis or inflammation of the gallbladder is present.

As heart failure approaches, the real symptoms of the heart ailment manifest themselves. At first these may not seem to be related to the heart. Shortness of breath on slight exertion is one of the earliest symptoms. Distress and an abnormal feeling of fullness after eating are common. In fact, the person with heart disease often comes to the doctor complaining about stomach trouble, not suspecting the real cause of his symptoms. A person past middle age who has never had stomach trouble, but who now finds that he has persistent indigestion or other stomach symptoms, should consult a physician without delay.

Other early symptoms of which people with developing heart diseases often complain are weakness and lack of endurance, particularly in the legs; dull pain and soreness in the region of the liver or over the heart; and palpitation of the heart, with fullness in the chest and a dry cough. Swelling of the ankles may be an early

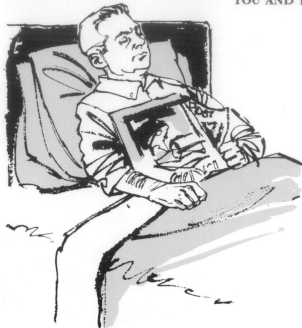

Treatment for heart symptoms typically includes bed rest.

symptom, and it may be present a long time before any other pronounced symptoms appear. Such swelling is usually worse in the evening and subsides during sleep. The person concerned also finds that he needs more pillows to raise his head higher than usual in order to sleep comfortably, and spells of difficult breathing during the night are likely to occur. Though bed rest at this stage may be advisable in order to relieve the strain on the failing heart, it is often hard to convince the person concerned that anything serious is wrong.

As the heart becomes weaker, the above-mentioned symptoms become more marked, and what is called congestive heart failure (a serious turn of events in which the heart is no longer able to pump the required volume of blood) becomes fully manifest. Weakness increases until the victim finds himself utterly exhausted on the slightest exertion. His legs become swollen, and his breathing grows increasingly difficult, until he cannot lie down. Pains develop through his chest and back. He is restless and sleepless; and at last, no matter how stoical he may once have been, he realizes that he is really sick and ought to be on a program of complete rest. Many people who have seemed to be at death's door from congestive heart failure have been brought back to a fair degree of health, and with care have been able to live on for several years.

What to Do

A patient with symptoms of heart failure should be placed under the supervision of a physician, and his instructions should be followed implicitly. Depending on available facilities and circumstances, the physician may prefer to have the patient in the hospital, or he may arrange for qualified nursing care in the home. There are three governing principles in the treatment of a patient with heart failure:

1. *Reduce the heart's work load.* The patient's physical activities should be reduced to come within his heart's limit of tolerance. This implies bed rest, often in a semireclining position, until the condition of the heart improves sufficiently to allow restricted activities otherwise. If the patient has high blood pressure, the physician will use medications to bring this within reasonable limits. The physician may also consider the treatment of other defects of the heart if these are adding to the heart's work load.

2. *Provide competent nursing surveillance.* The nurse must be in constant attendance, both as a means of detecting changes in the patient's condition and to sustain the patient's morale. In heart failure there is a tendency for fluid to accumulate in the body's tissues. The nurse must keep the doctor informed on the patient's "water balance." At times it may be necessary to administer oxygen to the patient. The doctor often specifies a saltfree or a salt-restricted diet.

3. *Improve the heart's function.*

The use of proper medications is thoroughly justified as a life-saving measure in the treatment of heart failure. The two kinds of medications most commonly needed are diuretics to facilitate the removal of excess fluid from the body's tissues and some form of digitalis to reinforce the action of the heart's muscle. The physician and the nurse work in cooperation to use these medications most effectively.

HYPERTENSIVE HEART DISEASE.

In this form of heart disease the heart gets tired and becomes inefficient because of being overworked for many months and years. It is not the patient's physical activity, as such, that causes this damage to his heart, but extra exertion by the heart in maintaining blood pressure higher than normal. In other words, hypertensive heart disease is one of the later complications of hypertension (high blood pressure). It is clear, therefore, that the way to prevent hypertensive heart disease is to prevent high blood pressure. Hypertension is considered earlier in this same chapter under *Coronary Heart Disease* and also in the following chapter (chapter 10) under *High Blood Pressure*.

An early result of hypertension (high blood pressure), especially in younger people, is an increase in the size and strength of the heart muscle, most noticeable in the walls of the left ventricle. If a moderate increase of this sort is enough to compensate for the degree of high blood pressure present, few or no symptoms of heart trouble may ever develop. As the years pass, however, the pressure tends to increase, the aging heart muscle becomes less and less able to carry its heavy load with safety, and heart muscle failure becomes more and more likely to occur. High blood pressure may also cause some leakage at the valves, especially the mitral valve, thus increasing the difficulty of maintaining an adequate circulation.

Death from this type of heart disease does not result from a "heart attack" but rather from a gradual development of what has been called "decompensation" or "congestive heart failure." This problem is considered in the previous part of this chapter under *Heart Failure*.

RHEUMATIC HEART DISEASE.

Whatever causes inflammation of the joints in rheumatic fever may also cause inflammations of the heart. These may be (1) *endocarditis*, or inflammation of the lining of the heart, or of the valves; (2) *pericarditis*, or inflammation of the covering of the heart; or (3) *myocarditis*, an inflammation of the heart muscle. Any of these may result in permanent damage to the organ. Rheumatic fever, with resulting heart damage, often follows an attack of streptococcic sore throat or some other form of streptococcal infection. Rheumatic fever tends to recur, but the use of suitable preparations of penicillin or other antibiotics helps to prevent these recurrences.

During the course of any one of these inflammations, the heart valves may become scarred.

If the primary streptococcal infection is allowed to persist until rheumatic fever develops, it will take a long and tedious course of treatment to prevent permanent heart damage; and even such a course of treatment is not always successful. More than this, a streptococcal infection may cause damage to the heart without first passing through the stage of rheumatic fever. Thus it is that the prevention of rheumatic heart disease requires the prompt and adequate treatment of primary streptococcal infections.

In cases in which rheumatic heart disease develops, the acute inflammation of the heart's lining eventually subsides and the valve ulcerations heal. Two permanent defects may result: (1) a narrowing of the valve opening caused by scar formation and irregular contraction, and (2) an incomplete closing of the valve because of this deformity. At the time of the heartbeat, the blood is hindered from flowing freely in the direction it should go, by the narrowing of the valve opening; and between beats it is permitted to leak back in the wrong direction because of the imperfectly closed valve. The narrowing of the opening is called "stenosis," and the reverse flow is called "insufficiency." Either defect alone, or a combination of the two to a more marked degree, increases the work of the heart and may lead eventually to heart failure if due care is not exercised. The mitral valve, between the left atrium and the left ventricle, is most frequently attacked, and what is called "mitral stenosis" is the most frequent of the damaging results. This condition can now sometimes be treated surgically with success. The aortic valve may be similarly affected, though not so often. Other valves are rarely affected.

(See also the discussion of *Rheumatic Fever* in chapter 28 of this volume.)

What to Do

1. Rheumatic fever is the underlying cause of rheumatic heart disease. Therefore, urgent consideration must be given to the treatment and to the danger of recurrence of the rheumatic fever. (See *Rheumatic Fever* in chapter 28 of this volume.)

2. Once the valves of the heart become damaged there is the possibility that the heart's efficiency will be so reduced that the heart becomes unable to keep up with the demands upon it. This may result in heart irregularities such as atrial fibrillation or in so-called "heart failure." (See *Heart Failure.*)

3. In the chronic phase of rheumatic heart disease it is often advisable to consider the surgical repair or replacement of the damaged heart valve. The counsel of a specialist in internal medicine or that of a cardiologist (specialist in diseases of the heart) should be sought.

Blood-vessel and Blood Diseases

I. Blood-vessel Diseases

This first subdivision on diseases of the blood vessels is essentially a continuation of the preceding chapter on heart disease. The heart is readily affected by many of the abnormal conditions of the blood vessels. Such conditions as arteriosclerosis and high blood pressure, although involving the blood vessels in definite ways, lay the foundation on which heart ailments develop.

ANEURYSM.

An aneurysm is a bulging of an artery because of a weakness of the arterial wall, increased blood pressure, or both. It is always a serious condition. Aneurysms occur most frequently in the aorta, in both its thoracic (within the chest) and its abdominal portions. Aneurysms of arteries within the skull rank second in frequency to those of the aorta.

Various possible causes account for the weakening of an arterial wall, such as injuries, infection, the degeneration accompanying high blood pressure or arteriosclerosis, and syphilis in its later stages. Aneurysms occur most often between the ages of forty and seventy, oftener in men than in women.

The symptoms of aneurysm of the aorta in the chest may at first be few and slight, such as mild shortness of breath and pain on exertion. If the aneurysm is located near the outlet from the heart, the symptoms may never seem severe to the person who has it, but a physician can detect its presence by physical and X-ray examinations. If it is located in the arch of the aorta, the symptoms, generally much more marked, are likely to include a peculiar brassy cough, hoarseness, much pain, difficulty in breathing, swelling of one arm or the face and neck, distended veins in the neck and upper chest, and bulging of the chest wall, this latter forming a pulsating tumor. In early or doubtful cases the X ray is the most reliable means of diagnosis.

If the aneurysm is located in the descending portion of the thoracic aorta, there may be no symptoms unless it becomes large enough to press on one or more ribs or on the backbone. Such a pulsating pressure causes bone degeneration to take place, accompanied by much pain.

Aneurysms located within the chest can be treated by the modern methods of vascular surgery. Unless success-

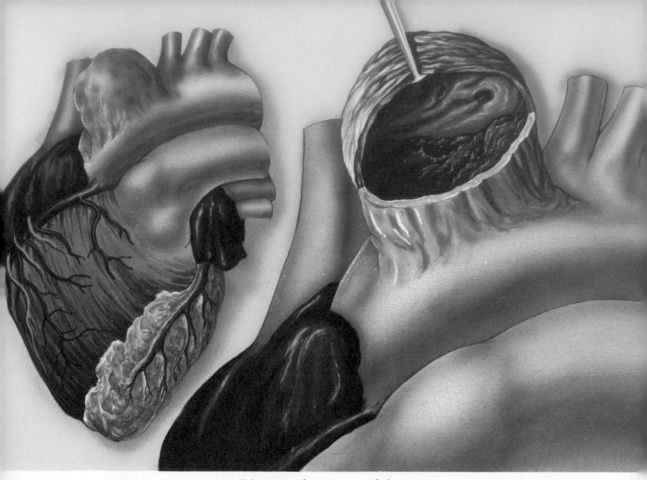

Diagram of aneurysm of the aorta.

fully treated, hemorrhage into the chest or the lungs, or even erosion through the chest wall with external bleeding, may occur, usually resulting in death within a matter of minutes. Physical exertion is likely to bring on such a hemorrhage.

Aneurysm in the abdominal portion of the aorta is usually the result of arteriosclerosis. It is indicated by a pulsating mass deep in the central part of the abdomen. There may be pain in the upper abdomen, lower back, or groin. There is danger of sudden, fatal hemorrhage. Treatment is by vascular surgery in which the involved portion of the aorta is replaced by a preserved artery (from the "artery bank") or by a section of a specifically fabricated synthetic tubing.

Aneurysms of arteries within the skull are likely to cause headache, especially on exertion. They also frequently hinder the normal action of some of the cranial nerves, especially the second, third, and fifth, giving rise to signs and symptoms that help the physician to determine what is wrong. An X ray of the head after an injection of a radiopaque dye into the arterial system will also help detect this condition. Rupture of and bleeding from an aneurysm within the skull is one of the conditions that can cause a stroke.

APOPLEXY (STROKE).
(See *Stroke.*)

ARTERIOSCLEROSIS (HARDENING OF THE ARTERIES).
(See also ARTERIOSCLEROTIC HEART DISEASE in the preceding chapter.)

This disease, which produces a gradual deterioration of the walls of

100

the arteries throughout the body, is the fundamental cause of the commonest form of heart disease (coronary heart disease which causes the usual kind of heart attack) and of the interruption of blood flow through the arteries of the brain, which occurs in strokes.

A certain degree of hardening of the arteries occurs in most persons as they become older. It may become noticeable earlier and progress more rapidly in some people than in others. Hardening of the arteries frequently develops so slowly and gradually that it is not recognized until a person reaches 50 or more years of age.

This "hardening" of the arterial walls may be caused by an increased proportion of fibrous tissue in them, by a deposit of calcium in them, by a deposit in them of a fatlike substance called cholesterol, or by any two or all three of these factors. It is the cholesterol deposits that are most likely to weaken the arterial wall so that they can more easily rupture, or to promote the formation of clots within the artery, thus causing what is called thrombosis.

Other factors besides advancing age believed to hasten the hardening of the arteries are high blood pressure, diabetes, overeating—especially of egg yolks, cream, butter, and other animal fats—infectious diseases, overweight, and excessive nerve strain.

It is significant that persons in whom the amount of cholesterol in the blood is higher than normal carry a greater than average risk of developing coronary heart disease—this being the complication of arteriosclerosis which takes the greatest number of lives. Furthermore, studies of human populations indicate that the cholesterol level in the blood is influenced by the kind of diet eaten and the amount of exercise done per day. Population groups which consume diets low in total calories and fat (particularly "saturated" fat) have low blood cholesterol readings and have a low incidence of coronary heart disease. The reverse is also true.

Among the other systemic effects of arteriosclerosis are impaired kidney function, a reduced blood supply to all parts of the body, especially the brain and the heart muscle, and an increased proneness to arterial rupture and hemorrhage into the surrounding tissues. Further and more manifest effects are attacks of severe chest pain, mental deterioration, pain in the muscles of the limbs on exertion, stroke, and paralysis.

In many cases the hardening of the arterial walls and the narrowing of the blood channels are particularly marked in the small arteries of the extremities, especially the feet, and near the body surface. This is a common condition in people who have diabetes. In such cases the extremities tend to be cold, and gangrene of the feet is likely to develop, especially if care is not taken to keep them clean, warm, and dry. Alternate warm and cold foot and leg baths may be helpful, if prolonged, and if the difference in the temperature between the warm and the cold is not great.

Gangrene in the extremities may result from arteriosclerosis.

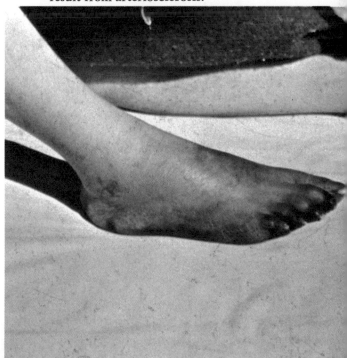

Preventive Measures. Treatment of arteriosclerosis is rather discouraging, for by the time the disease is recognized, damage to the body's tissues has already been done. Emphasis, therefore, should be on prevention more than on cure.

In view of the demonstrated relationship between the level of cholesterol in the blood and the development of arteriosclerosis and its complications, prevention is aimed at those measures that tend to keep the concentration of blood cholesterol within normal limits. There are two principal aspects of the daily life that must be considered.

1. *Diet.* An excess of calories in the diet (eating too much food) predisposes both to overweight and to the development of arteriosclerosis. Therefore, overeating should be avoided. It is even assumed that arteriosclerosis, once it becomes established, can be reduced somewhat, by cutting down the amount of food eaten. Also the fat content of the diet should be low, and the type of fat eaten should be mostly unsaturated rather than saturated. In ordinary language this means avoiding hydrogenated vegetable fats as well as fats derived from animal sources (fatty cuts of meat, dairy butter, cream, and hard cheeses). Also, concentrated sugar in the diet (as in desserts, sweets, soft drinks) should be kept to a minimum.

2. *Exercise.* A program of physical fitness, including daily exercise (preferably outdoors) is of benefit in maintaining the cholesterol in the blood at safe levels. Admittedly, the elements of recreation and freedom from nervous tension associated with the exercise also probably exert other beneficial influences.

Several epidemiological studies have indicted cigarettes as a major factor in causing arteriosclerosis. This explains the high incidence of coronary heart disease among smokers. The use of cigarettes should therefore be avoided.

What to Do

1. Presently the cure for arteriosclerosis is unknown. Hardened arteries can probably not be restored to their former condition even though their condition may be improved somewhat by following a suitable diet as mentioned above.

2. To prevent rupture of the arteries, especially those of the brain, avoid overexertion; but moderate exercise may help to maintain or even improve the circulation.

3. To avoid overburdening the heart, the digestive organs, and the kidneys, take an easily digestible and not too abundant diet which is low in fats derived from animal sources.

4. If the blood pressure is above normal limits, ask your doctor for help in bringing this under control.

5. Abstain from the use of cigarettes.

CARDIOVASCULAR ACCIDENT.
(See *Stroke.*)

EMBOLISM.

A blood clot, or thrombus, may form inside a vein, an artery, or the heart itself; and a portion of such a clot (called an embolus) may break off and be carried along by the bloodstream. In a vein, the embolus moves toward the heart, then through the right side of that organ and out into the pulmonary artery, finally lodging somewhere in a lung. The classic symptoms of pulmonary embolism (when an embolus lodges in a lung) are sudden pain in the chest with each breath, difficulty in breathing, and coughing up blood-tinged sputum. A few small emboli, lodging in one or both of the lungs may produce no symptoms and therefore may pass unnoticed unless specific tests are made. However, when a large number of small emboli move into the lungs, the patient's condition is potentially serious; for often a larger embolus, originating

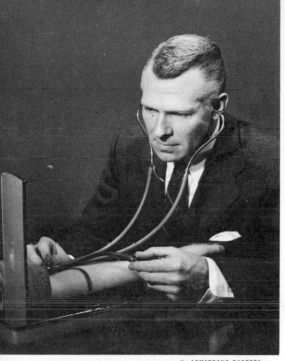

H. ARMSTRONG ROBERTS

the clot from the artery may save both life and limb. If the arterial embolus lodges in the brain, one type of stroke occurs; if it lodges in some artery in the trunk a variety of distressing symptoms occur, severe enough in most cases to prompt the calling of a physician.

What to Do

All cases of embolism require emergency treatment. Hospitalization is essential. The physician will decide on the appropriate methods of treatment, basing his judgment on the location of the embolus, the size of the area of damage, and the patient's general condition. The methods include the administration of oxygen, the use of anticoagulants (blood thinning agents), and surgery to remove the embolus.

HIGH BLOOD PRESSURE (HYPERTENSION).

In measuring a person's blood pressure, the doctor takes two readings, the high and the low. The highest pressure which the heart produces as it pumps blood into the arteries is called the systolic pressure. The low reading (the diastolic) is a measure of the pressure that remains in the arteries just before the next heartbeat takes place. The readings are traditionally expressed in millimeters of mercury—indicating the height of a column of mercury that this much pressure would support. The reading is usually written in this fashion: 120/80.

Average normal blood pressures are lower in children (90/60 at age six) than in young adults (120/80). The normal range for blood pressure in a healthy young adult is 90 to 140 for the systolic and 60 to 90 for the diastolic. A popular belief persists that an adult's blood pressure normally increases as he becomes older. The fact is that average blood pressure does increase with age, but this is not normal. Persistent readings above 140 systolic

at the same site, may soon follow. Medium-sized and larger emboli lodging in the lung cause symptoms to develop suddenly and threaten the patient's life. If the patient's life is to be saved in the case of a large pulmonary embolism, appropriate treatment must be carried out within the first 30 minutes. The treatment may consist of the administering of oxygen, the prompt use of some anticoagulant such as heparin, or a quick trip to the operating room where a large embolus may be removed by the surgeon. Very large emboli, lodging in a lung, may cause sudden death. (See *Pulmonay Infarction* in chapter 17 of this volume.)

When an embolus originates in the left side of the heart or in an artery, it is carried in a direction away from the heart and may lodge in any of the smaller arteries in any vital or nonvital organ of the body. If it lodges in an artery in an extremity, severe pain suddenly develops, and the limb is likely to become cold, pale, and numb. The pain tends to increase, the limb becomes dark colored and blotchy, and gangrene may soon set in; but immediate surgery to remove

103

and above 90 diastolic actually represent a corresponding degree of hypertension.

Many factors may cause a person's blood pressure to become abnormally high, any one of which or any combination of which may be to blame in a given case. Overeating with resultant obesity is a common causative factor, also heredity and racial background. Stress—physical, social, and business—is a factor in producing high blood pressure. It is among city dwellers, where such stress is greatest, that high blood pressure is most common. The condition may be made still worse by the use of tobacco. The smoking of a single cigarette may temporarily raise the systolic blood pressure between five and ten points.

Symptoms of high blood pressure do not often occur much before the age of thirty-five, in spite of the fact that unhygienic habits and other causative factors may have been in operation since the earlier years. A wise person will take warning from the experience of others and will correct his habits before disaster strikes.

Acute infections, such as tonsillitis, scarlet fever, and typhoid fever, sometimes lead to kidney disease, which may bring with it high blood pressure. In such cases the increased pressure is a natural compensatory mechanism to maintain a normal filtration rate through the hardened walls of the small arteries in the kidneys. Kidney disease of the slowly progressive type is often accompanied by hardening of the arteries, high blood pressure, and enlargement of the heart. Sudden attacks of convulsions in pregnant women (eclampsia) and other kidney disorders of pregnancy are associated with an increase in blood pressure.

Therapy for high blood pressure includes abundant fruit in the diet.

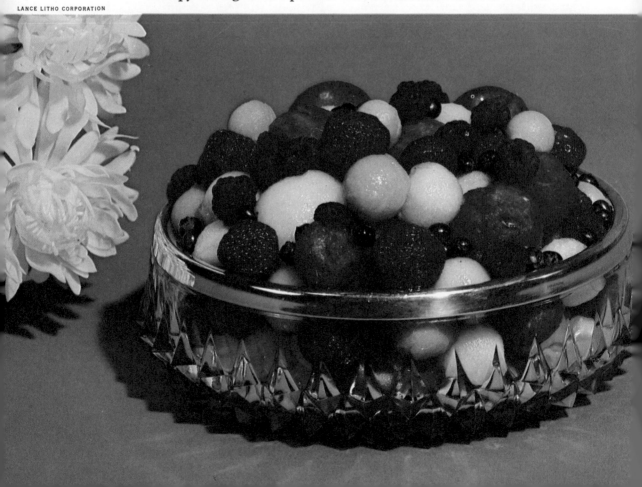

The signs and symptoms of high blood pressure may vary greatly. Overweight, a ruddy complexion, and apparently robust health may be the only outward manifestations in a man fifty or sixty years of age. In such cases, the systolic pressure may be as high as 200 or more, and yet the individual may suffer no discomfort. On the other hand, there may be dizziness, aching or throbbing of the head, ringing in the ears, and other disagreeable sensations.

Much can be done for high blood pressure before hardening of the arteries occurs or before it becomes extreme. Diet is of first importance, especially for obese people; and he who would keep his pressure down must control his appetite and maintain his weight at normal or even slightly below normal. Excessive protein foods, sweets, rich pastry, desserts, and all beverages containing caffeine should be omitted, and very little salt used.

Rest, both physical and mental, is a valuable remedy in all cases of markedly high blood pressure, though mild exercise is beneficial to people with moderate hypertension. In severe cases the usual business, professional, and social duties and cares must be entirely laid aside. Even the visits of friends and relatives may have to be restricted or prohibited for a time. No vigorous or tonic hydrotherapy or even massage should be administered. The neutral bath and complete bed rest give the best results.

Several drugs quite effective in lowering high blood pressure have been developed recently, but these need to be taken under a physician's supervision. The search for better remedies still goes on. It is well for a high-blood pressure patient to remain under a physician's care so that he will have the benefit of new discoveries as soon as they have been proved effective.

If the blood pressure has been above normal for a considerable period of time before the fact becomes known, which is often the case, the heart muscles and the kidney filters have already adjusted themselves to the increased pressure; and lowering it too rapidly or too much may do more harm than good. If a person has only a moderately high pressure, it is often more important for him to learn how to live with it safely than to try to lower it too much.

What to Do

1. Give attention to diet, abstinence from smoking, and rest, as discussed above.

2. Consult a physician and follow his instructions. He may prescribe one of the modern medications that serve to lower the blood pressure. He will need to check your condition at regular intervals and possibly modify your treatment program from time to time.

3. It is extremely important that the person who is taking medication for high blood pressure follow the directions implicitly by taking his medicine regularly and on time. He should not discontinue the medication except on his doctor's recommendation.

LOW BLOOD PRESSURE (HYPOTENSION).

In a large majority of people with low blood pressure the condition should not be considered a disease at all. These are normal healthy individuals whose lives will not be shortened by low blood pressure. Actually the life-span may be lengthened by low blood pressure, and few or no noticeable symptoms are likely to be caused by it. Such people should look upon low blood pressure as a blessing rather than as a disease.

In some cases, however, low blood pressure is caused by an impoverished diet, by the presence of some chronic wasting disease, or by some other condition that needs treatment on its own account. Occasionally low blood pressure is accompanied by a marked feeling of weakness and fatigability, which can possibly be corrected by dietary or other treatments. Headaches, shortness of breath, dizziness, inability to concentrate, and digestive disturbances—any or all of these may be present, though generally they result from causes other than hypotension. It is for such reasons that it is important to search for the cause or causes of low blood pressure when it is known to exist, but it is not important to do anything about it unless symptoms persist, indicating that health may be below par.

What to Do

1. Have a physician make a search for the possible causes.

2. See that the diet is adequate, especially that it is not deficient in protein.

PHLEBITIS.
(See *Thrombophlebitis.*)

RAYNAUD'S DISEASE.

Raynaud's disease most commonly affects the extremities, the hands more often than the feet. It occurs much more frequently in women than in men. Attacks are accompanied by numbness, tingling, pain, and blanching—all of these manifestations resulting from constriction of the small arteries under the influence of sympathetic nerves. Anything that stimulates these nerves to act—nicotine or an emotional upset, for instance—may have a causative effect. In severe cases the skin and subcutaneous tissues become somewhat dry and shrunken and may become gangrenous in spots.

What to Do

1. When an attack comes on, immerse the affected member or members in warm (not hot) water.

2. As far as possible, avoid exposure to cold, nervous or emotional strain, and participation in those types of work or exercise that previous experience has proved

may precipitate this kind of attack.

3. Use no tobacco in any form, especially cigarettes.

4. If the attacks continue to recur, consult a neurologist—a physician who specializes in diseases of the nervous system.

STROKE (APOPLECTIC STROKE).

An apoplectic stroke is caused by severe damage to some part of the brain because of an interruption of the blood supply to this part. The exact symptoms in a particular case are determined by the particular part of the brain affected.

The demands of the brain for a continuous supply of fresh blood are so great that one-fifth of the blood pumped by the heart is delivered to the brain. An interruption of blood supply to any part of the brain causes permanent damage to the brain cells within about five minutes.

Stroke of one kind or another accounts for about one fifth of the deaths in the broad category of cardiovascular disease. About 80 percent of the deaths from stroke occur in people sixty-five years old or above. Four out of five persons survive their first attack of stroke, but these are usually handicapped to a greater or lesser degree, perhaps by a paralysis of some muscles resulting from permanent damage to the brain.

Although the onset of a stroke is sudden, the underlying disease condition has usually been of long standing. Stroke may be caused when the formation of a blood clot (thrombus) at the site blocks a vessel—a complication of arteriosclerosis. It may be caused by the lodging of a floating fragment of blood clot (embolus) in one of the arteries of the brain. Or it may be caused by a rupture of the wall of an artery in the brain with consequent escape of blood into the brain tissue. The rupture may be brought about by high blood pressure forcing blood through a weakened vessel wall, as in arteriosclerosis or in aneurysm of the involved vessel.

For a discussion of arteriosclerosis of the blood vessels in the neck as a cause of some cases of stroke, see chapter 25 under the heading of *Stroke*.

The symptoms of stroke may develop instantly or over a period of several minutes. The patient usually collapses and may lose consciousness. His face may be red and congested. There may be vomiting or convulsions. Paralysis may cripple the muscles of one side of the face, causing the mouth to be pulled to the strong side. There may be a muscle weakness of one entire side of the body. In some cases the pupil of one eye is larger than that of the other.

What to Do

1. Call a physician or arrange for the patient to be taken to the hospital.

2. Keep the patient at complete bed rest, preferably with head and shoulders elevated slightly.

3. Apply cold compresses (cloth wrung out of ice water) or an ice bag intermittently to the patient's forehead and face.

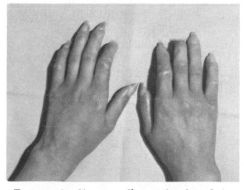

Buerger's disease affects the hands and feet, often causing ulceration.

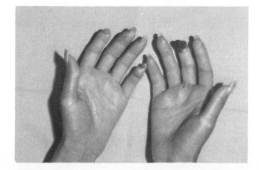

4. Give no stimulants except on a physician's order.

5. If the patient vomits, turn his head to one side to prevent his choking.

6. If convulsions develop, place a tightly rolled cloth between his teeth to prevent injury to his tongue.

7. Do not attempt feeding by mouth while the patient is unconscious. Feeding can be accomplished by tube-feeding or by intravenous injection.

8. It may be necessary to empty the patient's bladder by catheter.

9. During convalescence it is necessary to arrange a progressive program in which the patient is guided in taking exercise, in self-care, and, eventually, in learning to walk.

THROMBOANGIITIS OBLITERANS (BUERGER'S DISEASE).

In thromboangiitis obliterans the lining membrane of the blood vessels of the extremities become inflamed, leading to a plugging of the vessels and a shutting off of the circulation. The plugging develops gradually rather than suddenly. All extremities may be affected, but usually one leg is most severely involved. This extremity is colder than normal, painful, tender, and often of a mottled red appearance. Little or no pulse can be felt in it. In severe cases, an ulcerated condition in the vicinity of the obstructed vessel or vessels, or gangrene of the part of the limb that has had its blood supply reduced, may develop.

Exercise intensifies pain of thromboangiitis obliterans, most markedly in the arch of the foot or the palm of the hand; but "rest pain," especially at night, is also a frequent characteristic. Ulceration develops easily, and tends to extend or, at best, to heal very slowly.

The causes of thromboangiitis obliterans are not well understood, but

107

there seems to be some hereditary predisposition, as Jews are especially susceptible. It affects men much more often than women and is most common in adults under forty. The disease seems to occur only in smokers. The use of any form of tobacco apparently has a causative influence, and its continued use makes the chances of a cure much less.

What to Do

1. **Arrange a well-balanced diet with an abundance of fluids.**

2. **If the disease is at all severe, it is best to stay in bed with the affected limb slightly lowered.**

3. **Avoid exercise that causes pain, also exposure to cold, or injury to the affected part. Keep it scrupulously clean and dry.**

4. **If no skin break is present, give the affected part a brief alternate hot and cold bath twice a day. (See volume 3, chapter 18.)**

5. **The circulation in the affected limb can be somewhat improved by applying heat to the corresponding unaffected limb, conveniently by means of an electric light cradle.**

6. **Avoid all use of tobacco.**

7. **If possible, have a physician make a careful examination periodically and direct in the treatment. He may use some apparatus for the application of alternate positive and negative pressure to the affected limb, or other measures aimed at restoring its circulation. Surgery may become necessary, even amputation.**

THROMBOPHLEBITIS.

In thrombophlebitis a vein not only develops a clot but also becomes inflamed. These involvements occur most commonly in the veins of the thigh and leg. They affect women more often than men.

Thrombophlebitis occurring in the thigh or leg is characterized by pain or aching just below the groin or in the calf muscles, by tenderness, frequently by swelling, and sometimes by a moderate rise in body temperature. It may occur during pregnancy, or it may follow childbirth, abdominal or pelvic surgery, trauma, or acute infectious fevers such as typhoid, scarlet fever, or influenza.

Massage or rubbing in acute thrombophlebitis may cause part of the clot to be dislodged and pass to other parts of the body, especially the lungs, causing serious damage or death. Even though the victim remains in bed until the swelling has subsided, a slight relapse of the swelling may occur when he gets out of bed. Little exercise or even standing should be allowed while any swelling persists. Often if the channel of the vein in the thigh is much narrowed as a result of phlebitis, and nearly always if it is completely obstructed, varicose veins will appear lower down in the leg.

Thrombophlebitis of superficial veins sometimes occurs, and this condition is not so generally limited to the thighs and legs as is thrombophlebitis of the deep veins. It may develop in varicose veins. It may result from injuries or from the hypodermic injection of irritating chemicals. It is sometimes a sign of cancer in some internal organ. Moderately swollen and painful areas on the skin of one or more limbs is the most common sign of this condition, which usually runs a brief course and ends in complete recoverey unless the inflammation spreads to deeper veins.

What to Do

1. **Rest in bed.**

2. **Keep the affected limb elevated with pillows, but do not let it become chilled.**

3. **Fomentations may be used for a few minutes three times a day, but they should not be extremely hot, and they should be applied very gently, with no cold application or rubbing at the end. (See volume 3, chapter 20.)**

4. **Do not massage the limb.**

5. **Do not use the limb at all until all pain and swelling have disap-**

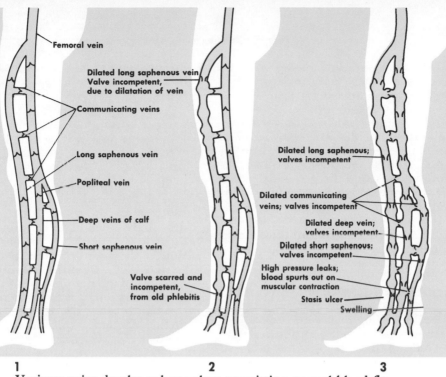

Femoral vein

Dilated long saphenous vein
Valve incompetent,
due to dilatation of vein

Communicating veins

Long saphenous vein

Popliteal vein

Deep veins of calf

Short saphenous vein

Valve scarred and
incompetent,
from old phlebitis

Dilated long saphenous;
valves incompetent

Dilated communicating
veins; valves incompetent

Dilated deep vein;
valves incompetent

Dilated short saphenous;
valves incompetent

High pressure leaks;
blood spurts out on
muscular contraction

Stasis ulcer

Swelling

1   **2**   **3**

Varicose veins develop when valves permitting normal blood flow
(1) become incompetent and allow blood flow to become retro-
grade (2), resulting in chronic venous insufficiency (3).

peared, and then return to normal
use very gradually.

6. When the use of the limb is
resumed, the wearing of a support
stocking or a properly applied
elastic bandage may prove beneficial.

7. It is important to have a
physician in charge of the case. He
may deem it advisable to use
anticoagulant therapy (medications
which retard the clotting of blood)
or antibiotics. Also, he will be alert
to the possibility of complications.

VARICOSE VEINS.

Varicose veins are most common in
the legs below the knees, but they
may appear anywhere from the pelvis
downward or even on some other
parts of the body surface. They show
up as large, tortuous blood channels
under the skin surface. Most cases
appear before the age of forty, but they
tend to persist indefinitely thereafter.

Some persons are more susceptible
to the development of varicose veins
than are others. This susceptibility is a
matter of heredity, being passed on
from parents to children. In women,
pregnancy and pelvic tumors predispose to the condition. The wearing of
tight bands or garters about the legs is
a possible cause. Occupations that
require long hours of standing cause
varicose veins in many people. Such
varicose veins usually appear along
the inner front side of the thigh and
leg or back of the knee and along the
back of the leg.

Aching in the leg, swelling, eczema
of the skin of the leg, and ulcers may
result from varicose veins.

The development of varicose ulcers
is the most serious complication of
varicose veins. The wearing of support hose in a case of varicose veins
may prevent the development of
varicose ulcers. When ulcers develop,
they are usually located just above the
ankle.

Varicose ulcers are hard to heal, and
may recur after healing. Strong ointments, lotions, or antiseptics may be

109

harmful. Some mild antiseptic ointment is the most that can be recommended as a dressing in the home treatment of a varicose ulcer. Any form of hydrotherapy that will improve the circulation in the affected limb or limbs is good, but whatever form is used, the skin should always be thoroughly dried immediately after the treatment, since a moist skin promotes the formation of ulcers.

Internal varicose veins occur very commonly in the rectum and occasionally in the tissues surrounding the esophagus near where it enters the stomach. These, of course, cannot be seen externally, and treatments useful for body-surface varicose veins are not suitable. Rectal varicose veins are commonly called hemorrhoids. They are readily detectable, and surgery is an effective cure. The varicose veins around the lower end of the esophagus are neither easy to detect nor easy to treat. Their presence is usually not known, or even suspected, unless something causes them to rupture, leading to a serious hemorrhage. They most commonly form as a complication of cirrhosis of the liver.

What to Do

1. If the condition is very severe, elastic hose, elastic bandages, or sponge-rubber dressings may put enough moderate pressure on the dilated veins to relieve the discomfort.

2. If occupation requires the patient to stand much of the time, he should change his occupation.

3. If swelling, eczema of the skin of the leg, or varicose ulcers are present, use alternate hot and cold foot and leg baths twenty minutes twice a day. Begin with two minutes in the hot and half a minute in the cold, and gradually increase the time of the cold until it is also two minutes, meanwhile decreasing the time of the hot somewhat. *After each treatment, it is essential to dry the skin thoroughly.* If you cannot do this, do not use this form of treatment.

4. Severe problems with varicose veins, such as varicose ulcers, often respond to adequate bed rest and elevation of the affected limb.

5. If ulcers are present, apply to them either 5 percent boric acid ointment or a paste made as follows:

Boric acid	6
Zinc oxide	6
Petrolatum	18
(Mix thoroughly)	

6. Have a physician make an examination to see if surgery may be necessary.

II. Blood Diseases*

Blood is composed of cells and plasma. (See the discussion of blood in the chapter on "The Body's Transportation System" in volume 3.) Plasma is largely water in which are dissolved minerals, proteins, gases, and other chemicals that assist in the work done by the blood. Whether all are in the right proportions or not depends on the state of nutrition and metabolism of the body and to a lesser extent on the activity of the blood-forming organs. Most commonly plasma abnormalities occur when something goes wrong with the respiratory, digestive, or excretory organs. Discussion of such problems in this chapter will be limited, however, to conditions which affect the protein of the plasma and thus directly alter blood clotting.

*The author and publishers acknowledge the significant contribution to the content of the remainder of this chapter by Irvin N. Kuhn, M.D., assistant professor of medicine (hematology), Loma Linda University.

Blood cells are produced in special tissues or organs. Bone marrow, the largest blood-forming organ, supplies red cells, certain white cells called granulocytes, and platelets. Other white cells (the lymphocytes and plasma cells) are formed in the spleen, lymph nodes, and other lymphoid tissues. Granulocytes once were considered the most important of the white cells because their activity could be easily observed in the laboratory. Recently, however, it has been discovered that lymphocytes and plasma cells are very important in overcoming infections caused by viruses and in maintaining immunity against certain diseases; e.g., measles, whooping cough, and smallpox.

Diseases of the blood may involve red cells, white cells, platelets, or plasma constituents. The effects of disease may result in too few or too many of the item concerned. When there are too many red cells, the condition is called polycythemia; when there are too few red cells, we speak of anemia. An increased number of white cells occurs in response to an infection or in a case of leukemia and is called leukocytosis. A decrease in white cells is called leukopenia. A condition in which there are too few platelets is known as thrombocytopenia. Conditions in which there is an excess of plasma protein are rare, but too little of the right kind of protein in the plasma may cause abnormal bleeding problems, as in hemophilia. Too little of the gamma globulin component of the plasma's protein causes a striking susceptibility to infection.

In the present chapter discussions of the characteristics, causes, and treatments of blood diseases are necessarily concise but are designed to be informative. Understandably, diagnosis of these conditions requires the facilities available in modern hospitals and clinical laboratories, and treatment demands the services of a physician.

The first part of our discussion of blood diseases pertains to the several conditions in which the red blood cells are affected in one way or another. As a preliminary, then, let us consider briefly the normal role of the red cells and the ways in which the body's functions become handicapped when the red cells are abnormal in composition or in number.

The primary function of the red cells is to carry oxygen from the lungs to the tissues. Each red cell (erythrocyte) is essentially a small elastic package of hemoglobin—a red, iron-containing substance capable of transporting oxygen from the lungs to the tissues.

All living tissues require a continuous supply of oxygen. The more active the tissue, the greater its need for oxygen. Three factors help to determine the amount of oxygen which the blood can bring to a tissue: (1) the amount of hemoglobin in each red blood cell, (2) the relative number of red blood cells in the bloodstream, and (3) the speed with which the red blood cells arrive in the tissue under consideration.

In anemia there is either a reduced amount of hemoglobin in each of the red blood cells or else the total number of red cells is less than usual. In either case the oxygen-carrying capacity of the blood is reduced and the tissues suffer on this account. Strangely, however, in the opposite condition of polycythemia, in which there is an excess of red blood cells, the tissues may also suffer for lack of oxygen. In this case the difficulty lies in the fact that with a high population of red cells the blood becomes syrupy and moves so slowly that it cannot deliver its oxygen as fast as necessary for tissue health.

Of all the tissues, brain tissue has about the greatest and most continuous need for oxygen. Headache is one of the symptoms that may herald the brain's need for more oxygen. (This is only one of the many possible causes of headache.) In the light of the explanation given above we can see that this kind of headache can occur either when the number of red blood cells is below normal (in anemia) or when the number is above normal (in polycythemia).

With this as an example, it becomes clear that the symptoms of blood diseases depend on what effects these diseases produce on the body's tissues rather than on what changes can be observed in the blood itself.

Now for a consideration of the various blood diseases.

AGRANULOCYTOSIS.

(See under *Bone-marrow Failure*.)

ANEMIA.

The term anemia applies to conditions in which the amount of hemoglobin or the number of red cells in a specified volume of blood is below normal. Normal blood is 40 to 45 percent red cells and 55 to 60 percent plasma. On the average there are 12.5 to 16 grams of hemoglobin per 100 milliliters of blood. The normal red-cell count is 4.5 to 5.5 million cells per cubic millimeter. All these values tend to be 10 percent lower in women. A person is considered anemic if his blood values are less than the lowest figures mentioned here.

Anemia may be the result of inadequate or improper formation of red blood cells by the bone marrow. A small amount of vitamin B_{12} is necessary for the cells to mature, and an adequate amount of iron combined with a proper arrangement of protein is needed so that each cell may receive its full supply of hemoglobin. Anemias resulting from failure of this system are called anemias of production. Other anemias occur when fully formed adult red blood cells are destroyed prematurely. These are called hemolytic anemias. When red blood cells are lost because of bleeding, the resulting anemia is called anemia of hemorrhage, or secondary anemia. Finally, anemias due to bone marrow damage are called aplastic anemia, the separate section discuss-

ing this problem to be found later in this chapter under *Bone-marrow Failure*.

A. *Iron-deficiency Anemia (Microcytic Hypochromic Anemia)*. Iron, an integral part of hemoglobin, is vitally important in the transport of oxygen from the lungs to the tissues and of carbon dioxide from tissues to lungs. When a deficiency of iron occurs, the production of red cells is less affected than is the formation of hemoglobin. But the deficiency causes the bone marrow to produce small cells. Then as lack of iron becomes more severe, red cells with less than optimal hemoglobin content are formed. Thus the red blood cells in this condition are both small (microcytic) and pale (hypochromic). In severe iron deficiency, the rate of red cell formation is curtailed, causing a low red cell count.

The most common cause of iron deficiency is blood loss, such as in prolonged bleeding. Women have iron-deficiency anemia more than men, one reason being that excessive menstrual bleeding may bring about the loss of more iron from the body each month than can be replaced by the iron contained in the usual diet. Pregnancy and loss of blood during delivery cause a tremendous drain on the iron reserves in women, and frequent pregnancies impose demands which the present-day American diet cannot supply. Hence a physician usually prescribes iron-containing medicine for pregnant patients.

Iron-deficiency anemia may be the result of unsuspected bleeding from the intestine. Often considerable blood loss can go on for a long time without the patient's suspecting anything wrong. Special chemical tests of the stool are often used to determine whether blood is present. Gastrointestinal bleeding can occur with ulcers, hemorrhoids, or small growths in the colon. Often the development of anemia is the first indication of a cancer of the colon. Intestinal parasites, particularly hookworm, can also cause severe iron-deficiency anemia.

Another cause of iron-deficiency anemia is lack of hydrochloric acid in the stomach, a lack which reduces the absorption of iron from food. Cancer of the stomach or the intestine, severe diarrhea from intestinal infections, and the surgical removal of most or all of the stomach or of the small intestine may also interfere with the absorption of iron. Certain vitamin deficiencies, such as that of pyridoxine (vitamin B_6), and the prolonged consumption of such poisons as lead, arsenic, or mercury prevent the efficient incorporation of iron into hemoglobin when red blood cells are being developed. Prolonged infections such as tuberculosis or prolonged inflammations such as rheumatoid arthritis prevent the movement of iron to the bone marrow where hemoglobin is formed.

Some of the common symptoms and signs of iron-deficiency anemia are fatigability, faintness, palpitation, shortness of breath with exercise, headache, pallor, and—in severe cases—deformed fingernails.

What to Do

1. Iron-deficiency anemia always has a cause. This must be discovered before any corrective treatment is begun. The patient can help the physician by taking special note of changes in the color of the bowel movements, by making a diet inventory list, or (in a woman) by noting a change in the amount of menstrual flow.

2. Strenuous exercise should be avoided in order to protect the vital organs from oxygen deficiency, thereby preventing discomfort or complications. Regular moderate exercise in the open air is encouraged as a means of maintaining general good health.

3. A pregnant woman should be under the care of a physician.

4. Women whose menstrual flow is excessive should seek medical help. Anemia may be corrected easily, but the underlying cause of the excess flow may be something serious. Abnormal bleeding is one of the seven danger signals of cancer. (See following chapter on cancer for complete list.)

5. A well-balanced diet is important.

6. The choice of which medicinal iron or iron tonic to take should be guided by the doctor.

B. *Macrocytic Anemia (Pernicious Anemia and Others).* Macrocytic anemias are characterized by red cells which are larger than normal. These anemias are caused by a deficiency of vitamin B_{12} or of folic acid. About 90 percent of macrocytic anemias in temperate climate countries are pernicious anemias. The rest are due to other causes of vitamin B_{12} deficiency or to lack of folic acid, a close cousin to B_{12} and also a member of the B vitamin group.

A lack of vitamin B_{12} may occur in several ways, one being failure of the stomach to absorb it. In order to absorb B_{12} properly, the stomach must secrete a substance called the intrinsic factor, which serves as a transfer agent locking itself to B_{12} and guiding it across the intestinal lining to enter the bloodstream. Without the intrinsic factor, vitamin B_{12} is absorbed poorly. Pernicious anemia refers to that anemia which occurs when the stomach is unable to secrete the intrinsic factor.

Macrocytic anemias may also be caused by insufficient B_{12} in the diet, or when certain germs living in the intestinal tract use up B_{12} before it can be absorbed. Vitamin B_{12} deficiency can develop in individuals on restricted diets, in persons who have had all the stomach removed, in persons whose stomach lining has degenerated so that it no longer produces sufficient intrinsic factor, or in special situations when certain tapeworm or bacterial infections in the intestines compete for and deprive the body of vitamin B_{12} before it can be absorbed.

Vitamin B_{12} and folic acid are necessary to form and mature the red blood cells, granulocytes, and platelets. Vitamin B_{12} is required also for the maintenance of nervous tissue. When the combination of anemia, nervousness, and peculiar sensations such as numbness and tingling in the hands and feet occurs, pernicious anemia may be present.

Folic acid is extremely important in the proper development of all rapidly growing tissue. It exists in abundant quantities in fresh vegetables. Folic acid deficiency is found most commonly in food faddism, alcoholism, chronic diarrheal states, and the later stages of pregnancy. In the latter condition, the mother needs especially large amounts of folic acid in order to supply adequately the baby's needs for its rapidly developing body tissues.

The pernicious anemia patient is usually over thirty. Typically he is of the Caucasian (white) race and likely of English, Irish, or Northern European descent. The onset of the disease is often subtle, the first likely symptoms being merely weakness, fatigue, pallor, and palpitation or breathlessness on exertion. Typically the patient has snowy white hair, a yellowish waxy complexion, and a smooth tongue. There is often a poor

Condition of the tongue figures in diagnosis of pernicious anemia.

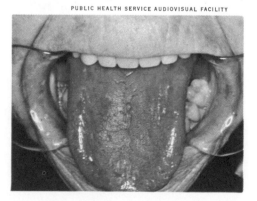

appetite, though weight loss is not frequent. Symptoms of indigestion are usually present. A striking change in behavior, and nervousness, numbness, and tingling of the hands and feet are commonly experienced. A peculiar inability to coordinate the feet when walking, especially in the dark, is characteristic.

Laboratory tests will show the patient to have a moderate to severe anemia, red blood cells extremely varied in size, shape, and color, no free acid in his stomach, and a low level of vitamin B_{12} in his blood. The average red cell size is greater than normal, hence the term macrocytic anemia. The white-cell count and platelet count are usually below normal.

The inability of the person with pernicious anemia to absorb vitamin B_{12} because of a lack of the intrinsic factor can be tested by administering an oral dose of vitamin B_{12} which has been marked with a tiny amount of radioactive cobalt. If no trace of this labeled B_{12} can be detected in the bloodstream or the urine, detectable with special instruments, the suspicion that the patient makes no intrinsic factor of his own is confirmed.

What to Do

1. Vitamin B_{12}, a specific remedy for pernicious anemia, must be given by injection at no greater than monthly intervals. If the diagnosis of pernicious anemia is confirmed, the injections must be continued for the remainder of the patient's life. When properly instructed, some member of the household can give the injections, but a physician must supervise the treatment program and arrange periodic physical examinations and laboratory tests.

2. The elderly patient under treatment for pernicious anemia should be advised to rest in bed until the hemoglobin level reaches 8 to 9 grams per 100 ml. of blood or higher depending on the general condition of his health.

3. Physiotherapy consisting of exercises to improve muscle strength and coordination should be instituted in patients with involvement of the nervous system. Patients with serious nervous system degeneration require expert nursing care to prevent bedsores and bladder infections. Progressive improvement of nerve dysfunctions may continue for a year or more after adequate treatment has been started.

4. Blood transfusions are rarely necessary except in the severely ill patient. With vitamin B_{12} injections and plenty of nutritious food the blood should return to normal within six weeks.

5. Folic acid deficiency may be treated by oral or injectable medication: but for the expectant mother, a special emphasis on fresh leafy vegetables in the diet will protect her unborn child in most cases.

6. "Blood tonics" by mouth without a doctor's advice should be avoided because some will correct the anemia but permit progressive degeneration of the nervous system.

C. *Hemolytic Anemia.* The destruction of red blood cells while they are in circulation is called hemolysis. Causes of destruction may be severe burns, chemicals of various kinds, or complications of certain infections or malignancies.

Red cells that normally "wear out" are removed from circulation by the spleen and, to a lesser extent, by the liver. Iron and protein from destroyed red blood cells are retained by the tissues and reused in the production of new hemoglobin. That component of the old hemoglobin which imparts the red color (pigment) undergoes chemical changes in the liver and is normally eliminated in the form of bile pigments, which pass through the bile ducts, gallbladder, and intestinal tract as part of the bile.

In the hemolytic anemias, in which there is an increased rate of red-cell destruction, the provision for eliminating the pigments derived from old hemoglobin may be overwhelmed, with the result that the bile pigments accumulate in the tissues, causing jaundice. Jaundice can be recognized by the yellow coloration of the skin and of the whites of the eyes plus a darkening of the urine.

D. *Congenital Types of Hemolytic Anemia.* Some persons inherit a condition by which red blood cells of poor quality are produced by the bone marrow. In some cases the red cells do not contain the right amount of enzymes. This may permit the cells to be destroyed by the spleen before they reach their usual life-span of 120 days. Or it may make the red cells more susceptible than normal to the damaging effects of certain drugs. The associated anemia is designated as congenital nonspherocytic hemolytic anemia.

In other situations, the walls or envelopes of the red cells are defective, resulting in peculiar shapes which appear to be more vulnerable to the incessant pummeling they receive as they pass through small blood vessels. Hemolytic anemias of this type may be recognized by observing the appearance of red cells on a blood smear and by discovering a family tendency to anemia and jaundice. One such disorder is chronic familial jaundice, or hereditary spherocytosis. In this particular difficulty, surgical removal of the spleen retards the rate of red-blood-cell destruction but does not improve the quality of the red cells produced by the bone marrow.

What to Do

1. The patient with congenital nonspherocytic hemolytic anemia should obtain from his physician a list of the drugs which may cause him to have a flare-up of severe anemia. He also must make sure that the physician in attendance during each hospitalization knows

115

of his problem and avoids prescribing drugs that may be harmful. The wearing of some identification with a mention of his disorder is advisable.

2. Congenital spherocytic anemia is best treated by removal of the spleen. This surgical procedure is usually postponed until the child reaches his early teens.

3. Transfusions may have to be given during a severe anemia phase of both kinds of hemolytic anemia.

E. *Hemoglobinopathic Hemolytic Anemias* (Sickle-cell Disease). A common disorder occurring exclusively in blacks is sickle-cell anemia. This hereditary disease causes the production of an abnormal type of hemoglobin by the bone marrow. This abnormal hemoglobin differs from the normal by a small change in the structure of the molecule.

Sickle-cell hemoglobin has peculiar sensitivity to a lowered oxygen supply such as occurs when climbing a high mountain, taking an automobile trip over high mountain passes, flying in an aircraft with an unpressurized cabin, or when suffering from pneumonia. Red cells with this type of hemoglobin form sickle or crescent shapes when subjected to lowered oxygen concentrations. These peculiarly shaped cells do not pass through the small blood vessels readily, and consequently may block the blood supply to vital areas.

There are all degrees of sickle-cell disease. Many persons become aware of the defect in connection with a routine physical examination. Others develop their first symptoms when they drive over a high mountain pass. Still others are severely handicapped from the time of birth.

Among the first symptoms to be encountered in sickle-cell disease is sudden, severe, abdominal pain, followed by the appearance of dark-colored urine. Also associated with it may be severe leg cramps, acute pain in the left side, and a yellowish discoloration to the eyes (jaundice). In the severest cases slight exercise may bring on the pain, there may be severe anemia, a huge liver, repeated fevers, recurrent bone pain, and chronic ulcers of the legs. Patients with sickle-cell disease show a marked susceptibility to infections. When patients with this disorder develop a cold or pneumonia they should seek medical help early.

What to Do

1. A person who suspects that he has sickle-cell anemia should present himself to the physician for examination.

2. If diagnosis is confirmed, the patient should place himself under a physician's care early in the course of any infection and follow his instructions.

3. Avoid situations where a lowered concentration of oxygen may be present, such as trips over high mountain passes, flights in unpressurized aircraft, skin diving without breathing equipment, and strenuous exercise.

4. In a crisis the patient should seek medical attention at once; but until help comes he may also obtain and breathe oxygen temporarily, lie down to conserve energy, and breathe deeply.

5. Obtain a highly nutritious diet rich in proteins and folic acid. Folic acid is found mainly in leafy green vegetables.

6. Blood transfusions, other intravenous fluids and intensive pain control medications are sometimes necessary.

F. *Mediterranean Anemia (Thalassemia).* Certain aberrations of hemoglobin formation may occur because of inherited tendencies. They have all the earmarks of a hemolytic disorder. Most of these are uncommon and beyond the scope of this chapter, but one disorder, Mediterranean anemia (thalassemia), an inherited defect, appears most commonly among the people who have originated from around the Mediterranean Sea, *e.g.*, Italians, Greeks, Turks, and southern Spanish. Patients with this disorder are unable to form enough normal adult type hemoglobin and consequently suffer from the continuous production of a fetal type of hemoglobin.

Fetal hemoglobin carries oxygen in postnatal life (after birth) much less efficiently than the so-called adult form of hemoglobin. In addition the cells filled with this fetal hemoglobin die much sooner than normal cells. The bone marrow responds to this low oxygen and rapid cell death by vigorously making more red cells. Such individuals will have large thick spongy bones filled with red bone marrow. They have large livers and spleens, are perpetually jaundiced, and continue to pass dark-colored urine.

Severely affected individuals often die before their tenth year of life. However, all degrees of severity, as with sickle-cell diseases, may exist.

What to Do

1. Physicians can do relatively little for Mediterranean anemia except to keep the patient comfortable. The degree of severity will determine the outcome. A few have responded remarkably to surgical removal of the spleen.

2. It is important to avoid infections and to take in plenty of nutritious food, particularly green leafy vegetables because of their folic acid content.

3. Blood transfusions may have to be used over an extended period of time.

G. *Autoimmune Hemolytic Anemia.* This anemia, the least understood type, may develop with amazing suddenness or with gradual progression. In some cases it appears spontaneously. In others it follows viral pneumonia. It may appear in association with other infections, with cancer, or with leukemia. It is similar to the reaction observed when the wrong type of blood is transfused inadvertently.

The body has a unique way of identifying its own tissues and defending them from invasion by foreign cells. This peculiar characteristic develops early, even while the child is still in its mother's womb. This defense mechanism may be set in motion when biologically active tissues are transplanted from one person to another, *e.g.*, kidney, heart, or liver. The simpler the transplant, the greater the prospect of success. Blood, being in this sense a simple tissue, is often transferred successfully in blood transfusions.

At times, under conditions not well understood, the body suddenly starts rejecting its own red blood cells, a situation brought about by the formation of a special type of protein which destroys red cells or makes them susceptible to destruction by the spleen. This protein is similar to gamma globulin which the body produces to fight infections. Autoimmune hemolytic anemia is such an example of a self-destroying disease.

Autoimmune hemolytic anemia is often ushered in with a chill, fever, vomiting, pain in the back or abdomen, and the production of yellow to reddish-brown urine. The spleen may enlarge rapidly, thereby aggravating the condition. Often other cells of the blood are affected.

The diagnosis depends on being able to demonstrate the abnormal gamma globulin attached to the red cells. This requires specialized laboratory tests. The treatment is first directed toward the associated disease, if present, which may have triggered the hemolysis. Then drugs may be prescribed which suppress the body's ability to produce anti-red-cell globulin. Finally the spleen may have to be removed. The treatment program may of necessity be conducted in a different order.

What to Do

This complicated disease requires expert medical care. To place oneself in the care of a good physician is most prudent. Cortisone in large doses is often required, or the doctor may elect to remove the spleen.

H. *Hemolytic Disease of the Newborn (Erythroblastosis Fetalis).* Much publicity has been given the Rh factor in human blood. Actually there are at least twenty different blood groups which have been positively identified, and more may yet be discovered. Of these, the ABO and Rh groups are of most significance in hemolytic disease of the newborn. The ABO group (blood belonging to this group is either A, O, B, or AB) is the most important when transfusion is considered; but for several reasons it is of less importance in the "baby and mother" disease.

If blood from a person with type A is transfused into a type B person, it will likely be destroyed because the type B person has antibodies (certain protecting proteins) antagonistic to type A red cells. In the Rh system antibodies do not develop until the foreign cells have once stimulated the recipient's defense mechanism. The first time Rh positive blood cells are introduced into the bloodstream of an Rh negative recipient, they will doubtless be tolerated. By a second time, antibodies will have developed which promptly destroy the foreign cells.

Identification of a blood group is done in a blood bank by mixing cells or plasma of known type with cells or plasma of the unknown type on clean glass slides or paper and observing whether "clumping" occurs. Anti-A plasma will agglutinate (clump) A cells, and anti-Rh positive plasma will agglutinate Rh positive cells.

Hemolytic diesase of the newborn occurs when red blood cells from a baby with blood of a type different

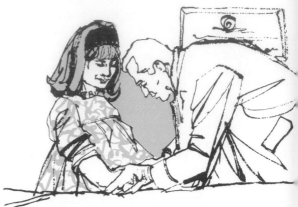

Prenatal consultation reduces risks.

from that of the mother seeps across the membrane of the placenta and enters the mother's bloodstream. Normally the membrane of the placenta separates the mother's blood from the baby's blood. If the mother is Rh negative and the baby also Rh negative, their blood is compatible and nothing will happen, providing the ABO group is compatible also. But if the baby is Rh positive and the mother is Rh negative, anti-Rh antibodies which can easily cross the membrane back into the baby's bloodstream begin destroying the baby's Rh positive red cells before the baby is even born.

Unless the mother has been previously transfused with blood which contained Rh positive cells, there is no problem with a first pregnancy. This is because the mother's production of antibodies has been so slow that their concentration never reaches seriously high levels. However, the danger of the child's being seriously affected by this problem of blood incompatibility increases with each subsequent pregnancy. Unless the mother receives proper treatment at the time of the delivery of her first child, there is danger that the second child may not even survive or, if it does, that it will be seriously handicapped with mental retardation and with abnormal control of its muscles.

As mentioned in volume 1, chapter 3, there is now available a method of preventing an Rh-negative mother who has just borne her first child from developing the antibodies that endanger the babies she may bear in the future. Giving her an injection of "Rh immunoglobulin" at precisely the right time suppresses her tendency to produce the harmful antibodies. But it is important that this injection be given within the first 72 hours after the termination of every pregnancy; that is, within 72 hours following the birth of every child, or following an abortion, or following a miscarriage.

When an Rh-negative mother does not receive the preventive treatment just described, her tissues begin to produce the antibodies that will have a damaging effect on the children she may bear later. The danger becomes greater with each succeeding pregnancy. Many of the babies born under such conditions die soon after birth. Subsequent treatment with "Rh immunoglobulin" will not restore the protection. The protective treatment must be carried out properly with the first pregnancy and with each subsequent pregnancy. Some babies who are born with this hemolytic disease of the newborn may be saved by the prompt use of "exchange transfusions" by which the blood of the baby which contains harmful antibodies from the mother is replaced by blood which does not contain the damaging antibodies.

What to Do

1. All complications of pregnancy can be reduced if the prospective mother will present herself for medical care early in the course of her pregnancy. If it develops that she is Rh negative and the unborn child is Rh positive, the physician will be prepared to use the proper methods of treatment and prevention of Rh disease in the child.

2. Babies from Rh-negative mothers should be closely followed by a physician after they are born.

POLYCYTHEMIA.

Polycythemia, either primary or secondary, is a condition in which there is an abnormally large number of red blood cells in the circulating blood.

The fundamental cause of primary polycythemia (polycythemia rubra vera) is not known. The immediate reason for the abnormally large number of red blood cells is that excess quantities are produced by the bone marrow. The total amount of hemoglobin is also increased, accounting for the deeply flushed appearance of the patient's face. With the excessive number of red blood cells the blood becomes "thick" and small vessels may be obstructed, producing corresponding symptoms of partial blindness and small strokes. The lips may appear purple because of the lessened speed of blood flow.

Secondary polycythemia occurs in individuals who have damaged lungs or who are born with false chambers or passages in the heart or large blood vessels. In these situations, the blood may become as thick as in patients with polycythemia rubra vera, but in secondary polycythemia the bone marrow keeps making red cells because the body tissues are suffering for lack of oxygen. A substance called erythropoietin, made by the kidney, is responsible for driving the bone marrow to make more red cells. When mountain climbers ascend to high altitudes, their total hemoglobin and the number of their red blood cells increases, in this case a normal provision by nature, to make it possible for more oxygen to be captured from the thin air and supplied to the tissues.

The signs and symptoms of polycythemia are headache, dizziness, fainting spells, unusual itching after a bath, a feeling of fullness in the head, frequent nosebleeds, and sometimes ankle swelling.

Various forms of treatment are acceptable for primary polycythemia, the simplest being repeated phlebotomy (bloodletting). Many individuals go on for years giving about six pints of blood a year and feeling quite well. Certain powerful drugs can be given to control the production of red cells. So far there is no known cure.

Treatment for the usual case of secondary polycythemia requires the correcting of the underlying defect of the heart or lungs if that is possible.

III. Bleeding Disorders

Blood circulates throughout the body through blood vessels. Since these are tubes made of tissue, any disruption of the tube will permit the escape of blood into the surrounding structures or to the outside in a never-ending stream were it not for an amazing mechanism which constantly seals tiny leaks or large breaks. It is hard to appreciate the value of this self-sealing mechanism until a person afflicted with bleeding problems is observed.

Hemostasis (the prevention of bleeding) is a cooperative effort on the part of tissues, blood vessels, platelets, and the clotting mechanism. The pressure of surrounding tissues acts to stop bleeding from puncture-type wounds. Cut ends of blood vessels retract like elastic bands, causing mechanical pressure to close the open ends. Substances released from injured vessels and tissues and from platelets stimulate the vessels to constrict and the blood to form clots. This amazing piece of jellied blood plugs vessel openings and pulls the ends of the broken vessel together. It hangs on until the vessel heals; then it disappears, often without a trace.

Platelets, previously mentioned, are formed in the bone marrow. The prime function of these little chemical packages of tremendous potency is constantly to plug the millions of tiny holes in the walls of blood vessels so as to constantly prevent blood from seeping into the tissues. When breaks appear, the platelets plaster themselves over the defect and quickly form a patch over the hole. Platelets also release chemicals which initiate blood clotting.

The process of blood clotting must surely be one of the most unusual mechanisms in nature. Of particular interest is the delicate balance between clotting at all and clotting too much; for if no clotting took place, man would die of hemorrhage, and if too much took place, he would become one big clot on the day of his birth. Defects in blood clotting do occur, and some of the most common will now be discussed.

THE PURPURAS.

Purpura is a condition in which numerous small hemorrhages develop within the skin. These small discolored spots may appear spontaneously or they may appear in areas in which there has been mild trauma as when bumping the arm against a door. Purpura results from toxic or chemical injury to blood vessels or from blood seepage due to a low platelet count. Sometimes changes in tissues from poor nutrition, hormonal imbalance, advancing age, or certain drugs may cause purpura.

A. *Non-thrombocytopenic Purpura.* Non-thrombocytopenic purpura (purpura in the presence of normal platelet levels) occurs most commonly in elderly people. A high percent of individials over eighty have purplish patches over the backs of their hands and arms. This is called senile purpura and is due to the loss of supporting tissue, through aging, around small blood vessels. It is not a serious condition, and no treatment is necessary.

Purpura also appears with vitamin C deficiency, following the administration of certain medicines, particularly cortisone, and in the presence of diabetes mellitus or chronic kidney failure. It accompanies severe infections such as erysipelas, plague, and sometimes measles and chicken pox. This is the cause of "black measles," "black pox," or "black plague."

What to Do

1. There is no effective remedy for non-thrombocytopenic purpura. The maintenance of the best state of health possible is advisable. Vitamin C in large doses produces no obvious benefits.

2. Purpura which accompanies measles or other infections is a

A patient with severe purpura must have strict bed rest.

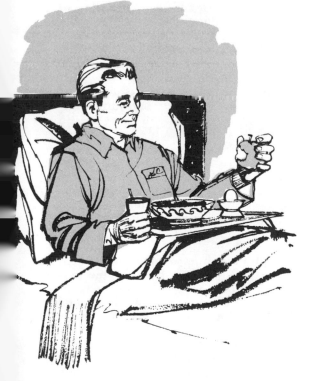

serious disorder and requires a physician's attention immediately.

B. *Thrombocytopenic Purpuras.* Thrombocytopenic purpuras result from reduced platelets and occur most commonly as the result of drugs, chemicals, infections, or malignancies. These agents may depress the formation of platelets by the marrow, may destroy platelets, or may cause them to be used up excessively. Some degree of thrombocytopenia is present in all pancytopenias due to marrow damage, and purpura is often seen.

Idiopathic thrombocytopenic purpura, for which no cause is found, may occur at any age, but it is most common in children and young adults. In children the condition is often temporary and disappears after a few weeks or months. Spontaneous cures in adults are less likely. Even though the disease is self-limited it may be deadly and should not be taken lightly. The onset of thrombocytopenia in children is often preceded by an infection which occurred several weeks previously. The greatest danger is not the bleeding into the skin or the nosebleeds but the possibility of hemorrhage into vital structures such as the brain.

Thrombocytopenia may come in repeated attacks. It is characterized by fever, often by nausea, vomiting, abdominal and joint pains, prostration, bleeding from the bowel, the mouth, or the bladder, as well as by the development of a crop of skin hemorrhages. Or it may appear without any associated feeling of ill health. The skin hemorrhages can be distinguished from tiny superficial varicose veins by the fact that purpura does not disappear when pressure is applied.

What to Do

1. In a severe case of purpura, strict bed rest may be advisable as a precaution to prevent hemorrhages into vital areas. Even with moderate thrombocytopenia, and perhaps

no purpura, children must be restrained from playing vigorously.

2. All purpuras should be under the care of a physician, both for diagnosis and appropriate treatment.

3. Patients with severe purpura should be prevented from straining at stool and from coughing.

CLOTTING DEFECTS.

Blood clotting depends on a complex series of chemical reactions involving proteins and enzymes in blood plasma and in tissues. In addition, calcium and phosphorus and perhaps other minerals must be present. Thirteen known factors interact when the blood clots, and perhaps more are yet to be discovered.

Many of the clotting proteins and enzymes are made in the liver from ingredients derived from the diet. If liver damage is present, as in cirrhosis or hepatitis, or if the liver is too young as in some premature babies, clotting factors may not be synthesized in adequate amounts to prevent bleeding. Some individuals are born with an inability to produce one or more of the clotting factors.

Clotting factors can be deliberately lowered by "blood thinners," better known as anticoagulants. These are used with patients who have suffered a heart attack or who have developed thrombophlebitis. The aim is to decrease the clotting tendency in order to prevent a recurrence of the heart attack or to prevent extension of the clot in thrombophlebitis. The taking of too much medicine can cause serious hemorrhage. Anyone taking anticoagulants should strictly obey the instructions of his physician and report to him the first sign of spontaneous bleeding.

A. *Hemophilia.* Persons with hemophilia are known as "bleeders." These may have all degrees of bleeding. In a child who has severe hemophilia, death usually occurs early in life as a consequence of some minor injury. With a less severe case there is a tendency to bleed slowly for prolonged periods from even minor cuts or scratches. Sometimes bleeding into the tissues begins without apparent tissue injury. A favorite site for large bleeds is the large muscles of the back and buttocks, but any part of the body may become involved. Bleeding into the joints is common in the severely affected cases. Following a joint hemorrhage there is inflammation, redness, and stiffness; and each hemorrhage causes more and more joint dysfunction until finally the whole joint may become useless. The shoulder, elbow, knee, and hip joints are the ones most commonly involved.

Hemophilia results from an individual's inability to make factor VIII (antihemophiliac factor, AHF). A congenital defect, it is passed on from father to daughter to son, but girls are rarely affected by the actual manifestations of the disease. It cannot be transmitted directly from father to son but must always come to the son from the mother. This means that a man who is a bleeder of this type will have sons and daughters who are not bleeders unless the mother also has a family background of bleeders of the same type. The sons of his daughters, however, could be bleeders.

Great advances in the last few years have been made in handling cuts, wounds, accidents, or surgery in persons with hemophilia. It has become possible to concentrate factor VIII (AHF) so that 10 c.c., when injected, will have the potency of a whole unit of fresh blood, and now hemophiliacs may look forward to the prospect of normal living.

What to Do

1. Prevention of bleeding is of the first importance. The afflicted person should protect himself as far as possible from any injury. No dental extractions or surgical operations should be attempted without careful preparatory treatment.

2. Hemophiliacs should acquaint themselves with centers stocking

factor VIII (AHF) concentrates where they may be taken in case of an accident.

3. If bleeding occurs from a surface wound, pressure should be applied and retained until a pressure dressing can be applied. There is a tendency for the hemophiliac to bleed for about eight to ten days after a wound is inflicted.

4. If bleeding persists or if bleeding has occurred into the tissues, a physician should be called at once. He may advise giving fresh frozen plasma or a factor VIII (AHF) concentrate.

5. It is wise for the hemophiliac to wear an identification tag or bracelet so that in case of an emergency where quick action may be necessary and when unconsciousness occurs, those administering care may institute quick and appropriate treatment.

B. *Vitamin K Deficiency*. Vitamin K is the parent substance from which the liver produces four of the thirteen known blood clotting factors. Vitamin K is present in small quantities in leafy green vegetables, but most of the body's supply is made by bacteria in the bowel from other food material. Bile salts promote the absorption of vitamin K. Body stores of this vitamin are so small that complete deprivation may result in bleeding within a week or two. Bleeding may appear from the nose, gums, throat, kidneys, bladder, or bowel.

Numerous clinical situations may cause vitamin K deficiency. When the bile duct is obstructed with gallstones or scar tissue, bile salts cannot get into the intestine and little absorption of vitamin K can take place. In severe prolonged diarrheas, changes in the intestinal lining and the rapid onward movement of the intestinal contents decreases the amount of absorption. When some of the strong modern antibiotics are prescribed for a week or more, enough of the bacteria in the intestine may be destroyed to stop or retard formation of vitamin K and therefore only that obtained from the diet is available.

What to Do

1. A thorough medical examination should reveal the problem. A generous intake of leafy green vegetables or vitamin K supplement administered by a physician will help to correct the difficulty.

2. Any non-induced bleeding condition of a serious nature should be referred to a physician immediately for treatment. The blood pressure, and thus the bleeding, decreases if the afflicted person lies down and rests quietly until help arrives or until he can be taken to a physician.

IV. Bone Marrow Failure

In order that the body may produce an adequate number of blood cells of all types, it needs a healthy marrow bed in which parent types of each cell may grow. There must be an adequate circulation of blood to the marrow to provide nutrients so that each kind of cell can mature properly. There must exist an adequate stimulus to accelerate cell growth and maturation when there is an increased need as in anemia. The young cells must have a place to grow and must be able to develop into normal adult cells. There must be enough stored food material for use during the most rapid growth phase. Parent cells in the marrow must be able to respond to a message of blood loss by increasing their production of young cells. They must also reduce their rate of productivity at the right time lest the blood become too thick and clog up the circulation.

Obviously this is a complicated system, wonderfully devised, delicately balanced with automatic controls of many types. This balance can be influenced by many factors.

PANCYTOPENIA.

When there has been damage to the bone marrow bed or the parent cell types or when their ability to produce new cells has been drastically reduced, pancytopenia develops. This term designates a decreased number of all types of blood cells.

Pancytopenia exists when bone marrow fails to produce the various blood cells customarily originating here, e.g., red cells, granulocytes, and platelets. It is a serious disorder carrying a high mortality rate. Many patients with pancytopenia give no history of exposure to X-ray radiation, toxic drugs, or the industrial chemicals known to cause this disease—chemicals such as chloramphenical, benzene, certain hair dyes, some insecticides, and some plant sprays. Still damage may have come from this source, certain people being peculiarly susceptible to ordinarily harmless concentrations of certain drugs or chemicals.

Symptoms of pancytopenia will depend on which cell type is most affected. The resulting anemia will cause lack of energy, a high pulse rate, and all the symptoms of anemia previously described. The depression of granulocytes (one kind of white cells), whose function is to combat infection, will of course leave the patient comparatively unprotected from germ invasion. Since the skin, the gums, the throat, the lungs, and the intestine are the first lines of defense against infections, a person with low concentration of granulocytes can be expected to develop repeated and protracted infections of these areas. Platelets are important in plugging tiny leaks in blood vessels. They prevent minor bumps from becoming big bruises and small cuts

from becoming major bleeding problems. Platelet depression or absence will be characterized by bleeding gums, repeated or prolonged nosebleeds, easy bruisability, and the development of a fine reddish rash—minor hemorrhages into the skin. In women, there is usually a sharp increase in the amount and duration of menstrual flow.

A person afflicted with pancytopenia may not recognize the true nature of his ailment, but he is usually aware that something is seriously wrong. He should consult his physician at once. The doctor can by appropriate examinations and tests discover the offending agent so that it may be avoided in the future. The recovery rate from pancytopenia is less than 50 percent, and much less when the patient experiences repeated exposure to the original insulting agent. Outlook for a cure depends on how severely the bone marrow bed or the parent cells have been damaged.

What to Do

1. When infections recur time after time, a physician should be consulted.

2. All use of solvents, headache remedies, or prescription drugs not recently prescribed should be halted. No further use of pesticides or garden sprays should be made.

3. It is especially important to protect against lacerations of the skin which may become infected and to avoid contact with persons who have colds, sore throat, or cough. It is best to stay out of crowds.

4. The maximum state of good health should be maintained with plenty of rest, good wholesome food, liberal amounts of water, and moderate exercise.

APLASTIC ANEMIA.

Aplastic anemia is caused by the complete failure of bone marrow to produce red blood cells. Commonly,

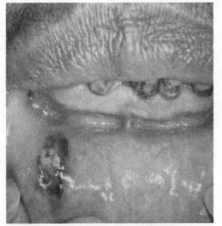

A symptom of aplastic anemia is canker sores on the lips or tongue.

the bone marrow deficiency is partial rather than absolute. It is then called hypoplastic anemia. This more common type is nearly always a temporary condition, while the aplastic anemia is likely to be of irreversible nature.

The symptoms of aplastic anemia are those of any severe anemia: easy fatigability, palpitation of the heart, pallor, shortness of breath on exertion, ankle swelling, and canker sores on lips or tongue. Commonly, the term "aplastic anemia" is used synonymously with pancytopenia, the condition described in the preceding section. If used in this sense, the symptoms will be those described under pancytopenia.

When no recovery of the bone marrow's ability to make red cells occurs, the patient will be dependent on repeated blood transfusions. He will need anywhere from two to four units per month to keep the red-cell concentration up. The level at which the physician elects to keep the red count or hemoglobin will depend on the activity needs of the patient. For example, a retired man can get along well on less than 50 percent of the normal red-cell count, whereas a workingman may need 75 percent. Additional treatment may be required if other cell types are also depressed.

What to Do

1. No attempt at self-treatment with iron or blood tonics should be attempted, because one of the problems in aplastic anemia is that the patient accumulates too much iron. Your physician should decide what medicines are needed.

2. A concerted attempt should be made to reduce excess activity, but regular light exercise should be taken.

3. All further exposure to cleaning solvents, pesticides, weed killers, or patent medicines should be stopped and strictly avoided. In some cases recovery has been prevented by a mild second exposure to the injurious agent.

4. A few medical centers are now prepared to treat selected cases of irreversible aplastic anemia by a procedure known as "bone marrow transplant." It involves taking marrow from a compatible donor (usually a brother, sister, parent, daughter, or son) and injecting such marrow into the afflicted person. With very close and careful medical management, the implanted marrow will grow and supply the cells which have been in short supply.

AGRANULOCYTOSIS.

Agranulocytosis is another blood condition resulting from marrow injury, known or unknown. Specifically, it is an absence in the bloodstream of granulocytes (often also referred to as neutrophiles), which is that variety of white cell most concerned with fighting disease germs. Granulocytopenia or neutropenia is a similar condition but of less severity. The terms agranulocytosis, granulocytopenia, and neutropenia are often used interchangeably. Granulocytopenia implies a reduction rather than an absence of the white cells. This condition is always present in pancytopenia also and may be present with aplastic anemia, or it may exist by itself.

Agranulocytosis may come as a single attack and rapidly progress to a fatal termination if not promptly and vigorously treated. It may also occur as a series of attacks with none severe enough to cause death, or it may develop a long-drawn-out course with frequency and severity of symptoms proportion to the degree of the reduction of the white cells below the normal level.

In the typical acute attack—always serious—the onset is abrupt, with chills, fever, headache, severe sore throat, and prostration coming on in rapid succession. Early delirium is common. Fortunately however, in the more common and less serious granulocytopenia, there is only a mild to moderate depression of granulocytes. The patient may then have only a slightly more than normal susceptibility to infection and may be able to lead a near-normal life. Still, any infection contracted by the patient is serious and should be promptly treated with appropriate antibiotics.

The cause of agranulocytosis is not always clear, but the drugs and chemicals likely to cause pancytopenia or aplastic anemia are also likely to cause agranulocytosis. Many more drugs have been incriminated as causal agents in granulocytopenia than in aplastic anemia, outstanding among them being some of the most valuable drugs for treating infections and heart, kidney and glandular conditions. Many tranquilizers cause trouble for a few people peculiarly sensitive to doses ordinarily harmless. Pharmaceutical companies and physicians have worked together to remove from use those drugs which can cause harm and for which other drugs can be used. However, no replacements have been found for some medicines valuable in the treatment of particular disease states. The possibility of developing such a serious disease as agranulocytosis is one of the reasons that taking drugs without a physician's supervision is a perilous practice.

What to Do

1. Whenever a rise in the frequency and severity of skin, throat, or lung infections is experienced, a physician should be consulted. He will likely order a complete blood count and tell you quickly whether agranulocytosis is the problem. If it is, he can identify the offending agent, start suitable treatment early, and prescribe precautionary measures against future infections.

2. As far as possible, avoid infections and exposure to infectious diseases by avoiding large crowds or public gatherings.

3. Take no drugs of any kind, including herbs, without the express permission of the physician.

4. Visit your physician regularly and have a blood count taken each time.

5. Keep the general state of your health at the best possible level by abundant rest, daily moderate exercise, and good wholesome food.

6. Promptly cleanse all open wounds with soap and water, and protect them from contamination.

LEUKEMIA.

Some forms of leukemia are among the most feared of all diseases, perhaps because nearly everyone remembers a child who died within a few weeks after becoming ill with leukemia, despite all that physicians could do. However, not all types have such a poor outlook.

Several different diseases which affect the white blood cells are grouped under the general term leukemia. They range in manifestation from vicious killers of children and adults to milder forms which permit older people, if afflicted by them, to carry on full activity without discomfort or treatment for ten to fifteen years. Nevertheless all are considered malignant. They are named according to the degree of cell change produced or according to the course of the illness and to the kind of cell involved. Leukemia therefore may be designated as acute or chronic, and then as lymphocytic, granulocytic (myelocytic), or monocytic; *e.g.*, acute granulocytic (myelocytic) leukemia.

In the normal course of events, parent cells (also called stem cells), located in the bone marrow or in the lymphoid organs, constantly produce younger cells destined to become mature and circulate in the blood. This is necessary in order that cells which wear out in the circulation may be constantly replaced. This multiplication of cells is accomplished by cell division—a biological process in which one cell is squeezed in two in the middle, thus producing two cells. In the early stages of their development, these young blood cells have the ability to divide again and again, each time producing offspring of the same order as themselves. As they mature they develop the capacity to carry out the function for which they were designed. For example, the mature granulocyte becomes able to combat infections caused by germs. Also they eventually lose the ability to multiply by dividing.

In leukemia, the parent or stem

Infection of the mouth and bleeding gums may be symptoms indicating acute leukemia.

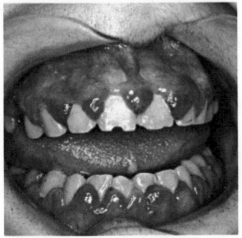

cells, or their immediate offspring, lose the ability to mature. In a sense they become "juvenile delinquents," as a famous leukemia expert describes them, retaining the ability to divide and thus go on forming many cells like themselves but being unable to take up their adult duties. The more immature the cells remain, the more acute the leukemia, the more serious the disease, and the less likely that the treatment will be effective.

The continuous division of daughter cells, all paying no attention to the usual controls effective on normal blood-forming tissue, may produce a fantastic number of cells in a very short time. This "runaway" cell growth uses up the nutrients and the space required by the remaining normal parent cells, and they die or do not proliferate. Often the abnormal young cells break out into the bloodstream and circulate as immature blood cells. The behavior of leukemia and its classification depend on the degree of maturity that the involved cells achieve. Acute leukemias have predominantly very young cells, while the chronic leukemias sometimes have cells almost normal in appearance.

A. *Acute Leukemias.* Acute leukemia occurs as commonly in an adult as in a child. In children it strikes more frequently below the age of six than above; and in children, too, it is more likely to be acute lymphocytic leukemia, while in the adult acute leukemia tends to be of granulocytic cell type. No race has been found to be exempt and no predilection of one sex over the other is seen.

The symptoms of either acute lymphocytic or acute granulocytic leukemia are indistinguishable except that lymph node enlargement is more common in the lymphocytic variety. The disease may begin suddenly, anemia being the first indication. Bleeding tendencies, infection of the mouth or throat accompanied by fever, extreme weakness, and headache are common. A white-cell count less than normal is the usual case in acute leukemia. In children there is often a history of an infection preceding the main attack by several weeks. Bleeding from the nose, gums, or rectum or excessive bleeding following tonsillectomy or a tooth extraction is common, indicating that the blood platelets are in short supply. At times, in the later stages of the disease, bleeding into vital areas such as the brain occurs. The spleen is enlarged more than the liver. Pain and tenderness in the bones and joints is common, probably because of the pressure of growing cells inside of the marrow cavity. Symptoms of anemia are usually present and may be severe.

A physician makes the preliminary diagnosis on the basis of a blood test. He sees young cells normally not present in the peripheral blood. He then performs or arranges for a bone marrow puncture so that a sample of marrow cells may be studied under the microscope. If he sees a disorganization of white-cell elements, he confirms the diagnosis of leukemia.

Treatment depends on the type of leukemia and the age of the patient. In some situations, one of the cortisones works best. In others, medicines designed to deprive cells of their ability to divide are given. Additional treatment, such as antibiotics for infections and transfusions for severe anemias, are used commonly. Great progress has been made in recent years in the development of drugs which relieve symptoms and in some cases cure the disease. The use of these powerful drugs deserves the best attention of a specially trained physician. The object of these medicines is to retard the growth of the abnormal cells without injuring the normal ones.

Cancer treatment is plagued by faddism more than all other areas of medical practice combined, except perhaps the "keep young" area. In spite of what some people would lead the patient to believe, physicians are as anxious as anyone can be to find a cure for leukemia. They have seen too many beautiful, talented children cut down at the threshold of life, to hold back on any medicines offering a cure, but they are equally anxious that the medicines used will do more good than harm. Do not trust individuals who promise cures in other countries or offer to sell medicines not handled by authorized drugstores.

What to Do

1. The parents of a child suspected of having leukemia should consult their family doctor, who will likely direct them to a specially qualified physician for the evaluation and initial treatment of such disorder.

2. During the periods of well-being, no favors should be shown to the child that the other children of the family do not enjoy.

3. It may be necessary to afford the afflicted child particular protection against physical injury because of his bleeding tendency.

4. A regular healthy diet and liberal rest are in order.

5. It is especially important that appointments with physicians be kept. Regular blood counts must be made.

B. *Chronic Leukemias.* Chronic leukemias always have an insidious onset, symptoms appearing commonly after several years of disease have elapsed. The same basic mechanism as occurs in acute leukemias is operative also in the chronic leukemias—an inability of the cells to mature, hence uncontrolled division of the cells and unimpeded accumulation. Since the process is slower and the abnormal cells more normal than in acute leukemia, higher counts of cells are seen in the bloodstream. Sometimes an abnormally high white-cell count is the only indication that something is wrong. After several months a person may have accumulated more than 100 times the normal number of leukocytes in his body. This extra tissue growth causes a drain on the body for nutrients and results in lassitude, weakness, and unexplained fatigue. These extra cells may infiltrate various organs and, depending on the degree of infiltration, may reduce that organ's function and efficiency. This is the cause of the enlarged liver and spleen.

Chronic granulocytic leukemia and chronic lymphocytic leukemia occur in the older age group, average age of onset for the former being forty-five and for the latter fifty-five. There is usually a larger spleen with chronic granulocytic leukemia and larger lymph nodes with chronic lymphocytic leukemia. Autoimmune hemolytic anemia is sometimes associated with chronic lymphocytic leukemia.

A person with chronic leukemia may experience the symptoms of anemia, may develop unusual lumps, may be unable to cope with infections as in agranulocytosis, or may have a bleeding tendency because of low concentration of platelets. Enlargement of the liver and spleen is an expected development. Nearly always a blood test shows an elevated white-cell count. At times, particularly with chronic granulocytic leukemia, there are nearly as many white cells as there are red cells, hence the term "leukemia" (white blood).

Treatment of chronic leukemia may involve the use of drugs or X-ray irradiation. No attempt is made to cure the patient, only to lessen the symptoms and treat complications as they develop. Chronic granulocytic leukemia more often than not changes to acute leukemia after about five years.

What to Do

1. Any patient with symptoms of a leukemia should be examined by a physician.

2. If diagnosis of leukemia is confirmed, the patient should ac-

cept the treatment program recommended and not seek so-called "cures."

3. He should follow the same precautions and instructions noted under agranulocytosis above.

POLYCYTHEMIA.
(See under "II. Blood Disease," *Polycythemia,* in this chapter.)

THROMBOCYTOPENIA.
(See under "III. Bleeding Disorders," *The Purpuras,* in this chapter.)

Hemotherapy

Hemotherapy is a comparatively new science of treatment, one in which whole blood or its products are used. Nearly four hundred years ago men knew that blood could be transferred from one person to another, but not until this century did physicians understand how to do it with safety. The greatest impetus to the therapeutic use of blood came during World War II, by which time the major blood groups were known and the art of cross matching had been perfected.

As has been alluded to previously, the human body has a fantastically complex code system by which it recognizes its own tissue. There are probably millions of individual code units in each person, so that perhaps no two people in the world have exactly the same code combination except indentical twins. Of course the closer the relationship between two individuals, the greater the likelihood that their codes will correspond.

The body also has a complicated defense system whereby tissue which doesn't "belong" is rejected. Such tissue is said to be incompatible. It is for this reason that skin grafts and kidney transplants from one person to another are likely to be destroyed, unless the people concerned are identical twins. It has been observed, however, that the simpler the tissue, the greater the possibility of its being tolerated. For example, the corneas of the eye can be transplanted from one person to another with little problem.

Blood is a comparativley simple tissue, but even so at least twenty different code systems have been identified in the red blood cells alone. Fortunately only two of them are strong codes, the ABO blood groups and the Rh blood groups. Determination of the group to which an individual belongs follow well-defined laws of heredity.

When "foreign" blood enters the bloodstream, the incompatible red cells are quickly destroyed, their hemoglobin being released into the bloodstream. Not only does such transfused blood fail to benefit the patient, but also the sudden tide of free hemoglobin is likely to damage the kidneys. It is this severe kidney damage that may cause death in a case of mismatched blood. For this reason, even in cases of severe injury, there must be a delay of at least half an hour before blood transfusion can be accomplished. It takes this much time to type the patient's blood (in most places at least four groups are checked) and then to mix it under controlled conditions with the blood intended for transfusion (cross matching). Only when the cross-matching test is favorable can the available blood be used safely for transfusion.

Young people can stand to lose more blood than older people and still recover. Even though blood substitutes will help to save some people who otherwise would die, they do not contain red cells which are necessary for the carrying of oxygen from the lungs to the brain. There is no genuine substitute for blood. Blood is absolutely necessary for most open heart operations, for organ transplant surgery (replacing a diseased organ like the kidney with a healthy kidney from another person), for many major

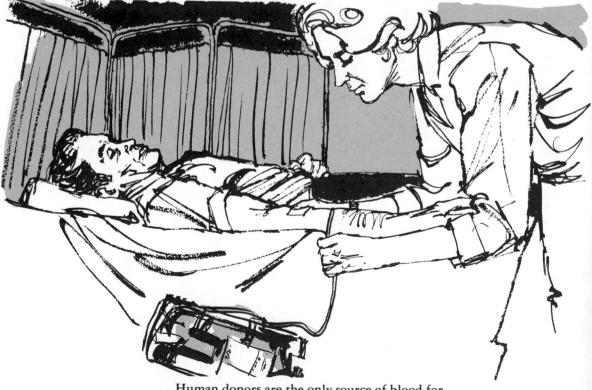

Human donors are the only source of blood for patients needing transfusions.

cancer operations, and in the use of some artificial kidneys.

The reception, preparation, and transfusion of blood or its components is not without hazard. Carelessness anywhere along the line from donor to patient could bring fatal consequences to the recipient. However, the number of lives saved through hemotherapy is many times greater than the number of serious complications induced. This fine record of safety does not mean that transfusions should be given indiscriminately as a tonic, to correct an undiagnosed anemia, or to supply iron in a case of iron deficiency.

Blood banks where blood is received, processed, and stored are set up all over the world. In these places specially trained technicians and physicians work constantly to improve the safety of blood transfusions.

The greatest need in almost every blood bank and in nearly every hospital is blood. Blood cannot be manufactured synthetically. It must come from people. At present only about 5 percent of the eligible donors are giving blood. People must have enough sympathy for their fellowmen to suffer the minor inconveniences of becoming blood donors. The rising need for blood or the blood components can be offset only by a rising recognition of responsibility on the part of those suitable to give blood.

Suitable individuals are those between twenty and sixty-five, who weigh over 100 pounds, who are in good health, who have not had hepatitis, malaria, or venereal diseases, and have not taken drugs—with the exception of aspirin—for the previous two months. A healthy person can safely donate four times a year; but if this is kept up for more than two years, the donor should take oral iron tablets daily for at least six weeks each time after donating. There are no known hazards of repeated blood donation at the above rate.

Cancer

Cancer is now the second most common cause of death in the United States. It accounts for 18 percent of the total number of deaths, being exceeded only by diseases of the heart. Take the two years 1970 and 1971. In those two years cancer killed more Americans than the total number who were killed in our four recent wars: World War I, World War II, the Korean conflict, and the Vietnam engagement. Cancer kills eight times more Americans each year than are killed in all automobile accidents.

Estimates indicate that 975,000 new cases of cancer were diagnosed in 1976. Almost one third of these were cancer of the skin. The estimate of cancer deaths for the same year (1976) totalled 370,000, which is slightly more than the population of the city of Miami. Slightly more than half of the cancer deaths occur in men. It is cancer of the lung that is responsible for the greater number of cancer deaths among men, cancer of the lung being more prevalent among men than among women.

Cancer is a tragic disease, not only because of the large number of deaths that it causes, but because of its high toll of human agony and suffering. The cancer victim who has received the best treatment that medical science can provide still continues in a state of uncertainty for weeks, and perhaps for many months wondering whether the treatment will have arrested the progress of the cancer. If such a person is still well after a year

Mortality for Leading Causes of Death: United States, 1973.

Rank	Cause of Death	Number of Deaths	Percent of Total Deaths	Rank	Cause of Death	Number of Deaths	Percent of Total Deaths
	All Causes	1,973,003	100.0	9	Certain Diseases of Infancy	30,503	1.5
1	Diseases of Heart	757,075	38.4				
2	Cancer	351,055	17.8	10	Suicide	25,118	1.3
3	Stroke	214,313	10.9	11	Emphysema	22,249	1.1
4	Accidents	115,821	5.9	12	Homicide	20,465	1.0
5	Influenza & Pneumonia	62,559	3.2	13	Congenital Anomalies	14,062	0.7
6	Diabetes Mellitus	38,208	1.9	14	Nephritis & Nephrosis	8,336	0.4
7	Cirrhosis of Liver	33,350	1.7	15	Ulcers	7,688	0.4
8	Arteriosclerosis	32,617	1.7		Other & Ill-defined	239,584	12.1

Source: Vital Statistics of the United States, 1973.

VOL. 26, NO. 1 JANUARY/FEBRUARY 1976, CA — *A Cancer Journal for Clinicians*, American Cancer Soc or two, he is haunted by the knowledge that the results of cancer treatment are commonly given in terms of five-year survival rates.

In a case in which the cancer resumes its growth after treatment, the patient knows that he faces a downhill course, every week bringing him one week closer to the time when his vital forces will no longer be equal to the devastating effects of the cancer.

What Is Cancer?

A cancer is a kind of tumor that threatens a person's life. But in order to understand the full meaning of the term cancer we must first explore the uses of the word tumor.

Used in its broad sense, a tumor is an abnormal enlargement of some part of the body. As usually used, tumor refers to a mass of tissue which is composed of unusual cells that have multiplied more than they normally should, that are not a part of the body's normal design, and that are serving no useful purpose. In this sense, the medical scientist prefers the Greek term *neoplasm* (new growth) to the word tumor. In the normal course of the development and growth of the human body, there is a precise control over the characteristics of the cells that compose tissues. This control is mediated through the mysterious DNA molecules that are found in the nucleus of each one of the body's cells. (See volume 1, chapter 2, and volume 3, chapter 2.) The DNA molecules are "coded" in such a way that they regulate the growth characteristics and activities of the cell in which they are contained, thus enabling this cell to work in cooperation with other cells. As the body grows, beginning at the time of conception and continuing to adulthood, the total number of cells increases tremendously. But this increase is carefully controlled so that only the proper number of each kind of cell is produced. Also the tissue boundary between one kind of cell and its neighboring cells is carefully preserved. But a developing neoplasm (tumor) is composed of cells which have multiplied irrespective of the body's normal checks and balances. Tumor cells are out of control.

There are two large classes of tumors: benign and malignant. The benign tumors are those in which the cells remain isolated from the surrounding tissues and grow within their own capsule. A benign tumor reminds one of a walled community surrounded on all sides by a large city. The word benign implies that this kind of tumor is harmless. But it occupies space, and it therefore may cause trouble by making pressure on surrounding tissues. A fatty tumor which develops under the skin and which may cause a bump on the body's surface belongs to this benign class of tumors.

Malignant tumors are composed of cells which are so far out of control that they continue to grow extensively and invade the surrounding tissues. It is such a malignant tumor that is properly called a cancer. As a malignant tumor grows, it sends its processes like tentacles in many directions. As it invades other tissues, it often destroys them, usually interfering with their supply of blood. Such destruction of the surrounding tissues may cause bleeding and ulceration.

The worst feature of malignant tumors (cancers) is that as their cells multiply and the tumor invades the surrounding tissues, small groups of these wild-growing cells may break away from their parent tumor and be carried either by the bloodstream or by the circulation of the lymph to some regional or distant part of the body. The colony of wild cells will there establish itself and develop a secondary tumor very much like the original one. The scientist speaks of this process of migration as lymphatic spread or as metastasis. Often the metastatic tumors may endanger the patient's life even more than the primary tumor.

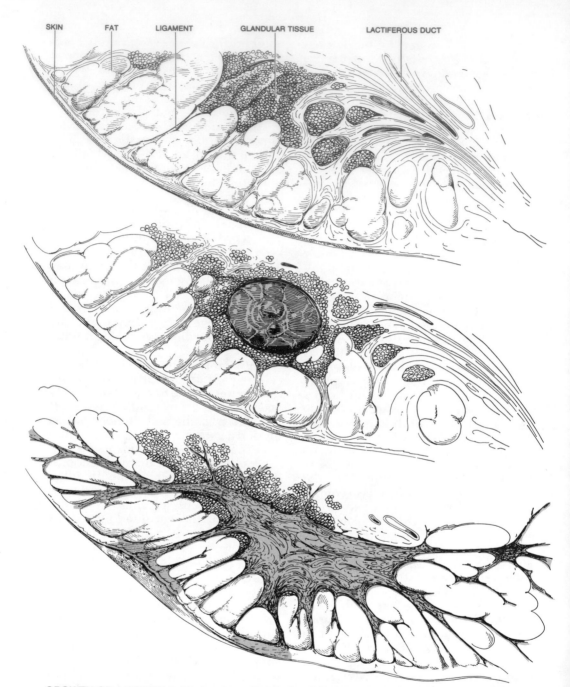

SKIN   FAT   LIGAMENT   GLANDULAR TISSUE   LACTIFEROUS DUCT

GROWTH OF A TUMOR in the breast ordinarily threatens life only when the tumor can spread to distant parts of the body. The normal breast *(top)* is organized into glandular tissue, fat, and other structures. Tumors arise almost exclusively in the glandular tissue. A benign tumor *(middle)* can grow rapidly and become quite large, but it cannot escape the tissue in which it develops. A cancerous tumor *(bottom)* can spread throughout the glandular tissue, can often involve ligaments and skin, and can sometimes penetrate the muscle underlying the breast. In addition cancers can in some cases migrate through the blood or the lymphatic system to establish new colonies of cells in distant, unrelated organs. This is the process known as metastasis.

From the "The Cancer Problem" by John Cairns; Copyright © 1975 by Scientific American, Inc. All rights reserved.

134

There are certain favorite routes that the colonies of cancer cells seem to follow as they move from one part of the body to another. For example, a cancer originating in the lung may metastasize to the brain or to other organs. A cancer of the prostate commonly migrates to the bones of the skeleton.

Notice that this tendency of malignant tumors (cancers) to metastasize distinguishes them from the less harmful, benign tumors. Notice, also, that most malignant tumors tend to grow for a while at the site of its origin before colonies of its cells break away and move to some other region. This latter fact explains the observation that the earlier a cancer is treated, the greater the prospect of success. That is, if a malignant tumor can be completely removed in the early stages of its growth, before it has metastasized, the prospects of saving the patient's life are relatively good. If, however, colonies of cancer cells have already broken away before the parent cancer is removed, the subsequent development of one or more metastatic tumors in other parts of the body makes a fatal outcome more certain.

Broad Classification of Cancers

As a cancer develops in any particular tissue of the body, its cells partake of the nature, somewhat, of the normal cells of the tissue in which it develops. True, the cancer cells are much distorted and have lost many of the normal characteristics of the parent tissue. This explains why there are so many kinds of cancers, for there are many kinds of normal tissue in which a malignant tumor may develop. Also, there are usually several patterns of abnormal development possible for every kind of normal tissue. Thus it would require several pages to list all the classes and subclasses of cancer that may develop in the human body.

For our present purpose we need only to mention the major kinds of cancer—the large groups of malignant

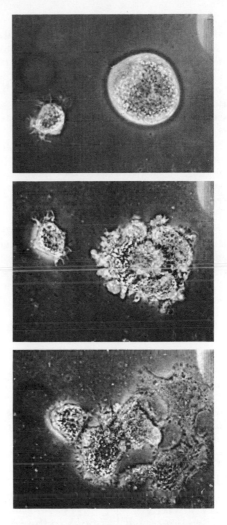

A time-lapse study of the division of a malignant cell, showing four stages of development and growth.

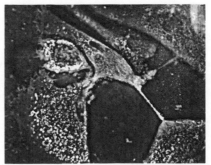

135

tumors as determined by the kind of tissue from which they take origin.

1. Carcinomas. The carcinomas compose the largest group of cancers. They are the ones that take origin from the epithelial cells that cover the body's surface, line its tubes and cavities, and compose the functioning cells of its glands.

2. Sarcomas. The sarcomas are the cancers that arise in the body's supporting tissues. Here we have the cancers that arise from fibrous tissue, from bone, from blood vessels, and from muscle tissue.

3. Leukemias. These are the cancers that develop in the tissues which produce blood cells such as the bone marrow and the lymph nodes.

4. Lymphomas. These cancers develop from the cells of the lymph glands.

What Causes Cancer?

Fifty years ago the answer usually given to this question was quite simple. It was assumed then that in most cases cancer was a result of hereditary fault. Instances were cited in which cancer developed in members of a certain family, appearing in one generation after another. Also, close relatives seemed to be vulnerable to the same kind of cancer.

Now, with a vast increase in medical knowledge, we understand something about what happens in the cells when they undergo the transformation to cancer cells. As mentioned earlier, there is a fault in the control mechanism so that the cells no longer conform to the normal pattern for the particular area of the body in which they reside. But the question still remains unanswered as to exactly what happens when cells lose their normal mechanism of control. Obviously, it has to do with the chromosomes and genes. But was this change in the control mechanism passed from parent to child as a hereditary fault, or did something happen during the present individual's life-span that damaged the control mechanism within certain of his cells? If the fault was passed from parent to child, we would blame the resulting cancer on heredity. If the cancer resulted from damage to the control mechanism during the individual's lifetime, we would say that environmental factors are responsible. Can it be that in some cases a cancer is caused by faulty heredity while in other cases it is caused by environmental influences? Or perhaps both, in some cases?

In a few instances of cancer the cause is almost purely hereditary. Probably, for the most part, these are the cases in which cancer occurs during early childhood. But it is estimated that in at least 80 percent of the cases of cancer some environmental factor triggers the changes that cause normal cells to become cancer cells. This understanding of the tremendous influence of factors in the environment is an encouraging development, for it logically indicates that the prevention of cancer is more important than is the prospect of cure, once the disease is established. The emphasis for the future should be on identifying the factors that predispose to cancer so that these can be avoided. Herein lies a real prospect of significantly reducing the number of cases of cancer.

But it is too simplistic to say that most cases of cancer are caused by some factor in the environment that insults the body's cells. Some persons are inherently more susceptible to these environmental insults than are others. Two persons can smoke the same number of cigarettes in a day and inhale just as deeply. One of these may develop lung cancer 20 years later and the other may not.

The factors which contribute to the development of a cancer are complex. Some cancers result from a combination of environmental factors acting together, reinforcing or even augmenting one another.

Among the many harmful effects of smoking is that by which tobacco smoke damages the cells that line the mouth. Thus cancer of the mouth occurs more commonly in smokers than it does in nonsmokers. Among the harmful effects of the drinking of alcohol is damage to the membranes which are bathed by the alcohol. So, cancer of the mouth is somewhat more common in drinkers than it is among those who abstain. But among persons who both smoke and drink, the incidence of cancer of the mouth is even higher than the figure obtained were we to add the effects of smoking and of drinking. The two factors in combination have a greater influence than the sum of the individual effects of the two factors (a so-called synergistic effect).

Another example of the intensified effect of a combination of environmental insults occurs among workers with asbestos. Nonsmokers who work with asbestos have about the same susceptibility to lung cancer that nonsmokers have otherwise. That is, contact with asbestos fibers, of itself, does not particularly predispose to lung cancer. But asbestos workers who are smokers have a much higher rate of lung cancer than do smokers in general. So the combination of smoking and the exposure to asbestos greatly increases the usual hazard of smoking as it relates to the development of lung cancer.

Predisposing Factors

By predisposing factors we refer to circumstances and conditions that increase the prospect of the development of a malignant tumor (cancer). We are not saying that these are causes of cancer; for, as yet, we do not know just what takes place within normal cells that causes them to lose their control factors and grow wildly. We will group these predisposing factors under four headings: (1) physical agents, (2) chemical agents, (3) biological agents, and (4) circumstances of life and health.

1. *Physical agents.* Excessive exposure to sunlight is an important predisposing factor in cancers of the skin. The solar keratoses which occur on those portions of the body exposed to the sun are the intermediate stage between normal skin and skin cancer. These occur commonly in farmers and sailors whose usual activities expose them to the ultraviolet radiation present in sunlight. The effect that sunlight has on the skin depends, of course, upon the individual's complexion. Dark-skinned persons are not so susceptible, because the pigment in their skin serves to screen the skin's tissues from the effects of the ultraviolet radiation.

Exposure to ionizing radiations (X ray, etc.) of various kinds greatly increases the risk of cancer. The incidence of leukemia (cancer of the blood-forming tissues) was significantly increased among the atomic bomb survivors in the three- to five-year interval following their exposure to the blast. In this same group of persons, those who smoked cigarettes developed lung cancer at a much higher rate than do smokers ordinarily. This provides another example of the synergistic effect

Pipe smoking can cause lip cancer.

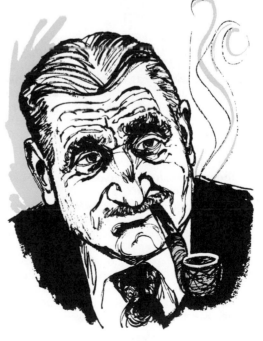

of two circumstances (exposure to the atomic blast plus the use of cigarettes) as compared with the effect of such influences acting singly.

In the early years of the development of X-ray technology, those physicians who worked with X-ray equipment were not so well informed regarding the hazards of the X ray or so careful in its use as are radiologists of the present day. Two scientific studies conducted about 1940 indicated that physicians who were concerned with the use of X ray had ten times the incidence of leukemia as did physicians in general.

Another significant observation was that the employees in watch factories who applied luminous paint to the watch dials were unusually prone to develop cancer. It was discovered that these workers followed the habit of touching the tiny paint brushes to their lips to straighten the bristles. The luminous paint contained a small amount of radium, which is a source of ionizing radiation.

It has also been observed that women patients who receive unusually large doses of radiation therapy for the treatment of cancer of the cervix of the uterus may later develop cancer of the vagina.

Smoking, particularly pipe smoking, is a recognized aggravating factor in the development of cancer of the lip, the tongue, and the lining of the mouth. It is apparently the heat of the pipestem against the tissues of the lip that makes these tissues more susceptible, eventually, to the development of cancer. With respect to the other tissues of the mouth it is difficult to know whether it is the heat of the smoke stream or the irritating effect of the smoke that make these more susceptible to cancer.

In various parts of the body, the tissues that are subjected to continuous irritation are more susceptible than usual to cancerous change. Scars resulting from corrosive damage to the skin may develop cancer. The irritating effect of gallstones on the tissues of the gallbladder may make this organ more vulnerable. Kidney stones may have a similar effect on the tissues of the outlet to the kidney. The long continued influence of ulcerative colitis makes the colon more susceptible to the development of cancer than it is under normal circumstances.

2. *Chemical agents.* It is not consistent to draw a sharp line between physical agents and chemical agents. Some of the substances to be listed as chemical agents in the discussion which follows may actually act by causing physical irritation in the tissues that they contact. Note the classic example of cancer of the scrotum which was so common among chimney sweeps of former decades, due to the local irritation of the soots and tars which presumably sifted through their clothing to irritate the skin of the scrotum. The modern counterpart is the occurrence of scrotal cancer among industrial workers with shale oil and with mineral machine oils.

Many industrial chemicals are known to predispose to cancer. Coal tar and creosote preparations are used in the experimental laboratory to produce skin cancer in laboratory animals. They have a similar effect on industrial workers exposed to these substances. Arsenic preparations, even when taken internally, cause skin cancer in humans. In the case of arsenic, the chemical passes through the tissues of the body and still causes skin cancer. Another industrial hazard involves the workers with aniline dyes who, after continued exposure, are particularly susceptible to cancer of the urinary bladder. It is presumed that the bladder is the vulnerable organ because the offending chemical substances are eliminated by way of the urine.

Considerable concern has developed recently because of the evidence that the use of synthetic estrogen hormones in women patients (such as diethylstilbestrol) has statistically increased the likelihood of cancer of the vagina and cervix of the uterus. Compounding this concern has been the observation that teen-age daughters of women who received this synthetic estrogen during the first three months of their pregnancy are more likely than usual to develop cancer of the vagina and cervix of the uterus. Thus there appears to be a carry-over of influence from one generation to the next.

Another line of evidence implicates the use of immunosuppressive drugs as being responsible for increasing the incidence of cancer in various parts of the body. These are the drugs which are used, in tissue transplants (e.g., a kidney transplant). The immunosuppressive drugs have the effect of dampening the body's mechanisms which normally bring about the rejection of tissues transplanted from another person. This observation does not mean that the immunosuppressive drugs should never be used, for not all persons, by far, who receive these drugs will develop cancer. The use of the drugs is often a life-saving procedure in a person who would otherwise die were he not to receive the transplant of a healthy kidney. Inasmuch as the body's immune mechanism is an important part of its ability to resist disease of various kinds, it is reasonable to assume that when the immune mechanism is depressed the tissues throughout the body are less able than usual to resist the changes that bring about the development of cancer.

Those who use alcohol have a higher incidence of cancer than do non-drinkers. The exact influence of alcohol is difficult to determine, for several reasons. One is that those who use liquor nearly always smoke cigarettes. Thus, when cancer develops in such persons, it is uncertain whether alcohol or cigarette smoke is the culprit. Some authorities class alcohol as a "co-carcinogen," meaning that its effect is to amplify the influence of other circumstances that are known to cause cancer.

Another reason for difficulty in evaluating the precise influence of alcohol is that the popular alcoholic beverages contain various additives. Is it the alcohol or some additive that has the damaging influence?

In spite of these difficulties in quantitating the effect of alcohol in predisposing to cancer, the evidence points clearly to an increase in cancer susceptibility in those tissues that come in contact with the alcohol: the mouth, the pharynx, the larynx, the esophagus, and the stomach.

The smoking of cigarettes is responsible for at least 90 percent of the cases of lung cancer, and lung cancer accounts for a greater number of deaths among men than any other kind of cancer. Furthermore, the incidence of and the number of deaths from lung cancer in women has been increasing alarmingly in recent years as more and more women smoke.

Dr. Brian MacMahon, of the Department of Epidemiology of the Harvard School of Public Health, made a very significant statement in this regard at a conference convened by the National Cancer Institute and the American Cancer Society at Key Biscayne, Florida, in December of 1974. He said, "No single known measure would lengthen the life or improve the health of the American population more than eliminating cigarette smoking.

The smoking of cigarettes increases the incidence of cancer in all the tissues that are bathed by the smoke stream as well as in some other tissues which have no direct contact with the cigarette smoke. It is difficult to know just which components in the cigarette smoke are responsible for the several effects which smoking has on the human body. Presumably it is the tars in cigarette smoke that dramatically increase the susceptibility of the lung tissues to cancer. The smoke is irritating, however, to all of the tissues with which it has contact: the mouth, the pharynx, the larynx, the trachea, the bronchi, and the delicate air sacs in which there occurs an exchange of gases between the inhaled air and the circulating blood. Smoking may also increase the risk of cancer of the esophagus, possibly because the saliva that is swallowed carries with it some of the constituents of tobacco smoke.

Cancer of the urinary bladder is also significantly more common among

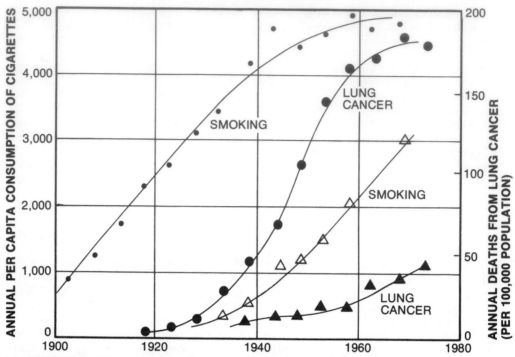

CIGARETTE SMOKING AND LUNG CANCER are unmistakably related, but the nature of the relation remained obscure because of the long latent period between the increase in cigarette consumption and the increase in the incidence of lung cancer. The data are for England and Wales. In the men (circles) smoking began to increase at the beginning of the twentieth century, but the corresponding trend in deaths from lung cancer did not begin until after 1920. In women (triangles) smoking began later, and lung cancers are only now appearing.

smokers than among nonsmokers. The probable explanation is that certain constituents of tobacco smoke are transferred to the bloodstream and eventually eliminated through the kidneys and the bladder. As the urine accumulates in the bladder, these constituents have a sufficient irritating influence there to predispose to cancer of this organ.

3. *Biological agents.* There has developed a considerable interest both among scientists and among intelligent people in general, in the possibility that some virus or group of viruses may be the agent responsible for causing cancer. The idea that at least some cancers are caused by viruses is attractive for at least two reasons. First, certain kinds of cancer can be induced in animals by inoculating viruses that have been derived from animals that have these kinds of cancer. Second, it has been dem-

onstrated that some humans who have cancer contain antibodies in their tissues and body fluids which, presumably, were developed there in the body's effort to combat cancer. Medical scientists cherish the hope that an antiviral vaccine may be thus developed to protect people from cancer.

A great deal of research has already been performed in the hope of clarifying the relationship of viruses to human cancer, but more needs to be done. As of the time of this writing, no clear scientific evidence proves that viruses are the active agents in causing the usual kinds of human cancer. Dr. John Cairns of the Mill Hill Laboratories of the Imperial Cancer Research Fund in London, stated in 1975, "As yet there is no unambiguous evidence that any class of human cancers is regularly caused by a virus." In a similar vein, Dr. Alfred G.

140

Knudson, Jr., of the Graduate School of Biomedical Sciences, University of Texas Health Science Center, Houston, Texas, stated in 1974, "Despite intense investigation, we still do not have one proven case of a human malignant tumor caused by a virus."

4. *Circumstances of life and health.* Certain circumstances of life and certain times of life alter a person's susceptibility to cancer. We will consider three broad categories.

Age. Here there are two important considerations: (1) the manifestations of cancer which are typical of early childhood and (2) the increasing susceptibility to cancer among adults as age increases.

Surprisingly, in the one-to-fourteen age group, cancer is the leading cause of death from disease. Before the conquest of the infectious diseases,

these caused more deaths among children, by far, than did cancer. But now that the infectious diseases are under control, childhood cancer takes first place except for the deaths caused by accidents.

It is true that the number of deaths from cancer among children is far less than the number of deaths from cancer among adults, totaling only 2,961 in 1973. Significantly, however, more deaths from childhood cancer occur during the first five years of life than during the next two five-year periods combined. This reflects the fact that many of the cancers affecting young children are unique in that they represent tissue areas in which the development of the component cells did not reach full maturity. Some of these tumors of early childhood, then, are a carryover from embryonic life.

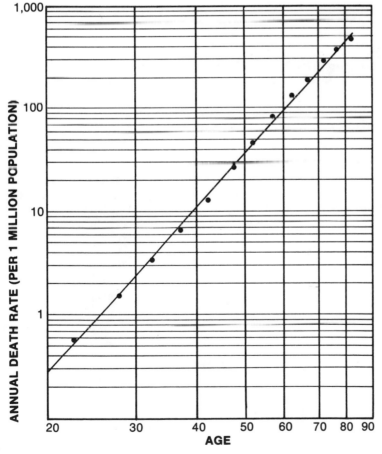

OLD PEOPLE compose the subpopulation that is most conspicuously at risk in the development of cancer. The incidence of almost all forms of cancer increases dramatically with advancing age. Here the U.S. death rate from a representative cancer, that of the large intestine, is plotted against age. It can be seen that the logarithm of the death rate is linearly related to the logarithm of age. The relation can be explained by the hypothesis that several mutations are required to generate a cancer, and that the probability of each mutation is proportional to age. The slope of the line suggests that the number of mutations required is five.

From *Scientific American*, November 1975, p. 67.

The tissues commonly developing childhood cancer are the blood-producing tissues (with resulting leukemia), the brain and other parts of the nervous system, the eye, the adrenal glands, muscle tissue, bone, and kidney.

During adult years, the likelihood of cancer increases, year by year. This steady increase reflects the circumstances that many of the predisposing factors to cancer require a more or less extended time in order to bring about malignant changes in normal cells. Thus the actual cancers resulting from the industrial hazard of exposure to chemicals may appear many years after the responsible chemical was encountered. The varied damaging effects of tobacco often appear more than 20 years after the individual began to smoke.

Sex. The manifestations of cancer are somewhat different among adult men as compared with those in adult women. The accompanying charts indicate that, for men, lung cancer is not only the most commonly occurring cancer, but also the one which causes the greatest number of deaths. For women, it is breast cancer that accounts for the greatest number of cases of cancer and also for the greatest number of deaths.

Marital state. Cancer of the breast is more common among unmarried women than among those who are married. Also, the age at which a woman bears her first child has its influence on her susceptibility to breast cancer. The woman who has her first child before age 25 has a much smaller risk of breast cancer than does the woman who has her first child after age 35.

With cancer of the cervix of the uterus, the influence of marriage is in the opposite direction. Women who are married in their teens or who have their first sexual intercourse while still in their teens, have a much greater prospect of cancer of the

Cancer Statistics by Site and Sex* 1976

*Excluding non-melanoma in cancer and carcinoma in situ of uterine cervix.

The *estimates* of cancer incidence on the following pages are based on newly available comprehensive data of the National Cancer Institute's Third National Cancer Survey. Carcinoma in situ of the cervix is first diagnosed in over 40,000 cases annually. Based on a special NCI survey, previous estimates of incidence of non-melanoma skin cancer may have been substantially understated. The survey indicates that the number is about 300,000 cases annually.

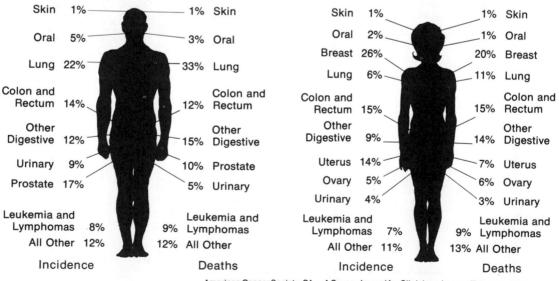

American Cancer Society, CA—*A Cancer Journal for Clinicians* January/February 1976

uterine cervix than those who are married when in their twenties or those who are never married.

Common Locations for Cancer

Every case of cancer is different and requires individual diagnosis and treatment. Furthermore, cancer occurring in any part of the body has unique characteristics. We will now list, in alphabetical order, the various parts of the body in which cancer commonly occurs and make brief mention of the typical features.

Bile ducts. The bile ducts may become involved either with cancer developing within the ducts themselves or with cancer in adjacent structures. The earliest significant symptom is usually jaundice (manifested by a yellowing of the whites of the eyes and of the skin), which results from continuous or intermittent obstruction to the flow of the bile. The surgical treatment of cancer in this location is difficult partly because there is no alternate route for the flow of bile and partly because the cancer is usually quite well advanced before the diagnosis is established.

Bladder (urinary bladder). It is now recognized that exposure to certain chemicals is the exciting cause of many cases of cancer of the bladder. These chemicals may be taken into the body by various routes but are eventually eliminated through the urinary system and thus appear in the urine as it is stored in the bladder. It was noted earlier that cancer of the bladder may be often caused by the use of cigarettes because certain irritating substances in tobacco smoke are eliminated from the body through the urinary system. Presumably these chemical substances serve as irritants to the tissues of the bladder.

The earliest significant sign of cancer of the bladder is blood in the urine, often unaccompanied by pain. Whenever this occurs, a prompt examination of the urinary system should be made to determine the cause of this bleeding. In some cases a growth somewhat like seaweeds develops within the bladder, and this may float over the outlet of the bladder to interfere with the flow of urine when the bladder is being emptied. This circumstance also deserves prompt attention by the physician. Usually the symptoms of cystitis appear, sooner or later, in connection with cancer of the bladder. (See chapter 22 on "Diseases of the Urinary System" in this volume.) Treatment of cancer of the bladder by surgery or by a combination of surgery and irradiation is relatively successful if the cancer is detected in its early stages.

Blood. The disease leukemia, in which the tissues which form blood cells become involved, is classed as a cancer of the blood-forming tissues. (See the discussion of *Leukemia* in chapter 10 of this volume.)

Bone. Cancer of the bone may originate within the bone itself, it may become involved by cancer of adjacent tissues, or it may develop secondarily when a colony of cancer cells is carried by the blood from a cancer in

Cancer of the bladder.

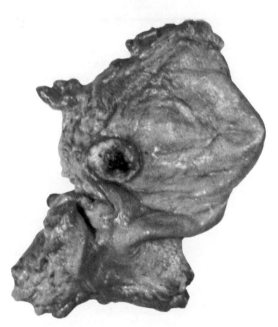

143

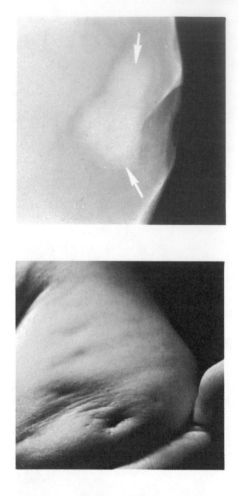

Top: X ray of axillary lymph nodes. A proven case of carcinoma of the breast with axillary metastases. Center: Adenocarcinoma, left breast. Below: Cancer of the breast, late stages of development.

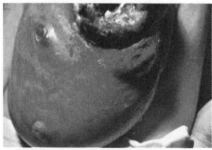

PUBLIC HEALTH SERVICE AUDIOVISUAL FACILITY

some other part of the body (by metastasis). Cancer of the bone typically causes considerable local pain and also a weakening of the structure of the bone so that it fractures easily (pathologic fracture). The treatment of cancer of the bone is difficult and may require radical methods, including X-ray therapy or chemotherapy.

Breast. The breast is the most common site of cancer in women, there being about 90,000 new cases a year in the United States and more than 32,000 deaths per year (data from the National Cancer Institute for the year 1974).

Cancer of the breast is treacherous because it tends to spread early in the course of the disease to distant parts of the body. When the cancer is detected early, before colonies of cancer cells have migrated to other parts of the body, the treatment by surgery and irradiation is quite successful. When the cancer has spread to other parts of the body before treatment is instituted, however, the outlook for eventual survival is grave.

Progress has been made in recent years in reducing the number of deaths from cancer of the breast, the progress being due mostly to early detection and to early and adequate treatment. The most successful treatment for these cases which are detected early is a surgical removal of the breast, plus in some cases irradiation therapy. The use of potent chemicals (chemotherapy) has not proved to be helpful in the primary treatment of cancer of the breast proper. It is used in selected cases, however, for the treatment of the tumors that develop in other parts of the body after having spread from the original site in the breast (metastases).

Women in general are becoming aware of the possible tragic outcome of a "lump in the breast." By reporting this finding at once to her physician a woman can receive the benefits of early treatment.

Not all lumps in the breast are caused by cancer. So the physician, in

144

Breast Self-examination

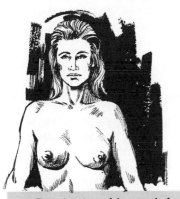

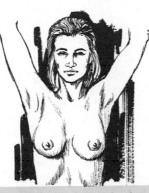

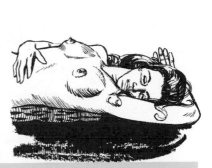

1. Examination of breasts before a mirror for symmetry in size and shape, noting any puckering of skin or retraction of nipple.

2. Arms raised over head, again studying breasts in the mirror for the same signs.

3. Reclining on bed with flat pillow or folded bath towel under shoulder on same side as breast to be examined.

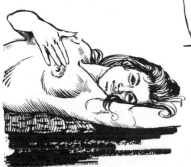

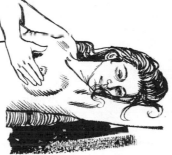

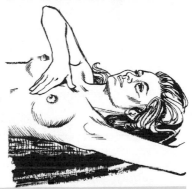

4. To examine inner half of the breast, arm is raised. Beginning at breastbone and working out, inner half of breast is palpated.

5. The area over and around the nipple is carefully palpated with flats of the fingers.

6. Continuing thus to palpate, examination of lower inner half of the breast is completed.

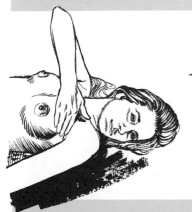

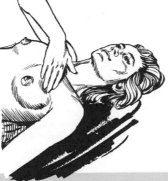

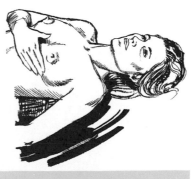

7. With arm down at side, palpation continues with examination of tissues extending to armpits.

8. The upper outer quadrant of the breast is examined with the flat part of the fingers.

9. The lower outer quadrant of the breast is likewise examined in successive stages.

dealing with an early case of a lump in the breast, has to differentiate between a benign tumor (relatively harmless) and a malignant one. When he is certain that the lump is benign, he removes only a small amount of the breast tissue.

In many instances it cannot be known before operation whether the growth is benign or malignant. In such a case, the surgeon removes a small portion of the abnormal tissue and then waits, with the patient still on the operating table, while a pathologist makes a microscopic examination and reports the nature of the tumor. If it is benign, the remaining part of the operation is comparatively simple. If it is malignant, the surgeon may need to remove the entire breast and, possibly, some of the tissues in the chest wall and in the armpit (axilla).

A lump in the breast may develop quite quickly and without attracting particular attention. It may easily develop between times as far as the yearly checkup at the doctor's office is concerned. So it is now generally advocated that women learn the method of self-examination of the breast (see page 145) and that they make such an examination once a month—this in addition to the yearly examination by a physician. Of course, if the woman discovers any questionable lump, painless though it be, she should report it at once to her physician.

In making this self-examination, a woman should lie on her back and should use the flat surface of the palm and fingers (not their tips) as she carefully and systematically presses the various parts of each breast against the muscles and ribs which lie beneath.

When a malignant lump in the breast is still small and when it receives adequate treatment promptly (within days rather than months), the prospects of five-year survival are at least 75 percent.

In an older woman, past the menopause, any discharge from the nipple (primarily bloody in nature) is a serious omen and should be reported promptly to the physician. It may be the first indication of a beginning cancer.

Cervix of the uterus. The cervix is the outlet of the uterus. It is situated so that it protrudes into the deepest part of the vagina.

Studies in recent years indicate that cancer of the cervix of the uterus, along with cancer of other parts of the female reproductive organs occur somewhat more commonly in women who have taken diethylstilbestrol for therapeutic reasons. Also, this type of cancer is one of those that occurs sometimes in young women still in their teens whose mothers have received diethylstilbestrol during the first three months of their pregnancy.

A second line of interest among medical scientists in this particular type of cancer stems from the possibility that an infection with herpes simplex virus II may somehow predispose to this cancer. At this writing this possibility is still under investigation and no final conclusion can yet be drawn.

Cancer of the cervix of the uterus becomes a dangerous cancer once it spreads to other tissues. If recognized and adequately treated in its early stages, however, it can be successfully eradicated.

The Papanicolaou test ("Pap" test) has made early detection of cancer of the cervix relatively simple. It must be emphasized, however, that the availability of the "Pap" test does not make cancer of the cervix any less deadly once it begins to invade the surrounding tissues. Now that this test is available, every woman should take it upon herself to report to her doctor as frequently as he suggests so that he may use this test to discover cancerous changes at their earliest stage. Some clinics perform the "Pap" test on all women 25 years of age or older, preferably at intervals no longer than one year.

The Papanicolaou test consists of

obtaining a small amount of mucous secretion from the depth of the vagina or from the cervix and making a microscopic examination to determine the type of cells present. Should there be a cancer of the cervix, the cells contained in this sample of mucus will reveal changes which indicate their beginning transformation into cancer cells.

Colon and rectum. Cancer in this terminal part of the intestine seldom occurs in persons younger than 40 years of age. This is one of the more serious forms of cancer; and, as is true of most other kinds of cancer, the best results occur when the treatment begins in the early stages of the disease.

In 1940 the five-year survival rate for cancer of the colon and rectum was only about 20 percent. Beginning then, a strong campaign was carried out to encourage people to submit for periodic examinations in the hope that early detection and treatment would improve the patient's chance of survival. This campaign has brought a favorable turn of events to the degree that at the present time the five-year survival rate is about 50 percent.

The examination procedure includes (1) an examination of the tissues surrounding the anus and inside the anal canal, (2) an examination of the inside of the colon by the use of the sigmoidoscope, and (3) an X-ray examination of the colon if the physician feels that this is needed.

The only successful method of treatment thus far for cancers of the colon and rectum is the radical removal by surgery of the affected tissues. In advanced cases, in which the cancer has already spread, some of the other methods of treatment such as irradiation and chemotherapy have their place.

Small growths (polyps) which protrude from the lining of the colon are considered to be harbingers of cancer in this area. These are easily detected by the examination with the sigmoidoscope or the colonoscope. They are readily removed and thus become available for examination by a pathologist. If this examination indicates cancerous change, the physician in charge will make his recommendations accordingly.

It is interesting to note that cancers in the colon and rectum are uncommon among people in the so-called underdeveloped countries. It is probably significant that the diet of these primitive peoples contains considerable roughage and very little sugar.

Esophagus. The combined use of cigarettes and alcohol predispose to cancer of the esophagus. It may occur in any part of the organ, but it is most common in that portion next to the stomach. Of course it causes increased difficulty in swallowing. The results of treating this type of cancer have, for the most part, been disappointing. More recently, surgical techniques for approaching the various parts of the esophagus have been perfected, and the survival rate has improved accordingly.

Face. (See under *Skin.*)

Gallbladder. The presence of gallstones in the gallbladder seems to be associated with most cancers of this organ. The symptoms include those of "indigestion," plus pain and tenderness in the region of the gallbladder (under the lowest ribs in the upper right part of the abdomen). Jaundice often develops because of an obstruction to the flow of bile. There may be an accumulation of fluid in the abdominal cavity (ascites). Cancer of the gallbladder tends to spread relatively early to the adjacent tissues and to the liver. Cancer of the gallbladder is a serious condition and carries a high mortality rate.

Hodgkin's disease. (See under *Lymph Nodes.*)

Kidney. Here we deal with two distinct age groups, infancy and later middle life.

The malignant kidney tumor that occurs in infancy (nephroblastoma, often called Wilms's tumor) typically develops before three years of age. It is one of the common cancers of early life. The first sign is usually the discovery of a firm, painless mass in one side of the abdomen. Seldom is there blood in the urine, but when it does occur, it has unfavorable import. Fortunately, the disease is usually limited to one kidney. Early surgical removal of the involved kidney, often followed by irradiation therapy, has improved the chances of survival to as much as 50 percent.

The adult type of cancer of the kidney occurs most commonly between the ages of 45 and 60. The significant warning is the appearance of blood in the urine. Such an occurrence is significant even though the blood appears only intermittently, and this should be promptly reported to the doctor.

Cancer of the kidney often spreads to other parts of the body—typically the lungs and certain of the long bones of the skeleton. The primary method of treatment is, of course, the surgical removal of the involved kidney.

Larynx. Cancer of the larynx (voice box) occurs more commonly in those who smoke than in those who do not. Some evidence of the damage that smoking does to the larynx is suggested by the rather typical rough quality of the voice of those who smoke. When the vocal cords proper are involved in the cancerous transformation, the telltale symptom consists of unexplained hoarseness. Persisting hoarseness should always signal a need for examination by a physician.

When cancer of the larynx is discovered early and when only one side is involved, partial removal of the larynx may result in a cure. More commonly, the entire larynx has to be removed. Then it becomes necessary for the patient to use one of the methods of artificial speech. Some persons use a mechanical vibrator placed against the skin of the face and then articulate the words with their lips and tongue. The newer method, which, in many ways is more satisfactory, consists of

swallowing a small amount of air, holding it in the upper part of the esophagus, and then expelling it gradually as the tongue, cheeks, and lips, articulate the words using the sounds that are produced by the air escaping from the esophagus. This method requires a bit of training and the development of considerable skill, but once the method is mastered, it works quite satisfactorily.

Lip. A sore on the lip which refuses to heal should always arouse suspicion. Cancer of the lower lip usually occurs in a case in which there has been prolonged irritation (as in pipe smoking). When cancer of the lip is treated early, the prospects of cure are good (90 to 95 percent). The end result in neglected cases can be quite tragic. Treatment is by the surgical removal of the involved area of tissue with the possible additional use of irradiation therapy.

Liver. Cancer of the liver is frequent, but it rarely begins in the organ itself. It is common for cancers to spread to the liver from neighboring portions of the stomach, the colon, or the gallbladder. Others are transmitted to the liver from more distant parts of the body. The symptoms of cancer of the liver will vary from case to case. Frequently there is jaundice and the accumulation of fluid in the abdominal cavity. The liver itself is usually tender to pressure, feels nodular on examination, and grows steadily in size. The prospect of survival is quite remote.

Lung. (See volume 1, chapter 53, for a more complete discussion of the relationship of smoking to cancer of the lung.) Cancer of the lung has increased so markedly in recent years and it is so highly malignant that it now accounts for more deaths from cancer in men than are caused by cancer of any other part of the body. Lung cancer has also increased among women, but at a slower rate. This is because fewer women than men smoke, the average smoking woman smokes fewer cigarettes per day than

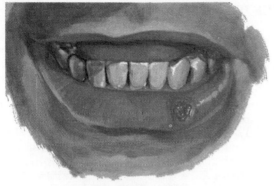

EARLY CARCINOMA OF LIP

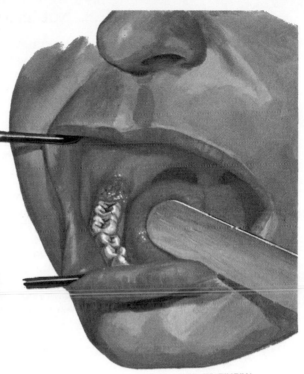

CARCINOMA OF GINGIVA
(RETROMOLAR SPACE)

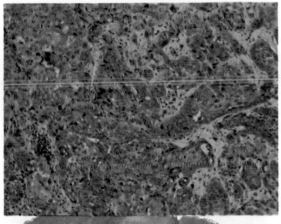

SQUAMOUS CELL
CARCINOMA

CARCINOMA OF TONGUE
(ON LEUKOPLAKIA)

CARCINOMA OF CHEEK

the average smoking man, and not so many women inhale as is true of men.

Cigarette smoking is the acknowledged aggravating cause of cancer of the lung. For the year 1973 in the United States there were 73,000 new cases of lung cancer among men and 20,000 new cases among women, making a total of 93,000 new cases of lung cancer in one year.

Cancer of the lung has such a high mortality rate that there are less than 20 percent of the stricken victims alive at the end of five years. In 1973 there were 59,000 deaths from lung cancer among men and almost 16,000 deaths from lung cancer among women.

Without treatment, the survival rate for the usual type of lung cancer is zero. Surgery offers the best hope for cure, meager though this hope is.

There are two reasons for the high mortality rate. First, cancer of the lung is highly malignant (very prone to spread). Second, it causes no distinctive early symptoms. Cough is often the first sign of lung cancer, but the average smoker has a chronic cough anyway; therefore, the first sign of the cancer usually passes unnoticed. By the time lung cancer is diagnosed, it has usually passed the stage of probable cure.

Lymph nodes. There is a group of closely related malignant diseases in which the lymph nodes are primarily affected. Hodgkin's disease is often placed in this group. Fortunately these diseases, until recently quite uniformly fatal, do not occur commonly. Intensive early treatment by irradiation therapy and by combination chemotherapy have greatly improved the prospect of prolonged remission in Hodgkin's disease until the five-year survival rate at some institutions is about 50 percent.

The lymph nodes are often involved secondarily, as cancers tend to spread from their original locations to other parts of the body.

Mole (pigmented mole). A nevus (plural "nevi") is a pigmented (colored) growth appearing on the skin, on a moist membrane, or in relation to the eye. Although nevi are supposed to be of congenital origin, many do not make their appearance until late childhood or about the time of adolescence. Occasionally one makes its first appearance during adulthood.

The importance of nevi is that occasionally one undergoes a sudden change and becomes transformed into a tumor with very malignant characteristics—a malignant melanoma—the mortality rate for which is very high. Fortunately, malignant melanomas are not common. When one does develop, however, its seriousness is so great that precaution should always be taken when a change occurs in any mole. Early surgical removal of such a nevus, including a rather wide margin of surrounding normal tissue, offers the best hope of avoiding the early death that a malignant melanoma otherwise causes.

The following rules should be of help in indicating when a nevus or pigmented mole should receive attention by the physician:

1. If a mole with suspicious characteristics should appear in infancy or childhood, it should be removed before there is time for a malignant change to occur.

2. Dark moles (deeply pigmented) in blond, red-headed, and freckled persons should be removed.

3. All moles that appear blue or black (rather than brown) should be properly removed.

4. Any mole that suddenly becomes elevated, that becomes suddenly darker, that ulcerates, bleeds, or crusts, that becomes painful, or that increases noticeably in size is potentially dangerous and should be removed by the physician.

Mouth. (See also under *Lip* and *Tongue.*) In response to long continued irritation of the membranes of the mouth there may appear one or more irregular, hard, milk-white, dry patches on the membranes of the lining of the mouth, of the tongue, or on the inner aspects of the lips or

Age-Adjusted Cancer Death Rates* for Selected Sites, Males, United States 1930-1973

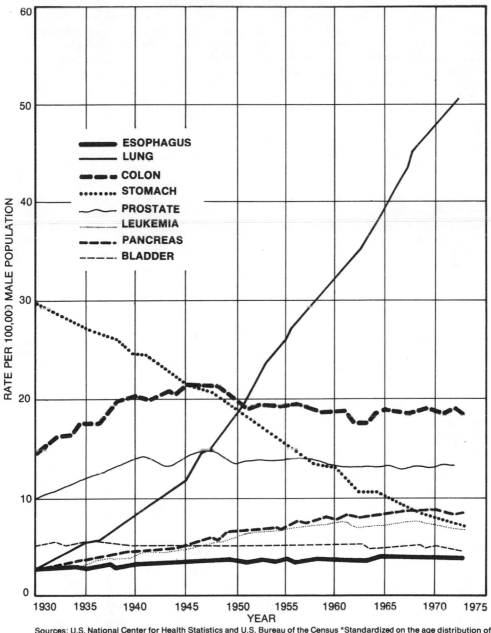

Sources: U.S. National Center for Health Statistics and U.S. Bureau of the Census *Standardized on the age distribution of the 1940 U.S. Census Population.

VOL. 26, NO. 1 JANUARY/FEBRUARY 1976, CA — *A Cancer Journal for Clinicians*, American Cancer Society.

Cancer of the lung has increased sharply during recent years in the United States, currently accounting for more deaths in men than from cancer in any other part of the body.

151

cheeks. Such a development is called leukoplakia ("white plaque" or smoker's patch"), and is recognized as a premalignant lesion (capable of transformation to cancer). It occurs most commonly in the mouths of smokers, although the use of alcohol and the use of an inadequate diet are also predisposing factors.

Such a lesion should be examined by a biopsy (removal of a small portion for microscopic study) and, if found malignant, treated either by surgical removal or by irradiation.

Nevus. (See under *Mole, pigmented mole.*)

Ovary. Cancer of the ovary is responsible for almost one-third as many deaths among women in the United States as are caused by cancer of the breast. It is difficult to diagnose cancer of the ovary in its early stages because the symptoms are indefinite. Surgery, often supplemented with irradiation therapy and chemotherapy are the methods of treatment. Because it is difficult to recognize this cancer while still in its early stages, the five-year survival rate averages less than 50 percent.

Pancreas. Cancer of the pancreas is a highly malignant disease in which the early symptom may be only abdominal or back pain. As the tumor progresses, there may be obstruction to the flow of bile with resulting jaundice. It tends to occur during the sixth and seventh decades of life.

Pigmented mole. (See under *Mole.*)

Prostate. Cancer of the prostate becomes progressively more frequent after age 55. Beyond age 75, it is the second most common cause of cancer death.

It can usually be detected in the early stages, before symptoms develop, by routine physical examination in which the physician palpates the prostate through the rectum. Early treatment consists of a combination of surgery, irradiation therapy, and hormone therapy.

Rectum. (See under *Colon and rectum.*)

Skin. (See also under *Cancer of the Skin* in chapter 12 of this volume and also under *Mole* in this listing.) Cancer occurs commonly in the skin, but offsetting its high incidence is the encouraging fact that the rate of cure is higher among skin cancers than in any other kind.

Skin cancer occurs most commonly in the parts of the body exposed to sunlight and weather: the face, neck, and hands. Actually, the most commonly offensive irritant to the skin, and thus a factor in the production of skin cancer, is exposure to sunlight.

Many persons in later life develop irregularly shaped brown blemishes on the skin of the exposed parts of the body, called keratoses. These are considered to be precursors to cancer even though they may lie dormant for years or may never undergo the actual change to cancer. These should be watched for evidence of change and then should be treated promptly by removal. The warning signs include a sudden tendency for the keratotic lesion to increase in size, a thickening of the skin of the involved area, the development of inflammation, and the formation of ulceration without healing. A safe rule is to regard any ulcerative lesion of the skin, especially that of the face, which persists

Skin cancer occurs commonly on exposed areas, such as the face.

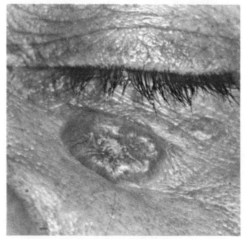

for longer than three or four weeks, as cancer. It should be completely removed at this early stage by whatever means the physician considers proper: surgical removal, electrocautery, or actual cautery.

Stomach. Cancer of the stomach is somewhat more common in men than in women. The number of deaths from cancer of the stomach has been declining in the United States until recently only about 3 percent of all cancer deaths stem from this cause in contrast to about 25 percent in 1930.

Some of the early symptoms of cancer of the stomach are loss of appetite, indigestion, and discomfort in the stomach region. These symptoms may be followed a little later by vomiting of "coffee-ground" material and by a loss of weight and strength.

In the early stages X-ray and gastroscopic examination of the stomach gives the most reliable information.

Prompt surgical removal of part or all of the stomach is the only satisfactory treatment. But even with surgical treatment, the five-year survival rate averages less than 25 percent. Cancer of the stomach tends to spread to the liver, and if treatment is delayed until after this has occurred, the outcome is uniformly fatal.

Thyroid. There are great variations from patient to patient in the characteristics of thyroid disease, it often being difficult to tell the difference between a malignant and a benign condition. Also, some cases of thyroid cancer are more highly malignant than others.

Enlargement of the thyroid gland, just below and on either side of the larynx (Adam's apple), or the development of nodules in the gland (especially in children and youth), calls for an examination and evaluation by a physician. If he considers surgery necessary, he will, during the time of surgery, have a piece of the affected tissue examined by the pathologist to determine whether there is actual cancer. If so, the surgeon will then proceed with a much more complete removal of the gland than he would if the tumor were benign.

Following the surgical removal of a cancer of the thyroid, the doctor will probably arrange for the patient to take appropriate hormone medication for the rest of his life. Irradiation therapy is of limited value in cancer of the thyroid.

Tongue. (See also under *Mouth.*) Cancer of the tongue is a serious disease and causes more deaths than any other cancer within the mouth. As for precancerous lesions of the tongue that result from persistent inflammation, these may disappear when tobacco and alcohol are eliminated and the diet is adjusted to provide an adequate nutritional balance. But when a lesion of the tongue is identified as actual cancer (as when it begins to invade the deeper tissues), it must be treated at once, either by surgery or by irradiation. Treatment of such a case by surgery requires the removal of the involved half of the tongue, the floor of the mouth on the same side, and also the lymph nodes on the same side of the neck. When performed in the early stages of the cancer, this is a life-saving procedure, and it is not as disfiguring or handicapping in the long run as the description makes it sound.

Uterus. (See also under *Cervix of the Uterus.*) In spite of a very encouraging reduction in the mortality rate in cancer of the uterus during recent years, a little more than one fourth of the 20,000 new cases per year in the United States will result in death. Much of the improvement in the mortality rate is traceable to the use of the Papanicolaou ("Pap") test, in which a small amount of mucus is taken from the vagina for microscopic examination. Many of the floating cells included in the sample of mucus have come from the lining of the uterus. Their characteristics as revealed by the microscope indicate whether the lining of the uterus is healthy or whether it has presumably become involved in a cancerous change. Such presumption should then be checked by microscopic examination of tissue taken from inside the uterus. As more and more women realize the importance of having periodic "Pap" tests, cancer of the uterus will be detected early in more and more cases, with the result that more lives will be saved because of the advantage of early treatment by surgery.

Curability of Various Kinds of Cancer

John Cairns, a noted scientist who has spent his life in research relating to the fundamentals of the cancer problem, makes a statement in the *Scientific American* for November 1975, which in a few words summarizes the hazards of cancer and at the same time implies the importance of prevention as well as early detection. He says, "Fewer than half of all cancer patients survive five years from the time cancer is first diagnosed. Death is almost always caused by metastasis: the spread of the cancer to distant sites."

As discussed at the end of this chapter, progress is being made in treatment of cancer. The five-year survival rate (prospects for an individual to be alive at the end of five years) are improving. A chart at the end of the chapter shows the rates for various kinds of cancer. The key for survival is early recognition and prompt treatment.

Early Recognition of Cancer

From the foregoing it is clear that the best way to avoid the tragedy of cancer is to prevent its occurrence in the first place. This is best done by avoiding those practices and circumstances that predispose to cancer. Following a health-building pattern of living is one's best insurance against the ravages of cancer.

It has been noted in the earlier part of this chapter that some persons are more susceptible to cancer than are others. There are hereditary factors in this by which some persons naturally have a greater vitality and greater resistance to the circumstances that break down the normal controls of the body's cells. So it is that some persons, even among those who are reasonably careful to avoid the predisposing factors, will develop cancer. As of the present time, there is no real "cure" for cancer, nor does there appear to be one in immediate prospect. There are treatments that are partially successful in eradicating a cancer that is established. And there are methods by which remissions may be brought about in the progress of cancer. But these are not cures. They are only means of interrupting or postponing the progress of established cancer.

These means of partially controlling a cancer and thus prolonging the victim's life are much more effective when applied early in the course of a cancer's development. As already emphasized, once a cancer begins to spread to other parts of the body, the battle for control is virtually lost. This is the reason that next to preventing cancer in the first place, the second most important item in the struggle against cancer deals with early recognition—the earlier the better—so that the available methods of therapy can be most effective.

In this effort at early recognition, a very important item is periodic examinations by the physician. These should be arranged at least once a year, and oftener if there are any indications of a special susceptibility. But some cancers develop in parts of the body that are not easily examined. Furthermore, in some cases the cancer develops quickly so that waiting until the next yearly examination would be disastrous. Therefore, the first responsibility rests with individuals to observe their own state of health. If questionable symptoms develop, these should be reported promptly to the doctor even though it is not yet time for another annual checkup. The American Cancer Soci-

CANCER DANGER SIGNALS

The telltale symptoms listed in the right-hand column suggest the possibility of cancer in the organs named on the left. When the symptoms appear, arrange promptly for an examination by your doctor.

Bladder	Blood in urine; increase in the frequency of urination.
Bone	Local pain and tenderness; unusual thickening on the bone; walking with an unexplained limp.
Blood (leukemia)	Vague symptoms: fever, pallor, bleeding into the tissues.
Breast	Lump or deformity in the breast or nipple.
Cervix	Abnormal bleeding, spotting with blood, or abnormal discharge.
Colon and Rectum	Bleeding by rectum, change in bowel habits.
Esophagus	Difficulty in swallowing.
Kidney (in adult)	Blood in the urine (usually without pain); loss of appetite, fatigue, and loss of weight.
Kidney (in three-year-old or younger)	Firm, painless mass in one side of abdomen.
Larynx	Sudden, unexplained, progressive hoarseness; later, difficult breathing.
Lip	Warty growth; crusting ulcer or fissure (resting on a disk-like, firm area).
Lung	Cough (particularly different from the usual smoker's cough); transient wheezing. Later, blood-spitting.
Mouth and Tongue	An area of roughening; mild burning when eating highly seasoned foods. Later, ulceration.
Skin	A "pimple" or small sore fails to heal and gradually enlarges; an old skin lesion now begins to grow; a persistent lesion crusts but bleeds when the crust is removed; an old wart or mole changes size or color.
Stomach	Persistent distress in upper abdomen, loss of appetite, loss of weight.
Uterus	Episodes of vaginal bleeding unrelated to menstruation.

NOTE:

Most cancers are not painful, at least in their early stages. Thousands of cancer victims have lost their lives needlessly because they waited too long before seeing their doctor—thinking that their lesion could not be cancer because it was not painful.

Some cancers do not give a warning signal; they develop "silently." In these the best prospects of cure have passed by the time the symptoms appear. Hence the advice: SEE YOUR PHYSICIAN FOR A CANCER CHECKUP ONCE A YEAR.

ety provides the following list of warning signals:

1. Change in bowel or bladder habits.

2. A sore that does not heal.

3. Unusual bleeding or discharge.

4. Thickening or lump in breast or elsewhere.

5. Indigestion or difficulty in swallowing.

6. Obvious change in wart or mole.

7. Nagging cough or hoarseness.

Kinds of Treatment Now Available

It should be emphasized once more that even though we have *treatments* for cancer, as yet there are no sure *cures* for cancer.

Surgery. Surgery is still the "old reliable" in the treatment of cancer. The attempt of the surgeon is to remove whatever tissue is affected by cancer before it has the opportunity to send colonies of its cells to the surrounding tissues or to some distant part of the body. Surgeons have become very knowledgeable on the best surgical approaches to the various kinds of cancer as they are found in one part of the body or another. Some persons hesitate to consult a physician when they fear that they are developing a cancer because of their thought that the surgery might be mutilating. Some women with a lump in the breast delay seeing their physician for fear he will recommend that the breast be removed. If only these persons could realize the greater hazards of delay, and if they could understand that allowing the cancer to progress will cause a much greater and more terrible mutilation of their body, if they even survive, they would consult their doctor at the first sign of difficulty. In some cases, the doctor's examination will indicate that the problem is not one of a cancer but rather of some benign lesion. This knowledge is surely reassuring. But in those cases in which the patient's fears of cancer are verified, the prospect of continued life and health are much better when the lesion is treated early than when it is neglected.

Irradiation therapy. The use of X-ray therapy and the other similar irradiation techniques have become important adjuncts in the treatment of cancer. In many cases they are used following surgery. In a few selected cases, they are used instead of surgery. Irradiation has a profound effect on the cells of the body, both normal and abnormal. The theory behind its use is that it will stifle the growth of the cancer cells. It must be used cautiously, however, lest it damage the normal cells.

Chemotherapy. Chemotherapy consists of administering powerful chemical substances to the person having cancer. The substances used are those that have proved to be toxic to the abnormal cells of cancer. Here again there is danger of damaging the normal cells, and so the selection of the chemicals used and the intensity and duration of the treatment program must be carefully regulated by a physician who is experienced in this method of treatment. Some of the most successful results are obtained by the use of "combination chemotherapy" in which smaller doses of the powerful chemicals are used with the thought of avoiding damage to the normal cells of the body. The combination of several drugs, each one of which is toxic to cancer cells, however, reinforces the effectiveness of the treatment program.

Immunotherapy. Immunotherapy is a recent proposal for the treatment of cancer. Interest in the possibility of immunizing a person so as to protect him from developing cancer or so as to treat the cancer already developed, is based on the assumption that cancer is caused, fundamentally, by a virus. Inasmuch as there has been success in developing vaccines for several diseases that are caused by viruses, it has been hoped that a similar breakthrough could be developed for the treatment of cancer.

Actually, in a few forms of cancer

the relationship to viruses is very close. Particularly in treating the leukemias, some treatment centers are now using the methods of immunotherapy as an adjunct to other methods of treatment. As previously mentioned, however, the scientific proof that cancers are caused by viruses is still lacking. Furthermore, the methods of immunotherapy are still in the experimental stage.

Summary. Inasmuch as we do not have an overall *cure* for cancer, we must still rely on a combination of the available methods of treatment—surgery, irradiation, and chemotherapy—with the exact application of these methods being adapted by experienced physicians to the needs of a particular case.

Nostrums

The situation just described in which there is no established cure for a disease that is responsible for taking many thousands of lives each year lends itself to exploitation by unscrupulous persons who claim to have discovered a "cure for cancer." "Cancer cures" have come and gone for as long as there has been a recognition of cancer. Cancer still persists, but, one by one, the promoted cures have run their course and disappeared.

It is very tempting to a person with cancer who has just listened to his doctor's explanation of the seriousness of his illness and of its uncertain outcome, to "grasp at a straw" by listening to the confident promises of some irregular practitioner who reports marvelous results from some "new discovery."

One such cancer "cure" has carried the name of Laetrile. This product is prepared from "ground, defatted apricot kernels and concentrates of apricot and peach pits." The United States Food and Drug Administration arranged for careful scientific inquiry and experimentation with this product, only to find that the claims of the promoters are not based on fact and

that the product itself has no curative qualities. The proponents of this product continued to smuggle it into the United States under the new name of "Bee-Seventeen" a supposed, "antineoplastic vitamin." Also it has been marketed under the trade name "Aprikern."

When a person becomes interested in any new "cancer cure," it is well for him to consult with his family physician. The ethics of the medical profession require a physician to be open-minded and to share his information whenever there is a possibility of benefiting human beings. Every physician has opportunity to keep up-to-date in his understanding of medical progress. He receives medical journals and attends lectures which are designed for this purpose. He has channels of communication by which he can make inquiry of the leading medical authorities on whatever subject he desires. He is therefore in a position to guide his patient in evaluating such matters.

The tragedy of the nostrums that relate to the cure of cancer is that oftentimes cancer patients develop such faith in these supposed cures that they neglect the accepted methods of treatment until the stage when these are no longer effective. Thus, some lives have been unnecessarily sacrificed—the lives of persons who could have been spared or at least relieved of suffering by the use of the accepted methods of treatment.

Progress in the Fight Against Cancer

Many facts contained in the present chapter may make it seem to the reader that medical science has failed in its effort to cope with one of life's major problems. In spite of the tremendous amount of research work that has been conducted in the effort to solve the problems of cancer, persons still develop cancer and persons still die from it. We should avoid an attitude of discouragement, however, and observe with gratitude the progress that has been made. There has been steady improvement in the five-year survival rate, with the result that many thousands of lives have been saved. Notice the improvement of survival rate in which the present rates are compared with those of the 1940's:

Some kinds of cancer would be largely preventable if individuals were willing to avoid the known factors which cause such cancers. Lung cancer is the outstanding example in that it would be almost completely eradicated if the use of cigarettes were abandoned.

Five-Year Survival Rates for Certain Kinds of Cancer

	1945	1970
Cancer of the prostate	35 percent	56 percent
Cancer of the body of the uterus	61 percent	74 percent
Cancer of the thyroid	64 percent	85 percent
Cancer of the kidney	26 percent	42 percent
Cancer of the bladder	42 percent	61 percent
Cancer of the larynx	41 percent	62 percent
Melanoma of the skin	41 percent	66 percent
Hodgkin's disease	25 percent	54 percent
Chronic leukemia	15 percent	30 percent

(Statistics published by the American Cancer Society, 1975.)

SECTION IV

Specific Diseases, Their Nature and Treatment

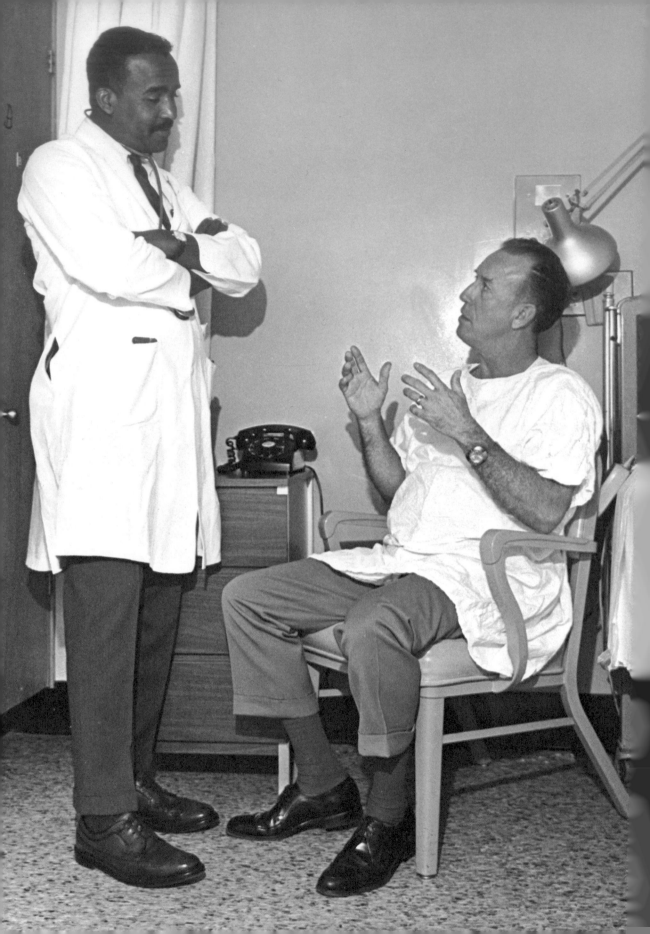

Skin Diseases

Diseases of the skin are usually unsightly, and are frequently the result of, or occasionally the cause of, ill health of other parts of the body. While they are often uncomfortable, few of them are a menace to life; but many of them may be quite persistent. Their visibility aids in their early recognition and in judging the effectiveness of treatment. But since they result from the widely differing hereditary tendencies, habits, environmental conditions, and diets of mankind, and are affected by both mental and physical powers and limitations, a great variety of skin abnormalities are exhibited by skin diseases. Some of these may be so unusual or malignant that only a competent physician or specialist is qualified to recognize their true nature or to treat them. In cases where any doubt exists regarding the nature of a persistent skin eruption, attempts at self-diagnosis or self-treatment are not wise. In such a condition, giving the wrong treatment, or delay in giving the right treatment, may be serious.

There are numerous skin disorders, however, which an intelligent person with little guidance can recognize and treat, at least temporarily, when he is out of reach of a skin specialist or is unable to afford professional medical care. In discussing the various skin diseases included in this chapter, we have tried to give the reader a reliable basis for judging what can safely be done without prior consultation with a physician, and what circumstances indicate such consultation necessary or at least wise.

Perhaps the most important warning that should be heeded by all, but especially by those who try to treat skin diseases without professional supervision, is this: Do not overtreat. While a skin disease is being treated, any increase in the signs of irritation or inflammation should be taken as evidence of probable overtreatment, or as an allergic reaction to the applied medication.

New remedies for skin diseases are being discovered or devised all the time. Furthermore, no two patients and no two physicians are exactly alike; and what a physician uses or recommends will depend to a considerable degree on his past experience in dealing with patients. It often happens that a remedy or treatment program that works well in one physician's practice does not work so well in the practice of another. Do not be surprised, therefore, if a physician prescribes remedies or treatments differing from those recommended in this book.

Most of the new effective remedies discovered in recent years cannot be purchased without a physician's prescription, and many cannot be safely used without a physician's supervision. We consider it unwise to recommend in this book a remedy that the reader cannot buy on his own, or that would be unsafe for him to use if he could buy it. We have limited our recommendations to remedies that have stood the test of time, to those that can usually be obtained without a physician's prescription, and to those that are not likely to be harmful if used as directed.

For information on routine self-care of the skin, plus other interesting facts about the skin, see volume 3, chapter 5.

To aid the reader in his search for a particular item in this chapter, we include a table of contents for the chapter.

Index of Skin Disorders

Allergy

Some people are abnormally sensitive to certain substances which may be present in the air they breathe, in the food they eat, or in something they get on their skin or may brush against. These same substances may be harmless to other members of the family and to other people in general. This sensitivity may be present from birth, in which case it is said to be atopic; but it is more often built up as a result of repeated contacts with the offending substance or substances. The sensitivity itself is called allergy; and, if comparatively prompt and violent, the reaction of the body when brought into contact with a substance to which it is sensitive is known medically as anaphylaxis.

Allergy might properly be discussed in relation to any or all of several different body systems. It is mentioned in this volume as a causative factor in the discussions of many diseases that have no relation to the skin. We discuss it in a general way in this chapter, however, because so many of its most common manifestations are in the skin. See also the chapter on "Allergy" which appears later in this same volume.

Almost every body tissue may show allergic reactions, and the reactions may take many different forms. Reactions associated with skin diseases will be discussed later in this chapter in their due order. Sometimes the reactions come on immediately after contact with the offending substance, but sometimes they come after a delay of one or more days. Delayed reactions are comparatively common when the digestive tract is concerned, and hence they may cause much perplexity. The person concerned may eat some of the offending food and not notice any trouble till considerably later. The tendency then will be to blame some food eaten shortly before the distress became manifest, and the true offender will not be detected.

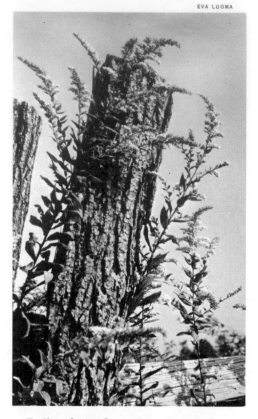

EVA LUOMA

Pollen from flowering plants often produces an allergic reaction.

A variety of diseases, at least in a large proportion of the people suffering from them, may be caused by allergy. Hay fever and asthma, acute vomiting or purging—especially in children—eczema, hives, and several other skin affections are prominent examples. Occasionally tests reveal that a single individual may at times suffer from more than one of these conditions.

Among the offending substances frequently affecting these abnormally sensitive individuals are these common ones: various pollens from plants; hair or dandruff; emanations from cats, dogs, or horses; various kinds of fur or feathers; such foods as milk, eggs, fish, shellfish, pork, fowl, wheat, oranges, and strawberries; and in children, some of the cereals and butter.

What to Do

1. Try to find out the identity of the offending food or other substance and avoid it. This may call for the aid of a physician, and one of the methods he may use in his detective work is a series of skin tests.

2. When an attack occurs, possibly caused by sensitivity to some food, discontinue all food for a few hours. As eating is resumed, try one food at a time in the hope of discovering the offending one.

3. Itching may be troublesome. The various skin diseases in which allergy plays a part are discussed later in this chapter in their proper order, together with suitable treatment. Further suggestions as to the relief of itching are given under "Miscellaneous Skin Ailments: Itching, General."

4. If the attack is severe and a physician is available, consult him. He may be able to give some injection that will give prompt relief, and he may be able to prescribe other remedies to fit the individual case.

Atrophies

KRAUROSIS VULVAE.

This is a malady peculiar to middle-aged or elderly women, characterized by atrophy, shriveling, and constriction of the skin and mucous membrane of the external genital region. While rarely present in a fully developed form it is a chronic and stubborn disorder, with surface changes, including hardening, drying, and graying of the skin, and sometimes of the underlying tissues, resulting in a narrowing of the vaginal opening. Itching in the affected tissues may be intense.

This is not a discrete disease but, rather, a manifestation of some other illness such as senile atrophy (see the following item) or one of the systemic connective tissue diseases (see chapter 13 of this volume under "II. Connective Tissue Diseases").

What to Do

1. Apply a soothing lotion or ointment such as calamine lotion or rose water ointment.

2. Consult a dermatologist (a physician who is trained in treating diseases of the skin) so that he may identify and treat the underlying condition.

SENILE ATROPHY (ATROPHIA SENILIS).

Senile atrophy is a skin condition accompanying advancing age, appearing as patches of tightened, dry and inelastic, or thin and shiny skin, abnormally discolored, especially in spots and frequently giving rise to more or less itching. It is not a disease with a specific cause, but only a manifestation of one of the body changes due to a reduction in hormones, which to some degree affect all elderly people. It seldom becomes noticeable before the fiftieth year, and is most pronounced in slender individuals.

This type of atrophy, when aggravated by exposure to sunlight through the years and resulting from a decrease in the amount of fat normally padding the deep layer of the skin, is characterized by spots or areas of skin that are usually yellowish or brownish in color, appearing most noticeably on the backs of the hands, the legs, the neck, or the face. Itching is most troublesome in cold or very dry weather.

What to Do

1. Remember that the character of this ailment is such that a restoration of the former normal skin condition is impossible.

2. Partial relief from discomfort may be obtained by avoiding the use of strong soap and by keeping the skin softened by the use of some simple ointment such as rose water ointment.

Bacterial Diseases

BOILS (CARBUNCLES, FURUNCLES).

Boils are hard, red, painful, and rather deep-seated swellings, usually beginning as pimples or nodules about hair roots. They increase rapidly in size and develop "cores" in their centers. Furuncle is another name for a boil. Carbuncles are unusually severe forms of boils, ordinarily characterized by more than one core or head, and accompanied by considerable systemic disturbance and general illness and debility.

Boils and carbuncles are caused by the same kind of germ—a more or less virulent strain of *Staphylococcus aureus* as a rule. To start a boil or carbuncle, the germs must gain entrance to an oil or sweat gland or to a hair follicle. It has often been noticed, however, that a general low level of resistance, a low metabolic rate, rubbing in of dirt by clothing, or the presence of diabetes mellitus paves the way for the development of boils or carbuncles—facts which emphasize the need for a physician to study cases characterized by a "run of boils."

The core of a boil consists of a collection of innumerable bacteria surrounded by and interspersed with white blood cells. It tends to soften

THE UPJOHN COMPANY

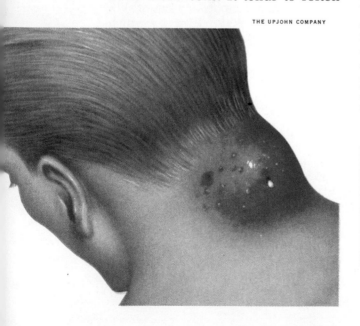

and form a thick liquid pus around it, which normally eventually escapes through a break in the skin. The pus, containing living germs, may spread the infection and cause other boils if it comes in contact with unprotected skin. Warmth and moisture hasten the formation and breakdown of the core, and help to keep the skin soft so that the pus may more easily break through. If the skin is kept wet continually, however, it may become soft enough to encourage the spread of germs through it. Dressings wet with strong solutions of salt or other suitable chemicals tend to stimulate the drainage of the pus out of the tissues and into the dressings. Boils are most painful if located on a skin area with but little soft tissue between the skin and the underlying bone. They continue to be painful until free drainage of pus is established. Following adequate drainage, a boil subsides quickly.

The danger of squeezing or picking at boils needs to be emphasized. The collection of germs in the forming core may be broken up and spread into surrounding tissues, thus making the boil larger than it would otherwise be. The germs may even spread into the bloodstream, causing septicemia or "blood poisoning," which may prove fatal. The most dangerous spot in all the body for a boil to be located is the area marked out by the bridge of the nose, the corners of the mouth, and the outer corners of the eyes. This includes the inside of the nostrils. Many cases of fatal septicemia or meningitis have resulted from improper interference with boils or pimples in this area.

What to Do

1. Immediately upon the appearance of a pimple which appears severe enough to develop into a boil—if it is not deep-seated and has a small yellow spot in the center—dip the point of a needle into tincture of iodine or carbolic acid and open the pimple by thrusting the needle sideways

through the yellow spot and lifting the needle. Do not press or squeeze. Wipe off the small amount of pus with a bit of sterile gauze or absorbent cotton. Apply 2 percent tincture of iodine to and around the opened pimple at once. This may abort the boil.

2. If the pimple is deep-seated, or if it does not have a definite yellow center, do not attempt to open it, but paint it and the surrounding skin twice a day with 2 percent tincture of iodine. Let the solution dry on the skin and apply no dressing of any kind for one hour. This will help to protect the surrounding skin from infection.

3. After the skin has been left dry for an hour as directed in (2) above, apply dressings of several layers of gauze kept wet with a warm saturated solution of magnesium sulfate (Epsom salts) on a repeat schedule of two hours on and one hour off. The dressings may be covered with waxed paper, oiled silk, or plastic to prevent their drying out. It is helpful to keep them warm by covering with a hot-water bottle with a layer or two of Turkish toweling between dressing and bottle. Other preparations have been recommended for dressings instead of magnesium sulfate. Five percent ammoniated mercury ointment is good.

4. The pain of the boil will be considerably relieved if the course of treatment outlined in (2) and (3) above is followed, and the boil will probably come to a head and break within a few days without other help. The boil should never be squeezed, and it should not be opened too soon. If instrumental opening becomes necessary, it is better to have a physician do it.

5. Penicillin injections and sulfadiazine by mouth are recommended for a carbuncle or a severe boil. The use of these requires the supervision of a physician.

6. From the start, but especially after the discharge of pus begins, it is wise to keep a wide area of skin surrounding the boil disinfected by frequent applications of rubbing alcohol or the mild tincture of iodine described in (2) above, to prevent the germs in the pus from getting a foothold in the skin and possibly starting new boils.

7. A "run of boils" should always lead to consultation with a physician. Special examinations and laboratory tests are necessary to determine the identity and nature of the causative germs and other possible causative factors, especially if diabetes happens to be one of them. Diabetes must be treated if found present, and sometimes it is advisable to build up resistance to the special strain of staphylococcus germ causing the boils by giving a long course of injections of "autogenous vaccine," which the physician can have made. Frequent changes of clothing, alcohol sponging, and frequent baths are also important and helpful.

CELLULITIS.

Cellulitis is a spreading, inflammatory infection, somewhat similar to erysipelas but usually less acute. It most commonly affects the skin, but it usually involves deeper structures as well. It is often found elsewhere than on the face, and the affected skin area does not show a distinct border. It may be caused by either streptococci or staphylococci, which gain entrance through a break in the skin but do not cause pus formation. The skin area concerned is hot, red, and painful. Without proper treatment, the condition is persistent and tends to recur. The involved area may become permanently swollen or thickened, especially after persistent or recurrent attacks.

What to Do

Call a physician at once. Home treatments are of little use, but treatments by a physician using

167

either antibiotics or sulfas or both is usually promptly effective.

CHANCRE (HARD CHANCRE, HUNTERIAN SORE).

(See under *Syphilis* in chapter 30 of this volume.)

CHANCROID (SOFT CHANCRE).

(See discussion of this item in chapter 30 of this volume.)

ERYSIPELAS.

Erysipelas is caused by a virulent strain of streptococci affecting the skin and the tissues immediately beneath it. It is characterized by redness, discoloration, small blisters, and swelling, most commonly attacking the face, and accompanied by high fever and other manifestations of acute illness. The skin shows a glazed appearance, and the affected area has a combined itching and burning sensation and shows a clearly defined margin. The swollen area feels firm and hot to the touch. There may be only a small patch of affected skin at first, but it tends to spread in all directions from the original site.

The victim of erysipelas feels extremely ill, with marked feeling of lassitude, chills, headache, vomiting, joint and back pains, and a rapidly rising fever, which may go even higher than 104° F. (40° C.). He is likely to have an unusually rapid pulse. In severe cases, delirium is common. In children, vomiting and convulsions often occur. The disease is serious, possibly even proving fatal in aged people, in babies, and in women who have recently given birth. It is likely to cause abortion in pregnant women.

The serious nature of erysipelas makes it impossible for a layman to administer effective remedies or treatments. Prompt attention by a physician is important, but the suggestions outlined below may be helpful in delaying the multiplication of germs and slowing the progress of the disease until a physician can begin

treatment. At present, penicillin and wide-spectrum antibiotics are the most successful known remedies, but there may be other treatments or remedies that the individual physician has found valuable.

What to Do

1. Call a physician at once, but until he comes keep the patient in bed and isolated from all except the person caring for him.

2. Give him a liquid diet. See that he takes at least three quarts (liters) of water or other fluids a day.

3. Keep the affected skin areas covered with ice bags or ice-cold

Typical manifestations of erysipelas.

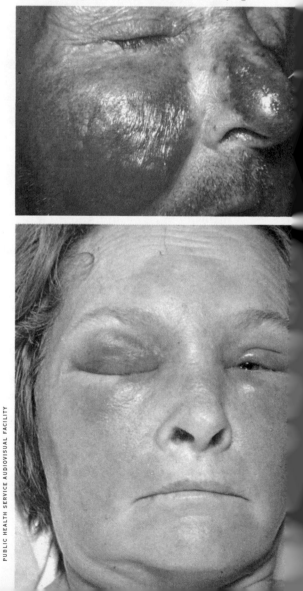

PUBLIC HEALTH SERVICE AUDIOVISUAL FACILITY

compresses (twenty minutes on and ten minutes off) until a physician takes charge of the treatment.

4. Cold compresses to the head are useful in relieving the headache, which is frequently distressing.

5. Remember that erysipelas is contagious. The person nursing the patient must wear rubber gloves, and should never come in contact with or care for children or other sick persons at the same time. Ice bags applied to the patient should be disinfected by immersion for five minutes in a solution of lysol—one teaspoonful to the pint (450 c.c.) of water. Cloths used for compresses should be soaked in the same solution for ten minutes before being laundered.

FELON (WHITLOW).

A felon is a condition of swelling, throbbing pain, and extreme tenderness, characteristically affecting a finger or a thumb. It may at first seem to be an infection or inflammation of the skin, and for this reason it is discussed in this chapter. The germs causing the infection are usually virulent staphylococci, carried in through the skin by a deep pinprick, a thorn, a splinter, or some other sharp object. The inflammation and pus are deep down among the tendons and tendon sheaths, or even near the bone. If thorough lancing is not done promptly, the tendons may slough or the bone be damaged, causing a crippled or deformed thumb or finger. If the pus is not drained, there is danger that the infection may travel to other parts of the hand, resulting in more serious crippling. Or the infection may reach the bloodstream, causing a possibly fatal "blood poisoning."

What to Do

Call a physician promptly and have the felon lanced. Because of the need for deep lancing and the extreme tenderness of the involved area, it is often necessary to use a local or general anesthetic. The physician will prescribe and supervise the aftercare.

FOLLICULITIS.

Folliculitis is caused by a staphylococcic infection of one or more hair follicles, with pustule formation. It is related to boils, but is a much milder infection, apparently caused by much less virulent germs. It is most common in men and tends to involve the bearded areas of the skin, but may attack any area in which hair follicles are found. When deep-seated and chronic, it is called sycosis; and the skin around the pustules becomes reddened and crusted. In most cases of sycosis, several to many follicles are involved. Symptoms are not usually acute, being limited to mild burning and itching, with pain only when an involved hair is pulled. Contamination of other skin areas by pus from a pustule is likely to lead to infection of other follicles.

If not properly treated, folliculitis may become chronic and persist for months or even years. It is sometimes confused with barber's itch, which it resembles to some extent (see *Fungous Diseases, Ringworm of the Beard*); but in this book the latter disease is considered to be limited to a fungous rather than to a bacterial infection.

What to Do

1. Apply 2 percent or 5 percent ammoniated mercury ointment several times a day, spreading the remedy onto the surrounding skin to help protect it from pus contamination.

2. If this treatment clears up the condition within one week, apply any antibiotic ointment except penicillin twice a day for another week to help prevent new infections.

3. If a pustule is on the upper lip, the nose, the eyelids, or the face on either side of the nose, or if it does not clear up within one week,

consult a physician. A deep or persistent infection, or one located in any of the indicated areas, may be dangerous.

IMPETIGO.

Impetigo is an acute, contagious disease, usually attacking the skin of the face, in children more commonly than in adults. It begins as a reddening of the one or more small spots on the skin, soon followed by small blisters. These become pustules, which dry into loosely attached, golden-yellow or honey-colored crusts, each with a narrow zone of reddened skin around it. All of these stages may develop within one or two days. If the crust is forcibly removed, a red area that oozes a little blood will be found beneath it.

Impetigo causes considerable itching, but no pain. It is so mild that there is seldom any feeling of illness. It is a pest, however, because it easily spreads from child to child, because it makes them look so repulsive, and because it is often resistant to treatment; but it is seldom dangerous to anybody but infants.

Both streptococci and staphylococci are often found in cases of this disease, but they are of only slight virulence. They work only on the skin or a short distance below the surface. Rarely are scars left after recovery.

What to Do

1. See that the patient's fingers are kept away from the crusts. Scratching the crusts is the usual means by which the disease is spread.

2. Twice a day use a soft cloth or a piece of gauze dipped in "alibour water" or magnesium sulfate (Epsom salts) solution to soak and loosen the crusts. Gently but completely remove the crusts. Then cover the raw area with Neosporin ointment or 2 percent ammoniated mercury ointment. Apply more ointment every one or two hours.

3. If the ointment gets rubbed off between treatments, put on more.

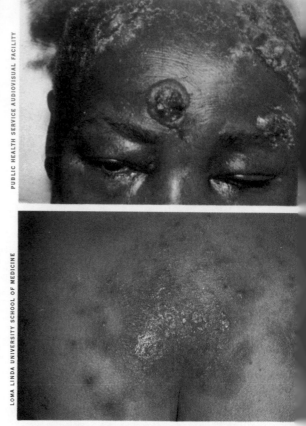

PUBLIC HEALTH SERVICE AUDIOVISUAL FACILITY

LOMA LINDA UNIVERSITY SCHOOL OF MEDICINE

Impetigo, a skin disease repulsive in appearance, spreads rapidly.

Except when the crusts are being removed, the affected skin areas should be kept liberally covered with ointment.

4. See that nobody else uses the towels and washcloths used by the patient. Boil them for five minutes after using. Disinfect them by soaking for thirty minutes in a solution of lysol—one teaspoonful to the pint (450 c.c.) of water—before laundering.

5. To protect the skin surrounding the crusts from infection, sponge it several times a day with rubbing alcohol.

6. Germs may become resistant to any remedy within a week or two, making it necessary to alternate remedies from week to week. If an

increase in inflammation should occur, it may be because the skin has become sensitive to the remedy being used at the time. In this case, do not use this remedy again.

7. When impetigo is allowed to run its course, infection of the kidneys is a frequent complication. For this reason a physician should supervise the treatment of every case. He will usually arrange for the use of an antibiotic such as erythromycin or penicillin to forestall damage to the kidneys.

8. Special care needs to be exercised incases involving young babies. Impetigo spreads rapidly on their tender skin, and their bodies seem unable to build antibodies against the germs. They are unable to do anything to cooperate in the treatment, and the disease may prove fatal.

WHITLOW.
(See *Felon.*)

Fungous Diseases

Fungous diseases may attack various parts of the body, but probably attack the skin most often. Fungi, a more complex form of vegetable organisms than bacteria, usually multiply by means of spores, a characteristic that classifies them midway between bacteria and seed plants. Diseases caused by fungi are rarely acute, but tend to be persistent. They seldom cause fever or result in true pus formation unless complicated by a secondary bacterial infection.

Many fungi are enemies of most of the common disease-producing bacteria, and other bacteria are enemies to them. This fact is the basis for the production of most of the antibiotic remedies. But these fungi are also enemies of certain bacteria which abound in the body and are friendly to it. This is especially true of certain bacteria commonly found in the intestine and/or the vagina of a normally healthy person. So, when antibiotic remedies have been used for a con-

siderable period of time, the friendly bacteria may have been killed off, and certain fungous diseases or yeasts which ordinarily are held in check by these friendly bacteria may take hold and begin to cause trouble.

Generally speaking, ordinary antibiotics are not only useless in treating fungous diseases, but may actually help prepare the way for their development. The outstanding exception to this rule is a special antibiotic —griseofulvin—an effective oral remedy for many fungous skin diseases. It may, however, give a variety of uncomfortable side reactions, so it should be taken only under the supervision of a physician. Also, since many fungous diseases may be caused by more than one variety of fungus, and different varieties of fungi differ in their response to treatment with griseofulvin, laboratory tests are often needed to determine what variety of fungus is present, as a guide to the physician in his use of this or perhaps some other remedy.

ATHLETE'S FOOT (DERMATO-PHYTOSIS, TINEA PEDIS).

Athlete's foot is caused by one or another of a group of parasitic fungi which almost always attack the skin of the feet. Many people are plagued by this malady, since the organisms which cause it are spread from contaminated floors surrounding pools, showers, and other public places. The skin between the outer few toes is most frequently attacked, but the disease may spread to any part of the feet, and it is possible for it to break out on the hands. However, what appears on the hands is usually caused by absorbed toxins circulating in the bloodstream rather than directly by the causative organisms themselves. Nevertheless, by scratching the sores on the feet, one may carry the infection on the hands or under the nails and spread it to other parts of the body.

As athlete's foot develops, blisters or cracks, or more often both, appear

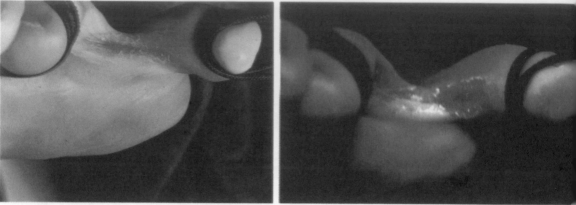

CHAS. PFIZER & CO.,

Athlete's foot between fourth and fifth toes, the view on the right being the same lesion, only under Wood's light. The orange color fluoresced by the secretion from the organisms identifies the disease.

in the skin, which softens, turns white, and tends to peel off in flakes. Pustules and ulcers may form in severe cases, and there is more or less itching and burning—occasionally pain. The disease is more severe in warm weather than in cool weather, and it is aggravated by any condition which keeps the feet warm, moist, and sweaty.

What to Do

1. Keep the affected skin areas as cool and dry as possible. Wearing sandals or open-toed shoes will help.

2. Protect other members of the household from infection by refraining from walking barefoot about the house, especially about the bathroom. Do not use the family shower, and before using the bathtub soak the feet for at least five minutes in a warm, saturated solution of boric acid.

3. Every night at bedtime wash the feet briefly with mild soap and warm water. Then soak the feet for 15 to 30 minutes in a warm, saturated solution of boric acid. If boric acid solution is not available, use instead a warm saline solution (one tablespoonful of table salt to a quart of water). Then with a bit of gauze pick and rub away all loose bits of skin, taking care not to get any of the contaminated material under your fingernails. Then apply Halotex cream or Lotrimin cream, working it carefully into all the affected skin, especially that between the toes.

4. Every morning, wipe away the remaining medicated cream with dry gauze and dust the skin area thickly with antiseptic powder. The following are two prescriptions for good powders to use in such cases:

I

Menthol	1
Thymol iodide	1
Zinc stearate	3
Boric acid powder	10
Talcum powder	100

II

Undecylenic acid	1
Zinc stearate	3
Zinc undecylenate	10
Talcum powder	50

5. Wear cotton hose, preferably white, changing to a fresh pair every day. To launder hose, boil for ten minutes to kill the organisms, or reinfection is certain and a cure may be impossible.

6. If sores appear on the hands, unless an examination has been made and the causative organisms found, do not use any treatment on them except mild and soothing ointments. If itching is severe, apply 1 percent phenol in calamine lotion. When the sores on the feet have healed, those on the hands will probably disappear.

7. To prevent a relapse after the infection appears to be cured, apply 2 percent ammoniated mercury ointment each evening, and talcum powder containing 1 percent of salicylic acid each morning, continuing the treatment for several weeks. Dust the same powder into the shoes daily.

8. In severe cases, keep off the feet as much as possible and use the soaks and medicated cream as in (3) twice a day instead of once.

9. In a persistent case of athlete's foot consult a dermatologist. One treatment which is usually helpful but requires a physician's prescription is the taking by mouth of griseofulvin, an antibiotic.

10. The person with athlete's foot should be considerate of others by not using public showers or swimming pools until his infection is completely cured.

BARBER'S ITCH.

(See *Ringworm of the Beard.*)

CANDIDIASIS (MONILIASIS).

Candidiasis of the skin, caused by the fungous organism Candida albicans, the same organism that causes thrush in the mouths of babies, may affect the mucous membranes of the digestive tract or the vagina in debilitated people or those who have been taking antibiotics by mouth for a long time. It most commonly attacks obese people, people who sweat freely, or people who have diabetes mellitus.

The skin areas most commonly involved are the regions around the anus or vagina, corners of the mouth, fingernail folds, and/or the body folds. The affected areas are red, raw, and beefy in appearance, but may have whitish, curd-like deposits on their surfaces. There may be mild burning sensations present, but itching is much more likely to be troublesome. Warmth and moisture make the condition worse.

What to Do

1. If the afflicted person has been taking antibiotic by mouth, this medication should be stopped at once.

2. Have a physician make the necessary examinations to detect the possible presence of diabetes mellitus, and, if found, to start vigorous treatment for it.

3. If the afflicted person is obese, continue a weight-reducing program until a normal weight is reached. (See volume 1, chapter 51.)

4. Keep the affected skin areas as cool and dry as possible.

5. Two fungicidal preparations usually very effective in the treatment of candidiasis are Mycostatin cream and Nystaform ointment. Griseofulvin is not of value in this condition.

RINGWORM OF THE BEARD (BARBER'S ITCH).

Ringworm of the beard is a contagious disease caused by a parasitic fungus, beginning with inflammation in and around the hair follicles of the beard. It is more persistent than either ringworm of the scalp or ringworm of the body, but fortunately it is not very common. It may be contracted in insanitary barbershops.

Small, superficial nodules appear at first. Later these become larger and more deep-seated because the parasites work down to the bottom of the follicles. Inflammation is general over the skin of the affected areas, but more marked over the nodules, which have a tendency to occur in groups. Usually a brittle hair projects from the center or each nodule. It is loose and can be pulled out easily. The follicles may discharge thin pus. The disease causes considerable itching and discomfort, and it is sometimes mildly painful.

A staphylococcic infection of the bearded area may closely resemble ringworm of the beard, except that the hairs do not loosen. It requires different treatment. Partly because of this fact, self-diagnosis is not easy, and self-treatment may not succeed, so in any suspected case of barber's itch a dermatologist should be consulted.

What to Do

1. The person who suspects that he may have barber's itch should carefully guard others from infection by not letting anybody else use his razor, toilet articles, washcloths, or towels; and each time after using such articles himself he should sterilize them.

2. Consult a physician.

3. Griseofulvin taken by mouth for four weeks under a physician's supervision is usually curative.

RINGWORM OF THE BODY (TINEA CIRCINATA, TINEA CORPORIS).

Ringworm of the body is a mildly contagious disease caused by a fungous infection affecting the skin of the face, neck, body, arms, and legs. It is characterized by reddened patches, round or irregular in shape, and usually scaly. It is uncommon in temperate climates. The patches are pea-size at first, but grow rapidly. They usually have a tendency to heal in the center, thus forming rings. The outer edges of the rings consist of tiny papules and a few small blisters. These are slightly elevated, causing the centers to look depressed. The rings may become as much as two inches (5 cm.) broad. Sometimes they do not heal in the center, but continue as inflamed and more or less scaly patches. This disease causes no feeling of general illness and only a mild itching, but it is quite unsightly. It is frequently contracted through contact

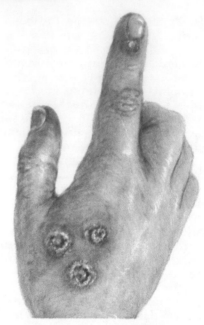

with infected domestic animals, especially cats.

What to Do

1. Apply calamine lotion to the affected areas every three hours during the day to help control itching.

2. Apply one of the following fungicidal creams to the affected skin area, rubbing it into the skin twice daily for two or three weeks: Halotex cream, Lotrimin cream, or Tinactin cream.

3. Griseofulvin taken under a physician's supervision is an effective remedy for ringworm of the body.

RINGWORM OF THE GROIN (CROTCH ITCH, JOCK ITCH).

Ringworm of the groin manifests itself as brownish or reddish, somewhat scaly patches, with tiny blisters at the spreading edges, commonly affecting the inner surface of the upper thighs, the scrotum, the groin, the perineum, and the anal region. This condition may be caused by different kinds of fungi, and by some is considered as only another variety of ringworm of the body. In many cases the person with this condition also has athlete's foot—the probable source of fungous infection which now affects the skin of the groin. Heat, moisture, profuse perspiration, and chafing by the clothing can prepare the way for the infection to take hold. It is more common and more troublesome in the tropics than in cooler climates. Mild itching or smarting sensations are the only forms of discomfort caused by it.

What to Do

1. Keep the affected skin areas as clean and dry as possible. Wear cool, soft, loose-fitting clothing.

2. Apply one of the following fungicidal creams to the affected skin areas, rubbing it gently into the skin twice daily for two or three weeks: Halotex cream, Lotrimin cream, or Tinactin cream.

3. In the morning, dust on talcum powder containing 10 percent of calcium propionate. Use this powder freely during the day to decrease friction when walking.

4. Griseofulvin taken under a physician's supervision is an effective remedy for ringworm of the groin.

RINGWORM OF THE NAILS.

This fungous infection causes the nails to become thickened, brittle, broken, white, and often ridged. It seldom, if ever, causes any pain, itching, or other discomfort, and frequently only one nail is affected. It is an exceedingly persistent infection, however, and only the expert attention of a skin specialist is likely to bring about a cure. It can be caused by one or more of the many kinds of fungi that cause ringworm of other kinds. In extreme cases, the nails degenerate into irregular masses of hard, crumbly material, with little or no resemblance to normal nails. Surgical removal of the diseased nails may be necessary for a cure.

What to Do

1. Nails affected by fungi are among the most difficult conditions to treat successfully. The application of any kind of medication to the nail surface usually does no good.

2. Occasionally painting the nail surface with tincture of iodine accompanied by scraping the surface of the affected nail is helpful.

3. The best results are usually obtained by the use of griseofulvin taken by mouth. This requires a physician's prescription.

RINGWORM OF THE SCALP (TINEA CAPITIS).

Ringworm of the scalp appears first as small, round, reddish, scaly spots with blisters. The spots enlarge rapidly, become grayish in color, show definite boundaries, and generally cause loss of hair. The infection seldom, if ever, attacks persons past puberty; and if it is present earlier, it tends to clear up by itself when puberty arrives.

When the affected spots are numerous, they may grow together, forming large, irregular patches. The hair in these spots becomes dry, lusterless, and brittle, breaking off and leaving short stumps which can easily be pulled from the scalp. Baldness may occur, but it is not likely to be permanent. There tends to be a constant mild itching of the scalp. The disease is usually curable within a few months.

Ringworm of the scalp may be caused by more than one variety of fungus. One form is caught by contact with pets, especially kittens or puppies, which may carry the causative organisms without showing signs of active infection. It may also be acquired through contact with an infected person or contaminated article, in a barbershop, by wearing somebody's contaminated hat, or by using somebody's contaminated comb or hairbrush.

What to Do

Griseofulvin taken by mouth for several weeks under a physician's supervision is usually curative.

TINEA VERSICOLOR.

Tinea versicolor manifests itself as small, rounded, velvety, flat spots, yellow or brownish-yellow in color, usually appearing on the chest, shoulders, armpits, and abdomen. The patient has an odd speckled appearance. The disease is discussed here, not because it is serious, but becasue it often worries people who do not understand its nature. The spots are covered with small dry scales, which are not always plainly visible. They may grow in size until they are an inch (2.5 cm.) or more in diameter. When they are numerous, they may grow together and form large, irregular patches. The skin of the affected spots will not tan.

This disease has no symptoms but mild itching, does not affect the general health, and is only slightly contagious. It is possible, however, to be reinfected by wearing underwear that has not been sterilized. People who sweat considerably are more prone to this disease and to having recurrences.

What to Do

1. Twice a day, wash the affected skin vigorously with soap and warm water, dry thoroughly, and apply a 15 to 25 percent solution of sodium thiosulfate in water, letting it dry on.

2. There are two commercial preparations that may be used in place of the above. One is Tinver lotion and the other is Akrinol cream. Griseofulvin is not helpful in this condition.

Inflammatory and Allergic Diseases

ACNE (ACNE VULGARIS).

Acne is a common inflammatory disease which affects the skin of the face and, often, that of the neck, shoulders, chest, and upper back. It appears in the early teens and often continues into the twenties. It has been described as the "scourge of adolescence." About 80 percent of teen-agers have some degree of acne even though it is usually nothing more serious than troublesome "pimples." About 20 percent of teen-agers are troubled with acne in its more severe forms which leave scars in the affected skin.

As a child reaches the age of adolescence, his or her glands produce sex hormones which circulate throughout all the body tissues. One of the effects of these hormones is to stimulate the tiny sebaceous glands (oil glands) which are associated with the skin's hair follicles. Under this stimulation the cells within the sebaceous glands multiply rapidly—so rapidly that in many cases the gland's outlet becomes plugged with impacted cells.

The gland continues to be active even though its secretion can no longer reach the surface of the skin. As

The unsightliness of acne makes it especially detestable to youth.

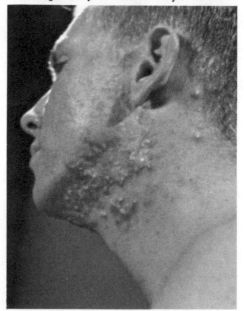

the tiny gland bulges, it stretches the surrounding tissue and produces a small white dot—a "whitehead." Some of the impacted secretion of the gland then undergoes chemical change which causes it to appear black. Thus a typical comedo ("blackhead") develops at the site of the hair follicle. As the sebaceous gland and its associated hair follicle are stretched even more, they rupture, producing a local inflammation. This rupture of the follicle gives rise, first, to a papule and then a pustule ("pimple"). In the more severe cases, the breakdown of the delicate tissues within the skin permits germs to enter so that an actual infection develops.

Acne occurs at a time of life when the teen-ager is particularly concerned over his personal appearance. The blemished skin, characteristic of acne, causes the individual to be sensitive and embarrassed. It is important, therefore, that treatment for acne, when it develops, be carried out early so as to avoid, as far as possible, the scarring of the skin that occurs in neglected cases.

The treatment of acne consists of two phases. The first consists of what the patient can do on his own. This requires him to do those things which build up his general health so as to make him more resistant to all kinds of illness. Also he must avoid those things that might aggravate the skin condition.

The second part of the treatment is the doctor's part. He must evaluate the particular case as to whether it is a mild form of acne or one of the more severe types. He must decide whether to use the newer types of medicines (such as Retin-A, benzoyl peroxide, and tetracycline or other antibiotics), as these may be indicated. He must advise the patient on what he should do and encourage him to persist in the program of treatment. The new kinds of medicine now available are powerful and must be carefully supervised by the doctor. But they have revolutionized the treatment of the severe cases of acne and made it much more successful.

What to Do

1. Cleanse the skin of the face and upper trunk twice daily, using warm water and a simple, non-irritating soap. Avoid excessive washing of the skin and the use of medicated soaps.

2. Abstain from using cosmetics during the entire period of treatment except for the moderate use of simple foundation lotions.

3. Avoid mechanical pressure on the skin such as resting one's chin in his hands and such as wearing a strap over one or both shoulders.

4. Obtain adequate rest. The person with acne should sleep not less than eight hours each night.

5. Use a well-balanced, wholesome diet. Avoid all between-meal snacks including sweetened drinks. Be moderate in satisfying all cravings of appetite. Most persons with acne benefit by abstaining from chocolate and from cola drinks.

6. Use no medicines or drugstore remedies except under the doctor's specific direction.

7. Correct any circumstances in the life program that cause anxiety or promote the spirit of competition.

8. Keep in close touch with the doctor, particularly if he prescribes some of the more powerful medicines.

9. Persist faithfully in following the treatment which the doctor prescribes. In many cases, the strong medicine which he uses will make the skin condition seem to be worse after three or four weeks of treatment. This is the usual response, and the treatment must be continued even so in order to derive the real benefits of the medication. Discontinuing the medication prematurely without the doctor's knowledge, even though the acne seems to be

improved, may cause the condition to become as bad as it was originally. The treatment program may have to be continued for many months.

BLACKHEADS (COMEDONES).

Blackheads are the small, black, unsightly dots that appear in the skin, usually of the face. Each consists of a tallowlike plug that fills the entrance into a hair follicle. The plug consists of inspissated sebum (secretion of a sebaceous gland) which appears black because of the chemical process of oxidation.

Numerous blackheads are characteristic of acne as described in the preceding item. Occasional scattered or isolated blackheads may occur in quite normal skin at most any time of life. These develop when the outlet to a sebaceous gland or the lumen of the associated hair follicle becomes plugged.

What to Do

1. When blackheads are numerous, treatment should be as in acne. See the preceding item.

2. For isolated blackheads, warm the skin thoroughly by enveloping it with a hot towel (a towel wrung from hot water), continuing the treatment for several minutes. Then use a metal blackhead remover (available at the drugstore) to assist in pressing out the plug of inspissated material from the hair follicle. This is accomplished by pressing the metal instrument firmly against the skin with the small opening of the instrument directly over the blackhead. The instrument is then moved sideways.

Do not squeeze this area of skin with the fingers, for this tends to injure the tissue and make it susceptible to infection. After removing the core of the blackhead, apply a disinfectant solution, or merely isopropyl alcohol, to the area that has been treated.

ACTINIC KERATOSIS (SOLAR KERATOSIS; formerly called SENILE KERATOSIS).

This is a skin condition which develops on those areas that have been repeatedly exposed to the sun (principally on the face, ears, and the backs of the hands) that occurs commonly in middle-aged and elderly persons, especially those of fair complexion. The skin lesions are patchy, poorly defined, slightly elevated, rough, uneven, dry, and often scaly. The lesions are skin-color or slightly red. Often the lesions itch and may bleed slightly when the scales are removed.

Actinic keratosis deserves serious consideration because of its tendency to develop into skin cancer. A person who has had one or more such lesions treated may protect himself from the development of other lesions by the use of a sunscreen ointment or lotion such as is used for preventing sunburn.

What to Do

1. Single lesions of actinic keratosis can be treated by the physician with his skilled use of liquid nitrogen or solid carbon dioxide to freeze the involved tissue.

2. For multiple lesions most physicians now prefer to prescribe a liquid preparation containing 5-fluorouracil (such as Fluoroplex) applied directly to the affected skin. Except where skin cancer has already begun, a course of this treatment usually restores the skin to its healthy condition.

3 If there is a question of whether a certain lesion is being transformed to skin cancer, the physician will arrange for a microsopic examination of a sample of the involved tissue.

ANGIONEUROTIC EDEMA.

Angioneurotic edema is characterized by rapidly developing extensive swellings, usually affecting the lips, eyelids, or ears, but not limited to these parts of the body. The swellings—similar to those of hives, but larger and more persistent—are accompanied by itching, burning, tension, and stiffness in the affected parts. They are caused by internal or external contact with some substance to which the person concerned is sensitive, though the identity of this substance cannot always be determined. They may lead to death by suffocation if they involve the larynx. Much that is included in the discussion of hives also applies to angioneurotic edema.

What to Do

1. If the affected areas are accessible, bathe them frequently with cool, thin starch water or a strong solution of baking soda.

2. Follow the advice given under *Hives*, What to Do."

3. Ephedrine sulfate by mouth, epinephrine by injection, or cortisone by injection, may be needed in severe cases. Such remedies require the supervision of a physician.

CHAFING (INTERTRIGO).

Intertrigo is a chafed patch of skin—red, moist, and somewhat raw in appearance, and characterized by smarting and burning sensations. It most often affects chubby children and fleshy older people. The rubbing of two skin areas together is the usual cause, but clothes rubbing on the skin can produce a similar effect. In some cases the smarting and burning become severe enough to amount to actual pain. Failure to keep the skin, especially folds in the skin, free from dirt and decomposing sweat makes chafing almost certain, particularly in warm weather. It is far better to prevent the condition than to make treatment necessary because of neglect. If the skin areas likely to become chafed are kept clean, dry, and well powdered, intertrigo will rarely develop.

What to Do

1. Carefully clean the affected skin areas with a soft cloth and warm water. Use a little mild soap at first, if necessary, but rinse all of it off carefully. Dry thoroughly, and apply a suitable powder liberally. A powder made of equal parts of talcum and zinc stearate, or of starch and zinc oxide, will usually be effective. Powders act as a lubricant and facilitate the movement of skin over skin. If the afflicted person is an infant or a young child, great care should be taken to prevent inhalation of any of the powder, particularly that containing zinc stearate.

2. If the affected areas are located where one rubs on the other, it may be necessary to keep them separated by cotton pads dusted thickly with powder. As far as possible, avoid any activity which produces rubbing.

3. In persistent cases, the treatment recommended under *Ringworm of the Groin* in the section on *Fungous Diseases* may be effective.

CHILBLAINS.

Chilblains are dark red or purplish inflamed areas of skin, usually on the feet, hands, face, or ears. They are caused by frequent or long-continued exposure to cold not severe enough to cause freezing of the tissues, together with a naturally sluggish circulation. They cause much discomfort from itching, smarting, and burning. With continued or repeated exposure to cold temperatures after chilblains have developed, ulceration, scarring, fibrosis, and atrophy of the affected tissues may occur.

The best plan is to prevent chilblains by protecting the susceptible parts of the body from exposure to cold, and by treatments that will stimulate the circulation, especially in those parts. After chilblains have once developed, it may take long treatment to bring about a cure; and subsequent exposure to cold is especially likely to cause a recurrence.

What to Do

1. Avoid vigorous rubbing or massage. Keep the affected parts dry, but not too warm. Wear enough clothing, or use any other practicable method, to prevent further chilling.

2. Immediately before bedtime, give alternate hot and cold baths or compresses to the parts (see volume 1, chapter 20) for twenty minutes, dry thoroughly, massage gently with olive oil, and apply the following ointment:

| Ichthyol | 3 |
| Lanolin | 27 |

3. Try to improve the general circulation by taking regular exercise and by taking a brief cold bath or shower every morning, followed by a brisk rub with a coarse towel.

4. Abstain from or discontinue the use of tobacco in any form.

CONTACT DERMATITIS.

Contact dermatitis consists of an irritation of the skin caused either (1) by direct contact with some irritating chemical substance or (2) by an allergic reaction in which the skin becomes reddened, swollen, and itchy because of contact with some substance to which the individual has become sensitized. The various forms of contact dermatitis cause considerable suffering and perplexity.

It is often difficult to determine just what the substance is that is irritating the skin or causing it to react unfavorably. Patience coupled with intelligent sleuthing are often necessary. Individuals react differently, and what bothers one person may have no detrimental effect on another. Once the offending substance is identified, the prevention and treatment consists, of course, of avoiding contact with this substance.

Many preparations which are useful around the house contain substances to which some people become sensitive. Common offenders are certain kinds of soap, detergents, bleaches, toilet bowl cleaners, oven cleansers, drain pipe cleaners, lye, and various ammonia preparations. For persons who work in industry, the list of things that may cause irritation of the skin is too long to be included here.

Prominent among the substances that may cause dermatitis are nickel and chromium. Nickel is contained in coins, jewelry, and watch bands, to name a few. Skin contact with articles containing this metal, especially when the skin is moist with perspiration, may cause the skin to become irritated. Chromium is used frequently in the tanning of leather and can thus cause a dermatitis of the skin of the feet or of other parts of the body exposed to leather that has been tanned by such a process. A construction worker may suffer from dermatitis because of the chromium contained in cement.

Modern technology has multiplied the number of chemical substances that are used in preparing fabrics. Some people become sensitive to certain dyes. Durable press finishes cause trouble in other cases. Some rubber products such as bathing caps, gloves, and the elastic components in stretch garments contain chemicals which are irritating to some people. Often, in such cases, the particular areas of the skin that are affected will suggest what article of clothing contains the offending substance.

Contact with the leaves of certain plants causes some people to have a severe skin reaction. See *Poison Ivy, Poison Oak* in this same chapter.

Diaper dermatitis illustrates how an infant's sensitive skin may react to irritating substances. The offending substance may be residues of detergent that remain in the fabric due to insufficient rinsing. Compounding the problem is moisture next to the infant's skin coupled with the ammonia resulting from the breakdown

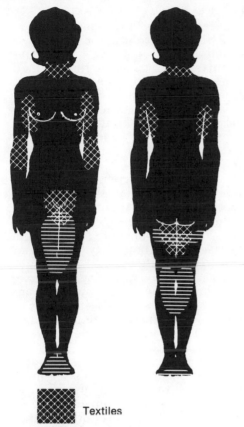

Textiles

Nylon stockings

Textured areas in the diagrams indicate location on the body where irritants contained in stockings and other garments may cause sensitive skin to react.

of the urea contained in the urine. Waterproof layers which exclude the air from the diaper area aggravate the situation.

The appearance of the skin in contact dermatitis may mimic that of several other skin ailments.

What to Do

1. Use all reasonable means of discovering the substance to which the skin is sensitive. Physicians often use "patch tests" to help in this discovery. The patch test is performed by strapping to the skin sample substances that may possi-

bly be responsible. These are left in place for 48 hours to determine whether the skin reacts unfavorably.

2. Once the responsible irritant has been discovered, ingenuity must be used to avoid contact with this substance or to protect the skin from it. Some persons must change employment in order to obtain relief. Others may benefit by switching to a different brand of clothing.

3. In many cases it is necessary to solicit the help of a physician who specializes in diseases of the skin. He will help to indentify the offending substance and to find ways to prevent contact with it.

DANDRUFF.
(See *Seborrheic Dermatitis.*)

DRUG RASH (DERMATITIS MEDICAMENTOSA).

Drug rash is caused by sensitivity to some drug being taken at or just before the time when the condition manifests itself. There are more than a hundred drugs known to produce rashes in people sensitive to them. Drug rashes are great imitators, and the rashes may look like skin eruptions from other causes. Suspicion of a drug rash is justified if a person, as far as can be determined, has no disease characterized by a rash, and at the same time is taking a drug. An investigation should be started at once to determine the true nature of the rash.

Among the common drugs that frequently cause rashes are: acetanilide, aminopyrine, arsenicals, barbiturates, bromides, chloral hydrate, ephedrine, iodides, novacain, penicillin, phenacetin, phenolphthalein, quinine, salicylates, various sulfas, turpentine, and many trademarked preparations the constituents of which may be unknown. Many of these drugs or their compounds are often taken without a physician's advice or knowledge; so if a physician is called to look at a rash, be sure to tell him if the person con-

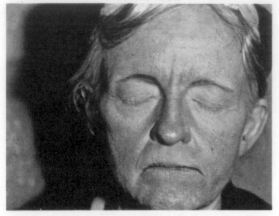

Above: Rash caused by iodides.
Below: Rash caused by penicillin.

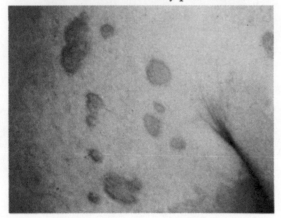

cerned is, or recently has been, taking a drug and, if so, what drug it is.

What to Do

Stop the use of the drug that may be causing the rash. It may be necessary to consult a physician to determine the true cause of the rash. Drug rashes vary so greatly in appearance that they are often hard to recognize, and the rash suspected of being caused by a drug may be from some other cause. In some cases of proved drug rash further treatment is needed after the drug is discontinued. No simple, general treatment will fit all cases. Many patients will be benefited by the use of cortisone cream, cortisone by mouth, or cortisone by injection.

ECZEMA (ATOPIC DERMATITIS).

Eczema is a mysterious disease which is very troublesome to those afflicted with it. It has some resemblance to contact dermatitis and some to those skin diseases which are caused by allergy. It consists of an inflammatory reaction in the skin characterized by itching, burning, and redness. Its severity and its particular manifestations vary a great deal from person to person.

Eczema occurs in persons who have inherited a type of skin which is hypersensitive. In about three-fourths of the cases of eczema, close relatives have been troubled with such allergic diseases as asthma, hay fever, and urticaria (hives).

Eczema runs a periodic course, there being times when symptoms are minimal and other times, especially in winter, when the condition becomes worse. There are three age periods—infancy, childhood, and young adulthood—in which eczema is most likely to occur. Eczema may appear for the first time in any one of these three periods. If it appears first in infancy, it may recur in childhood and, again, in early adulthood. In other cases it may appear in only one of the age periods.

Infantile eczema appears between the ages of two months and two years. Childhood eczema is common between ages five and ten. For young adults, eczema often appears during the early teens and lasts into middle life.

The skin of persons who are susceptible to eczema reacts unfavorably to certain conditions. Cold weather increases the susceptibility. So does heat and excessive humidity. Physical exertion, especially when this involves perspiring, tends to break down the skin's resistance to this tendency. Contact with wool is an aggravating factor. Emotional stress, a respiratory infection, excessive bathing, or the use of harsh soap will increase the susceptibility.

The characteristics of eczema differ

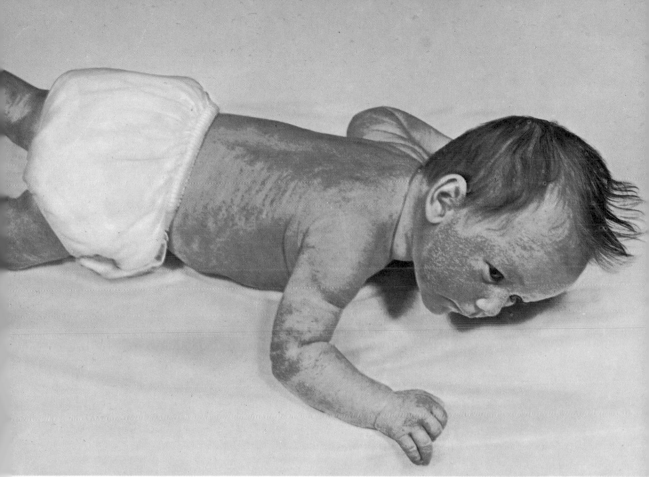

somewhat from one age group to another. In the infant, the skin involvement is particularly on the face and scalp, and on the extensor surfaces of the arms and legs. The involved skin exudes moisture with the subsequent formation of crusts. As at other times of life, itching and excoriation are major problems.

The eczema of childhood may occur on any part of the skin's surface but, particularly, on the extensor surfaces of the arms and legs. The lesions are in the form of papules (pimples) and plaques.

In the adult group, the common sites of involvement are the flexor areas of the arms and legs, the eyelids, and the sides of the neck. The skin is dry in contrast to that of the infant with eczema. The skin appears muddy with variations in the amount of pigment.

In the acute phase of eczema the skin becomes reddened and swollen.

Papules develop on this swollen skin and then merge into vesicles containing fluid. The fluid escapes as the vesicles break and the area continues to ooze. Crusts then form in this oozing area.

As the condition becomes more chronic, which is typical of the older age groups, the skin tends to form scales and the skin markings become accentuated. Because of the intense itching, there are obvious scratch marks and the skin becomes fissured. The lesions are not sharply demarcated from one another or from the surrounding normal skin.

Eczema is not the kind of disease that can be "cured" by any certain treatment. The aims of treatment are to give the patient relief from his discomfort, to prevent secondary infections of the involved skin areas, and to reduce the inflammation as much as possible.

183

What to Do

A. *Infantile Eczema.*

1. The infant with exzema should be spared from contact with the following: (a) domestic pets; (b) wool in clothing, blankets, etc.; (c) feathers; and (d) dust such as may accumulate in draperies.

2. Certain articles of food may aggravate the condition. The ones which should be omitted from the diet are wheat, orange juice, chocolate, and fish. In eliminating these items, however, care should be exercised, preferably with the help of a dietician, to make sure that the infant's diet is nutritionally adequate.

3. Abandon the traditional daily bath in which soap is used. A thirty-minute, tepid bath into which a tablespoonful of corn starch to the gallon of water (or a similar amount of powdered oatmeal) has been stirred into the water, will be soothing to the infant's skin.

4. The infant's clothing and diapers should be thoroughly rinsed after washing in mild soap. No detergents should be used.

5. In cleansing the infant's skin, use soap substitutes such as Soydome Medicated Skin Cleaner or Aveeno Soap Subsitute.

6. After cleansing, a soothing ointment should be applied to the infant's skin. Suitable preparations are rose water ointment USP, hydrophilic petrolatum USP, hydrophilic ointment USP, or such prepared ointments as Lubriderm, or Velvachol.

7. In severe cases that do not respond to the procedures mentioned above a corticosteroid ointment may be used as directed by the doctor.

B. *Adolescent Eczema.*

1. Living in air-conditioned quarters is usually of help in adolescent eczema, because the person is not subjected to the extremes of temperature which tend to aggravate the skin condition.

2. Moist compresses applied to

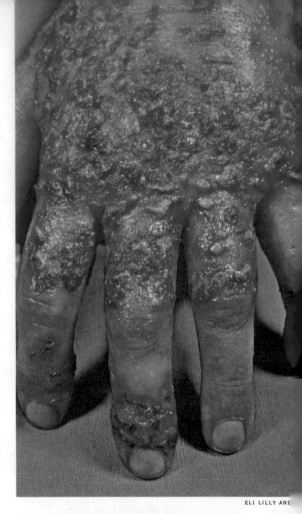

ELI LILLY AND

the affected skin areas for one hour, four times a day, help to relieve the discomfort. The compress consists simply of cotton cloth wrung out of cool tap water.

3. When bathing, the patient should avoid the use of soap and also of hot water, both of which tend to aggravate the skin condition.

4. Some cases are made more comfortable by the use of tub baths into which a cup of corn starch or of powdered oatmeal has been stirred into the water. Such a bath should continue for 30 minutes or longer as the patient may desire.

5. At times when the skin is not being kept moist by compresses or by tub baths, oil emulsion creams may be used on the affected areas. Suitable commercial preparations are Nivea Oil, Lubriderm Lotion, and Keri Lotion.

6. In the more difficult cases, corticosteroid creams, used under a physician's direction, may be applied to the involved skin areas.
C. *Adult Eczema.*

1. Because the skin is typically dry in the adult type of eczema, the patient is often made more comfortable by oil tub baths. The bath is prepared by adding to the bath water one-half to one tablespoonful of such commercial preparations as Alpha-keri, Domol, Mellobath, Lubath, or Avenol. *Caution: the bathtub is slippery when such preparations are used.*

2. Soap substitutes should be used in place of regular soap. Satisfactory commercial products are Soy-dome Medicated Skin Cleanser and Aveeno Soap Substitute.

3. Corticosteroid creams are often beneficial. These should be used under a physician's direction.

4. When secondary infections develop, the physician may find it advisable to prescribe appropriate antibiotic preparations to be applied directly to the skin.

ERYTHEMA MULTIFORME.

Erythema multiforme is an acute, inflammatory condition of the skin, characterized by flat or raised spots of a reddish color, commonly affecting the backs of the hands, the upper surfaces of the feet, the face, the sides of the neck, and sometimes the legs and the backs of the forearms. It occurs most commonly in the spring or the fall, and young adults are most often attacked. The eruption develops within twelve to twenty-four hours, the spots of various sizes being accompanied by little or no itching or pain. There may be headache, backache, and some fever. The flat or elevated spots may develop into blisters and pustules, which sometimes become ring-shaped. Pressure on a spot with a fingertip will cause the red color to fade, but it returns quickly when the pressure is released. Within ten to fourteen days, the red color

PUBLIC HEALTH SERVICE AUDIOVISUAL FACILITY

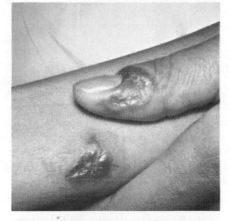

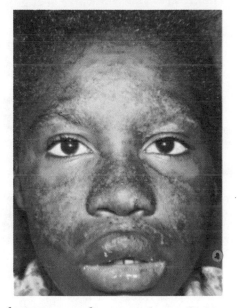

Cases of erythema: Above, erythema multiforme; below, erythema nodosum.

changes to a faint purple, and eventually all abnormal color disappears, leaving no scars.

Erythema multiforme rarely attacks a person in good health. It is most often observed on the skin of people who have rheumatism, some acute or chronic infection, sensitivity to certain foods or drugs, or a general run-down condition. In some people, damp and chilly weather seems to bring out the eruption.

The remedies that may prove useful

185

depend on the underlying causes. Since these causes may vary so widely, a course of treatment suited to one patient may do another very little good. All but the simplest cases, which show prompt improvement when a good hygienic program is begun, should if possible be carefully studied by a physician, who can recommend treatment aimed at the correction of general debility or any other specific condition revealed by his study as a possible cause of the skin eruption.

What to Do

1. Wet dressings, using cotton cloth and lukewarm tap water, are applied to the affected skin areas. Baths of lukewarm water also give some comfort.

2. After the bath or between the use of wet dressings a mild skin lotion such as calamine lotion may be applied gently to the affected skin.

3. In some stubborn cases the physician may prescribe a corticosteroid preparation to be taken by mouth.

ERYTHEMA NODOSUM.

Erythema nodosum is an acute inflammatory skin disease, marked by very tender red nodules which appear in successive crops, usually on the front surfaces of the legs but sometimes on the forearms, accompanied by intense itching and burning sensations. The nodules are from one-half inch to two inches (1.2 to 5 cm.) in diameter. Their appearance is often accompanied by mild fever, a general feeling of lack of energy, and rheumatic or joint pains. On careful examination, a patient who develops erythema nodosum will usually be found to have infected tonsils, rheumatic fever, tuberculosis, valley fever, or some other infection needing medical care. This makes it doubly important to consult a physician, if possible, as soon as the characteristic eruption appears.

What to Do

1. The patient should take no exercise for at least two weeks, and if possible should stay in bed.

2. The bowels and kidneys should be kept active, preferably by means of suitable diet and abundant fluids.

3. Local applications of any kind will not do much toward curing the condition, though they may reduce the discomfort. An ointment made according to the following prescription may be applied liberally to the nodules three times a day:

| Ichthyol | 3 |
| Lanolin | 27 |

4. Have a thorough medical examination to detect if possible the underlying cause of the skin condition. It may well be some infection or disease which itself needs treatment.

EXFOLIATIVE DERMATITIS.

Exfoliative dermatitis is not a specific skin disease, but an inflammatory condition of a serious nature, characterized by reddening and scaling or peeling of much of the skin surface, and accompanied by fever and various other signs or symptoms of general illness. The name means an inflammation of the skin resulting in the peeling off of pieces of considerable size. Sometimes the patient loses the whole outer layer of the skin before the attack subsides.

Because of the variety of possible causes, no definite group of symptoms characterizes the condition. Neither is there any characteristic appearance, though rather large blisters and pustules are found in many cases. In others there may be at first a severe redness and a burning sensation in comparatively large skin areas, followed a few days later by the aforementioned peeling.

Bacterial or fungous infections, spread of psoriasis, seborrheic dermatitis, toxic effects from arsenicals or other drugs, dietary upsets, malignant diseases of lymph and blood-forming tissues, vitamin deficiencies, external irritants, or any one of several other possible conditions may lie at the root of the skin inflammation that is the first step of this disease. Obviously it is the underlying condition that needs the most attention, and applications of lotions or ointments to the skin can do little more than help relieve itching or other unpleasant sensations. Since, however, the condition can become rapidly worse and put life in peril, expert attention should be sought as soon as exfoliative dermatitis seems to be developing. Do not waste time in trying to see what local applications will do.

What to Do

Without delay, consult a dermatologist or experienced physician. Hospitalization is often advisable.

HIVES (NETTLE RASH, URTICARIA).

An attack of hives appears as a local reddening of the skin which itches intensely and presently develops firm, elevated wheals. The condition may be temporary and fade away within minutes or a few hours, or it may become chronic and last for long periods of time.

The cause of hives in most cases is an allergy to drugs, to certain foods, to insect stings, or to protein substances such as pollens that are inhaled. However, in more than 20 percent of the cases of hives the skin reaction is brought on by some emotional crisis rather than by an obvious allergy-producing contact. In certain cases the occurrence of hives is precipitated by such physical factors as exposure to cold, to heat, to sunlight, to pressure, and even to water.

The swollen spots appearing in hives resemble those that come from contact with nettles. The area around each one of the spots is usually reddened but the spot itself may appear almost white. A typical spot is from one-quarter inch to one inch (0.6 to 2.5 cm.) in diameter.

Of the many drugs to which a person may become sensitive, penicillin and aspirin are the most common offenders. Inhaled protein substances that may cause the reaction of hives include pollens, molds, the dust from feathers, house dust, and animal dander. The insect stings that are most commonly productive of hives are those of bees, wasps, and hornets. In the case of a person who is sensitive to the substance which the insect injects into his skin, there may be a rather generalized appearance of hives over large areas of the skin.

It was formerly thought that a large number of cases of hives are the result of sensitivity to certain foods. It is now recognized that food sensitivity causes only a small percentage of such cases. Even so, when a genuine food sensitivity is present, the only permanent relief is to determine the offend-

A case of urticaria, showing the red swollen spots on the skin.

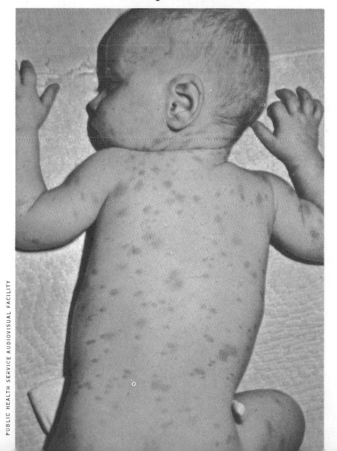

ing food and then omit it from the diet. The foods which may cause trouble are eggs, fish, shellfish, chocolate, certain nuts, tomatoes, cereals, berries, citrus fruits, pork, beef, and sometimes certain food additives.

Unsolved emotional problems, operating through the autonomic nervous system, render the tiny blood vessels within the skin more responsive to the various kinds of insults. Many cases of persistent hives are benefited by appropriate alterations in a person's way of life which relieve one's emotional crises.

What to Do

1. Identify, if possible the substance or circumstance which prompts the development of hives. Then avoid the offending substance or remove the troublesome circumstance.

2. For the immediate relief of the itching, the application of a thin paste of baking soda and water to the involved skin may give some comfort. The application of a 1/10 of one percent solution of menthol in alcohol may have a similar soothing effect. A prescription which may be used in this same way is:

Thymol	1
Glycerine	8
Alcohol (95%)	110
Water	100

3. Antihistamine drugs taken by mouth are often helpful in relieving a person's sensitivity to pollens and other protein substances which are contained in the inspired air. There are many brands of antihistamines; and it may take some experimenting, even under the direction of a physician, to find the one that works best in the individual case.

4. For the relief of severe acute attacks of hives, the physician may inject a dilute solution of epinephrine or may prescribe ephedrine to be taken by mouth or may administer corticosteroid by mouth or by injection.

5. In persisting chronic cases of hives, the physician's last resort is to use a corticosteroid medication. Such is very effective in relieving hives, but the side effects of the corticosteroids are troublesome; so this type of medication is to be avoided as much as possible.

LICHEN PLANUS.

Lichen planus is an inflammatory skin disease characterized by small, frequently angular, violet-colored, raised spots with flat, shiny tops, occurring singly or in patches, and appearing chiefly on the flexor surfaces of the wrists, on the ankles, genitals, and lips, and on the mucous membranes of the mouth or vagina. In some cases the eruption may appear elsewhere, or even become generalized, but the face and scalp are rarely attacked. If the rash is found on one limb or one side of the body, the opposite limb or side of the body will also show it. Sometimes the mucous membranes only are affected. Cases are not uniform in appearance. Spots on mucous membranes are characteristically covered with a lacy network of white lines.

Though the onset is sometimes gradual and the course chronic, in the typical acute case of the disease there is usually a general feeling of illness immediately before the rash begins to appear. Then within one or two days the eruption is complete, the slightly raised, red or light-purplish spots usually causing intense itching.

The exact cause of lichen planus remains unknown, but it is believed that mental or physical strain or a general run-down condition may give rise to it. It may be accompanied by a considerable degree of general debility, and it will often call for the attention of a skin specialist for recognition as well as treatment.

What to Do

1. Give the patient the benefit of good, plain food, hygienic living, and, when possible, outdoor life

with freedom from worry or care.

2. Apply the following lotion frequently and remove it by using any convenient kind of oil.

Sol. coal tar	12
Zinc oxide	24
Starch	24
Glycerin	36
Water. q.s. ad	120

3. In severe or persistent cases, consult a skin specialist, who can give more effective treatments.

LICHEN SIMPLEX CHRONICUS (LOCALIZED NEURO-DERMATITIS).

Lichen simplex is a chronic skin disease characterized by a slight inflammation but much itching. The eruption occurs in comparatively large patches, of which there may be from one to several present on the back of the neck, the inner surfaces of the thighs, the external genital organs, the ankles, eyelids, and ear canals. The affected skin areas are dry, thickened, leathery, and pigmented. The condition may be a late stage of any chronic or irritative skin inflammation, or it may develop on normal skin. It often affects people of Oriental extraction and women past forty. Scratching gives temporary relief, but the itching is likely to return later in a more intense form. The itching causes the skin to swell, and this produces more itching. The disease tends to be very persistent, but it may disappear from one area without any apparent reason, only to appear in another.

What to Do

1. Avoid stress or emotional upsets.
2. Avoid scratching the affected areas.
3. Avoid the use of soap.
4. Try applying the following lotion four times a day:

Menthol	1
Phenol	2
Glycerin	15
Alcohol, 35%, q.s. ad	240

5. Consult a skin specialist if possible. The most effective treatments or remedies cannot be given in the home or by people without medical training.

LUPUS ERYTHEMATOSUS

Lupus erythematosus is an inflammatory disease of unknown cause. Its manifestations vary a great deal from one case to another. It may affect any organ of the body either individually or in various combinations. Classically, two forms of the disease are described: (1) cutaneous or discoid lupus erythematosus which primarily affects the skin, and (2) systemic or disseminated lupus erythematosus which affects the body's organs, one or more.

Only about 5 percent of the cases of cutaneous lupus erythematosus develop into the systemic variety of the disease, but 50 to 80 percent of the cases of systemic lupus erythematosus develop skin involvements at some time during the course of the disease. In the present chapter we are concerned only with the cutaneous type of lupus erythematosus. The systemic type is considered in the following chapter (chapter 13) in the section on "Connective Tissue Diseases."

Cutaneous lupus erythematosus is a chronic recurring disorder of the skin which most frequently begins between ages 20 and 30 and is more common in women than in men. The skin lesions are red, rounded, slightly raised, scaly patches which appear typically in a "butterfly" pattern involving the bridge of the nose and the cheeks. Other areas of the face and scalp are often involved. Occasionally the lesions may appear quite widely distributed over the trunk, arms, and legs. Often the lips and the membranes of the mouth are involved. The lesions tend to spread at their borders and heal at the center. The healing may involve the formation of conspicuous scars. The skin involvement may disappear, sometimes permanently. More commonly, however, it

189

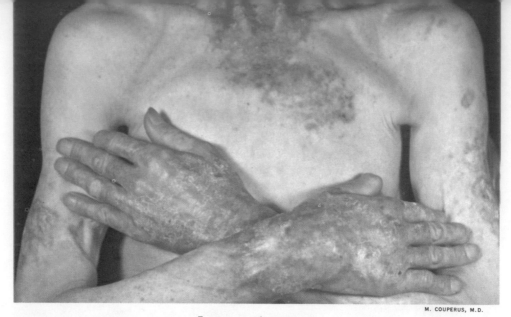

Lupus erythematosus.

M. COUPERUS, M.D.

recurs from time to time. The condition is typically aggravated by exposure to sunlight.

What to Do

1. **This is a serious disease, and the patient should be placed promptly under the care of a qualified physician.**

2. **Avoid excessive exposure to sunlight. Apply a sunscreen ointment to the exposed portions of the skin before being outdoors (as for preventing sunburn).**

3. **Avoid fatigue. Obtain adequate rest during each 24-hour period.**

4. **Apply corticosteroid cream to the affected skin areas as may be directed by the doctor.**

5. **Some cases are benefited by the use of the same medications as are used to control malaria. Of course this must be under the supervision of a physician.**

PEMPHIGUS.

Pemphigus is an uncommon but very serious skin disease. Untreated cases are usually fatal. It is an autoimmune disease in which the body produces antibodies that bring about serious changes in the structure of the skin. In cases that end fatally, death comes either as the result of infection or of starvation because of inability to eat on account of the involvement of the membranes of the mouth. The disease occurs in both men and women of all races. It usually begins after age 40.

Blisters develop on the skin and, in about 60 percent of cases, on the lining of the mouth. The blisters break easily, and the raw areas thus produced heal poorly and tend to spread.

Modern methods of treatment have greatly reduced the mortality rate and even permit those who develop this disease to continue to lead useful lives. But the medicines used in the treatment are powerful drugs and often produce unpleasant side effects. The treatment program must be modified to suit the individual needs of each patient

What to Do

1. **Best results follow when the disease is recognized and treated early. A physician should be consulted promptly once the typical skin lesions appear.**

2. **The treatment program, under a doctor's direction, requires the use of several medicines. A corticosteroid taken by mouth is the essential item. The reason for the other medicines is to prevent, as far as possible, the unfavorable side**

190

effects of the corticosteroid.

3. Local treatment of the affected skin has no effect on the course of the disease, but oatmeal or starch baths often make the patient more comfortable. (Stir a cup of corn starch or powdered oatmeal into the bath water.)

4. Compresses of 1:5000 solution of potassium permanganate may soothe the involved areas.

PHOTOSENSITIVITY REACTIONS.

The reaction of the human skin to sunlight varies from person to person. The skin of most light-skinned individuals is susceptible to "sunburn" when exposed directly to sunlight. Normally, tolerance to sunlight can be developed gradually by increasing the daily exposure. See the discussion of "Sunburn" later in this same subdivision of the present chapter and also the item on "Sunbaths" in chapter 19 of volume 3.

Unrelated to sunburn, the skin of some persons reacts in an unfavorable manner when exposed to sunlight. The reaction may occur after an exposure of only a few minutes. These unusual cases of hypersensitivity to sunlight fall into three categories: (1) those related to other skin diseases, (2) those in which certain drugs that have been taken into the body have caused the skin to become sensitized, and (3) those in which the application of certain substances to the skin have made it sensitive to sunlight.

The skin diseases which should be considered when a person's skin reacts unfavorably to short exposures to sunlight are: lupus erythematosus, and ichthyosis (see descriptions in this chapter), porphyria (see under *Disorders in Pigment Metabolism* in chapter 20 of this volume), and cold sores or herpes simplex (see under *Herpes Simplex* in chapter 28 of this volume).

There are several drugs which, when taken into the body either by mouth or by injection, may cause the

G. HANS, M.D.; PUBLIC HEALTH SERVICE AUDIOVISUAL FACILITY

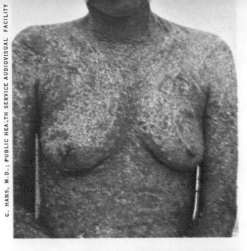

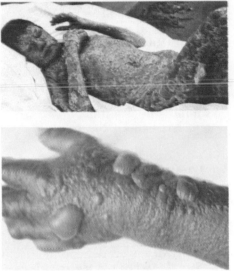

Characteristic manifestations of pemphigus.

skin to become hypersensitive to sunlight. This occurs in only a small percentage of persons taking these drugs. The possible offenders include sulfonamides, tetracyclines, thiazides, and griseofulvin.

Substances which, when applied to the skin, may cause sensitivity to sunlight include certain toilet waters and perfumes, sulfonamides, coal tar, and certain medicated soaps.

The particular type of skin reaction that results from exposure to sunlight in a person who is hypersensitive may mimic any one of other skin manifestations. There may be a simple reddening of the skin, an actual inflammation, hives, large blisters, or thickened scaly areas.

191

What to Do

1. Have the doctor check for the possibility of other skin ailments as mentioned above.

2. Take note of any medications that are being used. If it seems urgent that these be continued, check with the doctor to see if any one of these may be causing the skin problem.

3. Discontinue the lotions, medications, perfumes, or medicated soaps that have been applied to the skin recently. Sometimes the sensitivity of the skin persists for a matter of days even after the offending chemical has been discontinued. After the skin ceases to be hypersensitive, these may be resumed, one at a time, to see which one has caused the trouble.

PITYRIASIS ROSEA.

Pityriasis rosea is an inflammatory disease. It is sometimes classed among the virus diseases because it runs a definite course of about six weeks and seems to build up an immunity, but the virus has not been definitely discovered. Second attacks are rare. It is not contagious. It will subside of itself eventually, in three to six months, even if untreated. It deserves attention here chiefly for two reasons: (1) It is fairly common, and (2) those who have it may fear that it is something serious. Unrelieved fear may do more harm than the disease itself.

This disease manifests itself as numerous small, oval, yellowish or fawn-colored, sometimes pinkish or reddish, slightly scaly spots or patches, scattered over more or less of the trunk and those parts of the limbs adjacent to it. As a rule, a single comparatively large patch appears first somewhere near the waistline. This is called a herald or mother patch. The general eruption comes a week or two later. The long diameter of the patches lies in the direction of the natural wrinkles of the skin.

Dry, crinkly scales usually form on the patches, beginning in their centers. The larger patches may clear in their centers, forming rings, which are not, however, raised as much at the edges as are those of ringworm of the body, with which it may be easily confused. Mild itching is usually the only symptom, and the eruption disappears in a matter of weeks or months, leaving neither scar nor any other sign of permanent damage. In fact, the symptoms are so mild and the ordinarily visible parts of the skin surface so rarely affected that the eruption may be present for several days before its presence is noticed.

What to Do

1. If pityriasis rosea is suspected, consult a skin specialist if possible, not because the disease is serious, but for two other reasons: (1) The eruption somewhat resembles that of other more serious diseases, and its true nature needs to be known. (2) A short course of cortisone, administered by the physician will usually clear up the eruption promptly.

2. If the eruption is noticeably uncomfortable, which is not often true, use starch baths, mixing one or two cupfuls of Linit starch to a tub of bath water.

POISON IVY AND POISON OAK.

What we are discussing here is an acute inflammation of the skin, typical cases of which are caused by contact with poison ivy or sumac in the East and poison oak in the West. There are other plants in other parts of the world that cause similar skin inflammation by contact, and there are substances other than plants that may cause a similar inflammation.

The inflamed, swollen, and intensely itching skin areas, thickly covered with tiny blisters in the early stages, are so familiar to most people that recognition of the condition is often easy. Characteristically there are linear blisters associated with scratch marks. The substance causing ivy or oak poisoning is a waxy or resinous material which can be dissolved by strong soapsuds or rendered harmless by strong oxidizing agents. Extracts of poison ivy or poison oak have been prepared for use as vaccines. These vaccines seem to have afforded some protection to a number of people, but for others they have proved useless.

There are so many substances causing inflammation of the skin by contact that it is impossible to discuss them all here. Some affect a large proportion of all persons exposed to them, while others only occasionally cause trouble. It is usually a matter of individual sensitivity to the particular material in question. Fur, feathers, leather, various dyes, some of the plastics, and numerous drugs and chemicals are common offenders. The effect may vary from a slight and temporary reddening of the skin with mild itching to a severe inflammation with blisters and pustules that may not clear up for months.

Skin specialists always keep in mind the possibility of contact dermatitis when a puzzling skin eruption comes to their attention. The same treatments and preventive measures are of value in most cases of this type of skin inflammation. Avoiding further contact with the offending substance is obviously the most important preventive measure.

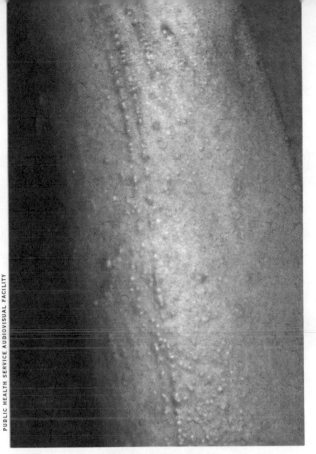

PUBLIC HEALTH SERVICE AUDIOVISUAL FACILITY

Characteristic linear inflammation of poison ivy or poison oak.

What to Do

1. If contact with the offending poison is recognized within a few minutes of the time it occurs, much of the poison can be removed or destroyed by washing the endangered skin areas with strong soapsuds, or by bathing them in a salt solution or a solution of Epsom salt (one tablespoonful of table salt or one tablespoonful of Epsom salt to the quart of water.)

2. During the stage of blisters and oozing, use cold (never hot) wet dressings as much of the time as practicable. For the dressings, use eight to ten layers of gauze, fluffed and crumpled, then wet with one or other of the following solutions: (1) saturated solution of aluminum acetate (Burow's solution) diluted 1 to 15, (2) saturated solution of magnesium sulfate (Epsom salt), or (3) 1 percent solution of zinc sulfate. Apply the wet dressings over the entire affected skin areas, cover with waxed paper, oiled silk, or plastic to keep in the moisture, and bind on snugly with bandages. The dressings should be kept wet, and the room kept warm enough to protect the patient from chilling.

3. When the blisters have dried and the oozing ceased, apply 1 percent phenol in calamine lotion three times a day.

4. As a preventive measure before going into places where there is danger of contact with poison ivy

193

or poison oak, apply to the skin a vanishing cream to which 5 percent of sodium perborate powder has been added. If you must stay in such a place very long, wash away the medicated cream and make a fresh application about every three hours.

PRICKLY HEAT (HEAT RASH).

Prickly heat is characterized by a red rash with many very tiny blisters appearing on the skin surface, most often affecting babies and stout persons, particularly those of fair complexion. The name is well descriptive of this familiar condition, for the skin feels both prickly and hot. The chief external causes of the rash are hot weather and the wearing of too much or too warm clothing. The use of alcoholic liquor encourages prickly heat to develop. With proper treatment, the rash should clear up in a week or less; but in severe cases with a large part of the body surface involved, body temperature regulation may be interfered with because the sweat gland outlets may have been damaged, and there may be a fatal outcome.

What to Do

1. Avoid the use of soap in cleansing the affected skin areas. Use thin starch water instead.

2. Apply the following lotion four times a day:

Menthol	0|3
Phenol	2
Glycerin	15
Alcohol, 35%, q.s. ad	240

3. Keep the affected areas cool and dry, as far as possible. When the acute stage of the rash is past, keep these areas thickly dusted with cornstarch.

4. If the causes of prickly heat cannot be avoided, dabbing on a small amount of a 10 percent solution of tannic acid in alcohol twice a day may toughen the skin and help

prevent further attacks; but this does not always succeed, and should never be done for more than a week at a time.

PSORIASIS.

Psoriasis is a serious, chronic, relapsing skin ailment in which the involved skin areas produce enormous numbers of silvery scales. The areas usually affected are the skin of the elbows, knees, back, buttocks, and the scalp. The lesions consist of large red plaques which are covered with overlapping, shiny, scales which are shed continuously.

It is estimated that there are no less than five million people in the United States who are troubled with psoriasis in one degree or another. In about one half million, the disease is of a severe, incapacitating degree. In about 5 percent of cases there is an associated arthritis in which the joints of the fingers and toes and also those of the spine become painful.

The fundamental cause of psoriasis is vague. It appears that heredity is a factor in about one third of cases. The essential alteration in the skin is an overproduction of cells in the epidermis. The cells composing this surface layer of the skin are normally shed continuously at such a rate that the average life of a cell is about twenty-eight days. In psoriasis the cells are produced and shed so rapidly that the average life of a cell is only three or four days. Taking this into consideration, the modern methods of treatment involve the use of strong chemical substances which inhibit the production of new cells. The ordinary over-the-counter or through-the-tube drugs available at the drugstore are usually not effective in the treatment of psoriasis.

Acute attacks of psoriasis usually end spontaneously but with the probability that the ailment will recur later. The effective treatments bring only temporary relief, for no method assures a complete cure of the ailment.

The number of persons with psoriasis is so great and the disease is so persistent that a National Psoriasis Foundation has been formed with headquarters at Suite 250, 6415 S.W. Canyon Court, Portland, Oregon 97221. This organization has literature available for those who make request. Another helpful pamphlet entitled "You, Your Dermatoligist and Psoriasis" may be obtained from the American Academy of Dermatology, 2250 N.W. Flanders Street, Portland, Oregon 97210.

The severity of the illness varies a great deal from person to person. It cannot be known, in the early phase of the illness, just how severe it is going to be in a certain case. It is advisable to consult a physician early, however, even though the skin problem is not very severe. Early in the course of the disease it is best to use the simpler forms of treatment, reserving the use of the strong medications for the future, if needed.

What to Do

1. Give attention to building up and maintaining the patient's general health by obtaining adequate rest each 24 hours; by using a simple, nutritious diet; by taking care of other health problems; by following a program of conservative outdoor recreation; and by developing a mental attitude of confidence and courage.

2. Each day remove the scales from the affected skin areas by using soap and water and a soft brush. Following this daily cleansing, apply an ointment such as the doctor may prescribe. The following prescription also serves satisfactorily as an ointment:

Sol. coal tar	12
Zinc oxide	24
Starch	24
Glycerin	36
Water q.s. ad	120

Reddish patches characteristic of psoriasis.

SPIRT & COMPANY, INC.

ELI LILLY AND COMPANY

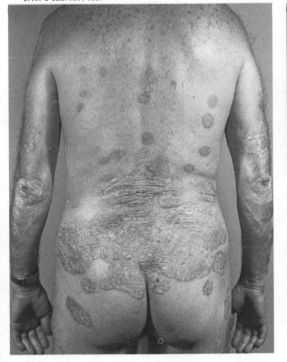

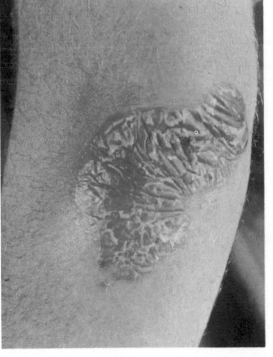

3. For the more severe, obstinate cases, a dermatologist (physician who specializes in diseases of the skin) should be consulted. He may recommend and supervise the use of one or more of the stronger medications such as the antimetabolites or the systemic corticosteroids. These often produce troublesome side effects, and their use must be constantly supervised.

ROSACEA. *(Acne Rosacea.)*

Rosacea is a chronic inflammatory skin ailment in which prominent areas of the face appear flushed. Rosacea is not a life-threatening disease but, rather, a cosmetic problem. The color varies from pink to a deep red to a purplish red. The areas affected are the nose, cheeks, brow, and chin. The skin of the affected areas is usually not raised or swollen. The skin surface is smooth, and the color fades under pressure. There may develop a permanent enlargement of the blood capillaries in the skin. Pimples, plaques, and thickening of the skin may appear in the more severe cases. The ailment is most common in women between the ages of 30 and 50.

The precise cause of rosacea is not clear, but it is known to be aggravated by the ingestion of alcohol, tea, coffee, cola drinks, and chocolate. Very hot or very cold foods may contribute, as may also exposure of the skin to sun, wind, or extremes of temperature.

What to Do

1. Give attention to eliminating the possible contributing factors (see above). This is more important in relieving the condition than is the use of lotions or creams.

2. Apply a 5 percent precipitated sulfur ointment to the affected skin areas one or two times daily.

3. For the more severe case, consult a physician who specializes in diseases of the skin. He will evaluate the case and prescribe more potent remedies as may be indicated.

SEBORRHEIC DERMATITIS (DANDRUFF).

Seborrheic dermatitis is a very common affliction, characterized by mild itching and free oily scaling, usually found on the scalp, but sometimes affecting the face, neck, chest, armpits, groins, or genital regions. It is included in the list of inflammatory skin conditions, first, because of its outward resemblance to certain other inflammatory conditions, second, because of a constant though very mild inflammation of the skin, and, third, because no proof exists that any infection is primarily involved.

Called "dandruff" when located on the scalp, it is so common that few people are completely free from it. When it appears on the body elsewhere, the eruption is more likely to be characterized by more or less oily crusts instead of dry scales. The skin beneath the crusts is somewhat thickened and mildly inflamed. The only unpleasant sensation is the mild itching.

A hereditary tendency, hormone imbalance, nutritional states, and emotional stress are possible causative factors. If any factor of infection is involved, it is probably secondary, and the causative organism or organisms cannot yet be definitely classified as either bacteria or fungi.

Seborrheic dermatitis tends to persist for a period of years, though it may come on in successive attacks, each of which may last from weeks to years.

What to Do

1. For "dry" dandruff on the scalp, proceed as follows:

Shampoo three times a week for four weeks—afterward once a week until a satisfactory cure is accomplished. Once a week, at bedtime, after a shampoo, apply Pragmatar ointment, which contains salicylic acid and sulfur and is available at any drugstore.

The following morning, wash away all traces of the ointment with mild soap and warm water, massaging the scalp well. After the washing and massage, rub into the scalp a little of the following lotion:

Phenol	5
Castor oil	1 5
Salicylic acid	2
Alcohol, 70%, q.s. ad	120

2. For "oily" dandruff, proceed as in (1) above, but make the morning washing rather brief and avoid all massage.

3. Though the condition is not primarily infectious, germs may be present and may make the condition worse, so sterilize your comb at least once a week. Use no hairbrush, because a hairbrush cannot be sterilized.

4. If the skin of the face or the body is affected, try the following:

Alternate nights at bedtime, rub in 5 percent sulfur ointment.

On the in-between nights, apply lotio alba.

5. For the more severe cases and for those in which larger areas of the skin are involved, the physician may direct the use of steroid and antibiotic preparations.

SUNBURN.

Sunburn is an inflammation of the skin characterized by burning and redness, due to overexposure to the rays of the sun. It needs little discussion; but sometimes one forgets that the redness and burning do not develop until some time after the exposure and that sunlight reflected from a glass or water surface can burn as well as direct sunlight. A person cannot tell by feeling alone at the time whether or not he is overexposing his skin. Every exposure to the sun produces some damage to the skin, especially to fair-skinned individuals.

Certain diseases that may be present, and a considerable number of drugs taken orally or applied to the skin, make the skin more sensitive to sunlight. Fair-skinned, blue-eyed people are more sensitive to it than dark-skinned. Severe sunburn over a large part of the skin surface is more dangerous than many people realize. It is well to remember that in extreme cases it can cause crippling or even death.

In severe cases involving a large fraction of the skin surface, there is likely to be pain, swelling, blistering with later peeling, a gastrointestinal upset, and considerable fever for several days. A toxic condition develops, probably because of some decomposition of the deeper skin tissues damaged by the sun's rays. If crippling develops later, it is likely to be the result of stiffening and contracture of damaged tendons. A still later possible effect is permanent hardening of the skin, or even the development of skin cancer.

What to Do

1. Apply continuous wet dressings of a saturated solution of aluminum acetate (Burow's solution) diluted with twenty times its volume of cold water. Continue until the pain and smarting are permanently relieved.

2. A similar effect may be obtained by getting into a lukewarm starch bath, prepared by stirring one or two cupfuls of Linit starch into a tub of bath water.

3. If large areas of skin are involved, and if the burning is severe, bed rest and the attention of a physician may be necessary.

4. In the most severe cases, application of a corticosteroid cream to the sunburned areas may be helpful.

5. Sunscreen ointments and lotions (available at the drugstore) are quite effective in preventing sunburn when applied to the skin before exposure to the sun. A 10 percent aminobenzoic acid ointment is effective for such use, as is a 15 percent titanium dioxide lotion.

Malformations

HEMANGIOMA (BIRTHMARK, VASCULAR NEVUS).

The ordinary birthmark of reddish or purplish color is composed of a mass or network of tiny blood vessels in the skin. In the simplest case the skin is smooth and normal in every respect except for the excessive number of the blood vessels in it. In more severe cases, the skin may be thickened or the area may show one or more "blood blisters." The birthmark may even be an irregular and unsightly tumor mass of one or more lobes. The unsightliness, however, is the chief disadvantage. Such tumor masses rarely become cancerous, but they may occasionally ulcerate. They do not injure the general health unless they become infected, which does not often happen. A large majority of birthmarks will disappear by age six even if not treated. It is usually only the very large birthmarks or those that are growing rapidly or that are ulcerating that need to be treated.

What to Do.

1. Do not try any home remedies.
2. In the case of an infant, arrange for an early consultation with a physician who is trained in diseases of the skin (a dermatologist). He will advise on whether this is the type of birthmark that will disappear spontaneously or whether it requires early treatment. For some of those that require treatment, it is disastrous to delay.
3. For those requiring treatment, whether infant or adult, the program should be chosen and administered by a specialist.

ICHTHYOSIS (FISHSKIN DISEASE, XERODERMA).

Ichthyosis is characterized by dryness, roughness, and thick, adherent scaliness of the skin. The outer layer or epidermis of the skin is thick and may show numerous shallow cracks, the surface tending to peel in rather large scales. In mild cases there is merely a persistent dryness and roughness of the skin surface. This condition appears early in life, and seems to run in families.

Ichthyosis affects only the outer layer of the skin and does not harm the general health. In occasional cases, however, the ability to perspire is lessened, and the afflicted person tends to become more readily feverish or overheated than he normally would. In most cases, the chief disadvantage is the more or less unsightly appearance, but, fortunately, the face, hands, and feet are rarely noticeably affected. During warm weather, mild cases will show improvement and the skin may appear practically normal. Dry air and cold weather make the condition worse.

What to Do

1. Do not expect a real cure, because the skin of the affected person is permanently short of sweat and oil glands.
2. Daily, but especially after each bath, apply some bland oil or ointment, such as petrolatum, cocoa butter, or oil of sweet almonds. Petrolatum to which 1 to 3 percent of salicylic acid has been added has some advantages over plain petrolatum.
3. Bathing should be restricted, as it adds to the dryness already present.
4. When a bath is taken, the water should be soft, preferably water that is naturally soft.
5. Use soap sparingly. It is advisable, however, to use it on body folds when bathing.

MOLE (NEVUS).

Moles are usually present at birth or appear early in life. In time they may grow and become considerably larger. In color most of them resemble the surrounding skin. Although they may never make trouble aside from their unsightliness, some of them may become cancerous, spreading cancerous cells through the bloodstream to other parts of the body, giving rise to a condition that may prove fatal. Moles which are black, bluish-black, or grayish-blue and flat, especially those located where they are exposed to irritation, are most likely to become malignant. Any mole which shows signs of irritation or which begins to grow rapidly, whatever its color, should be considered suspicious.

Moles showing any signs or symptoms suggesting possible developing malignancy should be promptly removed. Small moles can often be effectively treated by using an electrical instrument that kills and dries the tissue.

What to Do

1. Do not attempt self-treatment.
2. Have a physician, preferably a skin specialist, remove the growth, particularly if it is dark-colored, begins to change color or grow, or begins to feel tender or irritated. He will know what to do and how to do it.

Miscellaneous Skin Ailments

BALDNESS, FALLING HAIR (ALOPECIA).

Loss of hair, alopecia, or baldness, may occur in patches or over the entire body. It may be caused by hormone imbalance, seborrheic dermatitis (dandruff), syphilis, or other bacterial, fungous, or virus infections. The type and time of onset of ordinary baldness, however, are largely hereditary. Baldness may also be caused by acute fevers, certain drugs or chemicals taken internally or applied to the skin surface, X-ray or other burns, disturbed action of certain glands (particularly the thyroid or pituitary), or emotional shock.

Nothing effective can be done about common baldness of a hereditary nature. Discovering the causes of other types of baldness in any individual case may be difficult. Local

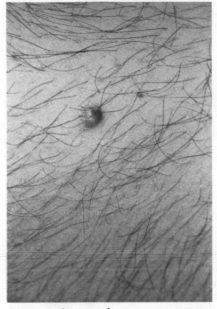

PUBLIC HEALTH SERVICE AUDIOVISUAL FACILITY

Some moles may become cancerous.

treatments of the scalp or hair in such cases, however, are likely to be useless until the causes are found. Some of the possible causes are diseases or abnormalities which need treatment as a protection to present or future health; therefore it is especially important that they be discovered and treated, whether or not the treatment brings about improvement in the condition of baldness. There is some basic cause, though not always curable which accounts for the baldness; and money spent on advertised "hair growers" is likely to be wasted unless this basic cause is found and can be corrected. In many cases finding the cause and treating it will call for a physician's attention; and even a physician may not be able to bring about much improvement.

What to Do

1. Do not expect a cure if common baldness of a hereditary nature has already developed.
2 The following program may have some value in delaying the onset or in slowing the progress of the condition:

199

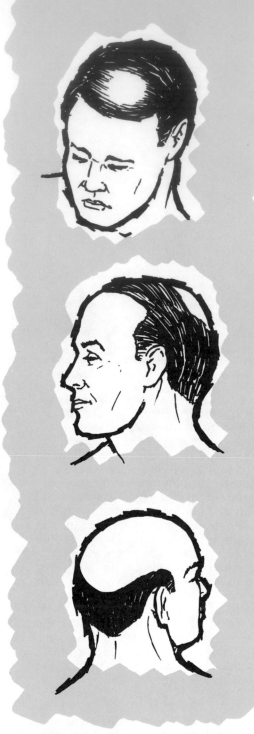

Development pattern of common male baldness: First, hair recedes from forehead and becomes thin around the crown (top and center); then the two balding areas merge (bottom), leaving a fringe.

Twice a week for oily scalps, or once a week for dry scalps, wash the scalp and hair with warm water and mild soap, rinsing and drying the hair thoroughly. Then apply a little bay rum.

Gentle massage may help, unless the scalp is very oily.

Avoid the use of others' combs or brushes.

3. If you are not sure the baldness is of the common hereditary type, have a physician make a study of the possible causes, and correct them if possible.

BEDSORE (DECUBITUS ULCER).

A bedsore is an ulceration of the skin and underlying tissue that occurs typically in debilitated patients who are confined to bed and remain in one position so long that pressure on the skin areas that bear the patient's weight deprives them of their normal blood supply. Gradually an involved area becomes dark in color, the skin breaks down, and an ulcer results. Prevention is much to be preferred, for cure is tedious and difficult.

What to Do

Prevention. Whenever a patient is confined to bed for a considerable period of time, the doctor in charge should be requested to give instructions on the prevention of bedsores for the particular case. The following are suggestions:

1. Turn the patient frequently from one position to another.

2. Use padding or inflated rubber rings to diffuse the pressure of body weight, particularly over the bony prominences.

3. If the patient has edema (swollen tissues), give attention to the appropriate means of removing the edema.

4. Maintain strict cleanliness of the skin.

5. After bathing the skin, use mild stimulation, such as gentle

massage with lubricating cream, or an alcohol rub, to increase blood circulation.

6. Use talcum powder and proper clothing to protect the skin from friction against the bed sheets.

Treatment once a bedsore has developed. The doctor in charge of the case should give detailed instructions. The following suggestions may prove helpful:

1. Use a special air mattress designed for this purpose, in which adjacent areas are alternately inflated and deflated automatically by mechanical means.

2. Clean and dress the ulcer daily, using sterile saline solution and sterile dressings.

3. Antibiotic ointments may sometimes hasten healing.

4. Continue (2) and (3) until the callus has been reduced to the thickness of normal skin.

CALLUS.

A callus is merely a patch of thickened and hardened epidermis, caused by long-continued pressure or friction. It is uncommon for a callus to be either very tender or very painful, or even to cause any marked discomfort. For a permanent cure, the cause must of course be removed.

What to Do

1. As far as possible, relieve the affected area from pressure or friction.

2. At bedtime apply a bit of the following mixture to the affected area only and cover with adhesive:

Salicylic acid	3
Lactic acid	3
Flexible collodion q.s. ad	15

An alternative is to apply small pads of cotton or gauze that have been dipped in 40 percent salicylic acid.

CAUTION: *Salicylic acid, as in the above, must not be used for a person who has diabetes.*

3. In the morning remove the adhesive and scrape off the softened skin tissue.

4. Continue (2) and (3) until the callus has been reduced to the thickness of normal skin.

CORN (CLAVUS).

A corn is similar to a callus in texture and has similar causes; but while a callus may be found on any one of several different parts of the skin surface, a corn is almost always on a foot, and usually on a toe, possibly on several toes. A corn is less broad than a callus, and is conical in shape with the apex of the cone directed inward. This shape accounts for the pain felt when pressure is applied to a corn. So-called "soft corns" are usually located between the toes where they are kept moist and softened by the perspiration.

ELSTON ROTHERMEL, D.P.M.

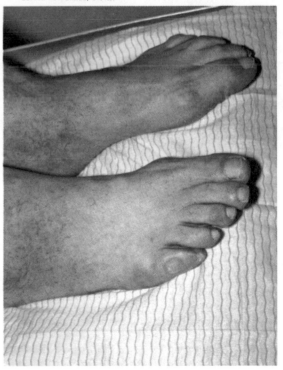

What to Do

1. Wear comfortable, broad-toed, "foot-form" shoes, made of soft and pliable leather, with heels not too high.

2. CAUTION: *The mixture mentioned herein, or any preparation containing salicylic acid, should not be used for a person who has diabetes.*

Surround the corn with a felt ring or corn protector. (These can be bought in almost any drugstore.) Each day, for three to five days, apply to the corn the mixture described under *Callus*, "What to Do," (2). Then soak the part for fifteen minutes in warm water and try to lift or pick the corn out. If it cannot be completely removed from its bed, continue the application for a day or two longer, and then try again. (Sometimes the application of this mixture will eventually make the tissues sore, even though a corn protector is worn continually. If this happens, the treatment should be temporarily discontinued.)

3. If the above treatment does not succeed, the corn may have to be surgically removed.

FRECKLES (EPHELIDES).

Freckles are merely spots of skin in which more than the usual amount of normal pigment has developed or has been deposited. They cause no distress and do no harm, except to the appearance of the skin. In many cases they are most numerous in childhood and tend to become less numerous or to disappear completely in later years.

What to Do

1. The prevention of freckles is the same as that for sunburn.

2. Avoid exposure to excessive sunlight and strong wind.

3. Freckles can be made less conspicuous by the application to the affected skin of certain lotions or creams that cause the skin to peel. These should be used, however, under a doctor's supervision.

GRAY HAIR.

Grayness of the hair is usually the natural result of aging, coming from a failure of pigment formation in the hair follicles. It may, however, be a symptom of endocrine disturbances, most often of the thyroid gland. It is known to accompany hyperthyroidism occasionally and to disappear after adequate treatment, the hair then regaining its natural color. In some cases of premature grayness, which is often familial, there are a few gray hairs in childhood, a sprinkling during adolescence, and complete grayness between the ages of twenty-five and thirty years. While worry, overwork, grief, anxiety, and nervous strain are contributing factors in the graying of the hair, stories of overnight blanching or whitening of the hair are contrary to physiological and anatomic facts. The graying of the hair is a slow process. In some cases early graying of the hair develops as a result of anemia, especially pernicious anemia.

The streak of white hair on the brow which many consider attractive is sometimes congenital and permanent, but is often acquired following the disease alopecia areata. It is typical for regrowth of hair following this disease to be white at first, but it usually regains its normal color in due course of time.

The person who chooses to conceal grayness of the hair by using hair dyes needs to be careful. Dyes which contain silver nitrate, pyrogallic acid, or paraphenylenediamine may be dangerous to the health; and if hair dyes are to be used at all, they should first be tested carefully for skin sensitivity.

What to Do

1. Try to determine the causes for the graying of your hair. Some of these may possibly be removed or corrected.

2. Do not waste time or money on any so-called "anti-gray-hair" vitamins.

HAIR, SUPERFLUOUS (HYPERTRICHOSIS, HIRSUTISM).

The tendency to an excessive growth of hair is usually considered to be hereditary. Men seldom object to an excessive growth of hair. Women object because of their natural desire to maintain a feminine appearance.

Superfluous hair develops more commonly in brunettes than in blonds. In women, the excessive hair often appears during pregnancy and increases with each successive pregnancy.

In about 1 percent of cases the excessive growth of facial hair is caused by some disturbance of the endocrine glands. But in these cases there are usually other telltale evidences such as the development of certain male characteristics.

There is no easy cure for excessive facial hair. The usual procedure is to remove the hair as it appears. The simplest methods are shaving and the use of depilatory wax. In either case the hair continues to grow and the removal must be repeated. Contrary to popular opinion, these methods do not cause the hair to become coarser.

What to Do

1. Shaving is really the most practical way for a woman to remove unwanted facial hair.

2. Depilatory creams that can be purchased at a drugstore are effective, but they often irritate the skin.

3. The use of depilatory wax is a rather tedious process.

4. More permanent removal of superfluous hair can be accomplished by the use of a galvanic current. This prolonged process requires the services of a skilled operator (an electrologist) as he treats one hair at a time.

ITCHING, GENERAL (PRURITIS).

The symptom of itching is not limited to any one certain disease. It is a symptom in several of the skin ailments. It occurs commonly as a symptom in some systemic diseases which are not primarily related to the skin. Among these are diabetes, obstructive liver disease, certain kidney diseases, and some instances of internal cancer. Itching may occur also in certain endocrine disturbances, at the time of menstruation, and in connection with the menopause. It often occurs in elderly persons in whom the skin glands are not as active as they were formerly.

What to Do

1. Bran, starch, or vinegar should be added to the bath water in the case of any warm, cleansing bath. Experience will prove which works best. Following the bath, the skin should be dried without harsh rubbing. Baths should not be more frequent than necessary.

2. Wear underclothing that will not irritate the skin. Launder it with care, making sure that all traces of alkali and soap are rinsed out.

3. Try applying 1 percent phenol in calamine lotion three times a day to the itching areas, if not too extensive. If this proves too drying to the skin, substitute for it a lotion made as follows:

Menthol	3
Phenol	2
Glycerin	15
Alcohol, 35%, q.s. ad	240

In the use of any lotion for the relief of itching, take care not to let any of it get into the eyes. This will not be difficult unless it is the skin of the eyelids that is itching.

4. Most important of all, try to find out the cause of the itching and avoid, treat, or correct it. This may call for the aid of a physician, especially in the case of persistent itching in the genital or anal regions.

5. For soothing the itching that is so troublesome to some elderly persons, commercial preparations may be used such as Nivea Creme

or Nivea Skin Oil, Keri Lotion, or Cetaphil Lotion.

ITCHING IN THE ANAL REGION (PRURITUS ANI).

Pruritus ani is a persistent itching, frequently with redness, maceration, and fissuring of the skin, occurring in the skin around the rectal outlet. The itching sometimes becomes so distressing as to demand vigorous treatment. It tends to be worse at night. There are many possible causes for this condition, but the commonest is an infection of the superficial skin layers by a yeastlike organism called "monilia" (candida). The constant moisture between the buttocks lessens the normal firmness of the skin. Germs and the yeastlike organisms, being always present, have a chance to grow in this softened skin.

Pruritus ani may accompany dermatitis from soap or douches, diabetes mellitus, diarrhea, intertrigo, leukorrhea, lichen simplex, seborrheic dermatitis, and nervous tension. Whatever the cause of the itching, the most important local treatment factor in controlling it is to keep the skin clean and dry. It may be necessary to keep a pad of dry absorbent cotton between the buttocks for this purpose.

What to Do

1. Avoid the use of soap, but keep the skin about the rectal outlet clean by washing it gently but thoroughly with warm water after each bowel movement and drying after each washing. Repeat at other times, if necessary to total at least two bathings daily. Soft, wet tissue or cotton rather than toilet paper should be used as an aid in washing.

2. After the washing and drying, apply a lotion made as follows:

Phenol	1
Glycerin	15
Rose water q.s. ad	120

3. After the lotion has dried, apply a generous amount of powder, and repeat the application of powder every two hours. A good powder is made as follows:

Salicylic acid	2
Talcum powder	58
Mix thoroughly.	

CAUTION: *Preparations containing salicylic acid, as in items 3 and 4, should not be used by a person who has diabetes.*

4. Each night at bedtime apply a small amount of a salve made as follows:

Salicylic acid	1
Sulfur ppt.	2
Cold cream q.s. ad	60

5. If the above treatment does not bring permanent relief within one week, have a physician make special studies to determine the underlying cause of the condition and to prescribe more appropriate remedies.

LIVER SPOTS (SENILE LENTIGINES).

Liver spots consist of small darkened areas that appear on exposed areas of skin in middle-aged and elderly persons. They occur in greatest numbers on the back of the hands.

What to Do

1. There is no completely satisfactory treatment.

2. The use of a bleaching cream, such as 2 percent hydroquinone cream, sometimes makes the colored areas less conspicuous. The cream should be rubbed into the affected areas twice daily for several months. If irritation results, discontinue the cream.

3. Exposure of the skin to sunlight should be avoided, as by the wearing of gloves.

MELASMA (Previously called CHLOASMA).

Melasma is characterized by pigmented blotches, brownish in color, which appear in women over the cheek bones, on the forehead, and, frequently, on the upper lip.

Melasma often develops during pregnancy. It usually disappears a few months after delivering the baby, only to reappear with any subsequent pregnancy. It sometimes appears, unrelated to pregnancy, in connection with some disorder of the ovaries. It is seen most frequently among women who are taking birth control pills. Strangely, it tends to persist in such instances even after the person discontinues the use of "the pill."

What to Do

1. There is no satisfactory method for causing the darkened areas of melasma to disappear.

2. Direct exposure to sunlight should be avoided.

3. The use of a bleaching cream, such as 2 percent hydroquinone cream ("Eldoquin"), sometimes makes the blotches less conspicuous. The cream is rubbed into the involved skin areas twice daily. If skin irritation results, the cream should be applied less frequently.

SEBORRHEIC KERATOSIS.

Seborrheic keratosis is a condition in which many, small, slightly raised lesions develop on the skin of a middle-aged or elderly person. The lesions are simple tumors, but they are not dangerous. They are not malignant and they have no tendency to become malignant. They are the most common type of skin tumor occurring in elderly persons.

The lesions of seborrheic keratosis are usually numerous. They occur on the face, including the forehead, on the neck, on the chest, and on the back. They vary in size, even in the same person, from a few millimeters in diameter to as much as several centimeters across. Most commonly they are only slightly darker than the surrounding skin, but some may be dark brown, even black. They are round in shape (or oval) and are sharply demarcated from the surrounding skin. They are covered with a greasy crust which is loosely attached. When the crust is removed, the base appears raw and pulpy and bleeds slightly. The surface of the lesion is smooth and shiny and may be crisscrossed by clefts. The lesion is soft and can be rolled between the fingers.

The lesions of seborrheic keratosis produce no symptoms except itching which, in some cases, is intense.

What to Do

1. It is important for the person with skin lesions of the type described above to see his doctor or a specialist in skin diseases to make sure of the diagnosis. In some cases the lesions may be mistaken for those of a much more serious skin disorder such as melanoma which is malignant.

2. Once the diagnosis of seborrheic keratosis is confirmed, then the only reason for the lesions to be removed is to relieve the itching, if present, or for cosmetic reasons.

3. The lesions can be removed by a rather simple surgical procedure which, when performed by a specialist, leaves little or no scar.

STASIS DERMATITIS AND STASIS ULCER

This disease involves a deterioration of the tissues of the skin in the legs which follows an interference with or slackening of the flow of blood through the veins of the legs. The condition frequently develops over a period of several years, often in the wake of known disease of the veins of the legs, such as varicose veins or thrombophlebitis. The skin itches, becomes reddened, and sometimes swells. Small injuries heal slowly, and the healed areas are scarred and pigmented (brown). As the condition worsens, injured areas fail to heal and ulcers form.

What to Do

1. Avoid standing in one position for long periods of time.

2. When seated, elevate the legs to the level of the hips.

3. In stubborn cases, elevate the foot of the bed about four inches above the level of the head of the bed to facilitate the return of blood from the legs during sleep.

4. If the veins of the leg are prominent, use elastic bandage or elastic hose to minimize the stagnation of blood in the veins.

5. Engage in exercise requiring the use of the legs as the general condition may permit.

6. Use leg baths with contrasting hot and cold water (three minutes of hot followed by a few seconds of cold, then repeat, up to fifteen minutes per treatment) two or three times per day.

7. Take precautions against bumps and injuries to the skin of the legs.

8. If an ulcer develops, a physician must use surgical techniques for removing fragments of dead tissue from the base of the ulcer. Use antibiotic ointment or powder to minimize the infection. Cover with a "pressure sandwich" type of dressing, gently applied, to minimize the stagnation of blood in the area.

VITILIGO (LEUKODERMA).

Vitiligo is a condition in which spots on the skin completely lose their normal pigment, or from birth have no pigment. The cause is not known, except that a hereditary tendency has been noticed in many cases. The condition, however, often accompanies psoriasis or arthritis. There is no known cure, but it is comforting to know that vitiligo causes no physical distress and does not harm the general health. The white patches on the skin are especially subject to sunburn, and tanning of the surrounding skin makes them more noticeable.

What to Do

1. Because the white patches are subject to sunburn, apply a sunscreen lotion to the exposed white spots before going into the sunlight.

2. Some persons with vitiligo receive benefit from a deliberate effort to tan the skin. A product called Trisoralen is first taken by mouth. Two hours later the skin is exposed briefly to natural sunlight or to ultraviolet light. The procedure is repeated on subsequent days as the physician may direct.

3. A skin dye is sold under the trade name of Dy-o-derm or Neo-Dyoderm. It is available in light and dark shades. It can be painted on the light skin areas to make them appear like the surrounding areas of normal color. For large areas, covering cosmetics such as Covermark or Erace are very useful.

WHITEHEAD (MILIUM).

Milia, or whiteheads, are small, comparatively firm masses of sebaceous material, similar to blackheads but never infected, and covered by the outer layer of the skin instead of extending up to or above the surface. They are usually located on the eyelids, cheeks, or temples, causing slight elevations of the skin which may be felt as tiny, hard nodules.

The development of whiteheads is hard to explain, but they are painless and harmless, though when numerous they give an unattractive appearance. They are usually associated with acne in teenagers or with aging skin in mature individuals.

What to Do

After sterilizing the affected skin area with 2 percent tincture of iodine, shell out the small masses by carefully opening the tops of the small nodules with a sterilized needle and gently squeezing them out. A blackhead remover will be helpful in this.

Nail Disorders

Nearly all abnormalities of the nails result from one or another of the following: congenital defects, accidental damage to the nail bed, bacterial infections, fungous infections, or some disease that affects the entire body or the skin in the region of the nails. Those abnormalities caused by systemic diseases usually correct themselves when these diseases are successfully treated. Until a study of the individual case is made by a physician, preferably a skin specialist, not much can be done about nail disorders of this sort.

Such a study is strongly urged, since some of the possible causative diseases—such as syphilis or psoriasis—should never go without treatment. This is especially true of syphilis, which may easily be present without the victim's knowledge. Syphilis, if present may have disastrous later results. See chapter 30 of this volume, "Venereal Infections."

Brittleness of the nails may be caused by sluggish thyroid action, hypochromic anemia, or long use of fingernail polish. Thyroid tablets will improve the nails if their brittleness is due to sluggish thyroid action, but they should never be taken without a physician's supervision. A blood count, with careful study of the blood cells, will either prove or rule out hypochromic anemia.

If the use of fingernail polish is the cause, discontinuing its use will be curative. Sometimes simply anointing the nails nightly with olive or castor oil will help toughen them, especially if dressings are applied to keep the oil from being rubbed off during sleep. The following cream, which should also be applied every night, is better than oil in some cases:

Lanolin	1
White wax	1
White petrolatum	3
Triethanolamine	4
Water q.s. ad	30

NAIL DISEASES.

The four involvements of the fingernails or toenails shown here relate to other skin diseases or in the case of koilonychia to a systemic disease.

Onychomycosis is considered elsewhere in the chapter under "Ringworm of the Nails." The patient should not attempt self-treatment of this disease because it is difficult to arrest. The physician may have to remove a considerable portion of the affected nail or nails and then prescribe medicated applications more potent than for usual manifestations of fungous disease.

The nails become involved in at least 15 percent of the cases of psoriasis (see under "Psoriasis"). The treatment of psoriasis of the nails is the same as for the disease in general.

Eczema often affects the nails when this disease involves the hands or feet. In such cases soothing lotions frequently prove helpful. The more heroic forms of treatment such as the corticosteroids are used only, of course, under the physician's supervision.

Koilonychia is usually associated with some such disease as anemia, thyroid disorder, or syphilis. It responds to the treatment of the parent disease.

INGROWING TOENAIL.

In this condition the skin and flesh at one or both corners of a nail, usually the nail of the great toe, become tender and often inflamed. Shoes that are either too short or too narrow across the toes may cause this trouble. High heels may also cause it by throwing the foot forward so that the toes are pushed into and pinched by the pointed front of the shoe. A faulty method of trimming the nails may also cause ingrowing toenails. The nails should be cut straight across and left long enough so there is no flesh in front of the corners. If they are cut short, especially if rounded at the corners, the skin and flesh are pressed inward in front of these corners, and as

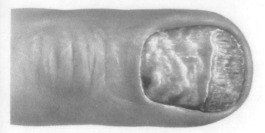

Onychomycosis. From fungi invasion.

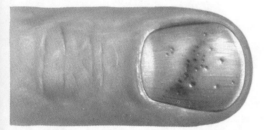

Psoriasis. Note typical depressions.

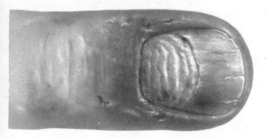

Eczema. Longitudinal splitting distinctive.

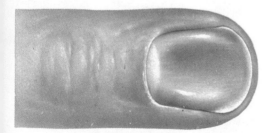

Koilonychia. Gives "spoon nail" effect.

the nail grows it cuts into the skin and flesh and makes the trouble.

What to Do

1. As a preventive measure, cut the toenails as suggested above.

2. If a toenail is already ingrown, proceed as follows:

Apply a strip of adhesive plaster, drawing it around *under* the toe and attaching the ends so as to pull the skin and flesh away from the corners and edges of the nail.

Gently pack a small amount of oiled cotton or a bit of oiled gauze under the buried edge and corner of the nail.

If the toe is inflamed, give alternate hot and cold foot baths twenty minutes night and morning. (See volume 3, chapter 20.)

Cut a V-groove in the nail near the sore side and parallel to it, going as deep as possible without drawing blood.

If all these treatments fail, consult a physician, who can cure the condition by a simple operation.

PARONYCHIA.

Paronychia is an inflammatory or infectious situation affecting the tissues which surround the fingernails, or occasionally, the toenails. The affected tissues become swollen, and extremely tender and may exude pus. In the most persistent cases, the nail plate becomes thickened and discolored with noticeable transverse ridges. Oftentimes several fingers are involved at the same time.

Paronychia develops in persons whose hands are immersed in water a great deal. In such, a slight injury to the finger allows bacteria or fungi to invade the tissues surrounding the nail. The susceptibility is greater in persons with diabetes or those whose nutrition is deficient.

What to Do

1. Guard the fingers against all kinds of mechanical injury (bruises, etc.).

2. Wash the hands only briefly and as seldom as possible. Dry the fingers gently and thoroughly after each washing.

3. Avoid all other contacts of the hands with water. When it becomes necessary to immerse the hands (as when washing dishes) wear cotton gloves next to the skin and cover these with rubber gloves.

4. If the infection becomes severe, consult a physician who may prescribe an antibiotic medicine to combat the infection.

5. For chronic (persisting) paronychia apply a medicated cream or solution designed to combat bacterial and fungus infections. Apply the medication to the affected areas at least twice a day. Suitable preparations are (1) Mycolog cream, (2) 2 percent gentian violet in isopropyl alcohol, or (3) Carbol-Fuchsin solution (Castellani's paint).

Neoplastic Diseases

CANCER (CARCINOMA) OF THE SKIN.

Cancer of the skin occurs more frequently in human beings than any other kind of cancer. Fortunately there is a higher rate of success in treating cancer of the skin than in any other kind of cancer—but it must be treated in order to avoid an unfavorable outcome. Persons between the ages of 40 and 60 are the most likely to develop cancer of the skin.

Skin cancers are new growths of epithelial cells of the skin, tending to spread into surrounding tissues, or giving rise to the transfer of such cells from one organ or part of the body to another. Some skin cancers begin as small scaly or warty spots called keratoses, from which thick scales tend to loosen and fall off from time to time. Others begin as waxy pimples or small, whitish, blackheadlike, nodules. Since they are of various types, it requires special training and experience to tell one type from another, or to tell whether or not some suspicious growth or nodule on the skin is really cancerous. Many that are cancerous are mixed or intermediate in type, so are not characteristic of either type.

Cancers which begin as scaly or warty spots tend to grow rather rapidly, becoming both broader and deeper and eventually forming large ulcers that bleed easily. These ulcers are surrounded by narrow zones of hard tissue. As they become larger, malignant cells often spread from them through lymph channels to surrounding and underlying structures. Rarely they spread through the bloodstream to distant parts of the body, especially the lungs. In the early stages, both pain and itching are slight or entirely absent, which may cause one to ignore the condition until it has spread far enough and deep enough to be really dangerous. Later there is more or less pain. After an extensive spread has taken place, no treatment can save life. Fortunately, the growth or spread is not so rapid that a really watchful person cannot seek for examination and treatment in time. Some skin cancers are up to 98 percent curable when treated properly. But some forms of skin cancer, such as the melanoma, have a far lower rate of cure.

Cancers that begin as waxy pimples or whitish or blackheadlike nodules are inclined to grow very slowly as a rule, forming small and comparatively shallow ulcers in the centers of broad, firm nodules. Causing very little pain, such cancers may spread over considerable areas before they begin to travel through lymph or blood channels. They are therefore less dangerous than the other type, but it is still not safe to let them go untreated.

Overexposure of the skin to sunlight is the principal cause of skin cancer, especially if the skin is dry, harsh, and of a complexion that does not easily tan. Repeated or continuous irritation of any kind also has a causative influence. Pipe smokers' cancer of the lip is a common form caused by irritation by pipestems. Irritation by

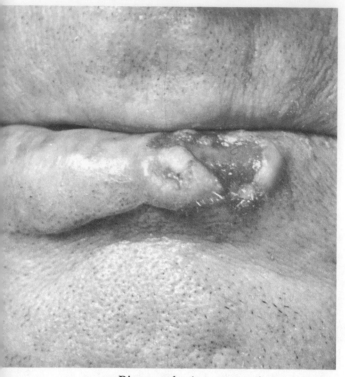

Pipe smoker's cancer of the lip is
a common form of skin cancer.

soot, paraffin, tar, or lubricating oils of
petroleum origin is especially likely
to cause cancer of the skin. Tampering
with the waxy pimples or the nodules
will hasten their malignant development.

Skin cancer occurs most frequently
on the face or on the skin of other
exposed parts of the head. The neck,
back of the hands, and genital regions
are also fairly common sites of skin
cancer. Other areas of the body
surface are rarely affected.

What to Do

1. If some waxy pimple or scaly or
warty spot appears on the skin, does
not itch, yet persists more than one
to three months, consult a physician, preferably a dermatologist,
without further delay. Let him
make a study to determine whether
or not the spot is, or may become,
cancerous. Nothing short of complete destruction or removal of the

seemingly simple but possibly
malignant growth is safe; and the
sooner the better. The physician
may use surgery, radiation therapy,
cautery, or cryosurgery (freezing of
the tissue) for treatment.

2. Do not try caustics, pastes, or
ointments on your own responsibility or on the recommendation of
others.

KELOID.

Keloids are overgrowth of scar
tissue or of tissue similar to that in
scars, which continue to grow and
form nodules or irregular tumors.
They usually result from injury such
as burns, surgery, or disease, the new
growth of tissue persisting and often
involving adjoining healthy skin.
Keloids, however, are not malignant,
and they do not endanger life.

The tendency to form keloids seems
to run in families and is more common
in blacks than in people with fair skin.
They may cause mild pricking and
burning sensations, and they are often
tender and painful. They are difficult
to treat successfully since they tend to
recur after removal.

What to Do

1. Do not try home treatment. It
will not succeed.

2. Consult a dermatologist (a
physician who specializes in diseases of the skin). The methods of
treatment with the best prospect of
success include radiation therapy,
cryosurgery (freezing), and the injection into the keloid of a particular kind of corticosteroid substance.
The simple surgical removal of a
keloid is not satisfactory because of
the probability that the keloid will
recur in the new surgical scar.

LIPOMA (FATTY TUMOR).

A lipoma is a benign and painless
tumor made up of fat cells and
developing in or close beneath the
skin. There is little danger that a
lipoma—a soft, slowly growing, freely
movable tumor—will ever become

malignant; but it may become the seat of gangrene or of fat necrosis. Even though this may not happen, if such tumors are large or numerous they may cause awkwardness of motion, discomfort from weight or from irritation, and a very ugly appearance. Surgical removal is simple and safe.

What to Do

1. Do not try home treatments. They will prove useless.

2. If the tumor is large enough to cause discomfort, to interfere with normal body movements, to be sore on account of irritation, or is located where it is unsightly, have it removed by a surgeon.

WEN (SEBACEOUS CYST).

A wen is an abnormally developed sebaceous or oil gland, resulting in a growth or sac filled with an oily or fatty material, usually appearing on the scalp, the neck, or the face, but sometimes on other parts of the body. The growth starts with a plugging of the gland outlet, or with some unusual activity of its secreting portion, resulting in a sac lined with the lining membrane of the gland and containing material similar to that secreted by the gland. Growth may continue for months or years, but eventually ceases, in some cases while the tumor is still quite small. Large wens, however, are not unusual. They may be from one to several in number, and from the size of a pea to that of an orange. They may be whitish, pinkish, or purplish in color. They may be either soft, doughy, elastic, or firm to the touch.

Wens seldom show up before middle age, and almost never during the growing years of life. They are rarely tender or painful, but may eventually become chronically inflamed and form pus. Very rarely, they may become malignant in elderly people. When located on the scalp—where they are most often found—the skin over a wen is usually bald, the hair follicles having either been killed or

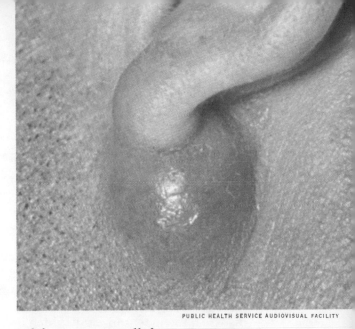

Sebaceous cyst, called a wen, commonly appears on the neck or face.

having their activity stopped by the pressure of the growing tumor. Surgical removal of a wen is advisable, not only for the sake of appearance but also for safety. The operation is simple and safe, and is permanently successful if care is taken to remove the entire sac as well as its contents.

What to Do

Have the tumor surgically removed. Any other treatment is useless.

Parasitic Diseases

GROUND ITCH (CUTANEOUS ANCYLOSTOMIASIS).

(See chapter 21 of this volume under *Roundworm Infections*.)

BODY LICE (PEDICULOSIS CORPORIS).

A body louse is slightly larger than a head louse, and it is usually grayish in color. It lives in the seams of the underclothing most of the time, particularly in the regions of the back, the chest, and the waistline, laying its eggs there. The eggs hatch in about six days, the young being ready to reproduce in about two weeks. They invade the skin of the body only when they wish to feed.

211

The presence of body lice causes severe itching. If the clothing has recently been changed, the lice may be hard to find on the body. The itching, however, the bloody spots or streaks which result from scratching, and the location of the same are enough to indicate the nature of the disease. The parasites themselves can usually be found in considerable numbers in the seams of underclothing worn for a few days or longer. The infestation is spread by body contact, by wearing infested clothing, or by sleeping in an infested bed.

Body lice are known to be able to transmit several different infectious diseases, the most serious of which is typhus fever.

What to Do

1. Do not sleep in underwear worn during the daytime. Underwear, hose, and bedclothes that will not be harmed by boiling should be boiled for ten minutes in soapsuds. Pressing the seams of clothing with a hot iron will kill many of the lice and their eggs.

2. Every seven days until the condition is cured, lather the entire body (trunk, arms, and legs) for four minutes in a shower with Kwell Shampoo. Rinse very thoroughly at the end of the four minutes.

3. If the skin continues to be inflamed, the doctor may prescribe corticosteroid ointments and/or antibiotic medication.

CRAB LICE (PEDICULOSIS PUBIS).

The crab louse, smaller than either the head louse or the body louse, translucent in appearance and nearly round in form, usually infests the hair-covered part of the pubic region. It may, however, be found on other

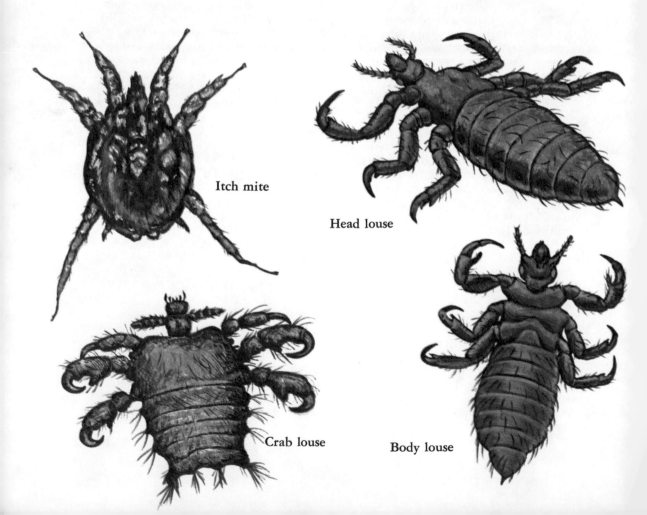

Itch mite

Head louse

Crab louse

Body louse

hairy regions of the body, though rarely on the scalp. The bite of this louse causes a sensation like a sharp pinprick. It produces intense itching and often a skin eruption, which may become severe enough to resemble eczema. The infestation is spread by body contact as a rule—most often at the time of sexual intercourse—though sometimes by means of infested toilet seats. The infestation is often considered a disgrace because of its being associated with promiscuity. It is frequently mentioned in connection with venereal disease because in both cases illicit intercourse is a common method of spread.

What to Do

1. Shave or clip the hair from the infested regions, burn this hair.

2. Wash the area or areas daily with soap and warm water. After washing, apply a 25 percent emulsion of benzyl benzoate or Kwell lotion each morning for three mornings. This kills the "nits" by dissolving them off the hair stumps.

3. When the eyelashes are involved, use a 0.25 percent physostigmine ophthalmic ointment (0.25 percent Eserine Ophthalmic Ointment) twice a day for 10 days.

4. Other persons who may have been exposed should be treated in the same manner. Clothing, toilet seats, and bedsheets should be sterilized.

5. If the skin continues to be inflamed, apply Crotamiton cream or lotion (Eurax).

HEAD LICE (PEDICULOSIS CAPITIS).

The presence of head lice on the scalp causes severe itching. Scratching, which is almost sure to occur, causes the oozing of fluid, watery at first, but later pussy or bloody. This fluid usually dries and forms crusts, but may remain sticky and mat the hair. It has a bad odor.

The lice live at the base of the hairs, near the scalp. They are quite dark in color and large enough to be seen easily with the unaided eye. During the short space of six days, a female louse can lay as many as fifty eggs. These are glued to the hair shafts and can easily be seen, being white in color. They hatch in from three to eight days, and the young lice are able to reproduce in two weeks. Infestation from one person to another is usually spread by personal contact or by the wearing of infested headgear. Since body lice are known to transmit typhus fever and certain other diseases, some medical authorities believe that head lice may also transmit them.

What to Do

1. Shampoo the scalp with ordinary shampoo preparation to remove oil and dirt, and rinse thoroughly. Then apply Kwell Shampoo and rub vigorously for four minutes; rinse thoroughly and dry.

2. Comb the hair with a fine-tooth comb to remove all remaining ova (nits). Brushes and combs should be treated with Kwell Shampoo after each use.

3. Shampoo the scalp again, as above, in seven days.

4. If the scalp becomes infected, the physician may prescribe antibiotic medication and/or corticosteroid ointment.

SCABIES (THE ITCH).

Scabies is a contagious skin disease caused by the itch mite, which bores beneath the surface of the skin, forming burrows. The disease is characterized by intense itching, especially at night, and by a form of eczema caused by scratching. The mite is yellowish-white and barely large enough to be seen by the unaided eye. The female, which is larger than the male, burrows into the skin to lay its eggs. The burrow may be either straight or crooked, is an eighth of an inch (3 mm.) or more in length, and looks somewhat like a very narrow and light pencil mark.

The itch mite seems to prefer the tenderest parts of the skin, such as the webs between the fingers, the inner surfaces of the forearms, thighs, and legs, the armpits, the breasts, the buttocks, and the navel. The face, scalp, palms, and soles are rarely attacked, but breast-fed infants are an exception to this rule. When one member of a family is infested, other members are very likely to become so.

Severe inflammation, with the development of papules, blisters, pustules, and crusts, may come as a result of infection from scratching. The disease may become fully developed within two weeks; the eggs hatch in about six days, and the parasites grow very rapidly. It may persist for months or even years if not recognized or properly treated. It is transmitted by body contact with others suffering from it, or by sleeping in an infested bed or wearing infested clothing.

What to Do

1. If the skin has infected scratch marks or pustules on it, this infection should be treated first before giving treatment for the itch itself. For this purpose, use Neosporin ointment rubbed into the affected skin four or five times a day.

2. Then every night for three nights apply an ointment such as mentioned in the next paragraph to the entire body from the level of the mouth and earlobes downward. Do not leave any area uncovered with the ointment, or the condition may recur. Be sure to apply it beneath the toenails and fingernails and all about the genital regions as well.

Many different ointments have been used in treating scabies. Some of the patent ointments have proved most effective. Among these, Eurax and Kwell may be mentioned.

3. Use the same underclothes, nightclothes, and sheets throughout the course of the treatment.

4. The first night, before applying the ointment, scrub the entire body with soap and warm water. Each night, apply new ointment without washing off the old ointment. If it is impossible to leave the ointment on during the daytime, wash it off each morning, but continue the treatment for five days instead of three.

5. The next night following the nights of the treatment, take a thorough hot bath and change into clean sheets, nightclothes, and underclothes. All clothes used before and during the treatment should be disinfected by dry cleaning, washing in cleaning solvent, sending them to a laundry, or boiling.

6. Immediately after completing the course of ointment treatment outlined above, apply 1 percent phenol in calamine lotion four or five times a day as a soothing and drying lotion.

7. If the skin still feels irritated, take starch baths for half an hour once or twice a day, mixing one or two cupfuls of Linit starch in a tub of bath water.

8. One week after completing the treatment program, if it seems that the condition is not entirely cleared up, repeat the treatment with ointment, et cetera.

Sweating Disorders

Three sweating disorders are common enough to merit discussion here: *anhidrosis,* or lack of sweat; *bromidrosis,* or foul-smelling sweat; and *hyperhidrosis,* or too profuse sweat.

Anhidrosis may be caused by sluggish action of the autonomic nerves. The condition may be present from the time of birth. It is a common symptom in ichthyosis, extensive psoriasis, and vitamin A deficiency. If the causative condition can be determined, the anhidrosis can sometimes be corrected, but this is often difficult. As a rule, the best that can be accomplished by way of relief is through care in adjusting to the weather. Cocoa butter, lanolin, or some other soothing creamy application may be used to relieve the dryness and harshness of the skin.

Bromidrosis is usually the result of fermentation, bacterial infection, or a chemical change in the perspiration after it has escaped from the sweat glands onto the skin surface. It is most obvious on parts of the body where perspiration is free but cannot readily evaporate, such as the armpits, or the feet if confined in poorly ventilated shoes. Certain foods, drugs, and germs give the perspiration characteristic odors, and some of these are unpleasant. As to this kind of bromidrosis, the only effective preventive measure is obvious. Bromidrosis affecting the feet or the armpits calls for more than usual care in cleanliness, with perhaps a change to better ventilated shoes or clothing.

Hyperhidrosis may affect the whole skin surface or only parts of it, such as the hands, feet, brow, et cetera. Nervous tension or fear may cause it. If small, circumscribed areas of the skin are affected, increased activity of one or more of the autonomic ganglia may be to blame. In such diseases as tuberculosis, malaria, undulant fever, exophthalmic goiter, and diabetes, profuse sweating is common at times. When the underlying cause of the hyperhidrosis is corrected, the excessive sweating is usually checked, but this requires effective treatment of any systemic disease that may be present.

What to Do

1. **Cleanliness is the first requisite in controlling the unpleasant features of either bromidrosis or hyperhidrosis. A daily bath, with change of underclothing and hose, is recommended.**

2. **A 5 percent solution of alum or zinc sulfate in 70 percent alcohol, dabbed on the surface of the affected skin areas and allowed to dry on, may be helpful. Commercial antiperspirant preparations available at the drugstore (such as those containing compounds of**

aluminum) **often work well when applied according to directions after a thorough cleansing of the skin. The use of such a preparation should be stopped, however, if skin irritation results.**

3. **A good powder for dusting on the skin of the feet and sprinkling into the socks or stockings is made as follows:**

Salicylic acid	1
Aluminum chloride	1
Powdered alum	3
Starch	15
Talcum powder	15
Mix thoroughly	

Virus Diseases

COLD SORE (FEVER BLISTER, HERPES SIMPLEX).

(See chapter 28 of this volume under *Herpes Simplex.*)

SHINGLES (HERPES ZOSTER).

Shingles is an acute and painful inflammatory virus disease affecting the skin overlying one or more sensory nerve trunks. The virus that causes shingles is the same kind of virus as causes chickenpox (varicella). The skin eruption of shingles is characterized by groups of small blisters on inflamed red skin areas. The skin eruption breaks out in crops, each succeeding crop tending to locate nearer the end of the related nerve trunk than did the preceding crop. The groups of blisters, each with a red base, dry and form crusts after a week or two. When the crusts fall off, scars are sometimes left. The blisters sometimes become pustules before drying. In severe cases they may turn into small spots of gangrene. The pain, neuralgic in character, may develop before the blisters appear; and it may persist for weeks, months, or years after all signs of the eruption are gone. This is especially true of elderly people, and outstandingly so when the forehead and face are involved.

The nerves which supply the skin of the chest are most likely to be affected. The eruption in a typical attack of shingles appears on one side of the chest, spreading from near the spinal column around almost to the breastbone. Nerves on both sides of the body, or more than one nerve on the same side, may be affected, with correspondingly widespread eruption. Occasionally nerves that supply the skin of the neck, arms, abdomen, or thighs are attacked; but second in frequency to the chest, shingles tends to appear on one side of the forehead and face, following the course of the supraorbital branch of the trigeminal nerve.

The usual course of the disease is four to six weeks. It is usually less severe in young persons than in old. Overwork, general debility, damp and chilly weather, or the absorption of certain drugs, particularly certain compounds of arsenic, or contact with a case of chicken pox, favor development of the disease. The specific cause, however, is a virus which affects both the nerve roots and the skin over them. One attack of shingles gives a high degree of immunity. Second attacks are rare.

Shingles. Note typical mini-blisters.

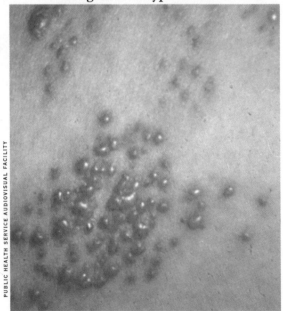

What to Do

1. The patient with shingles need not stay in the hospital. However, he should remain inactive for seven to fourteen days while the discomfort is severe.

2. An electric heating pad applied to the painful area or areas will relieve some of the discomfort.

3. Compresses moistened with Burow's solution (5 percent aluminum acetate solution) may be applied to the affected skin areas for fifteen to twenty minutes per day. At other times, calamine lotion may be applied sparingly.

4. Do not open the blisters that appear on the skin. If the skin breaks, the use of Bacitracin topical ointment will help to prevent the development of infection.

5. It is best to consult a physician in all cases of shingles, but especially in sever cases. Pain may be so severe that home treatments will not give relief.

6. In persons above 60 years of age who have shingles, there is the possibility that the pain will persist for long periods of time. This possibility is reduced by the administration (under a physician's supervision) of corticosteroid medication during the acute phase of the illness.

WART (VERRUCA).

A wart is an overgrowth of certain structures of the skin. There is conclusive evidence that warts are caused by a virus, and they are contagious under certain circumstances. They appear most commonly in the early years of life, rarely after the age of twenty; but they sometimes persist for years. While they must be distinguished from skin cancer, there is no proof that they never become cancerous. Though the largest and most troublesome warts occur on the soles of the feet or the external genital organs, they are most common on the hands. Small, slender, threadlike forms occur on the neck, the eyelids, and the bearded areas. This latter form may be spread by shaving.

What to Do

CAUTION: *Preparations containing salicylic acid, as in items (1) and (2) which follow, must not be used for a person who has diabetes.*

1. If located where they are readily accessible, common seed warts or flat warts may be safely treated by repeated applications of the following:

Salicylic acid	4
Acetone	15
Flexible collodion	15
Mix thoroughly	

CAUTION: *Take care not to smear this paste on the healthy skin.*

2. A 3 percent solution of salicylic acid in 40 percent alcohol may be used in the same way, with the same caution.

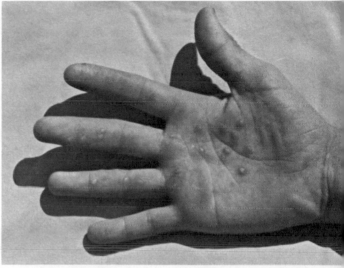

ELIAS PAPAZIAN

3. If the wart is large, not readily accessible, subject to irritation, or has persisted a long time, have it removed by a physician, preferably a skin specialist.

Disorders of the Skeletal Structures

I. Disorders of Bones, Ligaments, Muscles, and Tendons

Disorders of bones, ligaments, muscles, and tendons are considered together because all of these structures are important and related parts of a system which determines the general shape and posture of the body and enables it to move. There are many diseases that affect these structures primarily, and some in other parts of the body that can affect them secondarily. Disorders of body *movements* are more often caused by diseases or defects of the nervous system than by anything which directly involves the bones, ligaments, muscles, or tendons. Such disorders will be considered in discussions elsewhere in this volume, particularly in chapter 25.

ACHILLES TENDON CONTRACTURE.

This is a condition in which the foot becomes weakened and the calf of the leg and arch of the foot become painful. The condition is more common in women than in men and the symptoms most severe when the patient wears low shoes or goes barefoot. The cause is a shortening of the Achilles tendon (at the back of the ankle), usually brought on by the persistent wearing of high heels.

What to Do

Mild cases are improved by manipulation of the foot and a program of exercises in which the shortened tendon is gradually stretched. In more extreme cases, the tendon must be lengthened by a surgical procedure.

ARCH STRAIN.

(See *Flatfoot and Arch Strain* in this chapter.)

BACK PAIN AND BACKACHE.

Discomfort in the back, in its various forms, is one of the commonest of symptoms. Some causes for back pain originate in the skeletal and muscular structures of the back. These are discussed in the present chapter. Other causes originate in various organs or even in remote structures of the body. These are discussed appropriately in other chapters.

DISORDERS OF THE SKELETAL STRUCTURES

Obesity is a common cause of backache, causing poor posture and thus straining and fatiguing the structures of the back. Pain in the back is often referred from structures within the pelvis. Thus it occurs during menstruation, in pregnancy, and disease of the pelvic organs. Pain in the back commonly occurs in kidney disease. Backache is often an early symptom of an infectious disease. It can even result from nervous fatigue.

Diseases which cause partial destruction of the vertebrae cause backache.

Osteoarthritis of the spine is another cause. (See the following chapter on "Joint Diseases.") Fibrositis involving the muscles and ligaments of the back can be very painful. (See under *Fibrositis* in this chapter.) Fractures involving the bony structures of the back can be very painful. (See *Fractures, Fracture of the Back* in the chapter on "Handling Emergencies," volume 3, chapter 18.) Traumatic involvement of one or more of the intervertebral disks can produce pain in the back and also in the arms or legs, depending on which level of the vertebral column is involved.

Intervertebral Disk Involvement. The vertebral column (spinal column) is the mainstay of the skeleton. It is therefore subject to tremendous mechanical forces, as in lifting, jumping, twisting, and carrying heavy weights. Between each vertebra and its neighbor there is interposed a cushionlike disk of fibrocartilage (an intervertebral disk). It is these disks, by way of their resiliency, that permit the bending and twisting movements of which the vertebral column is capable.

Also between the body processes of each vertebra and its neighbor there emerges a pair of spinal nerves—nerves leading from the spinal cord to some particular part of the body or the extremities.

Under recurring forces of pressure the substance of the intervertebral

Herniations of the intervertebral disk.

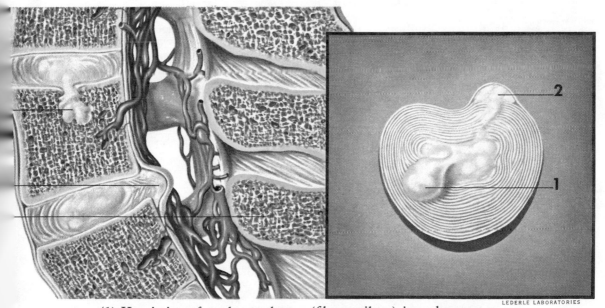

LEDERLE LABORATORIES

(1) Herniation of nucleus pulposus (fibrocartilage) into the spongiosa of the vertebra. (2) Herniation of nucleus pulposus beneath the posterior longitudinal ligament. (3) Spinous process.

disks may deteriorate and permit a portion of the disk substance to push its way against the root of an emerging spinal nerve, thus causing injury to the nerve and interfering with its function. This condition is often said to be caused by a "slipped disk" or a "herniated disk." The problem may occur at any level in the vertebral column, but most commonly it develops in the lower back where the nerves emerge that go to the thighs, legs, and feet.

Oftentimes the nerve that suffers is the sciatic nerve that passes down the back of the thigh. The painful symptoms occurring when the sciatic nerve is involved are often designated as "sciatica." A "slipped disk" is the most common, but not the only cause of sciatica.

The pain, usually limited to one side, is typically made worse by coughing, sneezing, and going to the toilet. It is aggravated by movement and by weight bearing. Often the muscles in the involved area go into spasm. There may be skin areas which lose their normal sensitiveness to pain or touch. Some of the muscles in the involved area may be weakened. Usually these symptoms will disappear completely in response to skillfull treatment.

What to Do

1. The victim of an injured intervertebral disk should be placed in a firm bed (as with a piece of plywood under the mattress) in the position of greatest comfort.

2. Local heat and massage to the painful areas may give comfort, as will also mild pain-relieving medicines and muscle relaxants (on a physician's order).

3. Pelvic traction may help to relieve the pressure of the nerve that has been compressed. This is accomplished most comfortably by the use of a pelvic belt to which weights are attached by means of cables and pulleys.

4 In obstinate cases surgical removal of the damaged portion of the disk and, possibly, a fusion of the vertebrae at the site of injury may become necessary.

BOWLEGS AND KNOCK-KNEES.

Bowing of the legs is normal in a newborn baby, and this condition tends to persist for at least a few months in most cases. The legs gradually become straighter as the child develops, so that bowlegs should not be considered a deformity except in cases where the normal straightening does not occur or is much delayed.

A child's legs are not likely to become permanently bowed from early walking *on his own initiative* if his diet contains adequate bone-building materials. Many children have walked at an age as young as nine months without prolonging or increasing the bowing of their legs. A knock-kneed baby is a rarity, but the change from early bowing may go on until knock-knees develop. This is more often true of girls than it is of boys.

Occasionally bowlegs or knock-knees are secondary to disorders of the growing centers of the bones at the knee, to brittle bones, or to such diseases as rickets, poliomyelitis, scurvy, cerebral palsy, et cetera. Overweight may be a causative factor. The habit of sitting on the floor with the knees flexed and the feet and legs to the outside of the thighs leads to knock-knees and "pigeon toes." In adults a recently developed deformity at the knee, usually on one side only, may be caused by osteomyelitis, a fracture, degenerative joint disease, or syphilis of the bones or the nervous system. There is no home remedy or treatment of value in such conditions. *Osteitis deformans* (Paget's disease), an incurable bone disease of unknown cause, sometimes results in the bowing of the legs of aged people. See more on this item in this chapter under *Osteitis deformans.*

What to Do

1. Prevention is of prime importance. If babies are given enough milk and foods containing an abundance of vitamins C and D and are are not urged to try to walk before they do so on their own initiative, bowlegs and knock-knees will not likely develop.

2. If, in spite of the above-advised preventive program, bowlegs do not correct themselves by the end of a child's second year, a physician should be consulted. He may advise the use of braces and/or modifications of the shoes to change the direction of weight-bearing thrust through the legs. In the meantime it may be helpful for a parent to stretch the child's legs in the direction of correction, applying barely enough pressure to make the child wince slightly, and repeating the pressure thirty to fifty times at least three times a day.

3. If the angle of deformity is 15 degrees or more and does not show improvement during the first few years of life, surgery is likely to be necessary for correction. This is more often performed for knock-knees than for bowlegs.

BUNIONS.

A bunion is a tender and painful enlargement of the joint tissues, including bone, at the base of the great toe. The enlargement appears greater than it really is because the entire great toe is now inclined to the side of the foot in the direction of the little toe. Bunions usually develop at the same time on both feet.

Bunions are the direct result of the wearing of shoes which are too narrow, too short, or too pointed. The narrow shoe subjects this joint to increased pressure and friction during walking. The short or pointed shoe does the same by bending the end of the great toe toward the others, thus making the joint more prominent and more subject to pressure irritation.

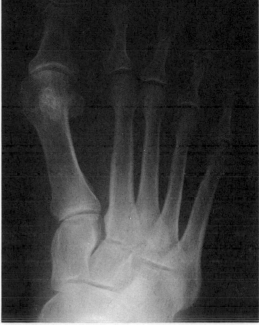

ELSTON ROTHERMEL, D.P.M.

The irritation of the injured structures stimulates overgrowth of all involved tissues. The longer the irritation continues, the greater the deformity will be. In severe cases, the great toe is virtually dislocated from the corresponding bone of the foot.

What to Do

1. Wear shoes of such a size and shape as to allow the great toe to assume its normal straight-forward position. This will relieve the pressure on the affected joint. Then, by using soft padding between the great toe and the second toe, try to push the great toe over into as nearly as possible its normal position.

2. Rest and a hot foot bath will bring relief in mild cases. Afterward, the callused skin may be pared away and the area protected by a bunion plaster.

3. Surgery is sometimes necessary for a cure, but it may leave the tissues as tender and sensitive as before.

BURSITIS.

Bursas are membranous sacs or pockets situated in many parts of the body, but chiefly near joints, especially the shoulder, elbow, or knee,

221

where tendons or muscles must slide over other tendons, muscles, or bony prominences, and where need to reduce friction occurs. The walls of the sacs are similar to thin ligaments in structure, and their lining secretes a lubricating fluid similar to that in joints.

When the lining of a bursa becomes inflamed, whether infected or not, the condition is called bursitis. There is pain on movement, tenderness on pressure, usually some swelling, and sometimes eventually a deposit of calcium salts in the bursa or its walls. Keeping the affected part quiet and improving its circulation are rational aims in treatment. To stop motion may involve putting the part in a cast or splinting it.

What to Do

1. Keep the affected part as quiet as possible. Apply fomentations or alternate hot and cold compresses to the painful area twice a day, whichever gives the most relief. (See volume 3, chapter 20.)

2. If shoulder stiffness is present, bending the body forward and making pendulum motions of the arms backward and forward and from side to side, will help restore the normal range of joint motion; but these motions must not be made too rapidly or with any force.

3. Diathermy, needling, or injections of a local anesthetic into the affected region may be given by a physician with benefit; or he may use one or more of several other treatments.

4. If healing does not take place with such a course of treatment, it may become necessary to use surgery to remove such calcium deposits as may be present or to obliterate the sac permanently.

CLUBFOOT.

The usual type of clubfoot with which an infant is born involves a malposition of the structures which form the foot's framework, but with the structures all present. If the foot is allowed to continue its development in this abnormal position, a crippling deformity results.

What to Do

Professional care should be arranged as soon as the condition is recognized. In many cases, a manipulation of the foot into normal position with a cast to hold it in this position for a few weeks or months will cause it to develop normally. Corrective exercises and corrective shoes may be necessary for a while during early childhood. In more serious cases, surgical correction is required.

CURVATURE OF THE SPINE (KYPHOSIS, LORDOSIS, SCOLIOSIS).

Spinal curvature in which the *hump* is toward the back (hunchback) is called *kyphosis;* that with the *hollow*

X rays of clubfoot.

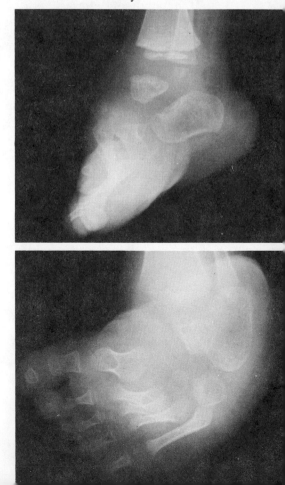

toward the back is called *lordosis;* and when the curvature is *side-to-side*, it is called *scoliosis*. Many cases of curvature are caused by long-continued faulty posture. Bad posture is more likely to cause spinal curvature if the muscles of the trunk become weak through lack of proper exercise.

Many cases of lateral curvature, or scoliosis, come from unknown causes. Some result from poliomyelitis, where imbalance of the back muscles results in the curvature. Malformations dating from birth are the cause of scoliosis in very few cases. Kyphosis used to be most often caused by tuberculosis of the spine, which is now quite rare. This type of kyphosis is usually sharp or angular—quite localized as compared with the gradual curve of the rounded back which results from irritation of the growing centers of the vertebrae during adolescence, or from the softening of the bone itself in elderly people.

What to Do

1. Watch children while growing up so that any faulty posture which seems to be promoting spinal curvature can be corrected in time. Such curvature may begin to develop as early as the age of ten or twelve years.

2. See that children in school are provided with seats and desks of proper height and adjusted so as to favor a normal sitting posture. The habit of carrying books always under the same arm or always on the same side of the body should be corrected.

3. If a noticeable curvature develops despite the above precautions, or as a result of neglect or disease, consult a physician, preferably an orthopedic specialist. Braces, plaster casts, special exercises, or even surgery may be needed to correct the condition.

Deformities of the spine: (1) Scoliosis, lateral curvature (observe the lowering of the right shoulder); (2) kyphosis (hunchback); (3) lordosis (note how curvature forms a hollow).

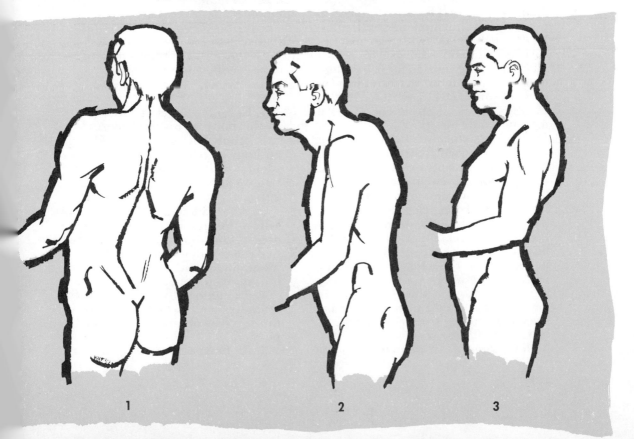

1   2   3

DISK, INTERVERTEBRAL.

(See *Back Pain and Backache* in this chapter.)

DISLOCATIONS.

(See under *Dislocations* in the chapter on "Handling Emergencies," volume 3, chapter 18.)

DYSTROPHY.

(See *Muscular Dystrophy* in this chapter.)

FIBROSITIS (MUSCULAR RHEUMATISM).

Fibrositis is an inflammation of white fibrous tissue anywhere in the body. Since tendons, ligaments, joint capsules, layers of fascia, the fibrous network underlying the skin, the covering of the bones, and the sheaths surrounding nerves, whole muscles, or smaller bundles of muscle fibers are all composed of this type of tissue, fibrositis may attack any or all of these structures. The inflammation often results in the formation of tender or painful nodules, cords, or bands in the muscles or elsewhere. Many physicians believe that focuses of infection occasionally, but more often allergies, have much to do with causing fibrositis. Probably the constitutional makeup of the individual is the chief deciding factor, as the tendency to develop fibrositis seems to run in families. Lack of sufficient exercise may be contributory.

When the sheaths of muscles or of bundles of muscle fibers are involved, the condition is also called myositis, myalgia, or muscular rheumatism. If the affected muscles are located in the lower half of the back, a commoner name is lumbago; if in the scalp or the back of the neck, a persistent type of headache results; if in certain muscles in the side of the neck, a painful but usually temporary variety of wryneck develops, though this condition is more often caused by neuromuscular spasms resulting from emotional upsets or conflicts. (See more on this under *Wryneck*, in this chapter.)

When structures in the vicinity of joints are affected, the condition is often, though mistakenly, called rheumatism. Many cases of neuralgia are in fact cases of fibrositis affecting nerve sheaths. This is also true of occasional cases of sciatica.

Acute fibrositis may start with a sudden sharp pain or with gradually increasing distress. There is aching in the affected areas, and sharp stabs of pain are caused by jarring the parts or by motions that stretch the inflamed tissues. The condition may entirely clear up in a few days or weeks, or it may become chronic. Attacks tend to occur again and again, often seeming to be aggravated by mental shock, nerve tension, or exhaustion, frequently associated with physical overexertion or exposure to a draft or to damp or chilly weather.

Chronic fibrositis is characterized by dull aching and stiffness of the affected parts, worse after periods of physical inactivity such as sitting still for a long period of time. Moderate exercise, applications of dry heat, and taking certain drugs usually give temporary relief. Many cases are characterized by marked fatigability. The distress varies considerably from day to day. Susceptibility seems to increase with advancing age.

What to Do

1. Keep the affected part or parts of the body at rest and *warm*.

2. Apply hot fomentations for half an hour or dry heat in any convenient form for an hour or two at least twice a day. (See volume 3, chapter 20).

3. After the acute stage is past, follow the applications of heat with gentle, kneading massage over tender and nodular areas, and arrange for gradually increasing exercise of the affected parts.

4. In unusually severe cases, remedies or treatments requiring the services of a physician may be needed.

5. In persistent cases, or if there

are frequently repeated attacks, have a physician search for possible focuses of infection or allergies, and give suitable treatments for such as may be found.

FLATFOOT AND ARCH STRAIN.

The normal human foot has two arches. One is a side-to-side arch, formed by the bones and ligaments in the ball of the foot. The other is a front-to-back arch, one end of which is the ball of the foot and the other end the heel. This one is made up of two parts: The inner side, which forms the true arch, is for resilience in walking, running, et cetera; and the other side, which is almost flat, is for weight bearing. The arches are supported by muscles, ligaments, and a strong layer of fascia which covers the sole of the foot.

There are two different types of feet that some might call "flat." In one, the forefoot and heel are in proper alignment and all the arches are present, but the inner side of the front-to-back arch is of less than normal height. This type is not likely to cause trouble. The other type, more properly called a "pronated foot," is the one that causes the most difficulty. In this type, the inner bulge of the ankle and the inner curve of the foot just in front of this bulge are more pronounced than normal, the sole of the rear part of the foot is tipped outward, and there is a loss of the normal alignment of the heel with the forefoot, the latter appearing to be swung outward. (See accompanying diagram.)

Undue strain on an abnormally *high* arch may cause pain in the ball of the foot and lead to the formation of "hammertoe" in some or all of the toes.

Flatfoot with arch strain is caused by anything that will weaken or unduly strain the muscles that normally support the arches, that will rapidly increase the load that these arches must support, or that will throw long-continued strain on the ligaments. If a person whose muscles are

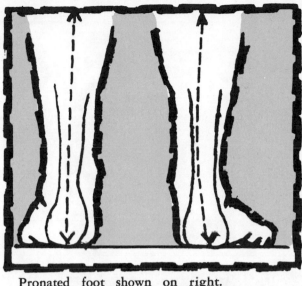

Pronated foot shown on right. Note the outward deviation of alignment, as compared with a normal foot, left.

weak from too little use suddenly begins to exercise his legs vigorously, the muscles are unable to support the arches of his feet. This throws an added burden on the ligaments, which stretch and allow the feet to flatten. The same result may come from a rapid increase in body weight. It may be caused by an occupation that involves the carrying of heavy weights, or standing for long periods without sufficient walking or active use of the feet to maintain the tone of the muscles. Flatfoot may also be congenital.

Discomfort from flatfoot usually begins when the strain on the muscles is great in proportion to their strength, and it is increased when the ligaments begin to stretch, allowing the bones to occupy an abnormal relation to each other. There is a sensation of weakness and strain about the inner side of the foot and ankle. After long standing, a dull ache in the calf of the leg, or a pain in the knee, the hip, or the back will be felt. Often, after overexertion, a sharp pain is noticed, radiating from the point of weakness. The victim finds it hard to buy comfortable shoes. Increasing discomfort from corns, bunions, enlarged great toe joints, and

225

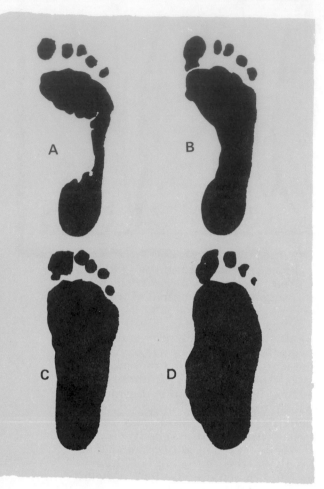

other deformities of the toes develops. Coldness, numbness, congestion, and increased perspiration of the feet, caused by weakness and a poor circulation, are very common.

Proper treatment of flatfoot gives good prospects for a cure, except in elderly people with arteriosclerosis. Cure, however, may take a long time. Perseverance is necessary. The advice and treatment which a good orthopedic surgeon can give are very helpful.

What to Do

1. Be sure that the shoes are correct. The following points should have attention:

a. Shoes should be long enough so that their tips are a thumb's breadth beyond the tips of the toes.

b. They must be wide enough to give complete freedom of toe action,

Left: Footprints on wet floor: A, of a normal foot; B, C, and D, of increasing degrees of flatfoot. Lower left: Diagram showing how arch support helps a patient suffering from flatfoot. Below: Normal distribution of body weight on the foot, the points bearing the major portion reflected in mirror.

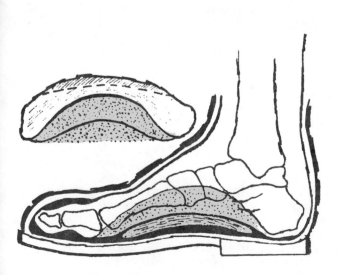

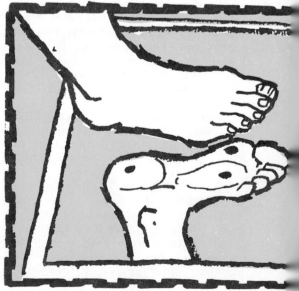

226

but not too wide, and should not have high heels.

c. The inner side of the shoe should form approximately a straight line from heel to toe.

d. It may help if the shoe heel is made about ³/₆ inch (5 mm.) higher on the inside and the sole raised about ¹/₈ inch (3 mm.) on the outside.

e. For a time, a properly fitting arch support worn inside the shoe is helpful, but this should either be fitted by a competent person or else not be worn at all.

2. In walking, do not turn the toes out, but try to throw the weight on the *outer* edges of the feet, and on *all the toes* at the "take-off" for each step.

3. Avoid standing a long time in one position, if possible; and, when this is not possible, stand "pigeon-toed" or with feet crossed.

4. When sitting down, cross the feet, but not the knees. This relieves strain on the stretched ligaments but does not impede the circulation to the feet.

5. In severe cases, massage and special exercises or appliances prescribed by an orthopedic surgeon will be necessary.

FRACTURES.

(See under *Fractures* in the chapter on "Handling Emergencies," volume 3, chapter 18.)

HEEL, PAINFUL (CALCANEAL SPUR).

Undue weight-bearing strain may cause the development of a bony spur in the tissues beneath the heel bone. This causes pain, of course, when weight is borne on the heel.

What to Do

1. Attach a ring-shaped pad of felt or sponge-rubber to the skin of the weight-bearing area of the heel, with the central area of the ring over the tender spot.

2. If the afflicted person is overweight, he should give consistent attention to bringing his weight within the normal range.

3. Hot foot baths followed by massage, once or twice a day, will increase the circulation of blood and help to relieve the discomfort.

HIP, CONGENITAL DISLOCATION.

Considerable progress has been made in recent years in the understanding of congenital dislocation of the hip. Formerly such cases were not recognized until the infant began trying to walk. When treatment was delayed this long, serious crippling defects resulted.

Now it is known that hip joints in these cases in which dislocation is in prospect are still in relatively normal position at the time of birth. The difference between one of these joints and a normal joint is that the process of ossification (formation of bone) in the structures that form the joint is delayed. The structures of the joint are of normal size and shape, but they still consist of cartilage rather than of bone. If such a joint is not treated before the age of two months, the muscles will have become sufficiently strong so that their pull begins to withdraw the head of the femur (the thigh bone) out of its socket. Often this pulling apart of the joint is not completed until the infant becomes old enough to attempt to stand.

What to Do

The secret of successful treatment in these cases of potential dislocation of the hip is early recognition and early treatment. That is, the abnormal condition should be recognized by two weeks of age or soon after. The evidence consists of a limitation in sideways motion of the affected thigh when the babe is lying on its back and the knees are flexed and drawn up partway toward the shoulders. Normally, at two weeks of age the thighs move sideways easily so that both can very nearly touch the bed at the same time. In a case of potential dislocation, the thigh on the affected side will move only partway in the sideways direction. Of course this observation should be evaluated by a physician, preferably a pediatrician or an orthopedic specialist.

Treatment at this early stage is relatively simple and consists of having the child wear a "Frejka splint"—a jumper-like device which keeps the infant's thighs spread apart. It is easily removed and reapplied whenever the baby's diapers are changed. When started early, the wearing of the splint need continue for only a few weeks.

HUNCHBACK.
(See *Curvature of the Spine* in this chapter.)

INTERVERTEBRAL DISK INVOLVEMENT.
(See *Back Pain and Backache* in this chapter.)

KNOCK-KNEES.
(See *Bowlegs and Knock-knees* in this chapter.)

KYPHOSIS.
(See *Curvature of the Spine* in this chapter.)

LUMBAGO
(See *Fibrositis* in this chapter.)

MUSCLE CRAMPS.
(See also *Cramps: C. Leg Cramps* in volume 3, chapter 22.)

Many persons are troubled with muscle cramps, particularly involving the muscles of the legs. Although this condition occurs more commonly in elderly people than in young people, the troublesome symptoms may occur at any age.

Painful muscle cramps are caused by any circumstance which interferes with a muscle's source of nutrition or its receiving oxygen or getting rid of carbon dioxide at the normal rate. It is the flow of blood through a muscle that brings energy food and oxygen and that carries away the carbon dioxide. It is the combination of energy food and oxygen within the muscle that produces muscle power. The by-product of this chemical action is carbon dioxide, which must be promptly carried away from the muscle in order for it to continue to function. Anything that interferes with the flow of blood through a muscle makes it susceptible to cramping. Overweight, anemia, poor nutrition, varicose veins, or diseases of the heart and arteries, if present, may reduce the supply of blood to the muscles of the legs. A person troubled with leg cramps should consult his doctor and ask for a complete physical checkup as a means of determining the basic cause of his symptom. The general health-building measures by which a person may overcome muscle cramps may be listed as follows:

What to Do

1. Ensure a sufficient quantity of milk in each day's diet. Milk contains calcium, which must be present in the tissues of the body if the cells are to function normally. Calcium, phosphorus, and sodium are particularly important for the normal functioning of the muscles. Though only about one part of calcium to 10,000 parts of blood is necessary, still when this small quantity is reduced by one half, the muscles become so irritable that they cramp readily. The diet should also include a supplement of vitamins and minerals, particularly vitamins B, C, and D.

2. Develop a good program of adequate physical exercise. For the person otherwise robust, walking (in preference to riding in a car), climbing stairs (in preference to taking the elevator), swimming, golfing, and playing tennis offer good opportunities to develop a

more adequate supply of blood to the muscles.

3. For persons not physically able to carry on active programs of exercise, other less rigorous means can be used to increase the circulation of blood and to develop the muscles. Warm baths followed by contrasting hot and cold showers serve to improve the general circulation. Muscle exercises which can be taken even by a person confined in bed, add their beneficial effects. Massage also helps to increase the circulation.

4. A heating pad (warm but not hot, placed next to the lower part of the back) will produce a reflex effect which enables the blood vessels of the legs to carry larger volumes of blood throughout the night. Often this simple procedure, with the heating pad left in place all night, will prevent leg cramps during sleep.

5. For the person whose work requires him to stand a great deal, the plan of sitting down or lying down for five minutes out of every two hours, meanwhile elevating the feet to a higher level than the hips, will serve to drain away the stagnant blood and thus to improve the circulation of blood to the lower extremities.

MUSCULAR ATROPHY.
(See *Muscular Atrophy* in chapter 25 of this volume.)

MUSCULAR DYSTROPHY.
Muscular dystrophy is an inherited disease characterized by progressive weakness caused by degeneration of the component fibers of muscle tissue.

Child Type (Duchenne form). This affects only boys. The weakness starts in the muscles of the hips, causing the boy to walk with a "waddling" gait. Sometimes the victim walks on his toes; he falls frequently and has difficulty in getting back to the upright position. The calf muscles often become enlarged and present the false appearance of being strong.

Adolescent type. The weakness usually begins during adolescence and affects both sexes equally. The weakness is usually first noted in the shoulders and then in the face and upper arms. Eventually muscles in the hands, feet, and back may become involved. There is a resulting tendency for the back to become swayed and for the arms and legs to assume abnormal positions. Occasionally the disease becomes arrested spontaneously and the patient becomes no worse. The diagnosis is best confirmed by removing a small sample of muscle tissue and examining this microscopically.

What to Do

1. There is no suitable treatment.

2. The patient's interests are best served by his being placed under the care of a pediatrician and an orthopedic surgeon. The cooperation of a physiatrist (a specialist in physical medicine) is also helpful.

3. The aim in caring for the patient is to prolong the time during which he can move about and engage in routine activities. The use of appropriate braces and the performing of surgical procedures to correct the deformities may help to keep the patient active.

MYALGIA
(See *Fibrositis* in this chapter.)

MYASTHENIA GRAVIS.
(See *Myasthenia Gravis* in chapter 25 of this volume.)

NECK, STIFF.
(See *Fibrositis* and *Wryneck*, both in this chapter.)

NECK SPRAIN (WHIPLASH).
This rather common type of injury is typically sustained by a person riding in a car that is in a rear-end collision. The impact of the collision causes the person's head to snap backward and then rebound forward.

The symptoms of neck sprain may begin at the time of the injury or within the next few hours. They consist of pain in the neck and back, muscle spasm, localized tenderness, swelling, guarding of the injured area, headache, and, possibly, sleeplessness. The fundamental cause is an overstretching of the ligaments and muscles that support and move the head.

What to Do

1. Arrange for an examination by a physician to determine whether there are any complicating factors such as injuries to the vertebrae or the nerves. If so, treat these accordingly.

2. Place a thin piece of plywood between the mattress and the springs of the bed used by the patient. This prevents sagging when the bed is occupied.

3. Wear an orthopedic type of collar support for about an hour three or four times a day or whenever the muscles of the neck are under stress as when riding in a car or walking over rough ground. This rests the neck muscles. The collar should not be worn for long periods, for this would allow the muscles to become weak.

4. Use a warming heat lamp directed toward the neck at a distance of about two feet for several treatments per day. The skin should become warm, not hot. A 100-watt bulb produces sufficient heat.

5. Exercise the neck muscles by moving the head in various directions. The range of motion and the extent of the exercise should be increased slightly each day. This strengthens the neck muscles.

OSTEITIS DEFORMANS (PAGET'S DISEASE).

This is a slowly progressive disease of unknown cause which usually appears only after age thirty and is said to affect about 3 percent of the United States population above fifty years of age. It consists essentially of a depletion of calcium in the bones with consequent alterations in their structure. Any bone or group of bones may be affected—commonly the vertebrae, the skull, and the bones of the legs. The bones become thickened, misshapen, and weakened. Extreme bowing of the legs is a common manifestation. Spontaneous fracture may occur.

Pain in the bones is a common symptom. The remodeling of the bones sometimes compresses certain nerves, causing symptoms referable to these nerves.

What to Do

Until about 1970 there was no satisfactory treatment for osteitis deformans. Beginning then, several medications have proved beneficial. The one which is least toxic is calcitonin, a little-known hormone produced in the thyroid gland. It is administered by the hypodermic route, under a physician's care, three or more times per week. It inhibits the loss of calcium from the bones.

OSTEOMYELITIS.

Osteomyelitis consists of an infection and partial destruction of some particular bone. It may be caused by a variety of germs but most commonly by the staphylococcus.

In osteomyelitis that occurs in the younger age group (most commonly between ages ten and fifteen) the germs usually come from an infection in some distant part of the body such as from a boil, from an infection of the middle ear, or from pneumonia. The germs are carried by the blood and lodge in the marrow of a bone where they cause a continuing destruction of bone tissue.

In the typical adult osteomyelitis the germs have migrated to the affected bone from a neighboring infection as in a compound fracture of a bone where the skin is torn.

The symptoms of osteomyelitis include sudden pain in the affected bone, with discomfort when that part of the body is moved. Also there are systemic evidences of infection such as chills and fever.

What to Do

1. Osteomyelitis is a serious condition, and the care of the case must be under the supervision of a physician.

2. Osteomyelitis is best treated by the precise and vigorous use of the proper antibiotic medication. The choice of the particular antibiotic depends on the kind of infection that is present. The medication must be continued for several weeks.

3. In cases in which the infection has made considerable progress, it may be necessary to intervene surgically to remove the fragments of devitalized bone and to permit drainage for the infected tissue.

OSTEOPOROSIS.

Osteoporosis is a condition in which bone substance throughout the skeleton is decreased. It may occur in a bone that is immobilized (as when in a plaster cast). It may occur in cases of malnutrition, of hyperthyroidism, diabetes, vitamin C deficiency, or when there is an excess of adrenal cortical hormones. It may occur in a woman, following her menopause. A certain degree of osteoporosis occurs almost constantly in old age in both sexes.

The possible complications of osteoporosis include pain in the bones, fracture of a bone that has become weak, kyphosis, and general debility.

What to Do

There are several possible basic causes of osteoporosis, as mentioned above. Therefore every case of this illness must be evaluated by a physician and the program of treatment designed accordingly. In general the four following items are recognized as being important in treatment.

1. Provide a high intake of calcium, either by the use of one quart of milk per day or by the intake of certain salts of calcium such as are contained in the pharmaceutical product Neo-Calglucon Syrup.

2. Administer estrogens (hormones) to women patients who are beyond the age of the menopause.

3. Provide intensive physical therapy to keep the major muscles in active condition and thus exert a stimulating influence on the bones of the body.

4. Arrange a program of active physical exercise, consistent with the individual's degree of vitality, and so planned as to continue for the remainder of life.

RHEUMATISM.

(See *Fibrositis* in this chapter.)

ROUND SHOULDERS.

Round shoulders are largely the result of early bad posture habits—wrong posture at school, in the home, or elsewhere. Another possible cause is tight or ill-fitting clothing that prevents a child from fully expanding his chest and extending his arms. In weak children, even the weight of too heavy clothing may bring on the trouble. Round shoulders or a round back may be a familial characteristic. They may be caused by disease of centers of bone growth, by softening of the bone structure in the vertebrae, especially in elderly women, by arthritis of the spine, et cetera.

What to Do

1. As soon as any tendency to round shoulders is noticed in a child, persistently train him to hold his body in a good posture.

2. A good corrective exercise is to lie on the back across a bed, with the rounded part of the shoulders at its edge, and the arms outstretched above the head, then have one

231

person hold the feet down while another presses the shoulders downward until the hands touch the floor. In a person no longer young, this may not be possible. Round shoulders in elderly people are incurable.

3. Prone lying hyperextension exercises (swan dive position) are helpful.

4. An upper back extension brace is often helpful, especially in the elderly.

SCIATICA.

(See under *Back Pain and Backache* in this chapter.)

SCOLIOSIS.

(See *Curvature of the Spine* in this chapter.

SPRAINS.

(See under *Sprains* in the chapter on "Handling Emergencies," volume 3, chapter 18.)

SPUR, CALCANEAL.

(See *Heel, Painful* in this chapter.)

STRAINS.

(See under *Strains* in the chapter on "Handling Emergencies," volume 3, chapter 18.)

STIFF NECK.

(See *Fibrositis* and *Wryneck*, both in this chapter.)

WHIPLASH.

(See *Neck Sprain* in this chapter.)

WRYNECK (TORTICOLLIS).

Abnormal shortness or contraction of one or more of the muscles on one side of the neck is the most common cause of wryneck. This condition may not be noticed until a child begins to try to hold up his head or to walk, because before this time his muscles are comparatively small and weak. In severe cases of long standing, there is a permanent underdevelopment of the face on the affected side. It is

shorter and flatter than the other side. Lines drawn through the mouth and the eyes converge instead of being parallel as they should be— characteristic of a condition called "facial curvature" or "facial scoliosis." A case slight in infancy may become more severe and more deforming as the child grows. Early treatment is of prime importance. It is tragic to neglect wryneck until incurable facial curvature has developed.

In the adult, torticollis may be a hysterical manifestation due to deep emotional conflicts. Treatment in such cases is frequently unsuccessful. For more on hysteria see chapter 6, in this volume.

What to Do

1. Since most cases of wryneck are present at birth and tend to

A typical case of chronic torticollis of muscular origin.

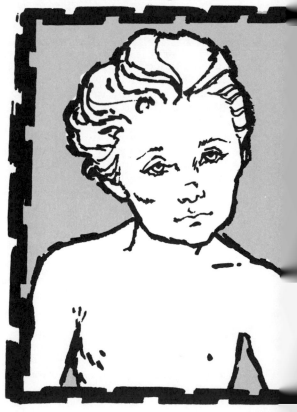

grow worse, begin corrective measures as soon as possible. If the condition is at all marked, the services of an orthopedic surgeon will be needed from the first.

2. If the condition is not severe, several times a day have one person hold the child's arms and shoulders firmly while another person draws the child's head and neck into as far

an *overcorrected* position as possible without causing severe pain, then massage the stretched muscles for a few minutes.

3. Surgery may be needed for complete correction. Following surgical release of the contracted muscle, correction is temporarily maintained by means of a plaster cast or by traction in bed.

II. Connective Tissue Diseases

The connective tissue diseases, formerly called the collagen diseases, are classed as a group because they all involve widespread inflammatory changes in the body's connective tissues and blood vessels.

SYSTEMIC SCLEROSIS (SCLERODERMA).

Systemic sclerosis is a chronic, slowly progressive disease of unknown cause which first affects the skin, causing it to become thick and inelastic. Later it produces scarlike changes in certain of the internal organs. It is at least twice as frequent in women as in men. It may begin at any age, but typically it appears first in persons between 25 and 55 years of age.

The changes in the skin usually begin in the hands and the feet. The skin becomes tight, smooth, and shiny. This interferes with movement and causes deformities and ulcer formations. The affected face becomes masklike.

The eventual involvement of the internal organs affects the organs of digestion most frequently. The esophagus or the intestine may become so narrow as to interfere with their functions. The lungs, the heart, and the kidneys may become involved as connective tissue encroaches on their functioning tissues.

Although there may be periods of remission, the disease is usually fatal within four to twenty years.

What to Do

1. There is no known cure for this disease. Various medications have been tried, but so far none have altered the progressive course of the disease.

2. The goal of treatment is to preserve normal functions and to prevent injury to the vulnerable hands. Passive and active exercises of the hands are helpful.

3. Local skin infections should be treated promptly before there is time for ulcers to develop.

4. Complications, as they develop, should be treated appropriately as directed by the physician.

POLYMYOSITIS AND DERMATOMYOSITIS.

This member of the group of connective tissue diseases affects primarily the skeletal muscles, there being inflammation and degeneration of muscle tissue. In the cases in which only the muscles are involved the disease is called *polymyositis*. In cases in which the skin as well as the muscles are affected the term *dermatomyositis* is used. The primary symptoms are weakness, tenderness, and stiffness of certain groups of muscles, most commonly those of the

233

shoulders and the pelvic region. In the cases in which the skin is also involved, there is redness and swelling of the skin followed often by a brownish pigmentation. The usual skin areas affected are those around the face and eyes and over the weakened muscles.

The cause of polymyositis and/or dermatomyositis is unknown although the manifestations often follow some specific infection. The disease may appear at any age. It is twice as common among women as among men. The course of the disease varies from case to case. Some cases improve spontaneously, even to complete recovery. In some the disease progresses rapidly, leading to involvement of the internal organs and death. In most cases the progress is slow to a certain point and then the condition remains at this level of disability.

What to Do

1. There is no specific cure for this disease. The aim of treatment is to preserve the patient's functional capacity and to make him reasonably comfortable.

2. Splinting of the affected parts may help to relieve the pain in the muscles. Local heat and gentle, passive exercises help to prevent contractures and deformities.

3. Many physicians are now administering the pituitary hormone corticotropin and/or a corticosteroid preparation. Although these medications are not curative, they do help to alleviate the symptoms. When used, they must be continued for long periods of time.

SYSTEMIC LUPUS ERYTHEMATOSUS.

Lupus erythematosus is the most prevalent of the connective tissue diseases. It occurs in two forms: (1) The cutaneous (discoid) form, which affects the skin primarily, is discussed in chapter 12 of this volume. (2) The systemic (disseminated) form is discussed here.

Systemic lupus erythematosus may first appear at any age but most commonly between the ages of 20 and 40. It is five to ten times more frequent in women than in men. The manifestations vary a great deal from case to case. Typically it produces fatigue, pain in certain joints, skin rash on the areas exposed to the sun, and fever. Beyond this the symptoms depend on which of the internal organs are affected: the kidneys, the heart, the lungs, the digestive organs, or the nervous system.

Although the cause of the disease is not known, it is described as an "autoimmune" disorder in which the normal balance between tolerance and immunity has become altered. Affected persons seem to have developed antibodies to some of the constituents of their own cells. The rate of progress of the disease varies from person to person. Usually there is a series of remissions and relapses. In the occasional, fast-moving case, death may occur within a few weeks. In the more usual case the illness becomes chronic with long periods of remission.

What to Do

1. The aim of treatment is to hasten a remission when symptoms are present and to avoid or postpone a relapse when the patient is free from symptoms.

2. Certain things which seem to predispose to a relapse should be avoided as far as possible: exposure to sunlight; use of drugs, especially the antibiotics and sulfa drugs; immunizations; blood transfusions; and elective surgery.

3. The patient should follow an easy pattern of living, as free as possible from stress and extremes.

4. Complications involving the various organs should be treated appropriately by a physician.

5. The use of a corticosteroid medication adapted to the circumstances of the individual patient is usually helpful.

PERIARTERITIS NODOSA (POLYARTERITIS NODOSA).

In this disease it is primarily the small and medium-sized arteries that are affected in various locations throughout the body. The processes of inflammation and destruction of the arterial tissue occurs in a particular spot along the course of each of the affected arteries. This accounts for the development of nodules (lumps) that can be felt by the examining finger; hence the term "nodosa."

In the course of the attempted healing at the site of destruction of an arterial wall, the artery becomes closed to the flow of blood, or it may rupture. In some cases an aneurism develops at this site of tissue damage.

An affected artery is no longer capable of conveying its usual quota of blood. Therefore the part of the body which the artery normally supplies is now deprived of blood. It is this complication—deprivation of blood to all or part of an organ or tissue—that accounts for the predominant symptoms and also for the fatal outcome (within about five years) in the majority of cases. The symptoms vary, of course, depending on what organs are involved.

The kidneys are the organs most frequently affected. Other frequently involved organs include the heart, the organs of digestion, the nervous system, and the skin.

Periarteritis nodosa may appear at any time of life but most commonly between the ages of forty and sixty. Women are more susceptible than men in a ratio of about three to two.

What to Do

1. As is true of the other connective tissue diseases, so with periarteritis nodosa, no known treatment can cure the disease.

2. The treatment program must be designed to fit the individual case with provision to ease whatever symptoms have developed on account of involvement of the various organs.

3. The use of a corticosteroid medication usually helps to control some of the symptoms and may prolong a period of remission. But the improvement is usually only temporary.

Joint Diseases

The chief structures we think of in relation to diseases or injuries of the moveable joints are the following:

1. The bones that form the joint.

2. The ligaments that hold the ends of the bones together, preventing motion beyond normal limits and forming or helping to form the joint cavity.

3. The cartilage that covers the surfaces of the bone ends where they touch each other.

4. The synovial membrane that lines the inner surface of the joint cavity and secretes the fluid that lubricates the joint.

The more important common diseases and affections involving joints and their neighboring structures are arthritis, sprains, dislocations, synovitis, and gout. Arthritis, of which there are several forms, means an inflammation involving some or all of the structures of a joint.

ARTHRITIS, ACUTE (SEPTIC ARTHRITIS).

Acute or septic arthritis may attack people who for some time have had tonsillitis, decayed teeth, pus pockets around tooth roots, infection in nasal sinuses or mastoid cells, or infection in the intestinal tract; but it is still a matter of argument whether or not these chronic so-called focuses of infection are actually the source of the germs present in the arthritic joints. Arthritis may be a complication of such acute infectious diseases as septicemia, rheumatic fever, erysipelas, scarlet fever, typoid fever, gonorrhea, bacillary dysentery, undulant fever, and several others, though the use of antibiotics is making such cases, especially gonorrheal arthritis, increasingly rare. The disease is most common among young adults, and males are affected more often than females.

Acute arthritis usually begins rather abruptly; the fever rises quickly, and, at the same time, one or more joints become swollen and very painful, especially when moved. But as a rule the infection finally localizes in one joint. The swollen joint is tender and hot to the touch and may have a reddish appearance. If not promptly and properly treated, permanent stiffness and deformity of the joint may be the end result.

What to Do

1. **During the first day or two at most, ice compresses or ice bags may be used thirty to forty-five minutes out of every hour. Wrap the compress or bag in a Turkish towel before applying. If such cold applications do not bring noticeable relief of the pain, discontinue them and proceed as in (2) below.**

2. Later, long-continued applications of heat are helpful, whether in the form of fomentations, hot-water bottles, or any other method that may be convenient to use. A heating compress, one with very little water, worn every night, may give some relief. (See volume 3, chapter 20.)

3. Protect the body against chilling.

4. Take a liquid diet as long as fever persists. Eat little or no meat, but plenty of fruit.

5. The services of a physician are essential in the successful treatment of acute arthritis, and they should be sought as early as possible. Antibiotics are likely to be needed. The joint may need to be splinted, put in traction or a cast, aspirated, or opened to drain the fluid possibly present. Later, surgical manipulations or other types of surgical or medical treatments or prescribed exercises may be needed to restore the usefulness of the joint.

ARTHRITIS, RHEUMATOID (ARTHRITIS DEFORMANS).

"Rheumatoid arthritis" is a name which leading authorities now prefer to apply to what is really a group of joint troubles sometimes called "arthritis deformans," "atrophic arthritis," or "chronic infectious arthritis." It is one of the most ancient of diseases, skeletal evidences of it having been found in Egyptian mummies.

Rheumatoid arthritis develops as the combined result of several factors. An infectious factor may be superimposed on a background of malnutrition, disorders of endocrine glands, or maladjustment to life, this latter now being increasingly considered an important cause. The disease may be due to a virus or viruses or to poisons or toxins produced by bacteria; but no pus or disease germs have been found present in the joint fluid of people suffering from it. Considerable evidence indicates that physical or emotional shock, injuries, fatigue, exposure to cold and dampness, and, especially, hereditary predisposition and climate may prepare the way for the development of this disease. It is considerably more common in women than in men.

Rheumatoid arthritis usually makes its appearance after childhood and before the age of forty. Occasionally it appears as late as the sixties and seventies. Its onset may be rapid but is more often gradual. At first there is a low-grade fever, headache, and a general feeling of debility. The knees and fingers are usually affected first, then the shoulders, wrists, ankles, and elbows. In extensive cases, nearly every joint in the body may finally be attacked. The joints are swollen because of active inflammation of the synovial membranes and other structures in and about them. The pain may be only moderate, but it is often severe. But while the disease manifests itself locally and outwardly in only the joints, it is really a systemic malady involving the whole body.

When large joints are affected, they are likely to be red, tender, and warm to the touch; and there may be an increase in the quantity of the joint fluid. X-ray examinations indicate that the joint cartilage tends to become thinned by absorption because of the infectious process and/or by pressure from the spastic muscles or tendons that cross the joint, also that the bone ends lose calcium and become rarefied. Contractures and atrophy of muscles and tendons about the joints may cause them to bend in an unnatural way or may even put the bones completely out of joint, giving rise to extensive deformity. In some cases the bone ends grow together, making the joints permanently stiff. The affected limbs, aside from the joints, are cold and clammy. The victims tend to be thin and anemic in severe cases.

Rheumatoid arthritis is sometimes apparently curable, especially in its early stages; but as a rule it recurs again and again after apparent cure, becoming more chronic with each recurrence. It is best for the person who has recently developed rheumatoid arthritis to face up to the prospect that he will be troubled with this handicap for the rest of his life. But with modern methods of treatment and by cooperating consistently with the physician the afflicted person will probably be able to live productively even though handicapped.

The particular manifestations of rheumatoid arthritis in one case may be quite different from those in other cases. There is so much individual variation from case to case that it is not practical to set down a detailed plan of treatment that will benefit every case. The physician who cares for a patient with rheumatoid arthritis must observe the manifestations of the disease in this particular case and plan the treatment accordingly.

When it comes to specific remedies, certain ones work well for one case but not for others. Unfortunately, the most effective medicines often carry the greatest hazards of side effects. The physician must therefore use his professional judgment in balancing

Modern methods of treatment enable many arthritic patients to carry on normal activities and live useful lives.

D. TANK

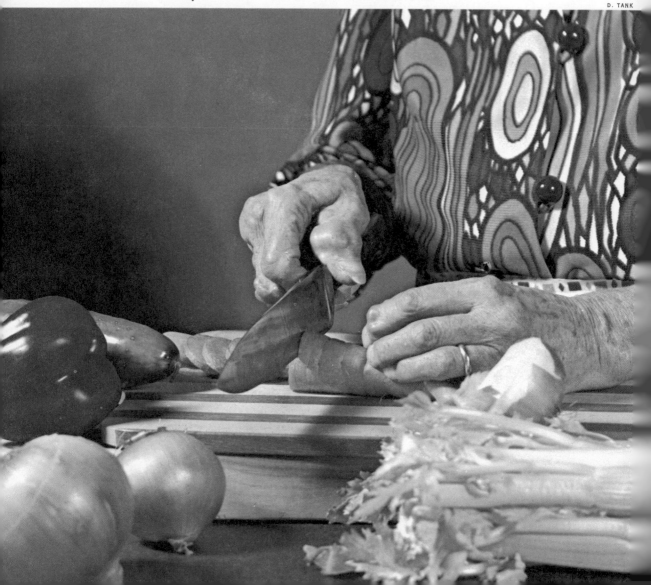

the benefits to be derived from a certain medicine against the possible unfavorable complications.

Even though there are times of remission in many cases, rheumatoid arthritis tends to run a progressive course. We may say that there is an early stage in which destruction of the joint tissues takes place, and a later chronic stage in which the patient retains whatever handicap he acquired during the early stage. The treatment of a given case will therefore be directed, first, toward preventing or at least reducing the amount of damage which occurs during the first stage and, later, toward rehabilitating the patient and restoring his lost functions as far as this is possible.

What to Do

1. One basic program of treatment for the early stage of rheumatoid arthritis serves to benefit all cases—those that are severe and those that are less severe. In the less severe cases, this basic program, by itself, may give adequate control of the disease for long periods of time. It consists of six items:

A. *Rest.* This requires that the patient avoid straining the joints that are presently involved and also that he reduce his general activities so as to conserve his quota of vitality.

B. *Psychological adjustment.* The patient should be provided with a fund of information regarding his disease so that he knows what to expect. He should receive encouragement to become reconciled to the handicaps which his disease produces. On the positive side, he should plan his future so that he can be productive and can experience the rewards of success. Appropriate literature may be obtained from The Arthritis Foundation, 475 Riverside Drive, New York, N.Y. 10027.

C. *Relief of pain.* This is accomplished, in part, by the use of dry heat to the affected parts of the body and otherwise by pain-relieving medicines as recommended by the doctor. The commonly used medicines for this purpose are the salicylates of which aspirin is the most popular and the least harmful. The use of pain-relieving medicines introduces the danger of anemia, for these medicines may have a damaging effect on the blood-forming tissues of the body.

D. *Measures to combat anemia.* The physician in charge of the case will arrange for frequent blood tests to determine whether anemia is developing and, if so, its degree. Based on this information he may recommend corrective measures as necessary.

E. *Therapeutic exercise.* The exercise program must be adapted to the particular case with the motives of keeping the muscles in good condition, preventing or reducing deformities, and helping the patient to maintain his general vitality.

F. *A well-balanced diet.* It is important for the person with rheumatoid arthritis to maintain his general health and vitality in as favorable a state as possible. His diet should be simple but liberal, with plenty of vitamins, vegetables, and fruits.

2. For the more severe and more rapidly progressing cases, a more drastic program of treatment must be added to the basic program outlined above. It includes the following:

A. *Intensive physical and occupational therapy.* This should be prescribed by the physician and administered by a paramedical person trained in these techniques.

B. *Orthopedic devices.* Splints and other aids may be used to prevent or minimize deformities.

C. *Potent drugs.* The more powerful anti-inflammatory and analgesic medicines are often used to arrest the destruction of tissue and to relieve severe pain. Certain other medicines are also used effectively in some cases of rheumatoid arthritis. Included in this combined group are the corticosteroids, phen-

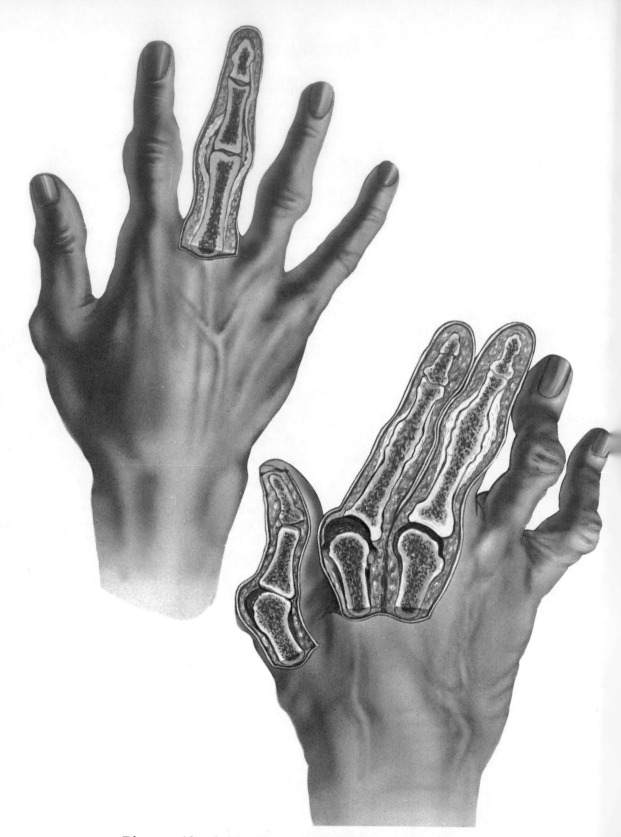

Rheumatoid arthritis. Note swelling of joints caused by synovitis and effusion. Right: Advanced case, showing deformity from stiffness and partial dislocation of joints.

ylbutazone, indomethacin, some of the "antimalarial drugs," and certain gold salts. These more powerful medicinal agents carry the risk of toxic reactions and other unfavorable side effects. Their use must therefore be carefully directed by the physician.

D. *Orthopedic surgery.* It is now recognized that the early use of orthopedic surgery in selected cases often helps to prevent devastating deformities and disability.

3. In the later stages of rheumatoid arthritis efforts are directed toward restoring the functions that were lost earlier in the course of the disease. The patient needs to be taught to carry on his activities in spite of his particular handicap. In addition, many cases are greatly benefited by appropriate reconstructive surgery in which the affected joints are replaced or reconstructed and in which tendons may be transplanted in a way to restore lost functions.

ARTHRITIS, TUBERCULOUS.

Tuberculous arthritis usually involves but one joint at a time, though sometimes more than one. The infection usually spreads from some primary focus in the lungs or lymph nodes. In many cases there is a history of injury of the involved joint a few weeks previous to the development of tuberculosis in it. The joints most commonly attacked by tuberculosis are the spine, the ankle, the hip, the knee, the elbow, the shoulder, and the wrist.

Joint tuberculosis is much less prevalent now than a generation or more ago. It used to be most commonly caused by a bovine type of germ transmitted by raw milk. Tuberculin testing of dairy cows and pasteurization of milk have done more than anything else to account for the improvement.

In the early stages of the disease the involved joint is not very painful, likely only to be considerably swollen but not noticeably inflamed. The infection begins in one of the bones at a point near the joint. If the process is not checked, the joint is invaded, the articular cartilage attacked, and the joint as a whole permanently damaged. It is possible, with proper treatment, for the active tuberculosis to be arrested at the earlier stages before the cartilage is damaged, and normal activity of the joint restored. As a rule, however, the disease continues until there is more or less destruction of the joint tissues. By then healing can occur only with solid bony union of the joint surfaces, which means a permanently stiffened joint. In untreated or improperly treated tuberculosis of the joints, deformities will be the result— hunchbacks, backward dislocation of the hips, and bent and outwardly rotated knees being the most common results. Having done such damage, however, the infection tends to terminate itself, so far as the joints are concerned, and does not end fatally.

The systemic symptoms of tuberculous arthritis are the same as in any other form of tuberculosis—anemia, daily rise of temperature, and loss of appetite, weight, and strength.

The local symptoms are pain on pressure or motion of the affected joint, with swelling or thickening of its tissues. The pain is often of such a nature as to cause the victim, usually a child, to cry out at night, especially when the disease is far advanced. There is also a spasm of the muscles controlling the joint, causing a limitation of its motion in either direction. This spasm causes stiffness in the early stage, while in the late stage the stiffness results from contractures of soft tissues about the joint or a growing together of the bones of the joint. Joint stiffness from this latter cause is called ankylosis. Characteristically, there may be abscess formation at any stage of the infectious process, and the abscesses may open through the skin or into the chest

241

cavity, the abdominal cavity, or the spinal canal, and discharge pus persistently. Surgical drainage of such an abscess may be advisable.

What to Do

1. Arrange for professional medical care. Self-treatment is useless; but proper remedies and treatments given by, or under the supervision of, a physician may result in a complete cure if begun early enough.

2. The affected joint must be put at rest, usually by means of splints, a plaster cast, or, if the spine is involved, a special frame.

3. Surgery, plus the use of new chemical remedies for tuberculosis, can bring about much improvement or complete recovery in many cases.

4. The same general program of diet and rest is needed as in any other form of tuberculosis. (See chapter 29 of this volume.)

DISLOCATION OF JOINTS.

(See *Dislocations* in the chapter on "Handling Emergencies," volume 3, chapter 18.)

GOUT.

Gout is usually defined as a special kind of arthritis. Actually, however, the involvement of the joints is just one manifestation of a systemic disease. The fundamental cause of gout is an inherited fault in the way the body handles certain chemical substances. Uric acid is one of the by-products produced in the body in the course of the digestion of food. In most persons this uric acid is readily eliminated by the kidneys. But in a person who has inherited the tendency to gout the uric acid is not eliminated as quickly as it should be, and so the body's fluids and tissues contain more than is normal. Because such an excess of uric acid is best detected by measuring the amount contained in the blood, this condition is called hyperuricemia (excess of uric acid in the blood).

Hyperuricemia is a relatively common condition, being present in 5 to 10 percent of American men above the age of 30, but in only about one tenth as many women. Many persons with hyperuricemia have no symptoms and do not know that they have this condition. But in a minority of this group (about three persons per 1000 population), one or the other of four possible complications develop. These are: (1) *acute gouty arthritis* on account of which gout is considered here with other involvements of the joints; (2) *tophaceous gout* in which hard masses of uric acid cyrstals develop in various parts of the body, often in relation to the joints: (3) development of *kidney stones* composed of uric acid crystals; and (4) *gouty kidney disease* in which the kidneys no longer function efficiently.

1. Acute gouty arthritis occurs in attacks which come unannounced and, if untreated, each runs a course of one or two weeks. The pain in such an attack is very severe and, if it be the first attack, usually emanates from just one joint. Often it is the joint at the base of the big toe that is first affected. The joint becomes swollen, warm to the touch, and extremely tender. The skin over the joint is tense, shiny, and red.

There will usually be a series of attacks which are successively more severe and more frequent. Various joints may be affected, such as those of the ankle, the instep, the knee, and even those of the hands and arms. With recurring attacks, there is often an involvement of more than one joint at a time.

2. Tophaceous gout is a chronic condition in which deposits of uric acid crystals, called tophi, make their appearance in various tissues of the body. One of the favorite sites for a tophus is the lobe of the ear. Commonly, however, tophi are situated in the vicinity of joints. The body's tissues react to these tophi as to foreign bodies with a resulting mild but persistent inflammation. When

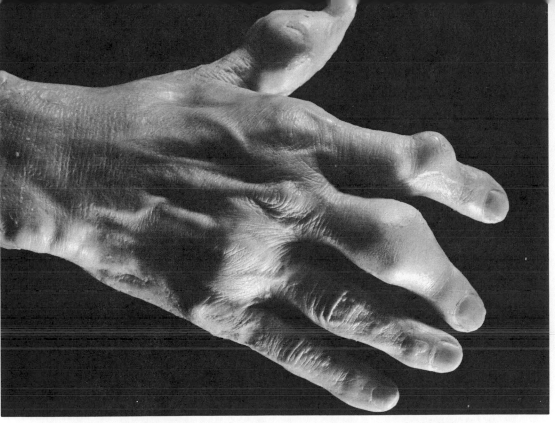

The hand of a person suffering from gout, one form of arthritis. Lumps on knuckles are caused by excess of uric acid leading to formation of urate crystals around the joints. See diagram below.

untreated, there develops a certain destruction in the tissues adjacent to a tophus. This destruction may involve the bones and the surrounding soft tissues.

3. Kidney stones. Gout is not the only condition in which stones develop within the pelvis of the kidney, but the development of kidney stones is much more frequent in persons with hyperuricemia (high concentration of uric acid in the blood). Kidney stones are discussed in chapter 22 of this volume.

4. Gouty kidney disease. There appears to be a two-way relationship between degenerative disease of the kidney and gout. About one third of the cases of hyperuricemia seem to be aggravated by or possibly even caused by the inefficiency of kidney function in which uric acid is not eliminated from the body as readily as it should be. On the other hand, the mere condition of hyperuricemia seems to have a damaging effect on the kid-

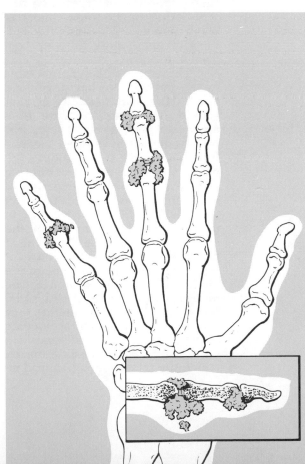

neys. Therefore in some cases kidney disease seems to contribute to the condition of gout; and in others, gout contributes to kidney disease.

What to Do

As mentioned above, many persons who have high levels of uric acid in their body fluids and tissues are not aware of this until one of the complications of gout develops. In case such a condition of hyperuricemia is discovered before any complication develops, it is well for the person to follow a program which helps to keep the concentration of uric acid in his body at reasonably low levels.

1. Eliminate from the diet those foods which contain substances that favor the production of uric acid within the body. The foods to be limited are flesh foods and animal fats.

2. If there is a condition of overweight, the weight should certainly be brought within "normal" limits. (See volume 1, chapter 51.)

3. Drink up to three quarts of water per day. This aids the kidneys in eliminating the uric acid from the body.

4. The person with hyperuricemia or the person who has developed one of the complications of gout should be under the care of a physician. Within recent years several medicines have been successfully used in the treatment of gout. Not only is it now possible to relieve and shorten the period of suffering in cases of acute gouty arthritis, but it is even possible to prevent the development of the complications of gout. This type of prevention requires the more or less continuous use of some of the medicines which influence the metabolism of uric acid within the body. The choice of medicines for a given case depends on the specific manifestations of the disease and on the stage of the disease during which the treatment is begun. The medicines which are particularly useful in gout include colchicine, probenecid (Benemid), and allopurinol. When the medicines are used selectively and discriminatingly, under a physician's direction, they can make the difference between intermittent or continuous invalidism, and a life which is essentially free from disability and deformity.

OSTEOARTHRITIS (DEGENERATIVE ARTHRITIS, HYPERTROPHIC ARTHRITIS).

Osteoarthritis usually develops slowly and gradually in the latter half of life. It involves degeneration and in one sense is a part of the aging process of the people afflicted with it. Impaired circulation is possibly a causative factor; and improvement of the circulation in general, as well as in the joints, is one aim in treatment. The condition shows a distinct hereditary tendency; but injuries, excessive body weight, and overexertion of a sort that brings increased pressure on the joint cartilages also have a causative influence. The joints of the spine, hips, knees, and fingers are most commonly affected.

Osteoarthritis is characterized by thinning or degeneration of bone in some parts of the joint, but an overproduction of bony tissue in other parts. It is this overproduction, a prominent feature of the disease, that gave origin to the name "hypertrophic arthritis." It takes the form of "spurring" or "lipping" around the joint margins. It may reduce the range of joint motion, or in time prevent motion entirely; but usually the bones do not actually grow together, even when the vertebrae are involved. The joint may be irregularly enlarged, but it is rarely inflamed. Many really severe cases may go on for years without any symptoms except limitation of motion. Attacks of pain are usually brought on by sudden strain, injury, or a direct blow that precipitates an inflammatory reaction of the local area. This inflammation involves the soft tissues about the spurs or lips of bone at the margins of the joints. Occasionally these spurs or lips may be broken, which also causes pain.

The X ray easily shows the abnormal bony growth in cases of osteoarthritis, and when this disease affects the spine it is often discovered by chance while an X ray of the chest or abdomen is being taken for some other reason. A surprising degree of osteoarthritis, even in the spine, may exist without causing any distress; but bony overgrowths along the posterior margins of the vertebrae may press on nerve trunks—one of the causes of sciatica in elderly people. Much can be done through physical therapy and/or orthopedic surgery to relieve distress and restore activity for the osteoarthritic individual, but there is no real cure for the disease.

What to Do

In addition to the specific things that can be done to help a person with osteoarthritis, attention should be given to the patient's mental attitudes. Such a person typically fears, even though he is still young in years, that he has passed the prime of his life. He thinks his symptoms mean that he is approaching old age. He resents this; therefore he disregards the symptoms as much as he can and tries to keep up his usual pace of activities. He needs help in becoming willing to establish a new pattern of life which is consistent with his reduced physical capacities. Following such a pattern will enable him to prolong his period of productive usefulness even to the normal lifespan.

1. If osteoarthritic joints are painful, apply dry heat in any form to them for half an hour or more at least three times a day.

2. Avoid injury to the involved joints, and limit their use enough to avoid bending them far enough to cause pain; but correct faulty pos-

Diagrammatic representation of osteoarthritis.

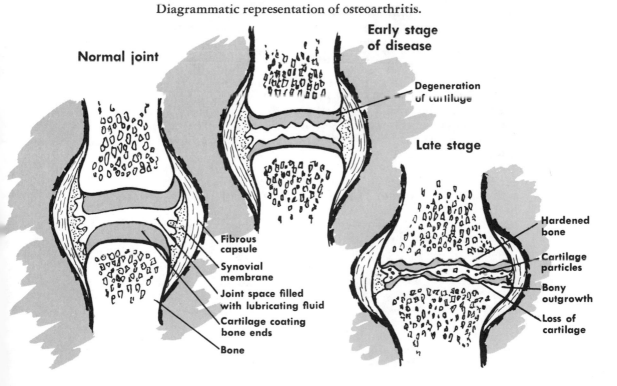

Normal joint

Early stage of disease

Degeneration of cartilage

Late stage

Fibrous capsule

Synovial membrane

Joint space filled with lubricating fluid

Cartilage coating bone ends

Bone

Hardened bone

Cartilage particles

Bony outgrowth

Loss of cartilage

245

ture as far as possible. Give massage and passive exercise with caution, taking care not to cause pain. In some cases splints or casts may be needed to prevent pain-producing motion.

3. Avoid fatigue and overexertion, especially in activities that involve use of the affected joints. This will be necessary for the remainder of life if the disease is fully developed.

4. If overweight, reduce the weight to normal. (See volume 1, chapter 51.)

5. If the joints of the lower spine and hips are involved, lying down for more hours of the day than usual may help bring relief by taking pressure off the affected joint surfaces.

6. Pay attention to all habits that influence the general health, including such correction of posture as will improve body mechanics, also such exercise as will increase muscle power.

7. The use of appropriate drugs helps to relieve the symptoms of osteoarthritis but does not alter the course of the disease. The most commonly used drug, the one which carries the least hazard and is the cheapest is simple aspirin. It should not be used indiscriminately, however. It is most effective in doses (for an adult) of 0.6 to 0.9 grams (10 to 15 grains) taken four times a day (total of 2.4 to 3.6 grams for the day): after each meal and with milk at bedtime. The reason for taking the medicine after meals or with milk is that this reduces the irritating effect of the aspirin on the mucosal lining of the stomach. The patient should report to his doctor periodically to have him check for possible side effects of the use of aspirin. Some physicians perfer to prescribe the more potent drugs, but these carry greater risk of side effects and therefore must be more carefully supervised.

SPRAINS.
(See *Sprains* in the chapter on "Handling Emergencies," volume 3, chapter 18.)

SYNOVITIS.
Synovitis is usually not simple or primary. It does not often occur alone, but usually accompanies some form of arthritis. It is an inflammation of the membrane lining the joint cavity. Since the function of this membrane is to secrete a lubricating fluid, irritation or injury causes distention and swelling because of an excessive secretion, together with the forcing of blood into the cavity. Without a history of any injury, however, there may first be a lowgrade inflammatory factor because of rheumatoid arthritis, tuberculosis, or any one of several other infections, in which case professional medical attention is needed at once.

There is another common cause of the synovitis that tends to occur intermittently; it is some metabolic disturbance, the nature of which may not be entirely clear, at least without the aid of special tests. There is usually pain and limitation of motion of the joint, mainly because of distention which stretches the ligaments and interferes with their normal freedom of motion.

Simple synovitis is most commonly the result of an injury associated with a sprain. The knee joint is most commonly affected; and if much fluid is present, the kneecap "floats" and may be felt to strike against the bone beneath it if it is pressed quickly backward with the leg held straight downward.

In any case of this kind a physician should be consulted, as it is not easy for a person without medical training to distinquish between a simple sprain and an injury involving a fracture of major or minor nature involving a joint. There is also the difficulty of discerning whether or not this apparently simple synovitis may be a symptom of a more serious joint disease.

What to Do

1. Rest the joint, preferably with the patient remaining in bed.

2. If the synovitis is possibly related to an injury, the use of ice packs for the first twenty-four hours may be helpful. Otherwise, or after the first day of treatment, it is helpful to apply hot fomentations to the affected joint three times a day. (See volume 3, chapter 20.)

3. Apply pressure to the affected part, preferably by the use of an elastic bandage.

4. It is wise to consult a physician. The true nature of the synovitis is not easy to determine and should be properly evaluated in order for treatment to be given.

Diseases of the Eye

Two other chapters in *You and Your Health* give information relating to the eyes and are recommended for additional reading in connection with the present chapter. Chapter 14 of volume 3 contains a subdivision on "Vision," which describes the structure and function of the eye in a way that will make the material in the present chapter much easier to understand. Chapter 22 of volume 3 consists of an alphabetical listing of the signs and symptoms of disease. There, under the heading "Eyes," are given the various symptoms of eye disease with mention of the possible causes of these symptoms. The person who has eye symptoms will do well to look in that chapter for the meaning of his symptoms and then consult the present chapter for discussions of the diseases perhaps causing his symptoms.

In the present chapter the common eye diseases are arranged in alphabetical order. Where a disease may be known by more than one name, cross-references are used.

AMBLYOPIA.

Amblyopia is a dimness of vision which cannot be relieved by glasses and for which examination of the eye shows no physical abnormalities. There are two principal types: (1) those in which the patient has subcon-

sciously trained himself to ignore the vision of one eye, and (2) those in which there has been chemical or toxic damage to the optic nerve.

A young child who has a crossed eye or a walleye often ignores the vision of one eye in order to avoid double vision (seeing two images) and therefore develops amblyopia. Also, in one form of hysteria the patient may actually believe himself to be blind even though his eyes are normal.

Toxic amblyopia may follow the excessive use of alcohol or tobacco or it may result from exposure to wood alcohol (methyl alcohol), carbon monoxide, carbon tetrachloride, arsenic compounds, lead compounds, or benzene. Amblyopia sometimes occurs and then disappears in the disease multiple sclerosis. It may occur in uremia and then disappear if the patient recovers from the uremia.

A patient with toxic amblyopia complains first of foggy vision, and then of a central blind spot which enlarges as the disease progresses.

What to Do

1. For children with squint (cross-eye or walleye) a careful treatment program should be carried on before the child develops a permanent habit of ignoring the vision of one eye. Do not wait to see if the child will outgrow the condition,

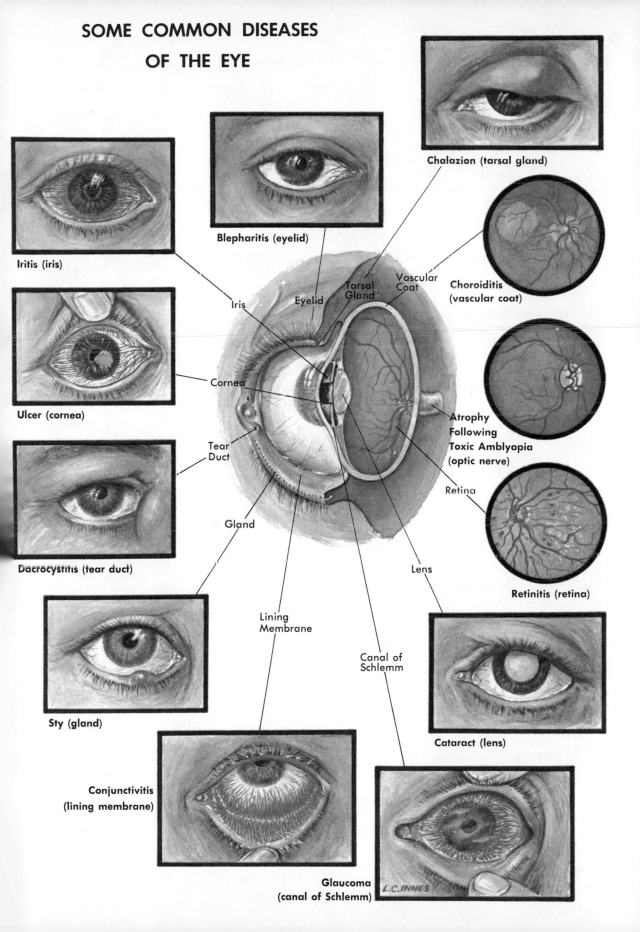

SOME COMMON DISEASES OF THE EYE

Iritis (iris)

Blepharitis (eyelid)

Chalazion (tarsal gland)

Choroiditis (vascular coat)

Ulcer (cornea)

Dacrocystitis (tear duct)

Atrophy Following Toxic Amblyopia (optic nerve)

Retinitis (retina)

Sty (gland)

Cataract (lens)

Conjunctivitis (lining membrane)

Glaucoma (canal of Schlemm)

Iris

Eyelid

Tarsal Gland

Vascular Coat

Cornea

Tear Duct

Gland

Lining Membrane

Canal of Schlemm

Lens

Retina

L.C. INNES

but consult an eye physician immediately.

2. For hysterical blindness, treatment should be directed to the fundamental cause of the hysteria.

3. For amblyopia associated with exposure to toxic chemicals, the actual cause should be sought out and removed. Administration of vitamin B complex should aid in the recovery.

BLEPHARITIS.

Blepharitis consists of an inflammation of the margins of the eyelids. The eyes itch and burn, and there is redness of the margins with swelling. There is an excess production of secretions, and the eyelashes may become glued together at night by a drying of the secretions.

In some cases blepharitis is caused by an infection with germs, but in others it seems to be an allergic manifestation. It is sometimes associated with skin diseases of the face or dandruff of the scalp. It often occurs in conjunction with a general reduction in vitality, in connection with some systemic infection, or in a person living on an inadequate diet. It occurs quite often in persons in need of glasses.

What to Do

1. Take steps to build up the general health.

2. Have the eyes examined for possible need of glasses or for a change of glasses.

3. The physician may prescribe specific remedies for infections, either for the infection of the eyelids or for an infection in some other part of the body which has predisposed to the blepharitis.

BURNS, THERMAL AND CHEMICAL.

Severe burns of the face often involve the eyelids. The treatment is the same as for burns on other parts of the face except that great care must be used to preserve all tissues that are still capable of healing.

Chemical burns involving the eye should be given prompt first aid by rinsing the eye with generous quantities of flowing water or milk. The eyelids should be separated so that the rinsing includes their under surfaces.

A physician should take over the care of the patient as soon as possible.

CATARACT.

In cataract the lens of the eye becomes progressively opaque. Early in the development of a cataract the patient notices a reduction in the acuteness of vision. As the cataract progresses, his vision continues to fail until he can perceive only the difference between light and darkness. Frequently cataracts develop at about the same time in both eyes.

Of the various types, senile cataract is the most common. It typically develops after the age of fifty.

Illustration shows defect in vision experienced by a cataract patient.

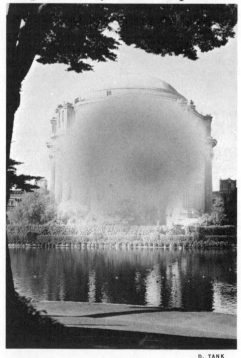

D. TANK

Left: How the lens in a normal eye brings light rays to a focus on the retina. Right: How in an eye from which the natural lens has been removed light is focused by an artificial lens worn in front.

Certain systemic diseases predispose to the early development of cataracts, notably diabetes. Sometimes a cataract develops following an injury to the eye. Long-continued exposure of the eyes to high temperatures, as with workers in glassblowing and iron puddling, favors the development of cataract.

What to Do

1 Consult a physician who specializes in diseases of the eye (an ophthalmologist).

2. The usual treatment for cataract is surgical removal of the lens which is now opaque. After recovery from surgery, light can enter the eye in the normal manner, but because there is no lens, the light rays do not focus on the retina. Therefore all visual images are blurred and appear distorted.

3. In order to have clear vision, the person who has had surgery for cataract must be supplied with artificial lenses for his eyes. These are provided in one of three ways:

a. The wearing of glasses fitted with specially adapted lenses. Such lenses which appear thicker than usual, provide reasonably good vision in a central visual field, although the lateral range of vision is somewhat limited.

b. The wearing of contact lenses which rest on the eye itself (beneath the lids) and are of proper size to enclose only the cornea of the eye. When properly fitted, contact lenses provide very satisfactory distant vision so that the person sees essentially as well as before his cataracts developed. For purposes of reading, such a person must wear conventional glasses in addition to the contact lenses.

c. The installation of implanted lenses ("implants"). In this instance, a small, specially prepared, plastic lens is inserted into the eye at the time of cataract surgery so that the artificial lens occupies the same part of the eye as was originally occupied by the natural lens. Implanted lenses have been in use in Europe for several years. Their use in the United States is relatively recent. Certain technical difficulties cause problems in a significant percentage of cases in which lens implants are used.

CHALAZION (TARSAL CYST).

A chalazion is a small tumor which develops on the eyelid when the outlet to one of the tarsal glands becomes plugged. With the normal outlet now closed, the secretion of the gland accumulates, and the size of the mass, composed of secretion and tissue debris, increases slowly over weeks and months. The condition occurs much more commonly in adults than in children.

By the time the little tumor reaches the size of a pea, it causes some disfigurement of the eyelid and some irritation of the moist membranes of the eye and eyelid.

What to Do

1. While it is still small, a chalazion may be treated successfully by applying hot compresses to the affected eyelid twice or three times a day, followed each time by gentle massage. After each treatment, a small amount of sulfa or antibiotic ophthalmic ointment should be deposited beneath the eyelid.

2. When larger, a chalazion can be removed by a simple surgical procedure in which the surgeon makes a small incision through the membrane of the underside of the eyelid and removes the entire mass of swollen tissue.

CONJUNCTIVITIS.

The moist membrane that lines the under surface of the eyelids and covers the "white" part of the eye (up to the circular margin of the cornea) is called the conjunctiva. Any inflammation of this membrane is therefore called conjunctivitis. Here we will describe three varieties of conjunctivitis.

A. *Acute Catarrhal Conjunctivitis.* The redness and swelling of the conjunctiva in this form of conjunctivitis is usually more pronounced on the under surfaces of the eyelids than over the "white" part of the eye. Early in the disease there is a watery discharge from between the eyelids. Later the discharge contains more mucus and, in severe cases, a mixture of mucus and pus. The patient complains of scratching, burning, and smarting sensations in the affected eyelids.

Because the infection is caused by a germ (any one of several carried by contaminated fingers, towel, or handkerchief) both eyes are often involved. Any age group may be affected, but the disease is more common in children and young adults. Often several in the same household or school are affected about the same time, the disease being easily communicated. The course of the disease when not treated is ten to fourteen days. The epidemic form of acute catarrhal conjunctivitis is commonly known as "pinkeye." The symptoms are intense.

What to Do

1. Take all reasonable precautions to keep the infection from being transmitted to other persons. Wash the hands with soap after each contact with the patient's face. Use paper face towels and handkerchiefs and burn these after use. Bed linen which has come in contact with the patient must be disinfected before it is laundered.

2. Apply a series of compresses wrung out of ice water to the affected eyes for a period of five minutes at least three times a day.

3. Consult a physician. He will prescribe the kind of eye drops or ophthalmic ointment that will combat the particular kind of germ involved.

B. *Chronic Catarrhal Conjunctivitis.* The symptoms here are about the same as in acute catarrhal conjunctivitis, only not so severe and usually worse at night. The disease tends to last for weeks and even months. Causes include a carry-over from a neglected case of acute catarrhal conjunctivitis, irritation from

252

polluted atmosphere, a poor state of general health, insufficient sleep over a long period of time, indulgence in intoxicating drinks, overuse of the eyes, the need for eyeglasses, chronic inflammation of the tear duct, and allergy.

What to Do

1. Correct all conditions that may have contributed to the disease.

2. Follow a general health-building program including the eating of an adequate diet with sufficient vitamins.

3. Cleanse eyelid margins and lashes at least twice daily with cotton applicators moistened with warm water.

4. Instill sulfa or antibiotic drops or ointment several times daily as recommended by your eye physician.

C. *Gonorrheal Conjunctivitis*. Gonorrheal conjunctivitis is one of the most severe of the infections that involve the eyes, and it can be the most tragic. It is caused by the same germ that causes venereal gonorrhea. The germ is carried to the eyes by fingers or towels that have been contaminated by contact with some of the discharge from a gonorrheal infection. It can also be acquired by a newborn babe at the time of birth from direct contact with the genital tissues of an infected mother. Without prompt and adequate treatment, gonorrheal conjunctivitis frequently causes blindness by destruction of the tissues of the eye.

The first symptoms appear from twelve hours to three days after the germs contact the membranes of the eye. There is extreme redness, swelling, and tenseness of the eyelids. A profuse discharge comes from between the eyelids, which is at first watery and bloody and soon becomes laden with pus. The eye burns and smarts and feels painful. It is tender to touch.

What to Do

1. From the very first, extreme care must be taken to prevent the infection from being carried to the other eye (if only one eye is infected) or to some other person. Anyone caring for the patient should wear a surgical gown, face mask, rubber gloves, and protective glasses while with the patient. All materials used in treating the patient, such as towels and compresses, should be placed at once in a disinfectant solution before being destroyed or laundered. Such a solution can be prepared by dissolving one teaspoonful of lysol in two quarts (two liters) of water.

2. The patient should be placed under the care of a doctor as soon as possible. Preferably, the patient should be treated in a hospital. Methods of treatment now available provide very good prospects of recovery with preservation of normal eyesight *provided* they are employed early in the course of the disease. Antibiotic and sulfa drugs properly administered usually control the infection promptly.

3. Cold compresses (wrung from ice water) applied to the eyes help to reduce the swelling and congestion of the eyelids and make the patient more comfortable. These can be used continuously at first and then intermittently as inflammation subsides.

CORNEAL ULCER.

The cornea is the transparent, front portion of the eye through which are seen the iris (colored portion) and the pupil. When circumstances permit certain germs to penetrate the front layer of the cornea, these cause a small, local destruction of tissue, and an ulcer results. Dangers associated with a corneal ulcer are: (1) The scar which follows healing of the ulcer will interfere with the passage of light into the eye (more serious when the ulcer is at the center of the cornea); (2) the ulcer may become so deep that a perforation of the cornea results; and (3) the infection associated with the ulcer may spread to structures within the eye.

In corneal ulcer the eye is painful and sensitive to light. Tears overflow the eyelids. The patient avoids all contact with light. On close observation of the eye, a small grayish-yellow opaque spot may be seen on the cornea. The white of the eye appears reddened immediately surrounding the iris and cornea.

The most common circumstance leading to corneal ulcer is injury, such as an accidental scratch of the cornea by a fingernail or penetration by a small piece of steel or other foreign body, which permits the entrance of germs. Corneal ulcer occurs commonly in elderly persons or those whose general health is poor. It may occur in cases in which the eyelid is persistently rolled inward so the eyelashes scratch the cornea. Injury to the nerve that supplies the cornea may predispose to corneal ulcer. The various forms of conjunctivitis may be complicated by the development of corneal ulcer.

What to Do

1. Consult a physician promptly.
2. The physician will try first to find the immediate cause of the ulcer. He will search for local injuries to the cornea such as penetration by foreign bodies, abrasions, or chemical irritation. He will consider whether there have been other eye diseases, taking steps to remedy any faulty condition which he may find.
3. The physician will use appropriate "drops" to dilate the pupil and thus draw the iris away from the area of the ulcer so that the iris will not adhere to the site of the ulcer. He may find it necessary to use gentle cautery on the base of the ulcer and may apply a soft contact bandage.
4. As soon as the immediate condition improves, the patient should cooperate in a program of improving his general health.

CROSSEYE.
(See *Squint* in this chapter.)

DACRYOCYSTITIS (INFECTION AND OBSTRUCTION OF THE TEAR DUCT).

In this condition there is an infection of the tear duct located at the corner of the eye next to the base of the nose. It occurs in about 1 percent of newborn infants and occasionally in older children and adults.

The ailment produces a pussy discharge at the inner corner of the eye, a redness of the membrane lining the lower eyelid near the inner corner of the eye, and a spilling of tears onto the cheek.

In most infant cases, the condition is caused by a failure of the lower portion of the duct to open at about the time of birth. In a few, there is a fault in development of the tear duct. In older children and adults the obstruction is caused by an injury, by some infection within the nose or sinuses, or, rarely, by a developing tumor. Once the tear duct is stopped up, it tends to become infected.

What to Do

1. In many infants the tear duct must be probed, and, in a few, reconstructive surgery performed.
2. In older patients the first problem is to control the infection. This is done by the use of sulfa drugs and antibiotics together with the use of cold compresses to the inflamed area. Once the infection is controlled, the route for the drainage of tears usually has to be reestablished by surgery.

ECTROPION.
Ectropion is a rolling outward of the eyelid (one or both) so as to expose part of its lining membrane. The exposed membrane is usually swollen and red; and, when the lower lid is

involved, there tends to be an overflow of tears. This may be caused by the contraction of scars following face injuries or burns. It may follow the chronic form of catarrhal conjunctivitis. In elderly people it may be the simple result of a general relaxation of the tissues. It is a common complication of facial paralysis.

What to Do

1. In elderly persons, placing the lids in normal position at bedtime and retaining them so during the night by the use of a bandage may be of some help.

2. Plastic surgery which loosens the tight scar of a previous injury or which shortens the margin of the eyelid may be necessary.

ENTROPION.

In entropion there is a rolling inward of the edge of the eyelid and the eyelashes. The rough edges of the eyelid, and especially the lashes, cause irritation of the cornea, with congestion, pain, a profuse flow of tears, sensitivity to light, and possible ulceration of the cornea. On account of the involvement of the cornea, vision is endangered.

Entropion often follows burns, injuries to the lids, and trachoma (a disease of the eyelids) in which the formation of scars pulls the tissues out of shape. In the lower eyelid, it may be due to spasm of the muscle. It may follow conjunctivitis.

What to Do

1. Temporary measures for preventing the eyelid from turning inward include the use of an adhesive plaster splint passing from the margin of the eyelid to the cheek, and the painting of collodion on the skin of the eyelid to stiffen it.

2. The only really satisfactory treatment in these cases is for an eye surgeon to reshape the eyelid so that the eyelashes are directed forward.

EYELID, INFLAMMATION AND INFECTION.

(See *Blepharitis; Sty;* and *Trachoma* in this chapter.)

EYELIDS TURNING OUT OR IN.

(See *Ectropion* and *Entropion* in this chapter.)

FOREIGN BODY IN THE EYE.

(See *Injury to the Eye* in this chapter. See also under *Foreign Body Injury,* volume 3, chapter 18.)

GLAUCOMA.

Glaucoma is a prevalent, sight-threatening disease in which the pressure of the fluid in the eye becomes so increased that, unless promptly and properly treated, the internal eye structures are permanently damaged.

Normally there is a constant production of clear fluid within the front part of the eye, which is drained away as fast as it is produced. In glaucoma interference with the drainage of this fluid develops increased pressure in the eye.

About 2 percent of the population above forty years of age are candidates for glaucoma. If these cases are not handled properly, about one million persons now living in this age group will become blind because of glaucoma. With early detection and proper care, however, vision can be preserved in 80 to 85 percent of all cases.

It is better for a person above forty to arrange for a routine eye examination every two years than to wait for the signs of glaucoma to develop before he consults an eye specialist. The prospect of favorable treatment is best in cases detected early.

When symptoms of glaucoma do occur, they may include: (1) a gradual decline in the acuity of vision (the person feels that he needs a change of glasses); (2) the seeing of "halos" around lights; (3) headaches; (4) pain in the eye which becomes throbbing in nature and, eventually, very in-

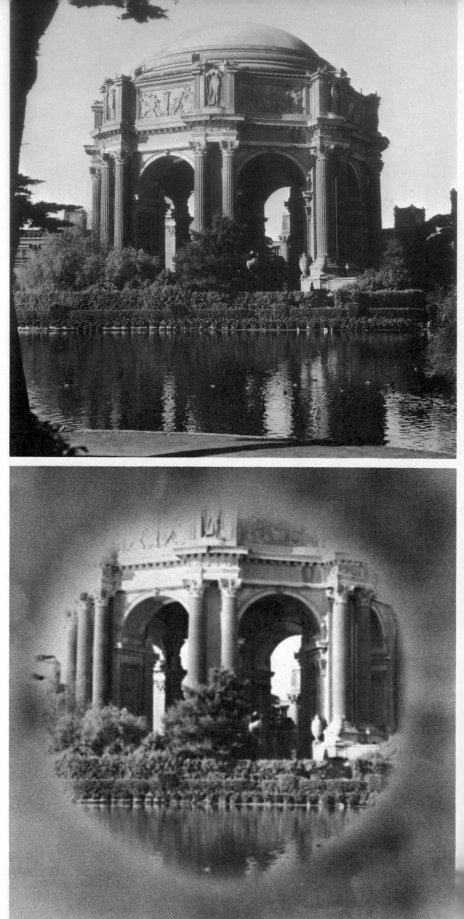

Upper: A scene as viewed by a person with normal vision. Lower: Same scene as viewed by a person with moderately advanced glaucoma.

256

tense; (5) redness of the eye, particularly in that part of the "white of the eye" which surrounds the cornea; (6) swelling of the eyelids; (7) tendency for the eyes to water; (8) enlargement of the pupil; and (9) a "steamy" appearance of the cornea.

Glaucoma may develop insidiously without any demonstrable cause, or it may follow some other disease of the eye. The acute type may develop very rapidly in a period of a few hours.

What to Do

1. **Even when there is no evidence of eye disease, it is advisable to have the eyes examined at least every two years. The examination should include a measurement of the pressure within the eye.**

2. **If there is question regarding the meaning of any symptoms relating to the eyes, consult a physician who specializes in diseases of the eye and carefully follow his directions.**

3. **Treatment of a case of glaucoma is of two types: (1) medical (using appropriate eye drops and medicines) and (2) surgical. In many cases, medical treatment alone will prevent progression of the disease and thus save the patient's vision.**

GLASSES—NEED FOR WEARING. (See *Refractive Errors* in this chapter.)

HORDEOLUM. (See *Sty* in this chapter.)

INJURY TO THE EYE. (See also *Burns, Thermal and Chemical* in this chapter, and C. *Foreign Body in the Eye* under *Foreign Body Injury* in volume 3, chapter 18.)

Most injuries to the eye involve penetration of the eye or one of its tissues by some foreign body. When the cornea is involved, symptoms of pain, excessive production of tears, and sensitivity to light call attention to the injury. The seriousness of an injury to the cornea depends on the depth to which the foreign body penetrates and on whether germs were introduced at the time of the injury.

Penetrations into the part of the eye behind the lens are even more serious than those involving only the cornea, iris, and lens. The seriousness of these deep injuries depends on the size of the object that penetrates and on whether it carried infection into the eye. These deep penetrations usually produce a severe inflammation which leads to destruction of the eye.

A sharp blow to the eye, even though there is no penetration of its tissues, may cause the retina to become detached. Unless successfully treated, this produces a loss of vision in part or all of the involved eye. A blow to the eye may cause hemorrhage into the front part of the eye and may predispose to acute glaucoma.

What to Do

1. **A physician, preferably a specialist in diseases of the eye, must be consulted at once.**

2. **When there has been penetration by a small foreign body lodged in the cornea, the procedure for removal is relatively simple. But the danger of corneal ulcer remains even after the removal.**

3. **Iron or steel foreign bodies in deeper parts of the eye can sometimes be removed by an electromagnet in the hands of a skilled operator. Other objects may be removed by small forceps introduced through the original opening.**

4. **In a severe eye injury the physician may recommend the prompt removal of the affected eye as a means of avoiding the tragic disease "sympathetic ophthalmia" in which the second eye becomes involved a few weeks after a serious injury to the first eye.**

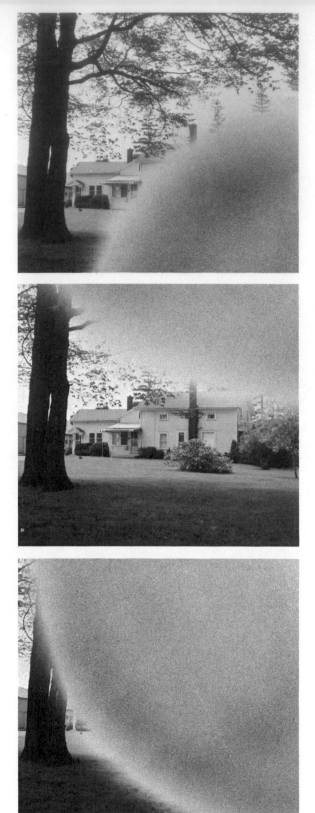

Different ways in which the visual field is partially obscured by a detachment of the retina.

IRITIS.

Iritis is a serious disease in which the iris (the colored circular curtain that surrounds the pupil) becomes inflamed. Usually only one eye is involved.

There is throbbing pain in the eye, with the pain radiating to the forehead and temple, also blurred vision, sensitivity to light, and an excess production of tears. The "white of the eye" around the cornea appears reddened, and the iris itself appears swollen and dull. The fluid behind the cornea may appear turbid.

Iritis often occurs in association with some other disease such as rheumatoid arthritis, tuberculosis, or diabetes. It may follow an infection in some other part of the body. It may complicate a disease of the cornea (as corneal ulcer) or be associated with an injury to the eye (either the same or the opposite eye).

The course of the disease varies from case to case. It may clear up in a few weeks or last for several months. Glaucoma and blindness may develop.

What to Do

1. Consult a specialist in diseases of the eye.

2. Give careful attention to the underlying disease or condition.

3. The physician may arrange for medicated eye drops and other medications.

4. Warm compresses to the eye may help to relieve the pain.

PTERYGIUM.

A pterygium is a wedge-shaped fold of membranous tissue containing small blood vessels which grows into the "white of the eye" and the cornea from the inner corner toward the pupil. It occurs especially in persons who are exposed to wind or dust. As it grows into the cornea, it destroys the clarity of the cornea and may interfere with vision.

What to Do

The only satisfactory treatment for pterygium is a minor surgical procedure. This should be done, preferably, before the pterygium has had time to grow far onto the cornea.

REFRACTIVE ERRORS.

The normal eye is so designed that the entering rays of light are brought to a precise focus on the retina, where the optical image is produced. In some eyes the rays of light are brought to a focus too soon so that the image on the retina is blurred. This condition is known as myopia or nearsightedness. In others, the rays have not focused by the time they reach the retina. This is hyperopia or farsightedness. In still other eyes, the optical system of the eye is slightly distorted so that rays entering in the horizontal plane focus at a distance different from those entering in the vertical plane. This is known as astigmatism.

The fitting of properly designed glasses compensates for the refractive errors of the eye so that all entering rays of light focus clearly on the retina. This not only provides a clear image but also relieves eyestrain caused by the muscles within the eye as they respond to reflex mechanisms intended to bring the visual image into sharp focus.

At about the age of forty-two to fifty, the natural lenses within a person's eyes may gradually lose their elasticity and therefore they cannot change shape sufficiently when vision at close range (as in reading) is attempted. We see such a person holding his newspaper farther and farther away from his face. This inability of the eye to adjust for near vision is called "presbyopia." Properly

In a person needing glasses light rays entering the eye do not focus sharply on the retina, hence the blurring of vision.

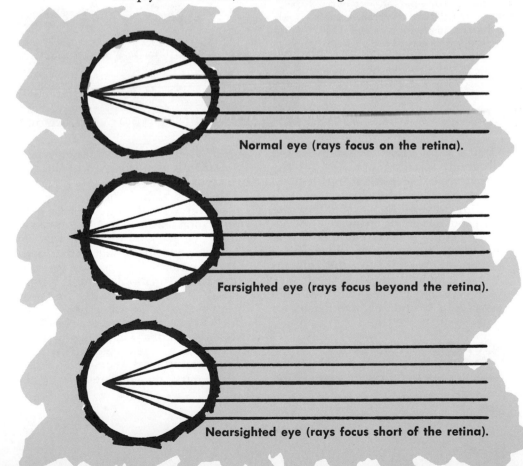

Normal eye (rays focus on the retina).

Farsighted eye (rays focus beyond the retina).

Nearsighted eye (rays focus short of the retina).

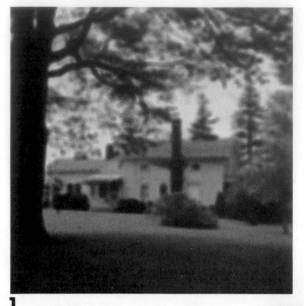

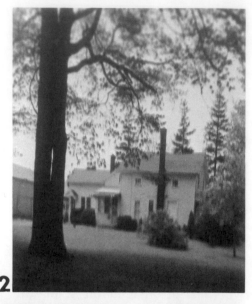

Differing views of the same house as seen (1) by a shortsighted person (blurred); (2) by a person with horizontal astigmatism (blurred, vertical dimensions heightened); (3) by a person with vertical astigmatism (blurred, horizontal dimensions widened).

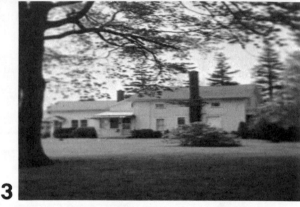

fitted reading glasses will remedy the situation, focusing optically on the retina what the normal eye focuses naturally. The difficulty is that with reading glasses the strength of the glass lens cannot be changed, as is true of the natural lens, to permit both near and distant vision. So the older person either removes his reading glasses when he looks at a distant object, or he wears double glasses (bifocals)—the lower lens for reading and the upper lens for distant vision.

SQUINT (STRABISMUS).

Squint is a condition in which the two eyes are not directed to the same object. There are two common types: (1) that in which the axes of the two eyes cross each other (cross-eye) and (2) that in which the axes of the two eyes diverge (walleye). A person with squint soon learns to ignore the vision of one eye or the other; otherwise he would see two objects rather than one.

In the normal course of events, during the early months of life, a child should develop the ability to direct the two eyes to the same object. The ability to fuse the visual images of the two eyes into a single, composite, three-dimensional image is a function of the cortex of the brain; and this ability must be acquired, if at all, during the first six years of life.

In squint, there is a lack of ability to fuse the two visual images. The basic cause may be refractive errors (a need for correction of optics by the wearing of glasses) or an inequality in the strength or nervous control of the muscles that move the eyes in the orbits.

What to Do

1. Consult a physician who specializes in diseases of the eyes. For a child this consultation should take place as soon as possible after the condition is discovered—by all means, well before the child reaches the age of six.

2. The physician will determine whether the child needs to wear glasses. He may arrange for the child to have exercises of the eyes which aid in the ability to fuse the two visual images. He may operate on one or both eyes to equalize the pull of the muscles within the orbits.

STRABISMUS.

(See *Squint* in the preceding paragraph.)

STY (HORDEOLUM).

A sty is a miniature pyogenic infection (like a small boil) which develops at the margin of the eyelid in connection with the opening of one of the glands contained in these tissues. It develops commonly in association with the need of glasses, in blepharitis, or in consequence of a lowered condition of general health, anemia, or diabetes. If the predisposing condition persists, sties tend to recur.

What to Do

1. Apply hot compresses for ten minutes at a time, at least four times a day. This relieves pain and hastens the time when the sty will rupture spontaneously.

2. If healing is retarded or if complications threaten, consult a physician at once. He may administer antibiotics or sulfa drugs.

3. Make a consistent effort to remove the cause and improve the condition of general health.

TEAR DUCT, OBSTRUCTION OF.

(See *Dacryocystitis* in this chapter.)

TRACHOMA.

Trachoma is an infectious, highly contagious disease, caused by a virus which affects the membranes lining the eyelids and covering the front of the eye. It is very common in Oriental countries and in districts where poor hygiene and overcrowding prevail. Once it becomes chronic, its principal manifestation is in firm "granulations" which develop in the membranes lining the eyelids. These scratch and injure the cornea with resulting blindness in many cases.

The initial symptoms are redness of the membranes, mild itching, the production of a watery discharge, swelling of the eyelids, and a sensitivity to light.

What to Do

1. Trachoma should be treated in its early stages before it causes damage to the cornea. The use of sulfa drugs and antibiotics, as supervised by a physician, usually brings cure within a few days.

2. Cold compresses to the eyes help to control the inflammation and thus improve the patient's comfort.

ULCER OF THE CORNEA.

(See *Corneal Ulcer* in this chapter.)

WALLEYE.

(See *Squint* in this chapter.)

Diseases of the Ear, Nose, and Throat

BOIL IN THE EAR.

A boil or furuncle in the skin lining the external auditory canal is similar to a boil elsewhere, except that it is rarely very large. The infection is usually caused by scratching the auditory canal with a fingernail, hairpin, match, or other contaminated object in an attempt to remove earwax. There is at first an itching within the canal, which leads to more scratching. Then the spot becomes tender and very painful. Deafness does not result unless the swelling is extensive enough to close the canal, and it is not permanent. When the boil ruptures, the pain moderates rapidly and soon entirely disappears. Possibly because it is hard to disinfect the skin inside the ear canal, one boil in the ear is likely to be followed by others.

What to Do

1. Make a thin wick of gauze, wet it with 5 percent phenol in glycerin, and gently push it into the ear canal, taking care to have the wick loose so that any possible pus drainage will not be obstructed.

2. Keep a hot-water bottle over the ear most of the time.

3. Without treatment the boil should rupture and discharge pus within four or five days. It is better to see a physician early. He may be able to give or prescribe antibiotics or sulfas that will abort the boil or shorten its course. Once the boil has developed, the doctor may find it advisable to lance it and thus hasten the process of healing.

4. After the boil has ruptured or has been lanced, keep a very loose wick smeared with 5 percent ammoniated mercury ointment in the ear, removing it every day and replacing it with a clean wick after a very gentle syringing with warm saturated boric acid solution.

5. After drainage has ceased, discontinue the wick and use a saturated solution of boric acid in alcohol as ear drops three times a day for several days.

6. If other boils come one after another, be sure to consult a physician.

DEAFNESS.

Most cases of deafness come under one of two types—conduction deafness and nerve deafness—though some cases combine the two. When conduction deafness is caused by foreign bodies, water, or wax in the external ear canal, it is easily curable in most cases. If it is from pus or exudate in the middle ear, it can usually be cured if expert treatment is not delayed too long. If it is the result

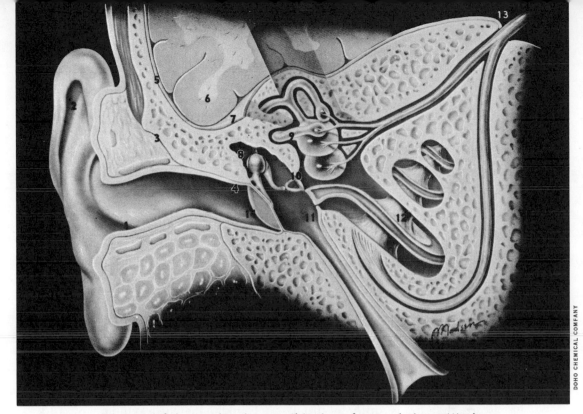

Diagram of the ear showing possible sites of severe lesions: (1) circumscribed furuncle of otitis externa; (2) infection of the cartilage of concha; (3) subperiosteal abscess in case of perforated cortex; (4) sinking of post-superior canal wall, during periosteal inflammation, as seen in acute mastoiditis; (5) epidural cerebral abscess; (6) circumscribed cerebral abscess; (7) subdural abscess; (8) cholesteatoma (pseudo) situated in the attic of middle ear; (9) circumscribed labyrinthitis; (10) fixation of stapes, involving the annular ligament; (11) fistula opening on roof of tympanic orifice of eustachian tube; (12) when these areas are involved, the labyrinth becomes seat of lesion; (13) by pressure on auditory nerve, especially the vestibular branches, symptoms of angle tumor develop; (14) perforated eardrum.

of a shortage of air in the middle ear because of a stoppage of the auditory tube due to enlarged adenoids, an acute cold, chronic catarrh, et cetera, a retraction inward of the eardrum will develop; but the condition is usually curable. If this condition is neglected, however, thickening of the drum and adhesions between the small bones in the middle ear tend to develop; and the hearing is likely to be permanently impaired, though not entirely lost. A rupture of the eardrum membrane so severe that it cannot completely heal will cause permanent partial conduction deafness.

Some cases of conduction deafness occurring in persons in the second and third decades of life are due to otosclerosis—an overgrowth of spongy bone which wedges the footpiece of the stirrup-shaped stapes bone tightly in the oval window leading to the inner ear. The cause of this overgrowth is unknown, but surgery can often restore the hearing.

Nerve deafness in people of any age may be the result of acute inflammation of the auditory nerve. This type is sometimes curable. If the nerve center becomes diseased and degenerates, however, the deafness will

263

become permanent. Arteriosclerosis in the blood vessels of the inner ear may lead to degeneration of its nerves and permanent deafness, but this is not at all likely to happen in early life. The sensory-neural structures may deteriorate from injury, infection, severe fever, tumor, or overuse of such drugs as streptomycin, quinine, or salicylates and result in varying degrees of permanent deafness. Nerve-type deafness may also be present from birth because of birth injury, German measles (rubella) in the mother during early pregnancy, hemolytic disease of the newborn, or abnormal development of the inner ear; but this type of deafness is not common.

Impairment of hearing in a small child may not be noticed. If it has been present from birth or develops soon thereafter, the child himself may not be aware that he is different from other people. Parents should be suspicious of impaired hearing if speech development and learning are slow, and if the child is uncooperative or inattentive. In such cases examination by an ear specialist will reveal the true condition; and the fitting of a hearing aid may remedy the situation. If not, the specialist's advice is a valuable guide in placing the child in a special school or institution for the deaf, if this is thought best.

An older child or an adult is likely to notice any increasing impairment of hearing, though this may not be true if the increase is very gradual. It is wise to be aware of this possibility and keep watch to detect any such impairment in its early stages. Tests by an ear specialist can detect its presence and can also determine the type and measure the degree to which it has developed. As a result of his examinations and these tests, he can give reliable advice on how to restore the hearing or at least to check the advance or the impairment. The condition may prove to be simple and easily remedied, or it may prove a cause of permanent loss of hearing if not treated properly and in time. There are no short or simple rules that can enable a person without special medical training and experience to arrive at an accurate judgment about the cause or the seriousness of a developing defect in hearing, and self-treatment is obviously not practical.

What to Do

1. If you are a parent or are responsible for a child, watch for signs of possible impairment of hearing. If any such signs appear, take the child to an ear specialist for examination and possible treatment or advice.

2. If you notice that you are becoming hard of hearing, do not delay in consulting a specialist.

EARACHE.

Earache may be a symptom of otitis media, or inflammation of the middle ear. (See *Middle-ear Inflammation* in this chapter.) Before proceeding with any treatment, read the discussion of that serious infection and follow the advice given there if it seems likely that the pain indicates infection. A physician may have to make an examination to determine the true nature of the case, and treatment without his knowledge is not wise. There are, however, cases of earache without infection, though infection is likely to develop if the earache persists very long.

Any congestion or inflammation in the nose may extend to the auditory tube and up that tube to the middle ear. Inflammation of the auditory tube and the middle ear may cause earache.

Many cases of ear trouble can be traced to violent blowing of the nose. Forceful efforts at clearing the nose are unwise. They are more dangerous when there is infection in the nose or sinuses. But whether there is infection or not, back pressure from forcible nose blowing may be communicated to the middle ear and cause earache.

264

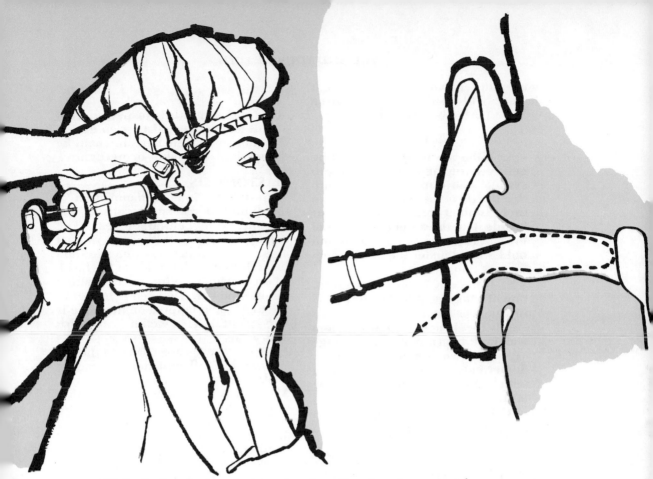

Method of syringing the ear, showing direction the water takes.

If there are repeated attacks of earache and the cause is not removed, serious and permanent damage to the ear and the sense of hearing may follow. In many instances loss of hearing can be traced to improper care of a minor ear disturbance. It may be the result of lack of medical attention in case of a persistent or recurrent common earache.

What to Do

1. At the first twinges of pain, apply to the ear a hot water bottle or some other source of steady heat.

2. Consult a doctor if attacks of earache are frequent or if any attack lasts more than a few hours.

3. Temporary relief from pain may be obtained by dropping two or three drops of a warmed "ear drops" preparation into the affected ear. A doctor's prescription is necessary for anything except unmedicated drops.

4. Olive or salad oil, gently warmed over the stove in a teaspoon and dropped into the affected ear, may give relief, and should be used if the remedies mentioned in (3) are not available. Take care that the oil is not too hot.

5. A nasal decongestant spray or nose drops used four times a day for two or three days will aid drainage and aeration of the nose and auditory tubes.

FOREIGN BODY IN THE EAR.
(See *Foreign Body in the Ear* in volume 3, chapter 18.)

IMPACTED EARWAX.
Impacted earwax is common. As a rule, the wax becomes quite hard and causes partial deafness. If proper care

is used in removing it, no permanent damage will result, and the hearing will be perfectly restored.

What to Do

1. If the wax is *soft*, remove it by gently syringing with a soft rubber syringe and warm water. Be sure that the tip of the syringe is held so there is plenty of room around it or beside it for the water to flow out of the ear. Have the patient sit up, and hold a bowl under the ear to catch the escaping water.

2. If the wax is *hard*, use a solution of a teaspoonful of baking soda in a glass of warm water and syringe gently for about two minutes. Then wait for fifteen minutes and syringe again for two minutes, and so on. Sometimes a peliminary softening with hydrogen peroxide or glycerine is necessary.

3. If the wax cannot be washed out without causing pain. consult a physician.

LABYRINTHITIS.

Labyrinthitis is an inflammation or congestion of the inner ear, especially that part of it having to do with the sense of equilibrium. It is usually onesided. It may be caused by infection. It is characterized by extreme dizziness, ringing in the ear, and a staggering gait. If no infection is present, the hearing is seldom seriously affected, and recovery is usually complete within a few days; but recurrences are common.

If infection is present, as may be the case when the labyrinthitis is preceded or accompanied by otitis media or mastoiditis, the condition tends to persist until extensive destruction of the tissue of the area occurs and permanent total deafness results on the affected side. It is important to know early whether infection is present or not, and whether there is need for prompt antibiotic and perhaps later surgical treatment to preserve the hearing.

What to Do

If labyrinthitis is suspected, consult an ear specialist for an examination and for such treatment as he may find advisable or necessary.

MASTOIDITIS.

Mastoiditis is an inflammation of the lining of the small cells in the mastoid bone behind the ear. The condition begins with pain in that area, which becomes intense and extends to the whole side of the head. There is usually redness and swelling behind the ear. The area is tender to the touch, and tapping on the bone is very painful. The victim is feverish and weak.

Nearly every case of mastoiditis is caused by inflammation spreading back from an infected middle ear. Mastoiditis is a common complication of those diseases which tend to cause inflammation of the middle ear. (See *Middle-ear Inflammation* in this chapter.) When not operated on, many cases formerly developed fatal complications, most commonly meningitis; but at present the early judicious use of antibiotics or sulfas usually aborts an acute mastoiditis that would otherwise require surgery to save life.

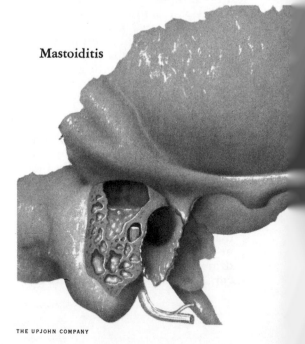

Mastoiditis

266

What to Do

1. If mastoiditis is suspected, consult a physician at once. He may be able to bring the condition under control by using antibiotics, sulfas, et cetera; but surgery may be necessary.

2. While waiting for medical care, keep a small ice pack over the affected side behind the ear.

3. Keep the patient's feet and legs warm. A hot footbath every few hours is helpful.

MENIERE'S DISEASE (HYDROPS OF THE INNER EAR).

This is a very troublesome form of illness characterized by attacks of extreme dizziness associated with nausea and vomiting. The nausea and vomiting may be so severe and so prolonged that the individual sweats profusely. There is no pain and no fever and no evidence of disease of the digestive organs. In addition to the attacks of dizziness, there is usually a more or less persistent ringing in the ear accompanied by progressive nerve-type deafness. In many cases only one ear is affected at first, but later both may become involved.

The attacks of dizziness associated with nausea and vomiting may last only a few minutes, or they may last several hours. The frequency of the attacks varies widely. Meniere's disease usually attacks those over 40 years of age, and it affects men somewhat more frequently than women.

The immediate cause of the attacks of dizziness is an increase in the pressure of the fluid contained within the inner ear (the endolymph). Because the inner ear is concerned with both hearing and equilibrium, both of these functions are affected when the fluid pressure in this organ is increased. It is debatable whether the increase in fluid pressure is caused by an excess production of fluid or a partial failure of the fluid to be reabsorbed at the normal rate.

In some cases Meniere's disease is aggravated or even precipitated by emotional stress. There are other cases in which allergy seems to be the aggravating factor. In still others there is some metabolic disorder, such as hypoglycemia, which seems to make the individual susceptible to this manifestation.

Some persons with this disorder experience relief from the symptoms after a few weeks or months. In other cases the symptoms persist for long periods of time. Perhaps the usual pattern is that the attacks of dizziness gradually become less frequent and less severe, but the deafness persists and even becomes more severe.

What to Do

1. The person with Meniere's disease should consult either a neurologist or an otologist (physicians who specialize in the nervous system or in diseases of the ear).

2. The specialist's first attempt will be to discover the basic precipitating cause of this illness, whether it be emotional tension, allergy, metabolic disorder, or arteriosclerosis. If he is successful in discovering the cause, then removing this cause should bring about an improvement in the patient's condition.

3. In extreme cases, the specialist may recommend surgery such as is performed at a few specialty clinics in certain medical centers. The surgical procedure is a delicate one and involves creating a bypass so that the excess fluid within the inner ear may escape into the fluid-filled space which surrounds the brain.

MIDDLE-EAR INFLAMMATION, ACUTE (ACUTE OTITIS MEDIA).

Inflammation of the middle ear is usually caused by germs that have spread from the nose or throat through the auditory tube to the ear. As a rule, it is a common cold that gets the germs started on this path. The infection may

Inflammation of the middle ear.

be forced into the ear by pressure in the nose and throat when the nose is blown. It is a bad habit to blow the nose forcibly. Middle-ear infection also occurs as a complication in attacks of scarlet fever, influenza, measles, or other diseases in which the throat becomes inflamed.

The attack begins with pain in the ear. The pain may spread over the side of the head. The victim may have chills and fever. The ear feels full. There may be ringing in the ear and partial or complete deafness. When the drum ruptures and lets the pus escape, there is prompt relief from pain, but a persistent discharge of pus begins.

Babies often have middle-ear infection. When a baby has this trouble, he cries constantly, turning his head from side to side, and unless he is too young to do so, placing his hand frequently upon the affected ear. He is almost sure to have fever, and he may have convulsions.

Two great dangers attend middle-ear infection. First, the infection may spread to the mastoid cells behind the ear, and from them to the covering of the brain or to the blood vessels of the brain, causing death from meningitis or from thrombosis of these vessels. Second, if the drum ruptures by itself, the ragged hole thus caused does not heal easily and may result in damage to the hearing.

Professional advice and treatment are important. The infection should be checked as soon as possible to keep it from spreading, and the physician may have to make an incision in the eardrum to prevent spontaneous rupture and to facilitate aftercare.

Some cases of inflammation of the middle ear are not caused by infection but by congestion in the air passages or by obstruction of the auditory tube. They may not cause fever or any severe pain, but there is often a sense of pressure or a snapping or ringing in the ears and an impairment of hearing. These cases, as well as the aftercare of many others that started as infections, often require special treatments that must be given by a physician experienced in handling ear diseases, if the victims are to be relieved of their distressing symptoms and to have their hearing saved from permanent impairment.

What to Do

1. **Drop three drops of warmed ear drops into the ear every three hours. A doctor's prescription is necessary for anything other than unmedicated drops.**

2. **Apply heat over the ear much of the time, preferably by means of a hot-water bottle.**

3. **If the pain persists more than three hours, consult a physician. He may be able to check the progress of the infection by using antibiotics or sulfas.**

4. **Another reason for securing the services of a physician, preferably an ear specialist, is that drainage of pus is important, and it is better to lance the eardrum than to let it rupture by itself.**

5. **If the pus begins to drain before the physician sees the patient, or in case it is draining as a result of lancing, the physician may**

268

give directions as to aftercare. If he does not, or if no physician is in attendance, clean the ear canal twice a day by the gentle use of a small, soft cotton swab. Do not syringe the ear. Continue the application of heat as long as there is pain or tenderness. It is well to protect the skin of the outer ear from irritation by keeping it anointed with a soothing ointment such as hydrophilic ointment or zinc oxide ointment. A loose bandage or a cap of several thicknesses of gauze will help protect the pillow from the pus.

MIDDLE-EAR INFLAMMATION, CHRONIC (CHRONIC SUPPURATIVE OTITIS MEDIA).

A chronic discharge from the middle ear may follow neglect or improper treatment of an acute middle-ear infection and is usually associated with a permanent perforation of the eardrum. It may be characterized by tissue degeneration or destruction as a result of the activity of some virus or other microorganism. The discharge may be simply mucus, but more often mucus mixed with pus. It is not often that any pain or fever is present.

What to Do

1. Very gently clean the ear canal twice a day with tiny dry cotton swabs, taking care not to go too deep. Then use eardrops of a saturated solution of boric acid in 70 percent alcohol. Do not irrigate the ear canal with water or any watery solution. It is best not to try to irrigate it at all in this condition or in any other condition in which the drum is perforated.

2. Avoid swimming or any other activity that involves danger of getting water into the ear canals.

3. If the discharge does not stop within a month, or if there is any persistent headache, dizziness, or pain on the involved side, consult a physician, preferably an ear specialist.

OTOMYCOSIS.

Otomycosis is really a skin disease rather than an ear disease, but it is a fungous infection of the skin lining the external auditory canal, so it is discussed here. It is quite common, usually very persistent, and needs treatment different from that for fungous infections of the skin of other parts of the body. Such an infection results in moist crusting of the skin, with a dirty coating on which there may be scattered moldy spots of yellow, green, or black. There is usually a foul smell and more or less itching, stinging, and pain.

What to Do

1. Clean the ear canal gently once a day with small cotton swabs wet with 95 percent alcohol, or dissolve one tablet of chloramine-T in an ounce (30 c.c.) of water and irrigate the ear canal.

2. Three times a day instill into the ear canal five drops of a saturated solution of boric acid in 70 percent alcohol.

3. More effective treatments may be given by an ear specialist or a skin specialist.

OTOSCLEROSIS.

Otosclerosis is a disease of unknown cause affecting the small bones of the ears or surrounding bone or other structures, but chiefly the footpiece of the stirrup-shaped stapes and the bone surrounding the oval window. It is characterized by progressive loss of hearing and is the causative factor in about half the cases of conductive deafness. There is no certain means of preventing this condition. In some cases an inherited tendency seems to play an important role. Expert surgical attention gives the best chance of help. Modern surgery may restore the hearing in most cases. In other cases not suitable for surgery, a hearing aid professionally selected may prove helpful.

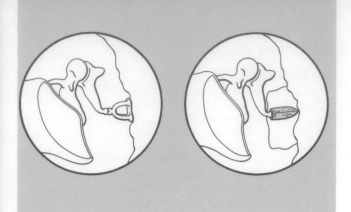

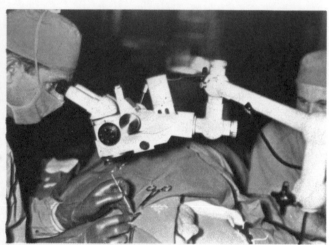

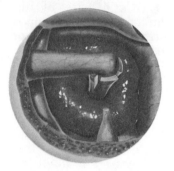

Top: Diagram of positions of normal stapes (left) and prosthesis (right). Center: Restorative surgery for otosclerosis. Bottom: Polyethylene prosthesis resting on a pad of gelfoam over oval window.

What to Do

Consult an ear specialist. He may outline a program that will delay the progress of the condition. A stapedectomy, a stapes mobilization, or a fenestration operation may become advisable.

RINGING IN THE EAR (TINNITUS).
(See also *Meniere's Disease* in this same chapter.)

Some people are troubled with noises in the ear. These may be pulsating sounds, continuous sounds, sounds like the ringing of bells, music, the buzzing of bees, and other noises.

Chronic irritation or inflammation of the middle ear is a frequent cause. Other causes are nervousness, high blood pressure, inflammation of the external auditory canal, foreign body in the ear, impacted earwax, Meniere's disease, disease of the auditory nerves, anemia, reflexes due to irritation of the nose or the teeth or the digestive tract, and the use of certain drugs such as quinine and the salicylates. The best hope for relief depends on finding the cause and correcting it, and an ear specialist's aid is usually needed in the search.

What to Do

No treatment is of any permanent value unless directed toward the cause. Ask an ear specialist to help you find it.

Diseases of the Nose

BOIL IN THE NOSE.
(See *Boils* under subhead "Bacterial and Rickettsial Diseases" in chapter 12 of this volume.)

THE COMMON COLD.
Everybody knows what a cold is from his own experience and observation. Being so common, colds are not considered as seriously as they should be. Neglected colds are often the forerunners of chronic catarrh, in-

fected sinuses, middle-ear disease, bronchitis, and even tuberculosis.

One or more viruses and several kinds of disease germs are the usual causes of the various symptoms associated with colds and their common complications, but they require favorable conditions in order to enter the tissues and produce their effects. Because of the virus causation, many colds are epidemic, affecting practically a whole community by contagion. Exposure to cold and wet, overwork, loss of sleep, or other debilitating conditions lower body resistance and prepare the way for the virus to begin its work. The virus, in turn, prepares the way for the disease germs already present in the nasal cavity and other respiratory passages to do theirs. Other predisposing factors are lack of resistance from living in overheated and poorly ventilated rooms, without sufficient outdoor exercise; lowered resistance due to errors in diet, including overeating, especially of such concentrated foods as sugar, fats, meats, and nuts; and diseased tonsils and adenoids. People who live truly hygienic lives save themselves from many colds.

What to Do

1. Consult a physician about the use of some of the remedies called, as a group, antihistamines, which may abort a cold or at least lighten some of its early symptoms if taken properly when the first sniffles and nose stuffiness appear.

2. If fever has already developed, put the victim to bed until the fever goes down.

3. Give hot fomentations to the face and chest, with a cold compress to the back of the neck and a hot foot bath, continuing the treatment until perspiration starts. (See volume 3, chapter 20.) Keep the victim well covered to prevent any chilling, and keep him in bed for at least twelve hours after perspiration has ceased.

4. Give the victim all the water and fruit juices he will drink, but no other food for twenty-four hours. After that, the diet should consist of soft or liquid foods, mainly fruit juices, until all acute symptoms have subsided.

5. Congestion in the head may be relieved by hot fomentations to the face and a cold compress to the back of the neck at the same time, three times a day. (See volume 3, chapter 20.)

6. Do not give drugs without a physician's orders.

7. When the fever and other acute symptoms have subsided, the victim may take moderate exercise in the open air and gradually return to a normal diet.

FOREIGN BODY IN THE NOSE.
(See *Foreign Body Injury in the Nose* in volume 3, chapter 18.)

HAY FEVER (ALLERGIC RHINITIS).

Hay fever is usually caused by the action of pollen from certain plants upon an oversensitive nasal mucous membrane. The disease may end in an attack of bronchial asthma; and the two are often associated, as both of them are caused by an unusual sensitivity of the afflicted person to certain proteins. So small an amount as two or three pollen grains may bring on an attack of hay fever in an unusually sensitive person.

The symptoms of hay fever are not unlike those of an ordinary cold in the head, but with more sneezing, headache, distress, and depression of the spirits, though less fever. The eyes are watery, red, and irritated; the nasal passages are red and swollen; and these distressing conditions tend to persist much longer than they would in case of a cold.

Local treatments may bring partial relief, but as a rule the symptoms persist until the passing of the season for the blooming of the plant that causes the disease, until a heavy rain or frost interferes with the spread of the pollen, or until the victim moves to a region where the offending plant does not grow. The dry air of a high mountain usually brings much relief, but any change that takes the victim away from the active cause will eventually bring about a cure of hay fever.

What to Do

1. The use of one of the group of antihistamine substances taken by mouth may be helpful.

2. If the victim can live in an air-conditioned house and breathe filtered air, his distress will be at least partly relieved while he is in the house.

3. Study the cause of the condition in consultation with a physician. He may carry out a program of desensitization that will give relief or prescribe remedies that will help control the symptoms.

NOSEBLEED (EPISTAXIS).

(See *Nosebleed* in volume 3, chapter 18.

OBSTRUCTION OF THE NOSE.

A common cause of nasal obstruction is the common cold already discussed.

Sometimes the turbinate bodies in the nasal cavities become enlarged and obstruct the nose. When they do, a part of them should be surgically removed so that air can get through. The bony partition, or septum, between the nostrils may be crooked and obstruct one or both sides. Relief calls for surgical straightening or partial removal of the deviated bony or cartilaginous septum.

A nasal polyp, a special kind of tumor that usually forms as a result of chronic infection in a sinus, or in people who have a tendency to allergic conditions, may obstruct a nostril. It also calls for surgical removal. When adenoids become much enlarged, the victim may be unable to breathe easily through his nose. Children who habitually breathe through

the mouth usually have enlarged adenoids and excessive mucus. Such enlarged adenoids should be surgically removed.

What to Do

Find out the cause of the obstruction and have it corrected. Doing so will probably call for the services of a nose and throat specialist.

SINUSITIS.

Certain cavities in the bones of the face and the floor of the skull are called sinuses. These cavities are lined with mucous membrane. All of them have openings communicating directly or indirectly with the nasal passages, and whenever an excess of mucus is secreted it must drain out through these openings into the nose or else build up pressure and create discomfort inside the sinuses. Such congestion often builds up in case of allergy or a common cold. If there is no infection present, the trouble may correct itself soon; but if pus-producing germs begin to work in the clogged sinuses, inflammation results.

The maxillary sinus, or antrum, is located in the cheekbone below the eye; the frontal sinus, in the frontal bone above each eye. Several small ethmoid sinuses are located in the ethmoid bone between the nasal cavities and the orbits of the eyes. The sphenoid sinus or group of sinuses is situated in the sphenoid bone at the base of the skull, deep behind the ethmoid cells. The ethmoid sinuses become infected easily, but they also drain easily, so they may be responsible for a more or less persistent discharge but rarely cause acute sinusitis. The maxillary sinuses also become infected easily, but they do not drain as readily as do the ethmoid sinuses. Acute maxillary sinusitis is, therefore, fairly common; and it also often progresses to chronic sinusitis with a slow but persistent discharge, which tends to dry into crusts inside the nasal passages. Frontal sinusitis is rather rare, but the drainage passages from these sinuses are long and narrow, so they easily become obstructed. As a consequence, frontal sinusitis is usually acute and painful and may require surgery for relief. Sphenoid sinusitis is very rare.

In general, acute sinusitis causes tenderness in the affected area, usually considerable pain, and a moderate fever. Heating for fifteen minutes at a time with a 100-watt electric globe held as close to the skin of the painful area as can be borne, or applying hot fomentations to the face, may give relief. (See volume 3, chapter 20.) Such treatments may be given from three to five times a day. It may require surgery to establish drainage of pus and to relieve pressure, especially in a severe case of frontal sinusitis.

Chronic sinusitis may produce few or no local symptoms; but, if there is no free drainage for the pus, toxic substances may be absorbed into the circulation, impairing general health and lowering general resistance to disease.

It is difficult and often impossible to apply any local treatment that will reach the germs inside the sinuses and clear up the infection. Suitable antibiotics taken by injection or by mouth are often beneficial, especially in acute cases. These, of course, must be ordered by a physician.

What to Do

1. If acute sinusitis causes pain or fever, and especially if it persists longer than a day or two, consult a physician for examination, advice, and treatment.

2. If the advice given above for the treatment of chronic sinusitis does not bring definite improvement, consult a physician.

3. Membrane-shrinking nose drops used sparingly may help to correct the drainage from the sinuses and improve breathing through the nose.

Diseases of the Throat

COUGH.

(See also under *Cough* in volume 3, chapter 22.)

The common cold often causes a cough. But a cough due to a cold should not last longer than a week. Any cough which lasts longer than a week, if the underlying cause is not already known and under treatment, should be carefully investigated to find out its true cause and to institute proper treatment.

What to Do

1. If the cough is a throat cough, use hot fomentations to the throat twice a day, and a heating compress to the throat every night. (See volume 3, chapter 20.)

2. If the cough is a chest cough, apply hot fomentations to both chest and throat twice a day, and a moist chest pack to the chest and a heating compress to the throat every night. (See volume 3, chapter 20.)

3. For a simple and harmless cough syrup, boil together 1 part lemon juice and 3 parts honey.

4. For a persistent cough, steam inhalations several times a day are often helpful. (See volume 3, chapter 20.)

5. If the cough persists more than a week, consult a physician.

CROUP.

(See *Croup* under "Handling Emergencies," volume 3, chapter 18.)

DIPHTHERIA.

(See under "Infectious Diseases," chapter 28 of this volume.)

ENLARGED TONSILS AND ADENOIDS.

The tonsils are located one on each side of the throat at the root of the tongue, and the adenoids are on the upper back wall of the throat behind the soft palate. Tonsils and adenoids are normal body structures; but when they become unduly enlarged, they cause obstruction in the throat and the back part of the nasal cavities. Enlargement of tonsils and overgrowth of adenoids are usually present together, and most often found in children. Mouth breathing may be present but not noticed because it may occur only at night. Because it interferes with normal oxygen intake, the child's growth and nutrition are deficient, and his mental activity may be slow.

Apparent mental slowness may be the result of defective hearing brought about by the partial closure of the auditory tubes by the large mass of adenoids in the upper and back part of the throat. Defective hearing in children is sometimes curable by the removal of enlarged adenoids. Acute earache may be caused by obstruction of the auditory tubes by enlarged adenoids; and the tendency to such a condition is usually checked by the removal of the adenoids. But the enlargement and consequent need for removal of the adenoids is not of itself a sufficient reason for removing the tonsils also. On the other hand, the adenoids may not be enlarged when the tonsils are.

The reason the tonsils and adenoids become enlarged is that this is their response to infection. The normal function of the tonsils and adenoids is to serve as part of the body's mechanism for resisting infection. These organs produce some of the lymphocytes, cell types designed to resist the invasion of germs.

When a person has a sore throat (pharyngitis), the tonsils and adenoids enlarge in response to the added demand for protection against the germs which are causing the sore throat. But when infections in this part of the body occur frequently or when the germs involved are particularly virulent, the tonsils and adenoids may themselves become infected and in this state remain enlarged for long periods of time. Such acute infection

274

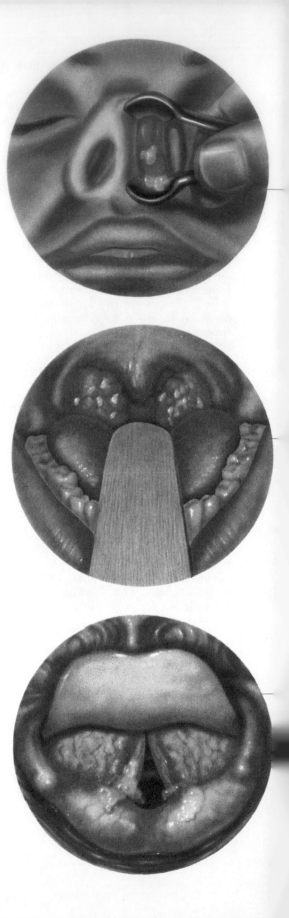

Upper respiratory
tract infections.
Shown in detail at
left are: (top) rhini-
tis, (center) tonsilli-
tis, and laryngitis.

of the tonsils constitutes tonsillitis which is discussed as a separate item later in this chapter. In the present discussion we are concerned with the problems of tonsils and adenoids which have become so large that they actually obstruct the passage of air from the nose into the lungs or of food from the mouth into the esophagus. In a given case, the physician must decide whether the advantages of removing these enlarged tonsils and adenoids outweigh the hazards involved in the surgical removal of these tissues.

Probably the best procedure for the physician to follow is to treat the child that has enlarged tonsils and adenoids with adequate doses of antibiotic medicines for a sufficient period of time to control whatever lingering infection may be present in these organs. If, in spite of such treatment, the child is still subject to frequent attacks of tonsillitis, and if either the tonsils or the adenoids or both are still so large as to interfere with the passage of air and of food through the pharynx, then it may be advisable for the tonsils and adenoids, one or both, to be removed surgically. It is preferable to wait until the child is past six years of age before removing the tonsils and adenoids. In some cases, however, the condition becomes urgent so that these tissues may need to be removed even before he reaches the age of six.

What to Do

In cases of chronically infected tonsils and adenoids and in cases in which these organs have become so large as to interfere with breathing or swallowing, the physician should be consulted to determine whether the tonsils and adenoids should be removed. Probably the physician will want to observe how the child responds to treatment with antibiotic medicines before he makes the final decision as to whether surgery should be performed.

FOREIGN BODY IN THE THROAT.

(See under *Foreign Body in the Throat* in volume 3, chapter 18.)

LARYNGITIS.

The larynx is the voice box. Externally, the front part of it forms a lump on the front of the neck commonly called the "Adam's apple."

The two most common symptoms of laryngeal disease are hoarseness and obstructed breathing. Hoarseness may progress to complete loss of the voice, and obstruction to breathing may become so severe as to cause death from asphyxia if not promptly relieved.

A. Acute laryngitis may be caused by overuse of the voice, an acute cold, eating too hot or otherwise irritating foods, breathing smoke or fumes, heavy smoking, or infection with various kinds of germs. It may be a part of some general acute-disease picture, as in case of scarlet fever, whooping cough, typhoid fever, influenza, or diphtheria. If so, the treatment will call for the services of a physician and will be part of the total treatment for the causative disease.

B. Chronic laryngitis is most often caused by chronic sinusitis or persistent wrong use of the voice. Persistent hoarseness in a case of supposed chronic laryngitis may develop as the only symptom of cancer of the larynx. A throat specialist should evaluate the situation.

C. Edema of the larynx, resulting in a swelling of its various parts and obstruction to breathing, causes no other marked symptoms than the difficulty of breathing; but this may become so severe that life can be saved only by having a physician make an opening in the trachea below the larynx—an operation called tracheotomy.

D. Chronic infectious diseases may affect the larynx. Among these, tuberculosis and syphilis are most common. They cause a characteristic interior appearance that is rather easily detected by an experienced physician. Early detection and suitable treatment are vital, but both of these require the services of a physician, and no home treatments of any kind will prove effective.

What to Do

1. In acute laryngitis, not known to be caused by any serious infectious disease, home treatments can be tried for a few days. The following are suggested:

A. Give the voice as nearly complete rest as possible.

B. Rest in bed in a warm room.

C. Use steam inhalations every three or four hours. (See volume 3, chapter 20.)

D. Apply a heating compress to the throat every night. (See volume 3, chapter 20.)

2. If relief does not result within two or three days, consult a physician for examination, advice, and treatment.

3. Chronic laryngitis calls for study by a physician.

PHARYNGITIS, ACUTE (SORE THROAT).

The pharynx or throat is that part of the body between the nose and the voice box. Any acute cold or catarrhal condition can readily extend to it and set up inflammation and soreness. Loss of sleep, breathing stale or smoke-laden air, neglecting exercise, or almost any other deviation from good health habits may bring a sore throat as one of the penalties. For the first day and night there is usually a feeling of increasing soreness and discomfort. For the second day the symptoms are usually worse if proper treatment is not being given, and the second night may be sleepless from the extreme discomfort.

An acute sore throat often occurs as a symptom of some other disease. (See *Sore Throat* under "List of Signs and Symptoms," volume 3, chapter 22.)

What to Do

1. If the sore throat is not known to be due to some other underlying condition which is already under treatment, proceed as follows:

A. Gargle every half hour with hot water to which common salt and baking soda have been added, half a level teaspoonful of each to a glass of water.

B. Apply hot fomentations to the throat for twenty minutes two or three times a day. (See volume 3, chapter 20.)

C. If fever is present, rest in bed as much as possible.

D. Apply a heating compress to the throat every night. (See volume 3, chapter 20.)

E. The diet should consist of liquid or soft foods, and not less than three quarts of liquid should be taken each day.

2. If the throat soreness gets worse, or if it persists more than three days in spite of the above treatments, consult a physician.

RETROPHARYNGEAL ABSCESS.

One complication of acute pharyngitis is the development of an abscess in the deeper tissues just behind the pharynx. Lymph nodes here function to control the spread of infection in the usual case of pharyngitis. When the infection is severe, these lymph nodes may be overwhelmed, allowing an abscess to form. This causes swelling and tenderness of the back wall of the throat, difficulty in swallowing and breathing, swollen glands in the neck, and a change to a nasal quality of the voice. In acute cases there may be chills, fever, and stiffness of the neck.

What to Do

1. When these symptoms develop, a physician should be consulted.

2. The use of antibiotic drugs as prescribed by the physician may bring the infection under control.

3. Once an actual abscess has

formed, the pus which it contains must be removed. If the abscess is allowed to rupture on its own, there is danger that the pus will be drawn into the air passages. Usually the physician will prefer to drain the abscess by making a surgical incision.

SEPTIC SORE THROAT.
(See under "Infectious Diseases," chapter 28 of this volume.)

TONSILLITIS AND QUINSY.
Acute tonsillitis is a common disease among young people, many of whom have repeated attacks. This condition may be associated with rheumatic fever. It may be followed by infection of the heart valves, by red and boggy swellings under the skin, by Sydenham's chorea (St. Vitus's dance), or by acute inflammation of the kidneys. These complications may also develop in connection with a tonsil infection that persists and becomes chronic, though no longer causing symptoms characteristic of acute tonsillitis. For these reasons, either children or adults who suffer from repeated attacks of acute tonsillitis or who have a persistent tonsillar infection without acute symptoms should have their tonsils removed. This is done, of course, after the infection has subsided.

In acute tonsillitis the onset is often accompanied by a chill and aching in the back and limbs. The fever may rise rapidly to as high as 104° F. (40°C.). There is intense soreness of the throat, with great difficulty in swallowing. The tongue is coated, and the breath is foul. The tonsils are swollen and red, and they may show yellowish or whitish patches on the surface. The neck glands are usually swollen. In some cases the entire throat is bright red, and there may be a red rash over the chest or the entire body. In such cases the infection is due to germs the same as, or similar to, those which cause scarlet fever.

Quinsy is often associated with tonsillitis. This consists of the development of an abscess in the bed of, or around, the tonsil. The throat on one or both sides is greatly swollen. There is much pain, and great difficulty in swallowing. The neck glands are swollen, and the victim can hardly open his mouth. There is high fever and great prostration.

What to Do

1. Apply hot or cold applications to the neck, whichever the patient tolerates best. For hot applications, narrow fomentations may be used. (See "Simple Home Treatments," volume 3, chapter 20.) Cold is best administered by an ice collar (an ice bag shaped to fit around the neck).

2. Apply a heating compress every night. (See "Simple Home Treatments," volume 3, chapter 20.)

3. Use a hot gargle every hour. A suitable solution is prepared by dissolving half a teaspoonful of common salt and half a teaspoonful of baking soda in a glass of very warm water.

4. The use of antibiotics or sulfonamides as arranged by the physician usually brings prompt improvement.

5. Plenty of water and fruit juices should be taken, preferably hot.

6. A liquid diet should be taken for at least two or three days.

7. When quinsy with abscess formation develops, it is advisable that the abscess be drained by surgical incision.

8. If there are repeated attacks of tonsillitis or quinsy, or if the physician finds evidences of a chronic infection, have the tonsils removed at a convenient season after the infection has subsided.

WHOOPING COUGH.
(See under "Infectious Diseases," chapter 28 of this volume.)

Diseases of the Respiratory Organs

Diseases of the Air Passages

ASTHMA (BRONCHIAL ASTHMA).
In asthma there is interference with the passage of air through the membrane-lined tubes that serve the lungs. The lining of the bronchi (the branches of the trachea that extend into the lungs) become congested and swollen. Also, there may be contractions of muscles which are in the walls of the bronchi and their terminal branches. Because of the resulting diminished caliber of the tubes, airflow is impaired. The patient has more difficulty in expelling air than in drawing it in.

Approximately half the cases of asthma are caused by sensitivity to certain pollens or dust contained in the inhaled air or to certain foods or drugs. The remaining half seem to result from infections of the organs of breathing in which the patient has become sensitive to the products of the germs responsible for the infection.

Asthma, a common disease which attacks the sexes about equally, may occur at any age from infancy to old age. It occurs in attacks in which the expiratory phase of the breathing cycle is prolonged and associated with a characteristic "wheeze."

What to Do

For Immediate Relief.
Persons who suffer recurring attacks of asthma usually carry with them the medicine that they have found gives relief. Often this is an aerosol of a bronchodilator or vasoconstrictor, such as epinephrin or isoproterenol, which they spray into their throats by a nebulizer as they inhale quickly. For the more acute cases, hypodermic injection of a small amount ($1/2$ ml.—less for children) of a very dilute solution (1 to 1000) of epinephrine usually gives prompt relief. Severe attacks may cause so much obstruction to air flow as to require prompt emergency treatment by a physician. Sometimes hospitalization is necessary.

When an attack is not too severe, a warm drink or the inhalation of vapor from a vaporizer or from a pan of boiling water may be helpful. A cone made of paper is useful in directing the vapor to the face of the patient. Care must be taken, however, to prevent the hot water vapor from burning the face or the membranes of the air passages.

Long-range Treatment.
1. Make careful observations of the contacts which seem to aggra-

279

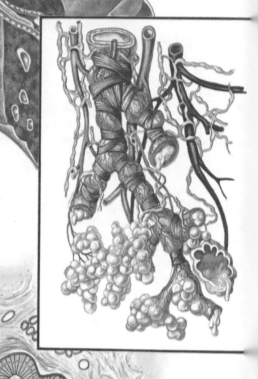

In asthma the membrane-lined tubes that serve the lungs (the trachea and bronchi) become swollen and congested with mucus. Upper left: Anatomical reconstruction of a primary lobule in a normal lung and a cross section through a small bronchus. Lower right: Anatomical reconstruction of a primary lobule of an asthmatic lung, showing constriction of bronchial walls and congestion of thick, tenacious mucus. Also a cross section through a small bronchus in bronchial asthma.

vate the asthma and to which, supposedly, the patient may be sensitive. Possibilities include pollens, house dust, feather pillows, pets, and substances used in connection with the patient's occupation. Avoiding contact with the offending substance is the most satisfactory way to prevent or relieve the asthma. In some cases the sensitization may be reduced by a series of desensitizing injections arranged by the physician.

2. For the asthmatic patient who has become sensitive to the chemical by-products of an infection within his own body, the physician will make a careful search for the infection and treat it accordingly.

3. Immunization with influenza vaccine annually may be beneficial.

4. Physical exercise should be limited to the individual's ready tolerance.

5. Extremes of cold and of humidity should be avoided by the asthmatic patient.

BRONCHIECTASIS.

In this condition the medium-sized and smaller bronchi, usually in the lower part of one or both lungs, dilate and become pockets in which chronic infection tends to persist with the formation of large amounts of more or less pussy sputum.

This disease is characterized by fits of coughing and the raising of much sputum, especially in the first hour or two after rising in the morning and immediately upon lying down at night. In severe cases the sputum is peculiar in that it tends to form three layers on standing—the lower layer purulent, the middle watery, and the top frothy. The color may be greenish, brownish, or blood-tinged, for mild hemorrhages are quite common.

Any condition that involves forcible coughing for considerable periods of time, together with occasional obstruction of the bronchial tubes, tends to stretch these tubes and produce bronchiectasis. The signs and symptoms—especially weight loss, weakness, night sweats, and fever—are much like those of tuberculosis, and a careful examination is needed to distinguish one disease from the other. In bronchiectasis, if free drainage of the bronchial "pockets" can be maintained, the disease becomes more a pest than a peril. However, patients with bronchiectasis are more vulnerable to attacks of pneumonia than they would be otherwise. Actual cure of the disease is rare, though in cases where the trouble is largely confined to part of one lung, surgical removal of that part may go far toward effecting a cure.

What to Do

1. Try to build up the general health by securing an abundance of rest, fresh air, sunlight, and an adequate diet rich in vitamins.

2. Have a thorough examination made by a physician, who will need to take chest X rays of the usual type, and possibly of some special types. He may also possibly do, or arrange for, a bronchoscopy, to detect the true condition of the bronchi. He can give advice as to the possible value of surgery, as well as give or supervise other treatments, most of which can probably be given at home.

3. Free drainage of the abundant sputum is highly desirable. Experience has proved that this can usually best be accomplished by having the patient assume and maintain some special posture, preferably one in which he lies across a bed with his face and chest hanging downward, his arms folded, the elbows resting on a pillow on the floor, and the most seriously affected side of the chest uppermost. The head and neck will therefore be at a lower level than the lungs. When by repeated trials it has been determined which position promotes the freest drainage, the patient should assume this position three or four times a day,

especially in the morning at rising time, and hold it for at least ten minutes each time. Coughing will probably be spontaneous, but this is desirable because it promotes drainage.

4. If the patient is a smoker, his smoking should be discontinued.

BRONCHITIS.

A. *Acute Bronchitis.* One of the most common ailments, especially among children and frail adults, is acute bronchitis. In most people myriads of germs lurk in the nose and throat, ready to find their way into the air passages and cause trouble there. In many cases acute bronchitis develops as a complication of the common cold. In children, enlarged adenoids and diseased tonsils may have much to do with the tendency to repeated attacks of acute bronchitis. In some adults there appears to be a peculiar lack of resistance to this condition. In others, allergy plays an important causative role.

Exposure to cold from improper clothing may be conducive to bronchitis. Along with the chilling there is a lowering of resistance, and the alert germs take advantage of the opportunity to overcome the existing natural resistance. Bronchitis is a common complication of measles, scarlet fever, whooping cough, influenza, typhoid fever, and other infections. Chlorine and some other gases or fumes accidentally encountered in chemical laboratories or manufacturing establishments can produce severe forms of acute bronchitis.

The early symptoms of a typical case of acute bronchitis are mild fever, mild headache, chilliness, some hoarseness and wheezing, a persistent but at first unproductive cough, and a "raw" sensation behind the breastbone. When the cough becomes productive, the feeling of distress behind the breastbone usually lessens or subsides. Ordinarily, acute bronchitis runs its course in a few days, but it may become persistent, lingering on

for months and finally becoming chronic bronchitis.

What to Do

1. If a fever is present, bronchopneumonia must be suspected and medical attention should be secured.

2. As long as there is any fever, keep the patient in bed in a moderately warm room, and keep the temperature in the room as nearly constant as possible.

3. If the patient is a smoker, his smoking should be discontinued.

4. If there is difficulty in breathing or a marked feeling of tightness in the central portion of the chest, give steam inhalations thrice daily.

5. Give the patient hot fomentations to the chest twice a day, and apply a moist chest pack to the upper chest overnight, taking care not to let him become chilled at any time. (See volume 3, chapter 20, "Simple Home Treatments.")

6. Once a day for the first two days, at the time of giving the fomentations, give a hot foot bath also, and continue the treatment long enough to produce free perspiration. Be especially careful not to allow any chilling of the patient as long as he is perspiring.

7. If definite improvement is not seen within two days, call a doctor. He may need to prescribe a cough remedy and to use some antibiotics or sulfas to combat infection.

8. If the bronchitis is a complication of some other disease, or if it was caused by the inhalation of irritating or corrosive gases or fumes, it is especially important to give the patient the benefit of a physician's care.

B. *Chronic Bronchitis (Chronic Catarrhal Tracheobronchitis).* Chronic bronchitis may develop after one or more attacks of acute bronchitis, but many cases that are thought to be chronic bronchitis may be something more serious, such as pulmonary emphysema, tuberculosis, or bronchiogenic carcinoma (in adults). It may complicate or follow any disease or condition which involves protracted or repeated irritation or inflammation of the lining of the bronchial tubes. In the 1964 report of the United States Surgeon General's Advisory Committee, which had been given the assignment of studying the relationship between smoking and health, it was stated that "cigarette smoking is the most important of the causes of chronic bronchitis in the United States, and increases the risk of dying from chronic bronchitis."

A dry cough, worse in the mornings, is characteristic. The cough is more severe and more likely to bring up sputum in the wintertime and following a cold. Wheezing and difficulty of breathing eventually develop in many cases. Fever is rare. The condition may become worse from year to year, but since the discovery of antibiotics it has proved possible to bring about improvement in many cases of chronic bronchitis in which secondary bacterial infection is a factor.

What to Do

1. Apply to a physician or to your local health department for an examination to determine whether or not what seems to be chronic bronchitis is really a more serious disease. Especially is this advice applicable to older people.

2. Do not smoke.

3. Avoid dusty air.

4. Correct the diet. Do not eat meat, fried food, greasy food, highly seasoned food, pastry, desserts, sweets, confections, or much starch. The diet should consist largely of fruits and vegetables.

5. In cool weather be sure to keep the limbs warmly clothed, giving special attention to the ankles and wrists.

6. Use steam inhalations once a day.

7. Hot and cold foot baths, fomentations to the chest followed by a cold mitten friction, salt glows, or revulsive compresses to the chest are good. (See volume 3, chapter 20, "Simple Home Treatments.")

8. Consult a physician. He can determine whether or not some underlying condition is causing the bronchitis or keeping it from being cured, and he can give or prescribe remedies aimed at the special needs of the individual case.

9. If other treatments fail, seek a warm, dry climate to live in.

COUGH.

(See under *Cough* in volume 3, chapter 22, "List of Signs and Symptoms.")

CROUP.

(See under *Croup* in volume 3, chapter 18, "Handling Emergencies.")

FOREIGN BODY IN THE AIR PASSAGES.

(See *Foreign Body in the Air Passages* in volume 3, chapter 18, "Handling Emergencies.")

Diseases of the Lungs

ABSCESS OF THE LUNG.

A lung abscess may develop as a complication of pneumonia, from inhaling infectious material at the time of or following nose or throat surgery, from irritation produced by an aspirated foreign body, from infectious material carried to the lung by the bloodstream, by extension of an infection in some neighboring tissue, or as a complication of a chest injury.

A patient with a lung abscess has a dry cough, chest pain, more or less difficulty in breathing, chills, irregular fever, and sweats. Also, as a rule, he has foul-smelling sputum which tends to be discharged at intervals rather than by constant drainage, if it is discharged at all. If expectorated and allowed to stand, it tends to form three layers as in bronchiectasis.

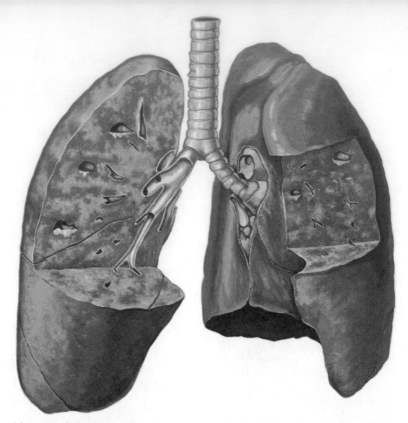

Abscess of the lung, showing accumulation of sputum in the tissues.

If the abscess is near the central portion of the lung, it may open into a bronchial tube fairly soon so that the pus will be coughed up. If it is near the outer part of the lung, it will probably need surgical opening and drainage. If not drained surgically, the pus is likely to break through into the pleural cavity and cause hemorrhage, emphysema (pus in the pleural cavity), or other serious complications. Without proper drainage, many lung abscesses eventually prove fatal.

What to Do

1. If a lung abscess is suspected, have a physician take an X ray and make a careful physical examination. If one is present, the fact should be known, because the condition is too serious to be left untreated and cannot be properly treated without medical help.

2. Follow the same general supportive program that is recommended for a case of pulmonary tuberculosis. (See first part of chapter 29 in this volume.)

3. If pussy sputum is being coughed up, try postural drainage, as recommended for a case of bronchiectasis.

CANCER OF THE LUNG.
(See under *Lung* in chapter 11 of this volume.)

COLLAPSED LUNG (ATELECTASIS).
Atelectasis, or lung collapse, is present in some newborn infants, in whom it may prove to be fatal. In others it occurs as a result of either an obstruction in a bronchus or pressure on the lung by some type of disease within the pleural cavity. Many cases are complications from a surgical operation.

Except in newborn infants, the onset of the condition is usually sudden. Difficult breathing, a dusky color, fever, chilliness, a rapid heartbeat, and pain in the chest are some of the symptoms. There are other signs which can be detected by a physician on examination of the patient, and which can guide in the treatment. Since the usual case develops in a surgical patient within from one to three days after the operation, a physician will almost surely be at hand to do promptly what needs to be done. In all other cases, if atelectasis is suspected, a physician should be called immediately, as death may come without immediate proper treatment. There is no home treatment of any use.

What to Do

1. The patient is likely to be in a hospital already. If not, obtain medical care immediately. Keep the patient as warm and comfortable as possible. Probably hospitalization will be necessary, because the doctor will need hospital equipment to use in treating the patient.

2. Emergency treatment will include every practical means of inducing the patient to cough and breathe deeply. One means is to give him a mixture of 5 percent carbon dioxide in oxygen to breathe. Other treatment will depend on how the case develops, and will be under the supervision of the physician.

EMPHYSEMA.

Emphysema is a disease of the lungs in which some of the walls which separate the thin-walled air sacs from each other have broken down, thus creating larger than normal air spaces within the lung. This condition reduces the efficiency of the lung in performing its function of exchanging oxygen and carbon dioxide.

Emphysema may develop from prolonged interference to the movement of air through the smaller air passages (as in chronic bronchitis or asthma) or from a condition which has increased the lung's fibrous tissue (as in pneumoconiosis). In many cases emphysema is associated with chronic bronchitis. As is also true of chronic bronchitis, the incidence of em-

Emphysema diffused throughout the lung. The enlarged alveoli, characteristic of the disease, may be observed on the surface.

physema has increased greatly in recent years, and it is now recognized that both of these diseases occur much more commonly among smokers. Emphysema usually occurs after the age of forty, and its mortality rate increases with the age of its victims. It is more common in men than in women in a ratio of about four to one.

The symptoms of emphysema include difficult breathing on exertion, wheezing when air is exhaled, severe cough with the expectoration of foul mucus, and a gradual change in the shape of the chest caused by the excessive activity of the muscles concerned with breathing (so-called "barrel chest").

Emphysema is a progressive disease with an eventually fatal outcome inasmuch as the changes in the tissues of the lung cannot be reversed. By following a health-promoting plan of living, however, the patient may be made relatively comfortable and his life prolonged.

What to Do

1. If the victim of this disease is a smoker, he should quit the habit. Smoking tends to aggravate the symptoms.

2. It is best for the patient to remain up and around as much as possible rather than being confined to bed. Strenuous exertion should be avoided, for this increases the work load of the lungs and aggravates the symptoms.

3. Great care should be taken to avoid infections, particularly those affecting the lungs. Here the physician's cooperation in administering antibiotic drugs as necessary is important.

4. Drugs which dilate the air passages and which make it easier to cough up the mucus produced in the lungs are helpful.

5. Some relief of the difficulty in breathing may be obtained by the patient's placing the palms and fingers of both hands just under the lower margin of the ribs in front and **pressing inward and upward as he exhales. This assists in emptying the lungs. This should be repeated with each breath for perhaps fifteen times. The procedure should be carried out three or four times a day.**

HYALINE MEMBRANE DISEASE.
(See *Respiratory Distress Syndrome* in this same chapter.)

INFLUENZA (FLU).
(See under *Influenza* in chapter 28 of this volume.)

PNEUMOCONIOSIS.
Pneumoconiosis is defined as a chronic fibrosis of the lungs, caused by inhaling irritating dusts. There are many varieties of such dusts, hence many varieties of pneumoconiosis, since the different varieties of dusts vary greatly in their effects on the lungs. Only a few varieties, however, are of much health significance, though no variety can be really cured. The most hopeful prospect comes from knowing the danger, avoiding the inhalation of dangerous dusts, and detecting the early warning signs of pneumoconiosis so that precautions against such inhalation can be taken.

Anthracosis is caused by inhaling coal dust, siderosis by inhaling iron particles, asbestosis by inhaling asbestos dust, and silicosis by inhaling particles of sand, quartz, or other forms of silica. Only the last two cause much damage to the lungs, with silicosis being a greater menace than asbestosis. Silica, and to a less extent other silicon compounds, have a severe irritating effect on lung tissue. Stonecutters, sandblasters, and hardrock miners are especially subject to silicosis. Anthracosis and siderosis may be complicated by more or less silicosis, however, because the causative dusts are often mixed with silicon compounds.

Silicosis develops gradually. The first noticeable symptom is like that of emphysema—difficulty of breathing on exertion. Later this difficulty may be present even during rest, and the complexion becomes dusky. There may be no cough at all, and coughing is rarely a prominent symptom. Tuberculosis is especially likely to develop in lungs that have been damaged by silicon. As silicosis progresses, there is increasing weakness, fever, loss of weight, and exhaustion; and death may come as a result of a complicating tuberculosis or bronchopneumonia.

If the early symptoms of silicosis are noticed in people exposed to suspicious dusts, that exposure should be terminated immediately; and subsequent exposure to tuberculosis should be carefully avoided. The disease will progress somewhat after the exposure is terminated, but in most cases not enough to menace life, and possibly not enough to prevent normal activity, except in occupations that require heavy muscular exertion.

The general treatment for silicosis is the same as that for tuberculosis, but no treatment can restore the lungs to a normal condition. The best that can be done is to check or slow down the progress of the disease, to help prevent the development of tuberculosis, and to conserve what lung capacity and physical strength are left. In some cases a late complication is threatened failure of the right side of the heart; and in these cases treatments aimed at this complication may give considerable relief.

What to Do

1. As soon as symptoms suggesting silicosis are noted, terminate all exposure to the dusts that may be harmful.

2. Have a physician make examinations to determine the amount of damage to the lungs and to advise on the future program for employment and living conditions.

PNEUMONIA.

Pneumonia is a disease of the lungs in which the delicate lung tissue becomes acutely infected. Several kinds of germs and viruses may cause such an infection. When the infection involves principally a certain lobe of a lung, the disease may be called lobar pneumonia. When the infection is scattered throughout the lungs and involves the delicate tissue closely related to the bronchi, it may be called bronchopneumonia.

Pneumonia is a serious disease for two reasons: (1) The toxemia is usually relatively great. (2) One's very life depends on the continuous functioning of the lungs. In diseases of the digestive organs a person may go without food for a while, thus giving the affected organs a rest from their usual functions during the process of healing. But the lungs must function continuously, day and night, whether they are involved with disease or not, in order that oxygen and carbon dioxide might be exchanged to satisfy the needs of the body's cells. If their involvement with disease curtails their function too much, death results.

Prior to the advent of antibiotic drugs, pneumonia in its various forms was one of the major killers. Infection of the lungs, once established, had to run its course as the body endeavored to build up resistance to the particular germ causing the pneumonia. If tissue resistance was developed soon enough, the patient got well, but if the infection overwhelmed the tissues, the patient died.

Now the picture is markedly changed. Pneumonia, untreated, is still a serious, even fatal, disease. But with the early and proper use of antibiotic drugs, most of the types of germs which cause pneumonia can be rendered harmless even while the tissue resistance to the germs is being developed. As for the care of the pneumonia patient, it is well to use general measures to build up his vitality while the antibiotic drugs are taking effect. The germs and viruses which cause the various forms of pneumonia are widely prevalent, and

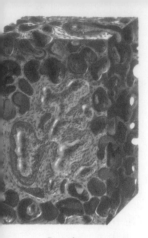

Bronchopneumonia

Purulent exudation in the terminal bronchiole is spreading into the attached alveoli, with a surrounding cuff of serous exudation and hyperemia.

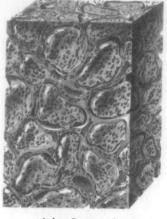

Lobar Pneumonia

Lobar pneumonia, showing alveoli filled with fibrinous exudate containing polynuclear leukocytes; the exudate traverses the alveoli and is of uniform composition throughout the section.

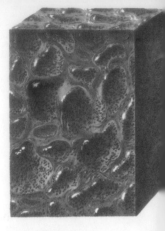

Friedländer's Pneumonia

The alveoli are packed with polynuclear leukocites and necrotic mucoid material; note necrosis of part of the alveolar walls, with early formation of microabscesses.

Lobar Pneumonia

Lobar pneumonia of the right middle lobe, gray hepatization, with acute fibrinous pleuritis.

Friedländer's Pneumonia

Lobar pneumonia of right upper lobe; Friedländer's bacillus; the pleura shows fibrinous exudate and the cut surface has a thick nucopurulent surface over a diffusely purplish-gray consolidation.

THE UPJOHN COMPANY

almost every individual is exposed to them repeatedly. The reason there are not more cases of pneumonia is that when the body's defenses are functioning well, the organisms which may cause infection of the lungs are disposed of before they become established in the lung tissues. Under conditions of lowered vitality and consequent lowered resistance to infection a person becomes ill with pneumonia. Understandably, pneumonia often follows the common cold. It occurs in alcoholism or in cases of malnutrition or general debility. It may result from exposure to extremes of temperature or may follow other injury to the tissues of the lungs.

A. *Pneumonia Caused by the Pneumococcus.* In inflammation of the lung caused by the pneumococcus germ there is a sudden onset of illness with violent chills accompanied by a rapidly mounting fever (up to 105° F. or 40.6° C.), chest pain on breathing (in which the pain may involve the abdomen or the shoulder), cough, and the spitting of rust-colored (blood-tinged) sputum. The breathing becomes rapid with respirations up to forty per minute.

When untreated, pneumococcic pneumonia runs its course in about two weeks, ending in death in more than 30 percent of cases and in prompt improvement (by "crisis") in the remaining 70 percent. Common complications are pleurisy, empyema, lung abscess, infection of the heart (pericarditis or endocarditis), and meningitis.

In cases treated early and adequately with antibiotic drugs or sulfonamides the mortality rate is less than 5 percent.

What to Do

1. Enlist the services of a physician and arrange for hospitalization if possible.

2. The physician will want to take samples of the patient's blood and sputum for laboratory study before he begins the use of antibiotics or sulfonamides. The laboratory findings will guide him in his treatment program. Penicillin is the drug of choice, but other antibiotics and the sulfonamides are useful in some cases.

3. For those patients who need it, oxygen to breathe (administered with appropriate precautions) may be lifesaving.

4. It is very important that the patient receive sufficient fluid—enough so that his daily output of urine is at least three pints (1,500 ml.).

5. As the patient becomes able to eat, his diet should be high in proteins, high in vitamins, and high in calories.

6. Hydrotherapy treatments are very helpful in building up the patient's resistance to the infection. These can be given two or three times a day during the acute phase of the illness. Make sure that the room is sufficiently warm. A hot foot bath in bed plus four or five hot fomentations to the chest, followed by a brisk cold mitten friction, constitute a suitable treatment. (See volume 3, chapter 20, "Simple Home Treatments.")

B. *Pneumonia Caused by Other Bacteria.* During recent years an increasing proportion of pneumonias are caused by a single bacterial organism other than the pneumococcus. These infecting germs include streptococcus, staphylococcus, and Friedländer's bacillus. Usually these cause bronchopneumonia; and among those who have a Friedländer's pneumonia, the mortality is relatively high. The illness in these cases may have either a sudden or a gradual onset. It usually develops secondary to some other illness such as a virus infection, viral pneumonia, influenza, measles, or some debilitating disease. Common complications in these cases include pleurisy, empyema, and lung abscess.

289

What to Do

It is important that laboratory tests be run as early in the disease as possible to determine what germ is causing the infection. Based on this information, intensive and appropriate antibiotic therapy should be instituted at once. The general care is the same as that described for pneumonia caused by the pneumococcus. (See above.)

C. *"Mixed Type" Bacterial Pneumonias.* A person whose general vitality has been lowered by such illnesses as measles, influenza, bronchiectasis, emphysema, heart disease, kidney disease, or cancer, or by a serious injury, can easily become the victim of a type of pneumonia in which several kinds of germs invade the lung's tissues. This type of pneumonia occurs commonly in older people.

The onset is usually gradual, and the symptoms may easily be masked by those of the other existing disease. They include fever, cough, difficult breathing, and expectoration. The mortality rate is relatively high because of the patient's previously existing debility.

In view of the several kinds of germs involved, the physician uses "broad spectrum" antibiotic drugs in the hope of retarding the infection while gaining time for improvement of the patient's general vitality.

D. *Primary Atypical Pneumonia.* There is a group of acute lung-involving illnesses which typically affect young adults who are otherwise healthy. These are so easily confused with diseases caused by viruses that many "atypical" pneumonias pass for "flu" without being recognized as forms of pneumonia.

The disease begins as a common cold. Not infrequently it reaches epidemic proportions, especially in schools and military camps, where many young people associate closely together. A dry cough develops which becomes severe. There is fever, hoarseness, headache, aching of the joints and muscles, and fatigue. Recovery is usually spontaneous in about ten days. Mortality in untreated cases is less than 1 percent.

Probably most primary atypical pneumonias are caused by the "Eaton agent" (Mycoplasma pneumoniae), which differs somewhat from a true virus. It is usually transmitted from one person to another by droplets produced by a patient's sneezing or coughing and inhaled by a susceptible person.

What to Do

As yet there is no specific drug treatment for the lung infections caused by viruses. For those caused by the Eaton agent, one of the tetracyclines (a group of antibiotic drugs) has proved to be quite effective. Other than this, general supportive care, including bed rest, adequate fluid intake, mild diet high in protein and vitamins, and hydrotherapy as outlined under pneumococcal pneumonia, is beneficial.

E. *Virus Pneumonia.* The virus pneumonias may be caused by one of a variety of viruses. Some of them are well-known to the virologist or physician, but others are very difficult to find and identify. For this reason, nonbacterial pneumonias frequently are labeled "virus pneumonia," even though a specific virus is not isolated. Usually the symptoms produced are somewhat similar to those of primary atypical pneumonia, but not infrequently they may be more severe and may produce symptoms and findings similar to a bacterial bronchopneumonia.

What to Do

Most patients with a virus pneumonia can be treated just as satisfactorily at home as in a hospital. The principal goals are to build up the patient's inherent vitality and make him comfortable.

1. The patient should be encouraged to rest in bed and to sleep as many hours per day as his inclination permits.

2. Patients often benefit by inhaling water vapor. We use the term water vapor rather than steam, because there is danger of injuring the delicate membranes of the air passages when live steam is inhaled. An improvised humidifier to provide the water vapor may consist of a kettle of water placed on an electric plate at the patient's bedside with the vapor from the boiling water conducted to the patient's face by a cone of rolled newspaper. If the patient's face is at least two feet away from the boiling water, there is little danger that the steam he inhales will be too hot.

3. Patients with virus pneumonia often have a productive cough which brings mucus from the lower air passages into the pharynx. Such coughing should be permitted so long as the patient shields his face when coughing so as not to contaminate the atmosphere in the room. The coughing serves to keep the air passages open and thus hastens the process of healing.

4. In the more severe cases where the patient's breathing becomes difficult, the best remedy is providing oxygen for the patient to breathe. The care of such a patient should be under the doctor's supervision.

PULMONARY EDEMA.

This is a life-threatening condition in which the lungs become waterlogged by an accumulation of serous fluid in the air sacs.

Pulmonary edema is almost always a complication of some other condition. It usually results from failing or weakening heart action; however, there may be other causes. It may come during a late stage of kidney disease. It may accompany some acute infectious disease. It may be caused by toxins or by the inhalation of acutely irritating gases or fumes.

The onset may be gradual, but more often it is fairly sudden. There is a sense of pain and oppression in the chest with rapid and difficult breathing. A persistent short cough is common; and a copious, frothy, sometimes blood-tinged fluid is raised from the lungs and tends to issue from both nose and mouth. There are typical signs of shock. Symptoms may begin to subside within a few hours, but without prompt and expert treatment any case of edema of the lungs may rapidly prove fatal.

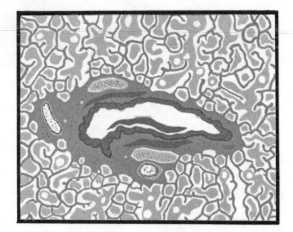

Microscopic section from a lung, showing pulmonary edema. The air sacs surrounding a bronchiole are nearly filled with a serous fluid (appearing pink).

What to Do

Consult a physician at once, for it is necessary that he evaluate the illness and give prompt treatment for the condition causing the pulmonary edema.

While awaiting instructions from the physician:

1. Keep the patient in bed and maintain body warmth. He may breathe more easily with head and shoulders elevated on pillows.

2. Give no fluids (except as in 3).

3. Mix a teaspoonful of aromatic spirit of ammonia with half a glass

View of the interior of the chest in a case of pulmonary edema. The lungs (right and left) are bulging because of their edematous condition. The incision into one lung shows serous fluid mixed with air bubbles.

of water and give the patient sips of this mixture.

PULMONARY INFARCTION (PULMONARY THROMBOSIS OR PULMONARY EMBOLISM).

Pulmonary infarction results from the plugging of a branch of the pulmonary artery (which carries blood from the right side of the heart to the lungs) by a clot that forms in the artery (thrombosis), or, more often, by a piece of a clot carried by the bloodstream to the lung from a thrombus located elsewhere. The involved area of the lung becomes functionless and tissue deterioration develops. The condition occurs as a complication of thrombosed veins, of certain forms of heart disease, or of severe injuries. It may also occur in predisposed persons following surgery.

The onset is marked by a sudden piercing pain in the chest which radiates to the shoulder, difficult breathing, an irritating cough, and blood-tinged sputum, or at least the spitting up of small amounts of blood. The patient may have persistent hiccup. He is anxious, has a rapid pulse, and usually sweats profusely. There may be an associated fever. In severe cases the patient may be in a state of shock.

Pulmonary infarction is a dangerous condition, the outcome of which is influenced by the size of the affected area of lung tissue. Prompt and expert treatment by a physician with the necessary equipment (preferably in a hospital) can save many lives that would otherwise be lost. Fortunately, in most cases patients are already in a hospital when pulmonary infarction occurs. Hospital treatment consists of the administration of oxygen, the use of anticoagulants, and the prevention of infection. Surgical intervention may sometimes be indicated.

What to Do

1. **If symptoms of pulmonary infarction develop while the victim is at home, consult a physician at once.**

2. **If shock develops, give appropriate first-aid treatment (See under *Shock* in volume 3, chapter 18, "Handling Emergencies.")**

RESPIRATORY DISTRESS SYNDROME (HYALINE MEMBRANE DISEASE).

The respiratory distress syndrome is an illness which affects some newborn babies, especially those who are born prematurely. Such a baby may have difficulty in taking its first breath. Then, when it does breathe, it becomes obvious that breathing is difficult. The infant may cease to breathe for a period of a few seconds. This cessation of breathing, up to ten seconds, occurs sometimes in newborn infants who are perfectly normal. If the cessation of breathing is for longer than ten seconds, however, and particularly if it is accompanied by cyanosis (dark blue coloration of the skin) it becomes clear that the child is not breathing normally.

The usual cause of the respiratory distress syndrome is that the walls of the tiny air sacs within the infant's lungs stick together just as though a membrane were interferring with the entrance of air into the lungs. Actually, there is no "membrane" present, and the term "hyaline membrane disease" which is sometimes used for this illness is a misnomer. When many of the tiny air sacs within the lung do not expand as they normally should, the child does not receive its full quota of oxygen and therefore is in danger of suffocation.

In the normal course of an unborn baby's development, certain cells within the lungs become active just before the child's birth and produce a chemical substance called surfactant. This substance reduces the surface tension of the fluid which the lungs contain prior to birth, making it easier for the tiny air sacs to balloon out as the child takes its first breath. In the case of many babies who are born prematurely, the cells which produce the surfactant have not yet become active, and so the walls of the tiny air sacs tend to cling to each other.

Formerly, only about 25 percent of infants with respiratory distress syndrome survived. Present methods of aiding the newborn infant with this problem to expand his lungs have greatly increased the prospects of survival. Recent scientific studies indicate that it is a delayed production of steroids by the unborn child's own adrenal gland that accounts for the insufficient production of surfactant and thus makes it difficult for the infant to expand its lungs. The newer methods of treatment therefore center around the use of resuscitation equipment adapted to the size and vitality of the newborn infant, and also on the appropriate administration of steroids.

What to Do

The survival of a newborn infant who is probably premature and who has the respiratory distress syndrome requires vigilance on the part of the obstetrician or pediatrician in charge of the case as well as the availability of proper equipment for infant resuscitation. Even under most favorable circumstances the risk is considerable.

TUBERCULOSIS.
(See chapter 29 in this volume.)

Diseases of the Pleura

EMPYEMA.
Empyema means the formation of pus in a cavity; but when the word is used without further definition, it is understood to mean the formation of pus in the pleural cavity, that is, between the lung and the chest wall.

The early symptoms are somewhat like those of lung abscess, pneumonia, or pleurisy; and one or more of these diseases will usually be present before empyema begins. The patient shows signs of a severe infection. The temperature is usually quite irregular, and there are copious sweats. Physical

examination and an X ray will detect the presence and the approximate location of the pus.

If the volume of pus is small, it can be removed by repeated tappings in which a needle is inserted between the ribs. Antibiotic drugs are usually instilled while the needle is still in place. When the accumulation of pus is large, an opening in the chest wall may have to be made—perhaps a piece of rib removed—in order to permit free drainage of the pus. Antibiotics are very useful in controlling the infection causing the formation of pus.

If empyema is suspected, consult a physician and have him arrange the program of treatment and supervise the nursing care.

PLEURISY.
Pleurisy is usually caused by infection, as with the tubercle bacillus (the most common cause), the pneumococcus, or the streptococcus. The two latter germs are usually present in pneumonia. Some pleurisy is always present with lobar pneumonia. Pleurisy is sometimes the result of an injury, as from a broken rib.

In pleurisy the pleural membranes are swollen and inflamed, and at first rub together with each breath, causing severe pain and making a sound that can be heard by a physician with a stethoscope. If the patient tries to take a deep breath or to cough or sneeze, the pain suddenly becomes more severe, feeling like a sharp stab.

Fluid may form in the space between the lung and the chest wall. When it does, the rubbing sound disappears, and with it much or all of the pain. The fluid may be small in amount, or it may fill half of the chest cavity, compressing the lung. A physician can detect and estimate its presence, location, and quantity by means of physical and X-ray examinations.

Pleurisy may be limited in extent. It may be on the surface of the diaphragm and give no signs which the

X ray of a pleurisy patient's thorax. The liquid produced by the pleurisy darkens one side of the lung.

physician can detect for several days. In such a case, the pain may be in the abdomen or at the pit of the stomach, or even be referred to the shoulder, and hence appear to be due to disease of the stomach, the liver, the gallbladder, or even of some structure entirely outside of either the chest or the abdomen. In children, the pain of pleurisy as well as the pain of pneumonia may seem to originate in the abdomen, and may lead to a suspicion of acute indigestion or even of appendicitis. It often takes careful and prolonged study by a physician to detect pleurisy under these unusual circumstances.

What to Do

1. If, during the course of any disease of which pleurisy is a common complication, suggestive symptoms develop, call a physician to try to determine the true condition.

2. If no physician is yet available, and if the symptoms are characteristic of pleurisy, proceed as follows:

A. Keep the patient warm, and in bed.

B. Move him and treat him very gently. Jars and quick motions make pleurisy worse and increase the pain.

C. Twice a day give him a hot foot bath and hot fomentations to the painful side of the chest. (See volume 3, chapter 20.) The fomentations should be large, thick, and hot, and be changed frequently. Use about five changes, but do not follow with any cold applications. Use a hot-water bottle on the chest following the fomentations. It may be kept on nearly all the time without harm. If the patient's chest is chilled at all during or after the treatments, the pleurisy will be made worse.

D. Give the patient nutritious food.

3. Antibiotics have shown curative value in many cases, but their use requires the supervision of a physician.

4. A physician may strap the affected side of the chest with broad strips of adhesive tape, giving the patient considerable relief from pain.

5. If fluid collects in the chest, the physician may remove it by tapping with a needle. When this stage of the disease develops, revulsive compresses do more good than hot fomentations, and a moist chest pack worn overnight may be helpful. (See volume 3, chapter 20, "Simple Home Treatments.")

Diseases of the Digestive Tract

For a description of the various organs that make up the digestive tract—those parts of the body concerned with the handling of food— turn to volume 3, chapters 9 and 10. There also mention is made of practices a person should follow to keep these organs functioning normally and efficiently—for instance, care of the teeth and the mouth so as to avoid dental decay. In the present chapter we are concerned primarily with the various diseases which may involve the organs making up the digestive tract.

The Lips, Mouth, Teeth, and Tongue

ABSCESS OF A TOOTH.

Ordinary dental decay, if not properly treated in time, may progress until the pulp cavity of the tooth is involved, resulting in infection of the pulp, which may spread into the tissues surrounding the end of the root of the tooth. Sometimes germs find their way between the gum and the tooth and cause an abscess to form around the root.

If the infection spreads until the bone is involved, the tooth may loosen, allowing pus to enter the surrounding tissues or ooze out beside the tooth. At this stage, the pain may become less. Without free drainage there may be swelling, pain, fever, and enlarged adjacent lymph nodes.

Antibiotics may help control the infection, but a cure of the condition calls for dental treatment. An abscess at the deep end of a tooth root may sometimes be drained by drilling into the tooth; and the tooth may then be saved by cleaning out, disinfecting, and filling the pulp cavity and root canals. Otherwise, the tooth must be extracted.

What to Do

1. Prepare a salt solution containing half a teaspoonful of salt to the glass of water. Heat this to as hot a temperature as can be reasonably tolerated in the mouth (about the temperature of a hot breakfast drink). Hold a sip of this hot solution in the mouth in the region of the aching tooth for a minute or so. Then expel the solution and replace with another sip until the glassful of solution has been used up. Repeat the procedure every hour or oftener as desired. In a small number of cases cold water or ice water will give more relief of pain than a hot solution.

2. Pushing into the cavity a small bit of cotton wet with oil of cloves may help.

3. Treatment by a dentist gives the best chance of controlling the abscess and saving the tooth, and the sooner the better.

297

ACCIDENT INVOLVING A TOOTH.

A tooth which has been fractured may need a protective covering which the dentist can supply until permanent repair can be made at a later time. Even teeth displaced by accident may gradually move back into their normal position, especially primary teeth ("baby teeth").

Surprising as it may seem, a tooth removed by accident may be successfully reimplanted, as several cases on record substantiate. For this reason a tooth which has been knocked out should be preserved in warm salt solution until the dentist has an opportunity to decide whether or not an attempt to reimplant it is feasible. Immediate care is of course essential.

What to Do

1. When a tooth is fractured, displaced, or knocked out, the victim of the accident should go as promptly as possible to a dentist for emergency care.

2. Even though the tooth is dislodged, it should be carefully preserved by placing it in a glass of warm water to which half a teaspoonful of salt has been added. It may even be possible for the dentist to reimplant the tooth.

3. When involved in accidents, primary teeth deserve the same attention as would be given to permanent teeth.

CANCER.

Several kinds of cancer may develop in the tissues of the lips, cheeks, mouth, and tongue. These may cause death if not treated early and properly. Cancer of the lip is much more common in the lower than in the upper lip. It often begins as a small lesion which passes for a "cold sore" but which becomes hardened and refuses to heal. It occurs commonly in men who smoke a pipe, the assumed reason being that the heat of the pipestem irritates the tissues of the lip sufficiently to make them susceptible to the development of cancer.

Any lump or ulcer developing in the lip, cheek, tongue, or palate which is not otherwise explained and which persists without progress toward healing deserves professional attention at an early date. Usually the physician will remove a small piece of the tissue in question and have it examined microscopically. If this indicates that a cancer is in progress, the usual treatments of radical surgery and radiation must be planned at once. Inasmuch as the tissues of the mouth and tongue are very active, some of the cells involved in the cancerous growth may break away and spread to other parts of the body. Early and adequate treatment of such lesions is imperative.

CANKER SORES.

Canker sores usually begin as small red swellings or tiny blisters on the mucous membrane of the mouth or undersurface of the tongue. They become painful as soon as an ulcer forms at the summit of the swelling. The lesion is usually one eighth to one fourth of an inch in diameter.

There appears to be no single cause for canker sores. They occur when one's general resistance to disease is

Canker sores in the mouth.

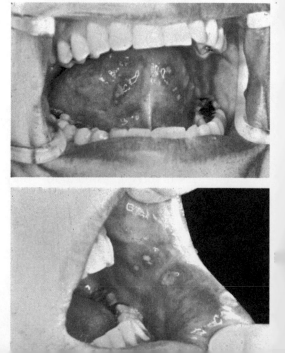

low. They also tend to occur when the membranes of the mouth are irritated by jagged teeth or by poor mouth hygiene. Allergy to certain foods, particularly those containing citric acid and acetic acid, seems to encourage the development of canker sores.

What to Do

1. Eliminate from the diet those foods to which the patient may be allergic: walnuts, strawberries, tomatoes, chocolate, citrus fruits, and pickled foods (containing acetic acid.)

2. The application of anesthetic ointments may serve to relieve the discomfort of canker sores. Suitable preparations are Dibucaine Ointment (1%) and Lidocane Ointment.

CARIES (DENTAL CARIES).

A broader background for understanding dental caries is given in volume 3, chapter 9, "The Mouth and Teeth." Three factors combine to cause the development of cavities in the teeth: constant presence of germs in the mouth cavity, protracted contact of food remnants with the teeth, and inherent susceptibility of the teeth to dental decay. The interaction of germs with food remnants in the mouth produces acids which dissolve calcium contained in the enamel of the teeth. When such destruction gives rise to a cavity in the surface of the tooth, the tooth deserves attention by a dentist.

Ninety-five percent of all Americans suffer some tooth decay at one time or another. One half of all children three years of age have one or more decayed teeth. The average child in the grades has three or more teeth in which dental cavities have occurred. The average sixteen-year-old youth has seven teeth which have either been affected by dental caries or have been filled or are missing. Nine out of ten high school students have suffered from some degree of dental caries.

A high content of sugar and refined food in the diet predisposes to dental caries.

The essentials for preventing dental caries are (1) prompt cleaning of the teeth after each meal, (2) an adequate diet consisting largely of natural foods, and (3) a limitation on pastries and confections because of the large amount of sugar they contain. Even under ideal circumstances the possibility of developing cavities still exists. It is wise, therefore, to consult a dentist at regular intervals so that he may treat any existing unfavorable conditions and may advise on better methods of caring for the teeth.

What to Do

1. The person who knows he has one or more cavities in his teeth should go at once to the dentist for treatment. A neglected cavity will grow in size and eventually penetrate the deeper layers of the tooth, causing permanent destruction.

2. Visit the dentist at least twice a year asking him to examine your teeth for cavities. If cavities are found, they should be properly treated and filled.

3. Clean your teeth promptly after each meal, preferably using dental floss or dental tape between the teeth, followed by gentle brushing with a toothbrush and thorough rinsing.

4. Avoid taking any food or sweetened drinks between meals.

5. Reduce the amount of candies, pastries, and highly refined foods in your diet, giving preference to whole grains, nuts, vegetables, and fruits.

CAVITIES IN THE TEETH.
(See the preceding item.)

COLD SORE.
(See *Herpes Simplex* in chapter 28 of this volume.)

CLEFT PALATE.
In cleft palate, a congenital defect, the two portions of the palate in the

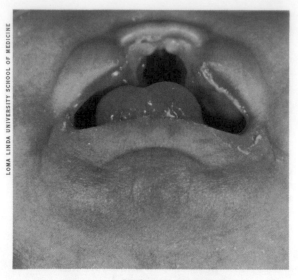

Cleft lip and palate.

roof of the mouth do not join as they should in the midline. There are various degrees of cleft palate, some involving only the soft palate and some involving the hard palate and upper jaw as well. Cleft palate is often associated with harelip. Cleft palate interferes with the infant's ability to nurse. Also, as the infant grows into childhood, a cleft palate interferes with his ability to speak. For these reasons, as well as for the sake of the child's self-esteem, a plastic surgeon should be consulted while the child is in early infancy.

Because the tendency to cleft palate is inherited, it is wise for parents who have one child with cleft palate to seek counsel from a specialist in genetics before planning for additional children in the family.

COATED TONGUE.

The appearance of the tongue's surface may vary a great deal according to the condition of general health. In simple anemia, the tongue may appear pale and small; in pernicious anemia, abnormally smooth. The user of alcohol commonly has a heavily coated tongue. This same appearance, however, may suggest nothing more than poor oral hygiene. The tongue commonly appears heavily coated in cases of high fever or dehydration. Deficient diet and allergic sensitivity to drugs or cosmetics may even influence the appearance of the tongue.

DECAY OF THE TEETH.

(See *Caries* in this listing.)

GINGIVITIS (INFLAMMATION OF THE GUMS).

In gingivitis there is swelling of the gums with redness and bleeding. Local causes include a lack of dental cleanliness, poorly positioned teeth (crooked or misplaced) which make oral hygiene difficult, the accumulation of hard deposits (tartar, or calculus) on the surface of the teeth, the accumulation of food residue between the teeth, jagged or poorly fitting dental appliances or restorations, and the custom of breathing through the mouth. Certain forms of ill health may cause gingivitis, as deficiency of vitamins (as in scurvy and pellagra)—also certain blood diseases, allergies, endocrine disturbances (as in diabetes and some instances of pregnancy), poisoning by certain chemical substances (notably those containing lead and bismuth), and chronic debilitating diseases.

What to Do

1. Discover and correct the underlying cause. A dentist or a physician can help in doing this.

2. For temporary relief, rinse the mouth with warm salt solution (one teaspoonful of table salt to the glass of water). The rinsing should be carried out several times a day and particularly right after meals.

GLOSSITIS (INFLAMMATION OF THE TONGUE).

Glossitis is a rather rare condition. When it does occur, the inflammation is usually caused by some infection which follows an injury to the tongue such as biting or burning. Following the injury, germs already present in the mouth invade the injured

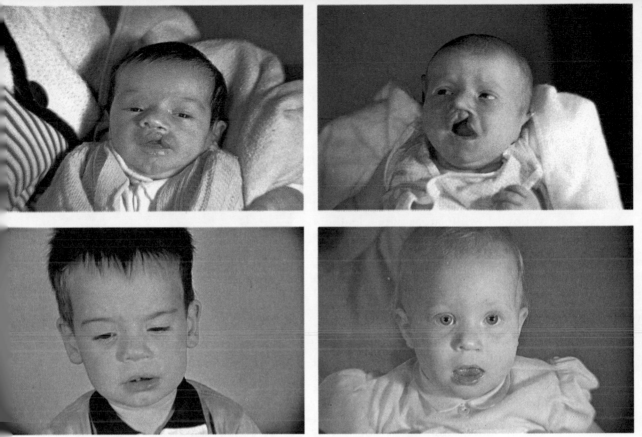

Harelip can usually be corrected by surgery. Upper (both cases), before surgery; lower, after surgery.

JAMES G. STUCKEY, M.D.

area and cause the tongue to become inflamed.

In glossitis the tongue becomes swollen, ulcerated, and very sore. The infection may proceed to the stage of an abscess. Because of the severe infection, the lymph nodes in the neck become swollen and tender. Frequently the flow of saliva may be so excessive as to be quite troublesome. There may be fever and other symptoms commonly caused by severe infection.

What to Do

1. Try to determine the cause of the inflammation of the tongue and eliminate this factor.
2. Rinse the mouth frequently with one of the following solutions:
 (a) Hexylresorcinol 1
   Glycerin   5
   Water   240
 (b) Alkaline aromatic solution (National Formulary).

3. Keep the teeth properly cleaned.
4. If an abscess forms, consult a physician. He may need to drain the abscess.

GUMS.
(See *Gingivitis* in this listing.)

HARELIP.
Harelip is a congenital defect involving the upper lip, sometimes on the right, sometimes on the left, and sometimes on both sides. It is sometimes associated with defects of the upper jaw and palate. A child with harelip should be taken to a plastic surgeon as soon as possible after birth. The results of carefully planned surgery are usually excellent. If a harelip is neglected, however, the child may form unfortunate speech patterns and suffer handicap in his personality development, being sensitive about his disfigurement.

301

HERPES SIMPLEX.

(See *Herpes Simplex* in chapter 28 in this volume.)

LEUKOPLAKIA.

Leukoplakia is a curious involvement of the membranes of the lips, cheeks, tongue, floor of the mouth, and palate. The disease is characterized by the appearance of yellowish-white areas with a leathery consistency. The size of the areas varies; and cracks, fissures, and even ulcerations may develop. Leukoplakia cerations may develop. Leukoplakia is considered to be the result of prolonged irritation of the membranes of the mouth and related structures. Tobacco smoking is given a large share of the blame for this development. Also, repeated and prolonged irritations by jagged teeth or dental restorations may cause it. Poor oral hygiene may be a factor, as may also the use of highly seasoned foods and the habitual drinking of hot beverages. Leukoplakia is considered to be a step toward the development of cancer; therefore patients suffering with this ailment are urgently advised to see a physician. Usually the condition will respond favorably to the avoidance of all irritating agents.

MOUTH, INFLAMMATION OF THE MOUTH'S LINING.

(See *Stomatitis* in this listing.)

MUMPS.

In mumps the parotid salivary glands (located above the back of the angles of the jaw) become swollen and very painful. This disease is described in great detail in the chapter entitled "Infectious Diseases" (chapter 28 of this volume).

PERIODONTITIS (PYORRHEA).

Periodontitis is related to gingivitis and consists of an extension of the inflammation into the tissues which support and stabilize the roots of the teeth.

As explained in volume 3, chapter 9,

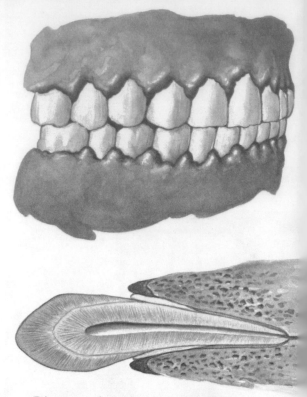

Diagram showing how pyorrhea in periodontal tissue initiates destruction in surrounding bone.

"The Mouth and Teeth," the root of each tooth is surrounded by a strong layer of fibrous tissue which binds the tooth to the bone and permits the tooth to move slightly without being fractured. As this periodontal tissue becomes involved in disease, it initiates destruction of the bone surrounding the tooth. Thus it may be said that as the soft tissues around the teeth become diseased, so does the supporting bone. It is for this reason that periodontitis, when neglected, results in the loss of the teeth.

The early signs of periodontitis consist of tenderness and redness of the gums with a tendency for the gums to bleed. As the disease advances and the surrounding periodontal tissues and bone become involved, the teeth become loose.

In advanced cases the dentist may find it necessary to use surgical procedures in removing diseased tissues and also to splinting certain of the teeth that have lost their bony support.

What to Do

1. Inasmuch as periodontitis endangers the vitality of the teeth to the extent that the teeth must be removed if the disease is allowed to persist, it is important that a dentist direct the treatment of this disease.

2. Arrange needed prophylactic care for the teeth. This includes removal of calcareous deposits that may have formed on the teeth near the gum margins.

3. Maintain an adequate program of home care for the teeth, cleaning them promptly and thoroughly after each meal. This will serve to remove the deposits of food which favor the development of periodontitis.

4. Follow the dentist's advice on the proper method of massaging the gums two or three times a day.

PYORRHEA.

(See the preceding item.)

SALIVARY GLAND INVOLVEMENTS.

(See also *Mumps* and *Tumors of the Salivary Glands* in this listing.)

All of the salivary glands are located in the vicinity of the mouth and discharge their secretion (saliva) through tubelike ducts which open into the mouth cavity. Occasionally one of these ducts becomes obstructed and the corresponding gland swells to produce a tumorlike mass. The common location for such an enlargement is under the tongue on one side or the other. The salivary glands may become involved in infections that develop within the membranes of the mouth.

STOMATITIS (INFLAMMATION OF THE LINING OF THE MOUTH).

Stomatitis is characterized by redness of the membranes of the mouth, a feeling of heat, and swelling of the tissues so marked as possibly to cause the cheeks to appear puffed. The flow of saliva is increased, and the saliva is more viscid than usual. The breath has an offensive odor. Usually there is fever and a feeling of weakness. Stomatitis may occur in connection with other diseases such as measles, scarlet fever, and stomach or intestinal disorders. It may result from a deficient diet, especially one low in vitamins. Contributing factors may be decayed teeth, deficient mouth hygiene, mouth breathing, the use of pacifiers by babies, taking food which is too hot or too highly seasoned, the excessive and continued use of tobacco, or the use of drugs containing certain of the heavy metals.

What to Do

1. In acute inflammation of the mouth, rinse or swab the mouth every half hour with a solution of baking soda (not more than 1 level teaspoonful of soda to a glass of cold water) or with alkaline aromatic solution (National Formulary).

2. Fomentations may be given every three hours over the mouth, cheeks, and jaws. (See volume 3, chapter 20, "Simple Home Treatments.")

3. The diet should consist of nutritious soups and soft foods.

4. Have a physician determine the basic cause of the disease and advise on more specific remedies.

5. Increase the vitamin intake both by using general-purpose vitamins and by including tomato juice, orange juice, and brewers' yeast in the diet.

THRUSH (ORAL CANDIDIASIS).

Thrush usually but not always affects babies rather than older persons. It is caused by a species of fungus (Candida albicans) which produces a white velvetlike growth on the tongue, the roof of the mouth, and the inside of the cheeks and lips. The lesions appear much like bits of curdled milk, which are firmly adherent to the membrane. General symptoms include fever and poor appetite, which in the case of a child may even involve a refusal to nurse. The patient becomes restless and may have diarrhea. This fungous infection often follows the use of some antibiotic medication. The antibiotic kills the germs which would otherwise inhibit the growth of a fungus.

What do Do

1. An effective treatment is the antibiotic nystatin. For use in the treatment of thrush it is prepared by the druggist in a suspension which contains 100,000 units per ml. One ml. (one-fourth teaspoonful) of this preparation is dropped into the patient's mouth four times a day. It should be held in the mouth a minute or so, for its local effect, before being swallowed.

2. By the use of general hygienic measures and an adequate diet, build up the patient's general resistance to disease.

3. If the patient is a breast-fed child, its mother's breasts and nipples should be washed with a saturated solution of boric acid and then rinsed with cooled boiled water, both before and after nursing.

4. If the patient is a bottle-fed infant, its nursing bottles and nipples should be washed and boiled after each using. Only bottles and nipples that have been thus sterilized should be given to the child either for its formula or for its drinking water.

TONGUE, INFLAMMATION OF.
(See *Glossitis* in this listing.)

TONGUE-TIE.
Underneath the tip of the tongue there normally occurs a fold of the mucosa (the frenum) which serves to anchor the undersurface of the tongue to the floor of the mouth. In an occasional case the frenum is abnormally short and restricts the movements of the tongue. If this situation is allowed to persist beyond infancy, the child is handicapped in his learning to speak. The treatment of tongue-tie, a very simple surgical procedure, should be performed during infancy or very early childhood.

TOOTH ABSCESS.
(See *Abscess of a Tooth* in this listing.)

TOOTH, ACCIDENTAL INJURY.
(See *Accident Involving a Tooth* in this listing.)

TOOTHACHE.
An aching tooth indicates that the tooth has been long neglected. Cavities that develop in teeth first penetrate the enamel, then the dentine, and finally into the pulp cavity where the nerve of the tooth is located. When the cavity penetrates all the way into the pulp, reaching the sensitive nerve, toothache occurs. Cavities should be discovered and treated while they are small and involve only the enamel and dentine.

Once dental decay has reached the pulp of a tooth, infection of the pulp usually follows, causing severe pain. Many a tooth even at this stage can be saved by a dentist's skillful work. He will usually find it necessary to make an opening into the pulp cavity and remove the pulp. The tooth then becomes "dead" in the sense that it is no longer sensitive to pain.

What to Do

1. When a tooth aches, the period of time during which home treatment would have been effective has already passed. Therefore the most important thing to do at this stage is to see a dentist at the earliest possible moment.

2. In the meantime, application of either heat or cold may help to relieve the discomfort of a toothache. Cold may be applied by holding either ice water or chips of ice in the mouth. Heat may be applied by the use of a hot salt water rinse (one-half

teaspoonful of salt to a glass of water).

3. If the cavity in the aching tooth is easily found, a small wick of cotton soaked in oil of cloves and introduced into the cavity of the tooth may give temporary relief.

TRENCH MOUTH (VINCENT'S DISEASE).

Trench mouth is a severe form of stomatitis characterized by painful bleeding gums, excessive production of saliva, a fetid breath, and small ulcers on the gums, particularly between the teeth. Swallowing and talking are painful, and the patient usually has a mild fever and feels ill. Among the causes, heavy smoking is listed in addition to those mentioned for stomatitis in this listing.

What to Do

1. Use a hot mouthwash every thirty to sixty minutes throughout the day. A suitable preparation is half-strength hydrogen peroxide (prepared by mixing equal parts of water and hydrogen peroxide as it comes from the drugstore).

2. The affected areas may be painted between mouthwashes with a paste prepared from sodium perborate powder to which a few drops of water have been added.

3. The patient should rest a great deal, and his diet should consist of bland, soft food.

4. Smoking should be eliminated, preferably for good.

5. Antibiotic therapy prescribed by a physician or a dentist may hasten recovery, but usually local treatment is sufficient.

6. As soon as the acute phase of the disease subsides (in a day or two), a dentist should institute measures to establish good hygiene of the mouth, gums, and teeth.

TUMORS OF THE SALIVARY GLANDS.

Malignant tumors (cancerous growths) sometimes develop within one of the salivary glands. These are serious because of their tendency to spread to other parts of the body. Any persistent swelling of the face at the angle of the jaw or beneath the jaw, especially when it involves only one side, deserves investigation by a physician.

VINCENT'S DISEASE.

(See *Trench Mouth* in this listing.)

The Esophagus

DIVERTICULUM OF THE ESOPHAGUS.

Food sometimes lodges in the narrower portions of the esophagus and by pressure causes the formation of a diverticulum—that is, a blind pouch or sac. Pouches may also be caused by inflammation in lymph nodes or other structures outside the esophagus. As these inflammations subside, the contracting scar tissue may adhere to the wall of the esophagus and pull it outward. The contracting scar following a burn by lye may also cause a pouch to form. As a pouch increases in size, more and more food may collect in it and decompose, causing a foul taste in the mouth and a foul odor, sometimes with difficulty in swallowing, pain, and vomiting, or regurgitation of undigested food.

Surgical removal of the sac is the only real cure for a diverticulum of the esophagus of such size and shape as to collect and hold food.

What to Do

If you have symptoms that make you suspect you may have a diverticulum of your esophagus, consult a physician, because you can do nothing to cure the condition yourself. He can have an X ray taken to determine the size and position of the sac. He can make a direct examination of the esophagus by use of the esophagoscope or can arrange for a specialist to make such examination. If these examinations

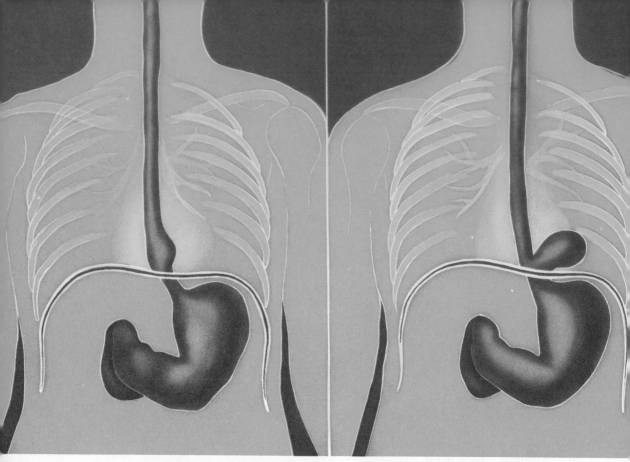

Hiatus hernia, whether the sliding type (left) or the rolling type (right), results in an abnormal pouch at the lower end of the esophagus just above the diaphragm.

confirm the presence of a diverticulum, he can arrange for removal of it by surgery.

HIATUS HERNIA.

While hiatus hernia concerns the stomach, because in this condition a part of that organ is pushed or pulled upward through the opening (hiatus) in the diaphragm, it is considered here because the fault is usually either a widely dilated lower segment of the esophagus, or an esophagus so short that it pulls the left end of the stomach upward. The result is an abnormal pouch, consisting of both stomach and esophagus tissue in various proportions, in which partly digested stomach contents and gastric acid may be present at least part of the time. In such a case, esophagitis or ulcers similar to a peptic ulcer may form. Whether or not this happens, there is likely to be a sensation or pressure, pain, or burning behind the lower end of the breastbone. Discomfort is caused by the backing up of acid-containing stomach contents into the lower part of the esophagus. The symptoms are made worse by lying down or by anything that will increase the pressure in the abdominal cavity—obesity, bending the body, lifting, or eating. In severe cases, cough, difficulty of breathing, palpitation, and a rapid heart rate may be caused.

What to Do

1. Avoid foods and drinks that irritate the lining of the stomach—particularly coffee, alcohol, and condiments.
2. Meals should be eaten "dry"—that is, without drinking any kind of fluid while eating. The person's quota of fluid should be

taken between meals, not at meal-time.

3. Use a non-absorbable, liquid antacid preparation (available at the drug store) for the control of discomfort.

4. If overweight, reduce the weight to normal.

5. Do not lie down or take vigorous exercise soon after eating.

6. Sleep with the upper part of the body somewhat elevated.

7. As soon as the condition is suspected, it is wise to consult a physician, who can have X rays taken and make other examinations and tests to determine the true nature and extent of the hernia. The physician will be able to give special advice for control of the esophagitis and to advise when surgery may become necessary.

NARROWING (STENOSIS) OF THE ESOPHAGUS.

A permanent and sometimes increasing narrowing of the esophagus can be produced by tumors growing within the organ or pressing on it from the outside, by contracting scars resulting from drinking caustic acids, alkalies (such as lye), or other corrosive substances, or as a result of esophagitis. A temporary narrowing is more likely to be caused by a spasm of the muscles in the walls of the organ—a condition commonly called cardiospasm because it nearly always occurs very near the place where the esophagus joins the upper, or cardiac, end of the stomach.

Permanent stricture usually causes an increasing sense of fullness under the breastbone when the patient attempts to swallow. He is compelled to eat slowly; and, as the condition gets worse, there is a return of food because it cannot enter the stomach. Seldom does the patient experience nausea, and the regurgitated food has no sour taste as it would if it had come up from the stomach. Pain may be troublesome, and danger of lung infections or even of strangling arises because some of the regurgitated food may get into the air passages. Sometimes the condition becomes so severe that nothing can be swallowed.

The first symptom of a narrowing of the esophagus due to the development of cancer is a painless difficulty in swallowing, sometimes described as a "feeling of fullness." This symptom deserves prompt evaluation by a physician. If he finds cancer present, he may be able to remove it completely by surgery. If this is not possible, temporary relief may be secured by using X-ray or radium treatments, or both. This treatment reduces the size of the tumor and retards its growth. It is sometimes necessary to make a permanent opening through the abdominal wall into the stomach so that enough food and fluids can be introduced to maintain life. (Cancer of the esophagus is further discussed in chapter 11 of this volume.)

If the narrowing is the result of contracting scar tissue, the esophagus may be kept open by stretching it with specially shaped instruments introduced in gradually increasing sizes. This may give the patient great relief and enable him to swallow as much food as he needs. By repeating the stretching treatments from time to time, the patient may have many years added to his life.

What to Do

1. If difficulty in swallowing persists, do not try any home treatment. It will be useless, and no medicine is of any use.

2. Consult a physician early. He can make such examinations and tests as are needed to determine the true nature and extent of the condition and can arrange such treatments as are necessary.

The Stomach

ACUTE GASTRITIS.

Gastritis is an inflammation of the mucous membrane which lines the stomach. Acute gastritis may result in no more than an uncomfortable feeling in the stomach, distention of the abdomen, headache, nausea, a coated tongue, and a bad taste in the mouth. In severe cases, all of these symptoms will be worse, and there will be severe upper abdominal pain, tenderness, vomiting, fever, and sometimes bleeding from the stomach.

Probably the most frequent cause of gastritis in recent years is the misuse of aspirin, such as taking large doses on an empty stomach. We ordinarily consider aspirin to be a "harmless drug," but one of its serious effects is damage to the lining of the stomach.

Other causes of gastritis are overeating, eating indigestible food, exposure to cold or wet weather, toxic infections, or some type of food poisoning or allergy. It may be a complication of any one of several common acute infectious diseases. Some cases seen in medical practice are caused by the taking of large quantities of alcoholic liquor accompanied by little or no food.

The most dangerous cases are those in which the irritation or inflammation is caused by the swallowing of corrosive acids or alkalies or other irritating poisons. Gastritis from such causes is likely to give rise to serious and persistent complications, calling for the longtime attention of a physician. Some cases of acute gastritis end fatally, but the ordinary case proceeds to recovery in a few days.

What to Do

In case of evidence that some corrosive or poisonous substance has been swallowed, take the patient at once to an emergency hospital. (See under *Poisoning* in volume 3, chapter 18, "Handling Emergencies.")

For other cases of acute gastritis:

1. Leave off all food for at least two days.

2. Give repeated doses of a nonabsorbable, liquid antacid (available at the drug store), following the directions for administering the antacid as printed on the container.

3. Apply hot fomentations over the stomach every three hours. (See volume 3, chapter 20, "Simple Home Treatments.") Continue this treatment no more than two days.

4. The first food taken should be thin broth in small amounts. Then add small amounts of white bread, mashed potatoes, and boiled rice. Return gradually to a normal diet.

5. Study the causes of the attack, and try to avoid them in the future. If symptoms persist, check with your physician to make sure there are no signs of stomach cancer.

CANCER OF THE STOMACH.

(See discussion of this item in chapter 11 of this volume.)

CHRONIC GASTRITIS.

Some of the most prominent symptoms of chronic gastritis are a bad taste in the mouth, a coated tongue, foul breath, belching of gas after eating, belching of food or fluid without a sour taste, discomfort in the upper abdomen after meals, tenderness over the stomach, nausea, and a general feeling of semi-invalidism, both physically and mentally. Sometimes the symptoms are so mild as to be hardly noticeable.

The malady may be caused by long indulgence in improper diet, eating too much greasy or fried food, overeating, too hasty eating, drinking large amounts of fluid at mealtime, cold beverages, irregular mealtimes, spices and condiments, the use of tobacco or alcoholic liquors, eating when worried or very tired, or any other habitual dietary error. It may develop from repeated attacks of acute gastritis. Whatever the cause, the result in a majority of cases has been to bring about more or less degeneration or atrophy of the stomach lining, especially of the glands which produce the hydrochloric acid and pepsin, active ingredients of the gastric juice. In some cases, the stomach lining is swollen and spongy rather than atrophic.

If the errors that caused the disease have been practiced for so long that the stomach glands have completely degenerated, a real cure is not possible. In the occasional case in which the lining of the stomach is swollen and spongy rather than atrophic, the symptoms may be much like those of peptic ulcer, and the treatment should be the same. (See *Peptic Ulcer* in this chapter.)

What to Do

1. Eat slowly, and masticate all food thoroughly.

2. Eat at regular times, and do not eat between meals.

3. Do not drink much of any kind of fluid at mealtime, and do not drink very cold or very hot beverages or alcoholic liquors at all.

4. Make your meals light, so that hunger is not completely satisfied.

5. Allow at least five hours between meals.

6. Rest for half an hour or more after each meal.

7. Avoid worry, anger, and other emotional upsets.

8. Study the effect of different foods on your stomach, and when you find that any particular food disagrees with you, let it alone forever.

9. If the above program does not bring about definite improvement within one month, consult a physician. Cancer of the stomach sometimes causes very similar symptoms.

HEARTBURN.

Heartburn is characterized by a sensation of "burning" in the upper middle part of the abdomen or along the course of the esophagus. It is caused by a stretching of the esophagus (usually the lower part) either by swallowing too much food or drink in a single swallow or by the regurgitating of stomach contents into the lower part of the esophagus. Heartburn does not indicate excess acidity in the stomach, for it has even occurred in persons who lack acid in their gastric juice.

What to Do

1. Do not eat again for at least six hours. A small bowl of bread and warm milk should be tried first.

2. If you are not sure whether your trouble is heartburn or perhaps gastric ulcer, consult a physician.

INDIGESTION (DYSPEPSIA).

Many people suffer from delayed digestion or occasional complete failure of the stomach to digest a meal. In such cases, food fermentation tends to occur, gas formation being a prominent symptom. Belching the gas from the stomach gives relief from the distress for a time. The gas may gurgle and rumble about in the bowels, causing bloating and abdominal distress. Intestinal irritation and gas formation may become so marked as to cause diarrhea. If so, the stools are at first broken up into segments, later becoming liquid and foamy. The patient may have headache and a sensation of mental dullness.

It is now recognized that an important cause of many cases of indigestion is a congenital deficiency of lactase—an enzyme which is needed for the assimilation of lactose, one of the carbohydrates contained in milk. When such a deficiency exists, milk taken into the digestive organs ferments instead of being digested and assimilated. The taking of more milk, even in combination, only makes the condition worse.

What to Do

1. The most effective treatment for acute indigestion is taking of repeated doses of a non-absorbable liquid antacid (available at the drug store). Do not exceed the dosage recommendation printed on the antacid container.

2. For the first 24 hours, take no food. Drink only water.

309

3. If the indigestion recurs when eating is resumed, try abstaining from milk in all forms—this because some cases of indigestion involve the intolerance for milk mentioned above.

4. If the attacks continue, have a physician study the case to detect and treat the underlying condition.

PEPTIC ULCER.

As used in medical literature, the term peptic ulcer includes (1) gastric ulcers that occur in the stomach and (2) duodenal ulcers which occur in the first part of the duodenum just beyond the stomach's outlet.

The term ulcer, as used for lesions in any part of the body, implies a raw area in which the normal covering of the underlying tissue is no longer present. So it is with peptic ulcers. A peptic ulcer consists of a relatively small area in the wall of the stomach or the duodenum which is no longer covered by the soft tissue that normally lines the stomach and duodenum. On examining the site of a peptic ulcer it appears that the lining tissue has been "punched out" at this site.

The gastric juice produced by glands in the lining of the stomach is composed in part of hydrochloric acid, hence it is a marvel that the lining of the stomach and of the duodenum is not all destroyed. The gastric juice also contains an enzyme, pepsin, which, together with the hydrochloric acid has the ability to disintegrate protein substances—and the soft tissues of the stomach consist, chemically, of protein. Normally the cells which compose the lining of the stomach and the duodenum possess some protective mechanism, as yet not fully understood, which prevents their being digested by the gastric juice. It must be, then, that at the site where an ulcer develops, this particular protective mechanism has failed. Beyond this, we do not know the precise cause of peptic ulcer. We do know, however, several of the factors that predispose to the development of peptic ulcers.

We often hear people say "I was so distraught that I almost got an ulcer over the situation." And it is true that persons under stress and persons who drive themselves beyond their reasonable limitations are in greater danger of developing peptic ulcers than are those who allow their lives to move along calmly and peacefully.

Presumably there is even a hereditary element in the predisposition to peptic ulcer. It would be hard to separate this, however, from the factor of psychic stress mentioned above. It may be that what the individual actually inherits is the tendency to work under pressure.

There are circumstances and customs in the environment that predispose to the development of peptic ulcer. The taking of aspirin into the stomach has a corrosive effect on the stomach lining. This has been demonstrated in animals and even in human subjects. Coffee, tea, and cola drinks increase the stomach's production of acid and thus favor the development of peptic ulcer. Also, persons who drink liquor are more subject to the development of peptic ulcer than are those who abstain. The use of cigarettes also has a detrimental effect on the lining of the stomach and duodenum. It is assumed that the effect of cigarettes is by way of the drug action which has an influence in constricting the tiny blood vessels in certain tissues of the body. At any rate, one recent scientific study indicated that among men ulcers are a little more than twice as frequent, percentage wise, among smokers as compared with nonsmokers. For women, the incidence of peptic ulcer is 1.6 times greater among smokers.

The incidence of gastric ulcer (ulcer in the stomach) is about the same for men and for women. Strangely, however, duodenal ulcer is ten times more frequent in men than in women.

The principal symptom of peptic ulcer is pain. Besides this, there may

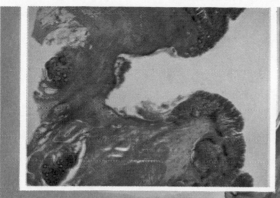

CHRONIC GASTRIC ULCER

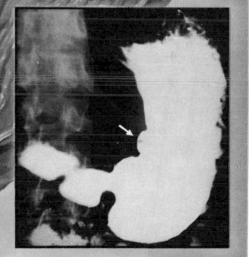

PERFORATED GASTRIC ULCER WITH
WALL ADHERENT TO PANCREAS

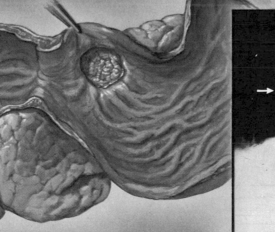

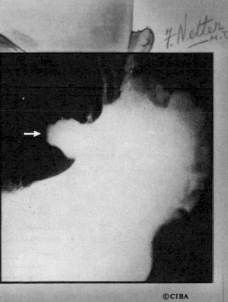

7. Netter M.D.

©CIBA

be a sensitive spot, especially noticeable on deep pressure, just below the lower end of the breastbone. Other symptoms of ulcer include heartburn, belching of acid, nausea, loss of appetite, and loss of weight. The pain of duodenal ulcer typically appears two to three hours after a meal. This pain is quickly relieved by taking more food or by using an antacid preparation, preferably in liquid form. This does not in any sense cure the ulcer, but only neutralizes the acid of the gastric juice which is otherwise causing the pain by irritating the raw bed of the ulcer.

Ulcers that occur in the stomach (gastric ulcers) frequently represent the early phase of cancer of the stomach. Duodenal ulcers, by contrast, are seldom malignant. It is because of this rather high probability of cancer that every ulcer which develops within the stomach should be carefully evaluated by a physician or by the members of a diagnostic clinic. It is now possible for the interior of the stomach to be viewed directly through the gastroscope and determinations made regarding malignancy.

In addition to the danger of cancer associated with gastric ulcers, there are three additional serious complications that may develop in either gastric ulcers or duodenal ulcers. These are obstruction, hemorrhage, and perforation.

The presence of an ulcer in either the stomach or the duodenum causes the neighboring tissues to become inflamed and swollen. In some cases the swelling is so great as to prevent stomach contents from passing through into the intestine. This constitutes what is called an obstruction. Vomiting is the principal symptom. The stomach becomes dilated. The treatment of this type of obstruction consists of passing a tube through the mouth or nose into the stomach and pumping out the stomach contents and secretions continuously for 36 to 48 hours. Meanwhile the body chemi-cals that are being lost by the continuous emptying of the stomach must be restored by intravenous injections. The obstruction usually subsides within the 48 hours so that liquid food by mouth can then be started.

We have already described a peptic ulcer as consisting of a raw area of tissue. Once the lining of the stomach or duodenum becomes eroded at the site of an ulcer, there is no longer any means of protecting the tissue at the base of the ulcer from the corrosive influence of the gastric juice. If the process of erosion at the base of the ulcer is allowed to continue, it may encounter a small artery. Even though this artery may be small in caliber, the normal pressure under which blood flows will cause it to bleed profusely, causing a serious, life-threatening loss of blood. The person experiencing such a hemorrhage may soon vomit a large quantity of fresh blood. Or, if the hemorrhage is not so profuse, the blood may clot and pass on through the intestinal tract to be discovered a few hours later as a dark substance in the stool. When the loss of blood from a hemorrhaging ulcer is rapid, the patient goes into shock, and his condition then constitutes a surgical emergency. In caring for such a patient, the surgeon must open the stomach, locate the bleeding vessel, and suture it so that it no longer bleeds. In the meantime, it is often advisable for the patient to be given a transfusion of blood to make up for the loss of his own blood.

The third serious complication—that of perforation—also requires surgical treatment. Perforation occurs when the process of erosion at the base of an ulcer continues until the wall of the stomach or the duodenum is actually perforated. This perforation allows the contents of the stomach or the duodenum to escape into the general abdominal cavity, thus producing the emergency condition of peritonitis (inflammation and infection of the membranes lining the abdominal cavity).

What to Do

There are two plans of treatment for peptic ulcer: the conservative "medical program" and the more radical surgical treatment. For most of the uncomplicated cases the medical program will bring relief and permit the ulcer to heal. In cases where the medical program is not adequate and in cases where the complications of hemorrhage, perforation, or pyloric obstruction have developed, the surgical treatment is used.

The medical treatment consists essentially of avoiding those things that predispose to ulcer.

1. Rest in bed for two or three weeks will often bring about definite improvement in the ulcer. The rest should involve freedom from mental taxation as well as from physical activity. At the end of this rest period, examination by gastroscope and by X ray should be made to determine whether or not there has been actual improvement of the ulcer. If this examination indicates that the ulcer is of the malignant type (cancerous), prompt surgical treatment is indicated.

2. During this initial period of rest, the diet should be simple, and excessive roughage in the food should be avoided. Taking frequent feedings in place of the conventional three meals a day often helps to prevent the accumulation of acid in the stomach.

3. The use of a non-absorbable, liquid antacid preparation with several doses per day, serves to reduce the amount of acid in the stomach and thus to prevent further irritation of the ulcerated area.

4. If the patient does not already abstain, he should now definitely discontinue the use of coffee, cola drinks, cigarettes, and alcohol.

The exact method of surgical treatment for peptic ulcer has undergone several changes during recent years. The procedure that most surgeons now prefer is designated as "vagotomy with pyloroplasty." This consists of removing part of the nerve supply to the stomach so that its production of gastric juice will be reduced, and of enlarging the opening at the stomach's outlet.

PYLORIC STENOSIS (PYLORIC OBSTRUCTION).

Pyloric stenosis is a condition in which the outlet of the stomach is narrowed and interferes with the passage of stomach contents into the intestine. Two manifestations of pyloric stenosis occur: (1) congenital pyloric stenosis in the first few weeks after birth, and (2) adult pyloric stenosis in later childhood or in adulthood. The latter may be a carry-over of inadequately treated congenital pyloric stenosis or may be associated with the development of peptic ulcer or with cancer of the stomach.

Congenital pyloric stenosis occurs on an average in one out of 200 newborn babies and is more common in boys than in girls in the ratio of three to one. It is the product of a faulty combination of genes at the time of conception (a polygenic problem). It involves an overdevelopment of the muscle in the wall of the intestinal tract at the junction of the stomach with the intestine. The symptoms appear first during the second or third week after birth and often become progressively worse until the child dies or until adequate treatment is given.

The symptoms are those that would be expected when the stomach contents are prevented from moving into the intestine: (1) vomiting after feeding, with the vomitus being projected as far as two or three feet, (2) the appearance of active contraction waves in the wall of the stomach, plainly visible through the infant's abdominal wall, (3) constipation, and (4) progressive loss of weight until the baby may eventually weigh less than at birth.

In the adult type of pyloric stenosis

the symptoms are comparable and may include those of a related disease such as peptic ulcer or cancer.

What to Do

The effective treatment for congenital pyloric stenosis is a surgical operation by which the muscle layer at the outlet of the stomach is cut through. The surgical procedure itself is relatively simple, and the prospects of a favorable outcome are good provided the case is taken relatively early and provided, of course, that the baby receives appropriate hospital care before and after the surgery.

For the adult type, the treatment consists of correcting the condition which underlies the pyloric obstruction.

VOMITING.

(See discussion under *Nausea and Vomiting* in volume 3, chapter 22.)

The Intestines

ACUTE APPENDICITIS.

The appendix is usually located on the right side of the abdomen, about midway between the point of the hipbone and the navel. Inflammation of this small organ occurs more frequently in children and young adults than in older people, but it may occur at any age. It is quite common, at least one in ten people having it at some time in life.

The first symptom of acute appendicitis is usually pain, and there may be tenderness on pressure. The pain quickly becomes severe. In many cases, however, the pain is not felt in the region of the appendix at first, but is distributed over the entire abdomen, and it may be most marked in the upper and central part. Somewhat later as the problem develops the pain and tenderness tend to localize in the region of the organ.

Cathartics (laxatives) should be avoided, for their use stimulates the intestines into activity and the appen-

dix may rupture, thus causing peritonitis. It is much more difficult to deal with a ruptured appendix than with one simply inflamed.

Pain alone is not enough to determine the presence of appendicitis. Neither is tenderness on pressure a certain sign. But if both rigidity and tenderness of the muscles of the abdominal wall appear together, especially on the right side, a little below the level of the navel, the condition is probably appendicitis.

Coughing and deep breathing tend to make the pain worse. More or less fever is likely to be present almost from the first, and there will be constipation, loss of appetite, nausea, vomiting, and a tendency while lying in bed to draw up the right leg to relieve tension on the sore side.

Such symptoms usually suffice to indicate that the trouble is appendicitis. In case of doubt, a doctor can give certain tests that will help confirm the diagnosis. A blood-cell count will give valuable information.

When the diagnosis of appendicitis has been confirmed by the doctor, the question of operation will be determined by the progress of the case and the general condition of the patient. If surgery is necessary and the delay is not too great, the chances are excellent for a speedy recovery.

What to Do

1. If appendicitis is suspected, consult a doctor at once. Surgery may be needed to save life, and delay may be dangerous.

2. In the meantime, keep the patient in bed.

3. Apply an ice bag to the painful area.

4. Give no cathartics, enemas, or food.

AMEBIC DYSENTERY (AMEBIASIS).

(See under *Protozoal Infections* in chapter 21 of this volume.)

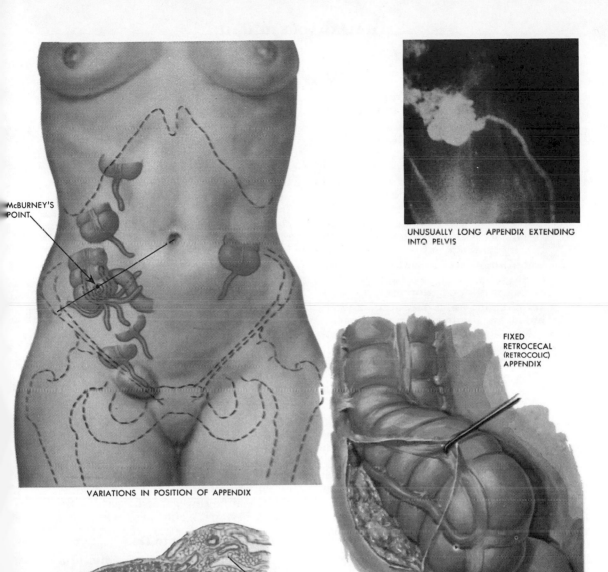

McBURNEY'S POINT

UNUSUALLY LONG APPENDIX EXTENDING INTO PELVIS

VARIATIONS IN POSITION OF APPENDIX

FIXED RETROCECAL (RETROCOLIC) APPENDIX

MESO-APPENDIX

SEROSA (VISCERAL PERITONEUM)

LONGITUDINAL MUSCLE

CIRCULAR MUSCLE

SUBMUCOSA

LYMPHATIC NODULE

CRYPTS OF LIEBERKÜHN

F. Netter M.D.

©CIBA

BACILLARY DYSENTERY.

(See in chapter 28 of this volume.)

CANCER OF THE COLON.

(See in chapter 11 of this volume.)

CELIAC DISEASE (IDIOPATHIC STEATORRHEA).

Celiac disease occurs most commonly in children between the ages of one and five. When it occurs in adults, it is considered to be a form of nontropical sprue. A fully developed case is characterized by frequent, large, loose, frothy, pale-colored, foul-smelling stools, anemia, emaciation, retarded growth and development, and a distended abdomen. The mouth and tongue are often sore, and the bones are likely to be fragile.

Causes of this common disease, more common than formerly realized, are not well understood. The mucous membrane lining the digestive tract tends to degenerate during attacks, and the walls of the intestine become very thin. They lose more or less of their ability to absorb fats, carbohydrates, proteins, water, calcium, and vitamins A, B_{12}, D, and K. Most medical scientists believe that celiac disease is an infantile form of sprue; and allergy to wheat protein (gluten) may be a factor in causing it. Also it may occur in connection with the disease cystic fibrosis.

What to Do

1. Give the patient a diet low in fats, but abundant in proteins, fruits, fruit juices, iron, and vitamins A, B_{12}, D, and K. Bananas may be helpful. Carefully avoid all foods made either wholly or partly from wheat.

2. Other treatment should be left to a physician to prescribe, the treatment being similar in principle to that given for sprue. (See chapter 32 of this volume.)

CHOLERA.

(For a discussion on this disease, turn to chapter 32 of this volume.)

COLIC.

Crying in young children is frequently a sign of colic (the word "colic" meaning a paroxysm of acute abdominal pain), though older children and adults can also have colic. The child may seem perfectly well and go to sleep as usual. Suddenly it starts from sleep and utters a cry. The legs are drawn up or kicked about in efforts to get relief from the pain.

There are many possible causes for colic, wrong feeding being the usual one. Giving too much sugar or sweets is a common mistake, also overfeeding or irregular feeding. Hasty drinking of milk or bolting of other food may be followed by colic. Undigested food in the intestinal tract can cause the trouble. Generally there is intestinal fermentation, but constipation rather than diarrhea. The resulting gas produces pain by distending the bowel walls.

Frequent attacks of colic demand correction of the feeding program. It is essential to select the right food, to prepare it properly, and to give it at regular times. Constipation should be overcome by right feeding and not by laxatives. At the time of the attack, the bowels should be emptied at once. A warm saline enema will as a rule speedily stop the cutting pain of colic.

What to Do

1. To prevent or treat colic in a baby, proceed as follows:

A. Feed regularly.

B. "Burp" twice after each feeding.

C. Lay the child on its abdomen awhile after each feeding, with a cloth-wrapped warm-water bottle under its abdomen if there are any signs of abdominal discomfort.

D. Give the child all the warm water it will drink if it cries between feeding times.

E. Keep the room warm, but the air fresh, carefully guarding the baby's feet and legs from chilling.

F. If an attack of colic comes, give

the baby a warm, 8-ounce saline enema. (See volume 3, chapter 20, "Simple Home Treatments.")

2. For *known* colic in older children or adults, proceed as follows:

A. Give a warm saline enema. (See volume 3, chapter 20.)

B. Apply fomentations or a hot water bottle to the abdomen. (See volume 3, chapter 20.)

Caution: If there is any *chance* that the trouble might be *appendicitis,* items A and B should not be performed: but a physician should be called to determine what the true condition is.

COLITIS.

The term "colon" is used as a very-near synonym to the term "large intestine." The term "colitis," therefore, refers to an irritation of the large intestine.

The colon (large intestine) is classically divided into four sections: the ascending colon (extending from the lower right part of the abdominal cavity to the upper right), the transverse colon (extending from upper right to upper left), the descending colon (from upper left to lower left), and the sigmoid colon (the terminal portion in the lower left which swings over to the midline to join the rectum). The exact length and position of the sigmoid colon varies from person to person even among normal individuals. This variation is shown well in the accompanying illustration.

A. *Irritable Colon (Mucous Colitis).* This is a condition of abnormal function of the colon, often involving constipation and abdominal discomfort, which occurs commonly in persons under emotional tension and stress. Symptoms include also the passing of a variable amount of mucus along with the stools, aching distress in the abdomen, occasional occurrence of diarrhea (alternating with the constipation), and other evidences of nervous tension such as headache, sleeplessness, and fatigability.

What to Do

1. The patient's way of life should be studied to discover the circumstances which produce stress and emotional turmoil.

2. Appropriate modifications should be made in the patient's pattern of living, perhaps reducing the excessive devotion to achievement or relieving his anxieties.

3. The physician should make a careful examination to determine whether any organic disease is present. If not, the patient should feel reassured that his symptoms are not the result of inflammation or malignancy.

4. A general program such as suggested under constipation (see below) will help in the relief of symptoms.

5. The use of a bulk laxative such as Metamucil provides bulk and at the same time reduces irritation.

B. *Ulcerative Colitis.* This is a condition in which the tissues lining the colon become inflamed and ulcerated, resulting in the passage of bloody, purulent, watery stools. The specific cause remains unknown although suggested causes include infection by bacteria and viruses, emotional tensions which interfere with the function of the colon and make its tissues vulnerable to inflammation, and allergy to certain foods. The disease may occur at any time of life but most commonly attacks adults in their third decade.

The symptoms usually appear gradually and include an urgency to move the bowels, discomfort in the lower abdomen, and the appearance of bloody mucus with the stools. Constitutional responses are fever, loss of appetite, nausea, and anemia.

The disease is not contagious. Typically there are periods of relative freedom from symptoms followed by relapses. Even after apparent cure, the illness may return quite suddenly.

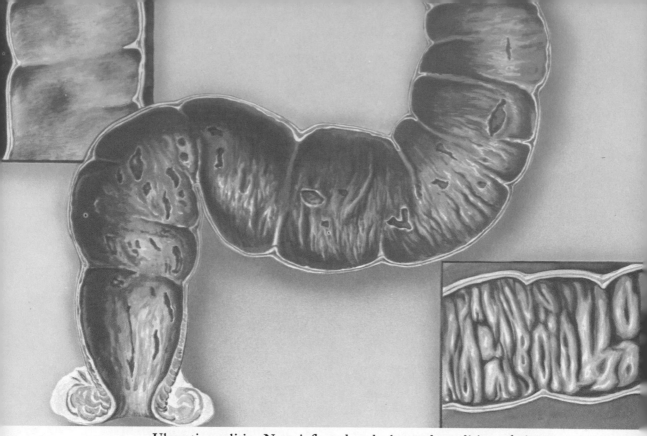

Ulcerative colitis. Note inflamed and ulcerated condition of tissues lining the colon. Inset above shows beginning stage of the disease; inset below, a more advanced stage.

What to Do

Successful treatment requires patience and persistence. It should be supervised by a physician.

1. A diet rich in protein and high in calories and vitamins should be provided. Items which aggravate the condition include iced foods and iced drinks, acid fruit juices, and uncooked and coarse vegetables.

2. The physician may deem it advisable to use antibiotics or sulfonamides to combat infection.

3. In case of anemia or abdominal cramping, he may prescribe medications for these conditions.

4. Psychotherapy to relieve emotional tension is often helpful.

5. In severe, persistent cases hospitalization may be necessary. Surgery has proved beneficial in some cases.

CONSTIPATION.

Before beginning to treat any case of constipation, its cause or causes should be known. Sometimes cancers or other tumors in the wall of the intestine or pressing on it from the outside, or adhesions, strictures, or displacements of the bowel, bring on constipation because of partial obstruction. To detect such conditions, much more to correct them, is beyond the skill of a person without medical training. The bowel itself may not be at fault; but improper action of the liver, gallbladder, or endocrine glands may result in sluggish intestinal action. Reflexes from a diseased rectum may affect the bowel higher up. All such conditions require study by a physician, and anybody afflicted with constipation should first make sure that he has no serious or dangerous condition beyond his own skill to remedy before he takes on the responsibility of trying

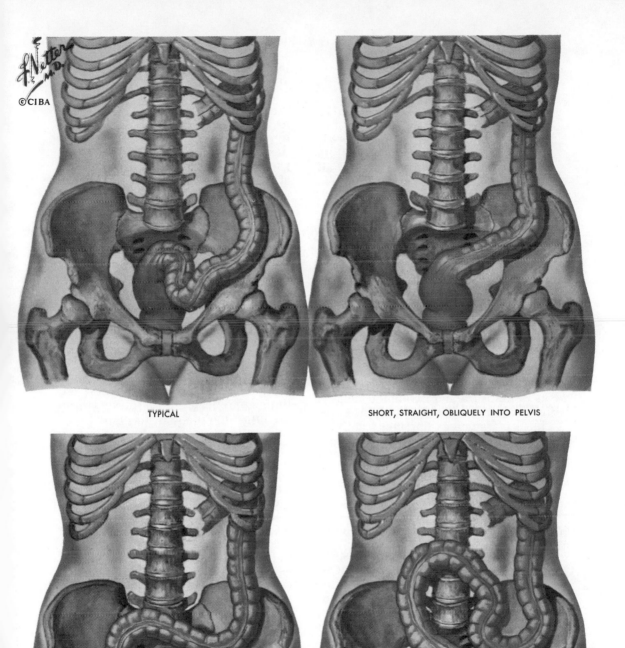

TYPICAL

SHORT, STRAIGHT, OBLIQUELY INTO PELVIS

LOOPING TO RIGHT SIDE

ASCENDING HIGH INTO ABDOMEN

NORMAL SIGMOID COLON, VARIATIONS IN POSITION

to solve his own problem along the lines discussed below.

A common cause of constipation is a lack of sufficient bulk in the diet. When a person eats milk, cream, butter, eggs, flesh food, refined cereals, and starchy vegetables, nearly all the bulk of his food is digested and absorbed, leaving little residue; but if he eats freely of fruits and green vegetables, a large residue of cellulose remains undigested and unabsorbed, which is useful in making the bowels act normally.

The mild acids in fruits are stimulants to the production of digestive juices. They also induce an antiseptic action in the digestive tract, and greatly assist in reducing fermentation. They stimulate the bowels to force the food onward and downward, and are nature's wholesome laxatives.

Neglect to answer the call of nature is perhaps the most common cause of constipation. Normally, when the fecal mass comes in contact with the mucous membrane lining the rectum, a message signaling need for evacuation is sent over the nerves to the brain. Habitual failure to give heed to such messages ends in obstinate constipation.

Among school children, and also among oversensitive people working in offices or other public places, the call to evacuation is frequently put off, or the teacher may unwisely refuse the children permission to go when the need is felt. Constipation due to emotional or nervous tension is also common.

In the absence of a natural call to evacuate the bowels, it is important to go to the bathroom at a regular, definite time anyway and to attempt a bowel movement. The best time for this is within an hour after breakfast. Taking of food into an empty stomach constitutes a powerful stimulant to peristaltic action, and the peristalsis which begins in the stomach tends to spread downward throughout the digestive tract. After eating, therefore, is the rational time for an effort at evacuation.

Fecal matter is collected slowly in the descending colon as it is delivered to that portion of the bowel by the upper portions. The lower part of the descending colon lies against the psoas muscle, which muscle contracts at each step one takes in walking or running. The action of the psoas muscle in walking or running, therefore, is stimulating to the bowel, especially when the bowel is full. Walking, running, or any other exercise that brings this muscle into activity, therefore, is a useful part of the treatment for constipation.

If their bowels do not move exactly when and how they think they should, many people resort to cathartics. Some take a cathartic regularly every ten days or two weeks, whether they are constipated or not. Many cathartics act by irritating the bowel. Continued or repeated irritation sets up an inflammation in the walls of the intestine and causes them to contract so firmly that the fecal mass has difficulty in passing. Hence what many people consider an effective treatment for constipation may only make the condition fundamentally worse.

The enema habit is also bad. Enemas tend to wash away normal intestinal secretions and may be irritating to the bowel. Plain water is a decided bowel irritant. Whenever an enema must be taken to clean out the large bowel, a heaping teaspoonful of common salt should be put into the water for each quart of water used. Such a salt solution is much less irritating than water alone.

Symptoms of constipation include, besides of course inability to evacuate, a feeling of fullness in the lower abdomen, a sensation of dullness, or even moderate pain in the head. Many people with chronic constipation think these latter symptoms are caused by toxins or poisons formed in their bowels and absorbed into their blood, but such symptoms seldom result from the absorption of poisons. They are caused by irritated mucous membranes and by reflexes from nerve endings in the intestinal tract. Dr. Alvarez proved by experimentation that such characteristic symptoms could be set up by packing a person's rectum with sterile absorbent cotton.

In many cases of chronic constipation there tends to be a spastic condition of the sigmoid part of the descending colon on the left side of the abdomen, with a dilated and inactive condition of the ascending colon on the right side; there are cases in which a considerably larger portion of the colon is spastic. These facts have led to the use of the term "spastic constipation" by many physicians, and the presence of this condition can usually be proved by X-ray studies. Because the spasticity may be made worse by too much irritation, if the constipation is known to be of the spastic type it may be well for a time to puree fruits and vegetables so they will be free from coarse fiber and harsh roughage. It may be inadvisable to take bran, so often recommended as a remedy for constipation. Later, when regular bowel action has been reestablished, such precautions will become less important.

Massage may be of value if properly given. It should be firm, deep kneading, not merely rubbing of the skin. It should begin low down on the right side, move slowly upward with a combined rolling and kneading motion to the lower margin of the ribs, then horizontally across the abdomen to the left side, and finally down the left side of the abdomen as far as possible.

What to Do

1. Try to learn the type and causes of your particular case of constipation. You may need the services of a physician in doing so, and he may need to use X ray and other kinds of examinations to get the answer. If he finds that surgery or any other special treatment is needed to correct or remove the cause, this should be arranged. The treatment program suggested below would be useless in certain cases, and it might cause dangerous delay in correcting conditions that should not be neglected. The program outlined in the following paragraphs is intended for use in ordinary cases where no tumors or organic defects complicate the situation.

2. Eat an abundance of fruit and vegetables, both fresh and cooked.

3. Drink at least eight glasses of fluid—chiefly water and fruit juices—every day.

4. Go to the toilet regularly every day—preferably soon after breakfast—whether you feel like having a bowel movement of not. Also go immediately at any other time when you feel the urge.

5. If not able to have a bowel movement otherwise, take a saline enema at the end of a regular stool visit, but not oftener than once in three days. (See volume 3, chapter 20, "Simple Home Treatments.")

6. Three times a day, take two tablespoonfuls of powdered brewer's yeast stirred into a glass of tomato juice or buttermilk. (This usually will not have to be continued more than a week.)

7. If possible, take half an hour to an hour of outdoor exercise daily, the exercise including running or walking and being vigorous enough to cause at least mild perspiration.

8. The use of a bulk laxative such as Metamucil helps to relieve constipation by providing bulk without causing irritation.

DIARRHEA (ACUTE CATARRHAL ENTEROCOLITIS).

Indiscretions in eating or drinking can be responsible for much trouble, especially in warm weather. One common ailment thus caused is inflammation or irritation of the lining membrane of the intestines.

The chief symptom is diarrhea. The first indication of trouble is usually pain in the abdomen—perhaps colicky in nature, coming and going, or perhaps sharp and continuous. In acute cases there may be fever, loss of appetite, and intense thirst. If long-continued, great prostration, loss of weight, and impairment of general health will result.

In infants and young children, the cause is usually contaminated milk or carelessness in preparing their food. In older children, overindulgence in candy, soft drinks, pastry, or unripe or overripe fruit may be responsible. In adults, the cause may be either these or other indiscretions in diet. Eating food that has been contaminated with disease germs by exposure to flies or other insects is a common cause of diarrhea in people of all ages, especially in warm climates. In the persistent cases due to emotional tension, the cause may not be easy to detect.

One important reason for calling a physician if home treatment does not check diarrhea promptly is the possibility of typhoid fever, amebic dysentery, or some other serious infectious disease that may begin with diarrhea as its first symptom.

Diarrhea is especially harmful to babies. To prevent diarrhea, give a baby particular care, especially during the hot season. Fresh air—all the time by ventilation and every day by outdoor life—is important. Sunlight is of great value in keeping a baby healthy at any season. It is safer to boil all water given to a baby. If he is fed from a bottle, it must be a sterilized bottle with a sterilized nipple. Some mothers may fear that their babies will starve if the advice given in (2) below is followed. Persistent diarrhea will do a baby more harm than will lack of food for a few days, but he will need plenty of water.

What to Do

Especially in the case of babies who have diarrhea it is important to determine at once whether the condition is mild or severe. Because of the loss of fluid from the body and with this the loss of some of the body chemicals, severe diarrhea in an infant can cause death very soon if not adequately treated.

1. For mild diarrhea in an infant, a temporary *reduction* in feeding by mouth will often cause the symptoms to subside. Caution must be used, of course, to make sure that the infant receives sufficient fluid so that he will not become dehydrated.

2. For severe diarrhea in an infant, the care should be supervised by a physician with the possibility that the infant should be placed in the hospital. Because of the rapid loss of fluid and body chemicals, it is usually necessary to replace these by the administration of intravenous fluid of proper composition. Also, in a case of severe diarrhea, the cause should be determined and proper medication given to remove this cause.

3. Some cases of diarrhea either in an infant or in an older child or adult are caused by the inability to assimilate milk. This is often due to an inherent lack of the enzyme lactase. In such a case milk must be eliminated from the diet and replaced by appropriate substitutes which do not contain the carbohydrate lactose.

4. As a baby recovers, he becomes able to take thin gruel. Except in those cases in which there is a sensitivity to milk, it can gradually be added to the gruel, day by day, until the baby is taking his normal food, within about a week's time.

5. For an older child or an adult, the first additions to the gruel diet should be toast, mashed potatoes, rice, bland vegetables that have been pureed or boiled soft, and later, milk and fruit. Raw food (except fruit juices), cold foods or drinks, and fried or greasy foods should be avoided.

FECAL IMPACTION.

A fecal mass that is hard and dry or puttylike may not pass easily through the lower parts of the large bowel and may become impacted there, interfering with the normal evacuation of feces and causing partial or even complete intestinal obstruction. In such a case, the bowel above the impaction is likely to become considerably distended. This most often happens with bedfast patients, with people taking a scanty or low-residue diet, with those who have taken drugs to quiet bowel action, or with those who may resist evacuation because of some painful rectal disease. Strangely, the usual indication of fecal impaction is the occurrence of watery diarrhea. This is because only fluid can pass the impacted fecal mass. This condition may be suspected, but not usually definitely detected, by a person without medical training and experience; but by physical and X-ray examinations a physician can be sure of it.

What to Do

1. Try large, warm, saline enemas, with the patient in the knee-chest position while the solution is injected *slowly*. (See volume 3, chapter 20, "Simple Home Treatments.")

2. If the impaction is near the outlet of the rectum, it may be broken up and picked out by rubber-glove-protected fingers.

3. It may be necessary to give oil retention enemas at bedtime every night, followed by saline enemas every morning. (See volume 3, chapter 20.)

4. In severe cases a physician's services may be needed.

FLATULENCE.

Flatulence consists of the accumulation of gas in the stomach or the intestines. Certain foods tend to cause the formation and collection of gas. This gas must be expelled from time to time in order to prevent distress or pain from stomach or bowel distention. Some people have the habit of swallowing air. This, as well as gases formed in the stomach, may be expelled by belching; but it may also pass on into the bowels. Nervousness, anxiety, and the chewing of gum tend to promote air swallowing.

Some cases of flatulence are caused by the inherent deficiency of the enzyme lactase which is necessary for the digestion and assimilation of milk.

What to Do

1. Eliminate foods known to promote gas formation in the individual case. In general, foods possibly to be avoided include raw vegetables and fruits such as cabbage, celery, cucumbers, onions, pears, peppers, and tomatoes. Among cooked vegetables, beans and broccoli are especially notorious. Do not use much sugar or concentrated sweets. Avoid fried foods, nuts, raisins, seedy fruits, spices, and carbonated or alcoholic beverages.

2. Take a bland, high-protein, low-fat, low-carbohydrate diet.

3. Do not take drugs without a physician's orders.

4. Elimination of gas from the stomach may be aided by taking half a teaspoonful of essence of peppermint in half a glass of water after each meal.

FOOD POISON.

(See section on "Poisonings" in volume 3, chapter 18, "Handling Emergencies.")

HEMORRHOIDS (PILES).

Hemorrhoids are swellings containing dilated or varicose veins situated in the mucous membranes of the rectum or in the skin around the anus. Veins, unlike arteries, have not sufficient strength in their walls to support much blood pressure. For this reason veins near the surface, without additional support muscles and other deep structures, often become distended.

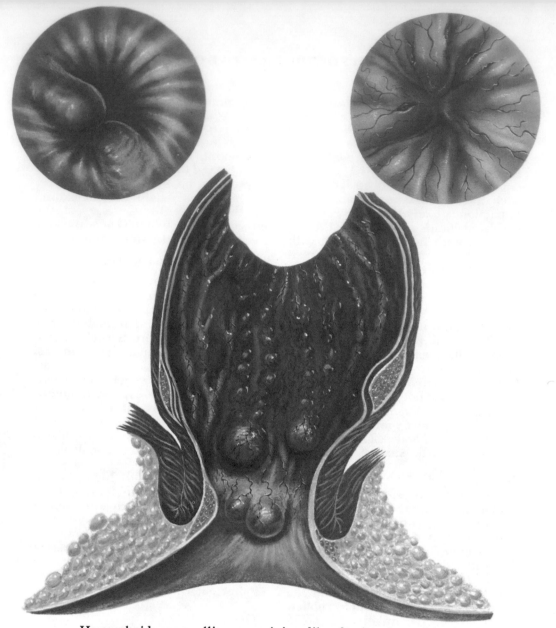

Hemorrhoids are swellings containing dilated veins situated in the mucous membrane of the rectum or in the skin around the anus.

Veins around the rectum do not have much support from any other tissue, so they distend easily. Constipation, and all conditions leading to it, are causes of hemorrhoids. Straining at stool is an important cause; and the straining associated with childbirth, together with pressure on the tissues surrounding the veins, is a common cause of hemorrhoids in women.

People with hemorrhoids may have pain in the rectum, with itching both inside the rectum and in the skin around its outlet. In many cases blood oozes from the hemorrhoids, usually in connection with the act of emptying the bowels. This is not the only cause for rectal bleeding, for it may also occur in connection with intestinal polyps or tumors involving the intestine. Piles may protrude from the rectum or they may not depending on how high up in the rectum the affected veins are located. When they protrude, the sphincter muscle of the rectum partially strangulates them and tends to prevent their return.

The most important point in the management of hemorrhoids is the correction of constipation so that the stools can pass regularly and with the least possible irritation. If the case is severe, the patient while waiting for surgery may have to keep off his feet much of the time so that the blood pressure can be reduced and the protrusion corrected by giving the hemorrhoids relief from the pull of gravity.

What to Do

1. **Take a diet adapted to prevent constipation. (See under** *Constipation* **in this chapter.)**

2. **Drink plenty of water.**

3. **If the hemorrhoids protrude, cleanse them very gently with pieces of absorbent cotton wet with a solution of a level teaspoonful of salt in a pint (450 ml.) of water, and** *gently* **press them back into place while lying down. A physician can prescribe pain-relieving ointments to apply after the cleansing if the hemorrhoids are painful.**

4. **Alternate hot and cold compresses over the rectum and perineum twice a day will help relieve pain. (See volume 3, chapter 20, "Simple Home Treatments.")**

5. **A daily hot sitz bath or a daily hot saline enema may do as well or better. (See volume 3, chapter 20.)**

6. **If rectal bleeding persists, a physician should be consulted.**

7. **In severe and long-continued cases, rest in bed and surgery are needed for a cure. After the operation the surgeon will direct in the aftercare, which is of much importance.**

HERNIA (RUPTURE).

An adult with a hernia was probably born with a weak spot in his lower abdominal wall. As he grew older, and perhaps had to perform heavy muscular labor, the weak spot slowly enlarged and became an opening through which a loop of intestine could protrude at times. Unless corrected, such a condition tends to grow progressively worse. A truss may bring relief, but in adults it seldom leads to a cure. The most effective treatment is surgery.

Care should be taken not to fall into the hands of a "rupture" quack who claims to cure all kinds of hernia by injection or some other nonsurgical method. Consult a properly trained and experienced surgeon. Once repaired by such an expert, a hernia seldom gives further trouble.

There is definite danger in allowing a hernia to go without attention. Sometimes a loop of intestine that has pushed its way through the abdominal wall becomes pinched, and the passage of fecal material through the intestine is stopped. This is called incarcerated hernia. The symptoms are unmistakable pain, vomiting, and abdominal distention. If the condition persists until the tissues begin to deteriorate for lack of blood supply, the hernia is then said to be "strangulated." Gangrene of the bowel, peritonitis, and death are likely to result if prompt surgical relief is not obtained.

What to Do

1. **If a hernia should protrude and resist being pushed back, have the patient lie down on his back, with his hips higher than his shoulders, and try gently to replace the protruding bowel loop. Sometimes a warm compress over the area for a few minutes will relax the tissues and make the loop easier to replace.**

2. **If it is impossible to replace the loop of bowel, a surgical operation should be promptly performed. Delay is perilous.**

3. **There is danger in reasoning that because a hernia is small, it does not need professional attention. Frequently the small hernias are the ones which carry the greatest hazard.**

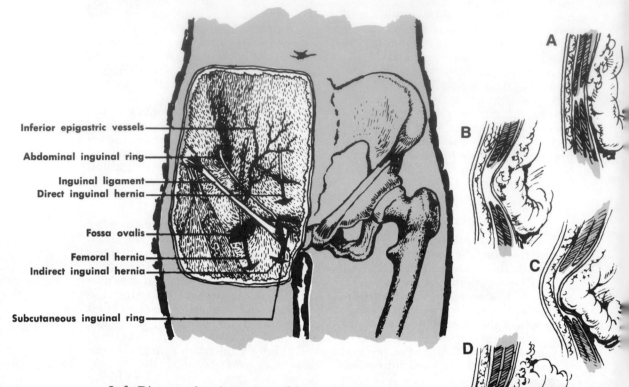

Inferior epigastric vessels

Abdominal inguinal ring

Inguinal ligament
Direct inguinal hernia

Fossa ovalis

Femoral hernia
Indirect inguinal hernia

Subcutaneous inguinal ring

A

B

C

D

Left: Diagram showing points of descent in the three common types of hernia. Right: Four stages in development of hernia—A. weak spot in lower abdominal wall, but intestine still in normal position; B. weak spot enlarges, allowing intestine to press abdominal wall outward; C. bulge increases, forcing a protrusion of the abdominal wall; D. loop of intestine becomes pinched, resulting in strangulated hernia.

4. Surgical repair is the only truly satisfactory remedy for hernia.

INTESTINAL DIVERTICULITIS.

The walls of the colon, especially the descending portion on the left side of the abdomen, sometimes form pouches called diverticula. When many of them are present, the condition is called diverticulosis. One or more of these pouches may become infected and produce symptoms and dangers much like those of appendicitis. Similar symptoms may be produced by a developing cancer of

the colon. It is advisable, therefore, to arrange with a physician for a careful diagnostic study.

What to Do

1. Follow the same general plan as advised in a case of acute appendicitis, varying the treatment according to the location of the most painful and tender areas. (See *Acute Appendicitis* in this listing.)

2. The use of a bulk laxative such as Metamucil is usually of considerable help.

3. As a preventive measure, follow the advice given for the treatment

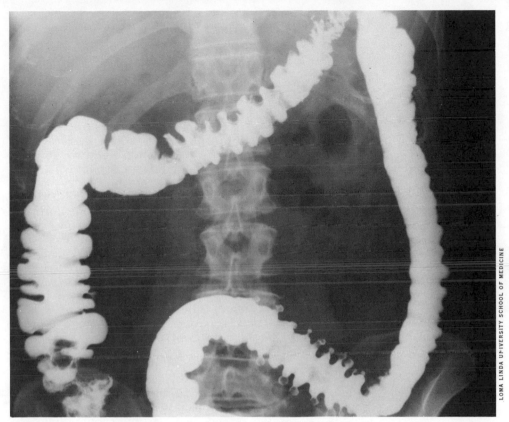

X ray of a case of diverticulosis.

of constipation of the spastic type. (See *Constipation* in this listing.) A daily intake of whole-grain cereals may help to prevent the development of diverticulitis.

INTESTINAL OBSTRUCTION.

Intestinal obstruction is produced by any condition which prevents the normal movement of intestinal contents. It may develop gradually and be unsuspected until an attack of severe pain strikes. At first the pain comes in occasional spasms. The paroxysms become more and more frequent, until finally the pain is continuous. Among common causes of intestinal obstruction are hernias, adhesions, volvulus (a twisting of the intestine), fecal impaction, foreign body in the intestine, gallstones, large intestinal worms, and cancer of the colon.

The pain of intestinal obstruction usually begins about in the midline of the body near the navel, not very low down; and it does not shift to one side or the other later. If the large intestine is involved, the pain is sometimes lower down; but even then it is usually in the midline of the body.

Complete constipation is to be expected. The enema solution may return with some fecal matter at first, but later it returns clear.

The third important symptom is vomiting. The material first expelled is like ordinary vomitus, but soon it is green with bile. Then comes a fluid brown in color and fecal in odor.

The obstruction dams up the intestinal contents. Gases accumulate and produce increasing painful distention of the abdomen. Soon there may be a mild fever and great thirst. It is impossible to do much in the home to relieve the thirst because of the

327

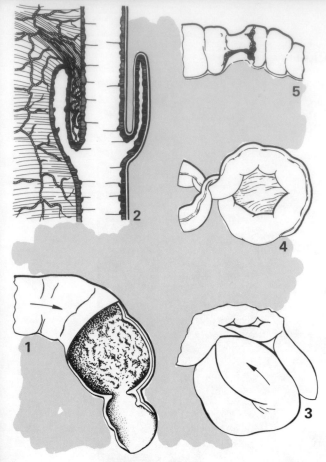

Intestinal obstruction is caused by (1) fecal impaction; (2) intussusception—intestine turns in upon itself; (3) restraint; (4) twisting of the intestine; (5) malignant tumor.

persistent vomiting. If the obstruction is not relieved, death results.

Intestinal obstruction sometimes occurs in babies or small children, many such cases being due to the telescoping of a portion of the bowel, a condition called intussusception. This disorder causes not only the ordinary symptoms of intestinal obstruction, but frequently bleeding from the bowel also. Intussusception occasionally occurs in older people too.

A form of intestinal obstruction called adynamic ileus is produced by an interference with the nervous control of intestinal peristalsis. This occurs most often following abdominal surgery, but may also result from disease or injury of one or more of the abdominal organs, injuries to the vertebrae or to the spinal cord, pneumonia or some other severe infection, uremia, diabetes, et cetera. In cases of adynamic ileus the severe symptoms tend to develop more slowly than in obstruction from ordinary causes.

The mesentery is a double layer of tissue which serves to attach the intestines to the abdominal wall. All the arteries taking blood to, and the veins taking it from, the intestines are embedded in the mesentery. If embolism or thrombosis occurs in any of these blood vessels, circulation throughout the corresponding part of the mesentery and the bowel is shut off. The affected tissue becomes engorged with stagnant blood and later becomes necrotic or gangrenous. Wherever this happens in a bowel area, intestinal obstruction occurs. The cause has been named mesenteric vascular occlusion.

What to Do

Consult a doctor as soon as intestinal obstruction is suspected. He can make such examinations and tests as may be needed to determine the true nature of the condition. He may possibly give treatments that will clear up the trouble, but usually surgery will be necessary to save life.

ISCHIORECTAL ABSCESS.

Sometimes the rectum becomes so inflamed through irritation that infection takes hold and comes to a head outside the rectum, forming an abscess, which is usually not very deep beneath the skin and not far from the anus. Such abscesses may be caused by inflammation from any source, as hemorrhoids, severe diarrhea, or the passing of foreign bodies that injure the mucous membrane of the rectum.

At first there is tenderness around the rectal outlet, which rapidly increases to severe pain. Redness and swelling soon appear, with a rising temperature and general ill-feeling.

328

Such abscesses may clear up and give no further trouble after they have been treated by a surgeon. They may, however, especially if the surgical treatment is long delayed, leave permanent fistulas—irregular openings or channels from the skin surface to the interior of the rectum—which will require more extensive surgery and which in some cases are never entirely cured.

Fistulas similar to those that come as a complication of ischiorectal abscesses may develop in the wall of the anus. Then there is a slow and sometimes intermittent leakage of fecal matter. (See *Rectal Fistula* in this listing.)

In other cases the membrane lining the anal outlet may be stretched and split by the passage of a large, hard mass of feces, forming a painful and intermittently bleeding fissure. All such conditions can easily be detected at the time of a physical examination and can be successfully treated; but a better plan is to try to prevent them by forming a proper bowel habit and choosing foods not likely to result in stools difficult to pass.

What to Do

As soon as evidence indicates an ischiorectal abscess is forming, see a physician and have the abscess treated. He will direct as to the aftercare.

ITCHING ANUS (PRURITUS ANI).
(See chapter 12 of this volume.)

PARATYPHOID FEVER.
(See chapter 28 of this volume.)

PERITONITIS.
Peritonitis is an inflammation of the membrane that lines the abdominal cavity and covers the organs within it, but the sufferer feels as if the trouble were in his bowels. A person with acute peritonitis has severe abdominal pain and tenderness, with rigidity of the abdominal muscles, not limited to any particular area. There will be a rapid pulse, fever, vomiting, sunken eyes, and a pinched expression of the face. It is a serious illness, and often fatal.

Acute peritonitis may be caused by blows, gunshot wounds, stab wounds, et cetera, or it may be a complication of surgical operations, perforated peptic ulcer, childbirth, appendicitis, or ovarian disease.

Chronic peritonitis is uncommon and is usually tuberculous in origin. People with tuberculous peritonitis do not have much pain or fever, and no other marked symptom except great emaciation, loss of strength, and often a collection of fluid in the abdominal cavity. All general measures used in treating people with tuberculosis of other parts of the body should be used with people who have tuberculous peritonitis. (See chapter 29 of this volume.)

What to Do

1. If acute peritonitis is suspected, make every possible effort to secure the services of a physician as soon as possible. No home treatments have enough value to be worth giving, and the condition may prove fatal if it does not receive expert attention promptly. Surgery will probably be needed.

2. Do not give the patient any medicine or any food or drink until he has been seen by the doctor.

RECTAL FISTULAS.
A rectal fistula is a narrow and often very crooked passage through the tissues from the rectal lumen to the skin surface. Fecal material oozes through this passage from time to time, soiling the clothing and giving rise to an unpleasant odor.

Ischiorectal abscesses are not the only causes of rectal fistulas—there are other less common causes—but whatever its cause, the condition is one that calls for careful surgery. Every vestige of the crooked fistulous tract must be operated on in such a way that the infection is adequately

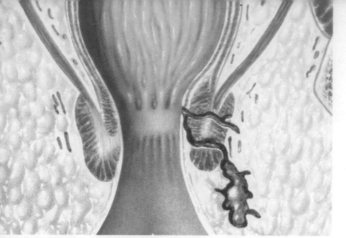

A common cause of rectal fistula is an ischiorectal abscess. Note fistulous tract leading from the abscess to the rectum.

drained, thus allowing the tissues to heal.

What to Do

1. Do not try any home treatment.
2. Consult a surgeon, preferably a proctologist.

RECTAL POLYP.

A rectal polyp is a small, rounded tumor, usually attached to the wall of the rectum by a short stalk or neck. Such tumors are rare in childhood and early adult life, but increasingly common later. Most rectal polyps do not cause symptoms aside from occasional minor bleeding. A small percentage of polyps are cancerous, however; and in consideration of this fact, it is best to have all rectal polyps removed.

What to Do

If you have passed your early adult years, have your physician do periodic rectal examinations, examining as high as he can with a sigmoidoscope. Such an examination can detect any rectal polyp that may be present; and removing one is a safe and simple procedure.

REGIONAL ENTERITIS (ILEITIS).

Regional enteritis is an inflammation of one or more loops of the small intestine, most commonly of that portion near its junction with the large intestine. The inflammation acts somewhat like a chronic, progressive, debilitating infection, though no specific germ has been found as its cause.

One or more segments of the intestine are affected, the intestinal walls becoming markedly thickened and infiltrated, and each affected segment tending to form a firm mass in the abdomen discernible to the touch. Between the inflamed segments the intestine may be quite normal. Fistulous tracts sometimes develop between the affected segments of the intestine and other abdominal structures or the body surface. Intestinal obstruction or perforation with localized abscesses may develop, making surgery necessary.

Among the characteristic symptoms are a mild diarrhea with pus and sometimes blood in the stools, a low-grade irregular fever, abdominal pain, anemia, and weight loss. The condition is better and worse by spells, but it often persists for several months, or even years. Complete recovery is uncommon without surgery, and even surgery does not prevent a recurrence.

What to Do

1. If the condition is suspected, consult a physician. X rays are usually needed for a correct diagnosis. The most effective remedies require a physician's prescription. Surgery may become necessary at any time.
2. Take a low-residue, non-roughage diet abundant in vitamins.
3. Follow every good health habit possible and thus build up your body's general resistance. Abundant sunshine, rest, and a mild climate are helpful.

SPRUE.

(See chapter 32 of this volume.)

TYPHOID FEVER.

(See chapter 28 of this volume.)

Bile Passages, Liver, and Pancreas

The Bile Passages

The bile passages include the gallbladder and the bile ducts. These passages, together with the liver and the pancreas, are really a part of the digestive system. They are considered here in a separate chapter because they are the seat of several characteristic diseases quite different from those of any other part of the system.

CANCER OF THE GALLBLADDER.

(See chapter 11 of this volume.)

GALLSTONES (CHOLELITHIASIS).

Gallstones may form in the tiny bile ducts of the liver, but only rarely. They usually form in the gallbladder as a sequel to infection or inflammation of the gallbladder wall. Flatulence is a common symptom.

A large proportion of all gallstones are partly or even largely composed of a solid, fatlike substance called cholesterol, found abundantly in many fats of animal origin but rarely in vegetable fats. This suggests that keeping the animal fats of the diet, including butter and egg yolks, low should help prevent the formation of gallstones. It is not certain, however, that this rule is important, because the body can manufacture cholesterol out of fats which do not contain it. The best dietary factor in preventing the formation of gallstones is to keep all fats low.

Gallstones may be present for years without causing symptoms. Some patients who have them never suffer pain, but most feel distress after eating, or a sense of fullness in the region of the liver. Others experience attacks of colic with these minor symptoms appearing between them. X-ray pictures taken after the administraton of certain dyes frequently show gallstones that can be detected in no other way.

A gallstone may be as small as a grain of sand or large enough to fill the entire gallbladder. The presence of these stones in the gallbladder may cause some pain, but this pain is never as severe as that caused by the passing of stones down the bile ducts to the intestine. Such pain is called gallstone colic and is usually extremely severe. With each paroxysm of pain the victim sweats profusely. The paroxysms last from a few seconds to a few minutes, and recur frequently for hours or days. Chills and fever may also accompany an attack of gallstone colic.

Medicines are of little use in treating people with gallstones except to relieve pain in case of colic. At present no medicine will dissolve gallstones

331

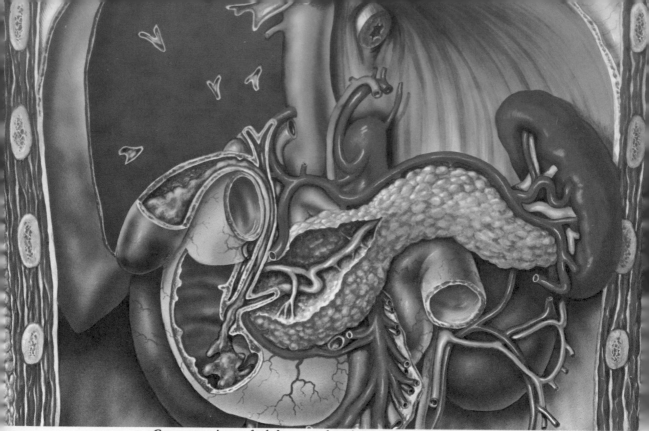

Cutaway view of abdomen, showing pancreas (yellow) and gallbladder (green). Note bile duct through which bile flows into
the duodenum. Gallstones sometimes pass through the bile duct,
causing severe pain.

inside the gallbladder or make them pass out of it, though comparatively small stones may pass out without any medication, causing colic when they do unless they are very small indeed. Recently, however, there has been some experimental work using large quantities of some of the bile salts in experimental diets where gallstones have been shown to decrease in size. Perhaps, someday in the future, medication or diet based on this experimental work may become practical.

What to Do

1. During an attack of what seems to be gallstone colic, keep the victim in bed.

2. Consult a doctor at once. He can give such treatment as is needed to control the pain and advise as to what further should be done. He will probably recommend an X ray of the gallbladder, which will be the best way to find out whether or not gallstones are present.

3. If gallstones are found, they should be surgically removed, and the gallbladder will usually be removed also to prevent further stone formation.

4. If surgery is not done, and if the person concerned is obese, he should go on a reducing diet. Whether he is obese or not, his diet should be kept low in fat of all kinds.

INFLAMMATION OF THE GALL-BLADDER (CHOLECYSTITIS).

Cholecystitis is an acute inflammation of the gallbladder. In the more severe and longer-persisting cases, the gallbladder may become filled with pus.

The onset of gallbladder inflammation is often sudden, with severe pain in the right upper region of the abdomen. There is a rapid pulse, fever, nausea, and vomiting. The abdominal wall may be rigid, and it is usually tender to pressure at or below the lower edge of the ribs on the right side. In a case with pus in the gallbladder there may be chills as well as fever.

Inflammation of the gallbladder may become chronic, in which case its symptoms are much like those of gallstones. (See above.) Careful study and special tests made by a physician are usually necessary to determine the real condition and to point out what should be done about it. Inflammation of the bile ducts (cholangitis) produces symptoms similar to those of inflammation of the gallbladder, and needs no further discussion here except to say that jaundice (see discussion on this item below) is much more likely to occur with this disorder than with cases of gallbladder inflammation.

What to Do

1. If acute inflammation of the gallbladder is suspected, do not attempt any home treatment.

2. Consult a physician at once, as the condition may rapidly develop into one that requires surgery.

OBSTRUCTIVE JAUNDICE.

Sometimes bile from the liver or the gallbladder is absorbed into the blood and circulates throughout the body, causing a yellow or greenish color of the skin, the mucous membranes, and the urine. It is most readily seen in the whites of the eyes. This staining of the skin or other tissues is what we call jaundice. It is often accompanied by rather severe itching.

Obstructive jaundice is not a disease of itself, but an indication of an obstruction to the outflow of bile from the liver or the gallbladder. The obstruction may be a gallstone lodged in a bile duct, especially the common bile duct. A tumor of the pancreas or cancer or inflammation of the bile ducts or of structures around them may cause obstruction. The resulting jaundice needs to be distinguished from jaundice caused by an inflammation of the liver substance or that caused by too rapid disintegration of the red cells in the bloodstream. Those two serious types of jaundice are not the result of obstruction of any sort.

Because of the variety of possible underlying factors and the seriousness of some of them, the appearance of jaundice is a signal for a thorough medical examination, an X ray of the gallbladder, and other tests to determine the location and nature of the obstruction, if obstruction is the cause of the jaundice. If it is not, still it is important to find out the cause of the jaundice.

An operation to remove gallstones usually includes removal of the patient's gallbladder also.

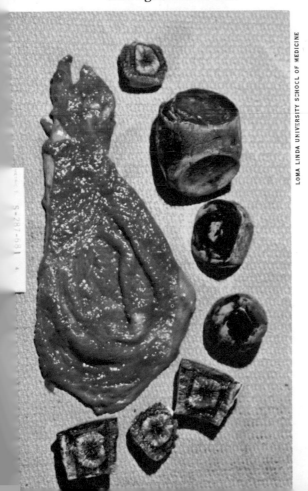

LOMA LINDA UNIVERSITY SCHOOL OF MEDICINE

What to Do

1. Do not attempt home treatment. No treatment will be likely to do good unless it is directed at the cause, and the cause must first be determined.

2. Consult a physician at the first appearance of what appears to be jaundice. His services and recommendations will be needed to determine the cause of the jaundice and to guide in the treatment.

3. In any case, free drinking of water is useful. It will help flush the bile from the blood through the urine.

4. Itching should be treated the same as itching from any other cause. (See *Pruritus* in chapter 12 in this volume.)

The Liver

ACUTE YELLOW ATROPHY OF THE LIVER.

This is not a separate disease, but an occasional terminal stage or complication of several liver diseases. It often begins with symptoms similar to those of viral hepatitis. It may occur following glue sniffing or exposure to carbon tetrachloride or insecticides. Jaundice develops rapidly or, if previously present, deepens rapidly. There is marked tenderness over the liver, which is enlarged at first but shrinks rapidly. At first the pulse is slow, but later both it and the breathing become rapid. The victim develops tendencies to hemorrhages, and is likely to be comatose or lethargic and to have tremors, rigidity, or convulsions. Kidney activity may entirely cease. There is a high mortality rate when this serious complication develops.

What to Do

In most cases, the victim will already be under a physician's care; but if suspicious symptoms appear while no doctor is present, call one at once.

AMEBIC LIVER ABSCESS.

This disease is a direct result of amebic dysentery, though not nearly all victims of amebic dysentery develop liver abscesses. (See chapter 21 of this volume.) A single large abscess is produced as a rule, destroying much liver tissue, sometimes so much that the liver becomes little more than a large sac filled with pus. The victim may have irregular fever, with drenching sweats and much prostration, or the abscess may produce but few symptoms, especially if it is not large. Sometimes the abscess ruptures into a lung, resulting in sudden coughing up of a large amount of somewhat thin, brownish pus. Surgical drainage of the pus is sometimes advisable; however, if there are several abscesses rather than only one, drainage is not likely to be practicable.

What to Do

If the victim is not already under a physician's supervision on account of the amebic infection, consult one as soon as any symptoms appear that suggest a liver abscess may be forming. Do not wait to try any home treatment.

CIRRHOSIS OF THE LIVER.

Cirrhosis is a hardening of the liver because of an increase in the fibrous tissue and a degeneration of the active liver cells. Certain conditions of malnutrition seem to cause it, also certain poisons. Considerable evidence indicates that alcohol is one of them, but there are many others. The poisons of infectious diseases may cause special types of liver cirrhosis. This is so outstandingly true of syphilis that syphilitic cirrhosis is considered as a distinct disease, though rare. It causes a peculiar nodular condition of the organ called *hepar lobatum*.

Cirrhosis of the liver is slow and gradual in its development. It is usually well advanced before its symptoms are noticeable enough to cause alarm. Weakness and loss of weight may be early symptoms.

Chronic disturbances of digestion usually develop. The liver may be either enlarged, normal, or even small in size. If enlarged, it is usually a general enlargement, leaving the organ with a smooth surface. The digestive disturbances may begin with a poor appetite, but they are likely to go on to indigestion, pain in the upper right quarter of the abdomen, and occasional vomiting of bloody material.

There are two general types of liver cirrhosis.

In one, obstruction of the portal vein occurs, resulting in a collection of fluid in the abdomen and dropsy (swelling) of the lower limbs. This type is the more common, and usually occurs in the middle-aged.

In the other type, there has been a previous inflammation of the liver tissue, and for this or other reasons the small bile ducts are obstructed, causing jaundice. This type usually occurs in younger people. The liver tends to be enlarged and smooth, there is no collection of fluid in the abdomen, and the other symptoms are more mild than in cases caused by osbstruction of the portal vein.

Either type of cirrhosis may run a course of several years. Large veins are often seen over the abdomen, especially in the region of the navel and across the body near the diaphragm. There are also enlarged veins in the rectum (hemorrhoids), the intestines, the stomach, and the esophagus, though their presence may remain unknown because they cannot be seen. Death from liver cirrhosis not infrequently happens as a result of a hemorrhage caused by the rupture of enlarged veins about the lower end of the esophagus.

Cirrhosis of the liver used to be considered an incurable disease, but with modern methods of treatment life may be considerably prolonged in most cases, and the progress of the condition may be permanently checked in many. This is particularly fortunate in view of the apparently growing incidence of the disease.

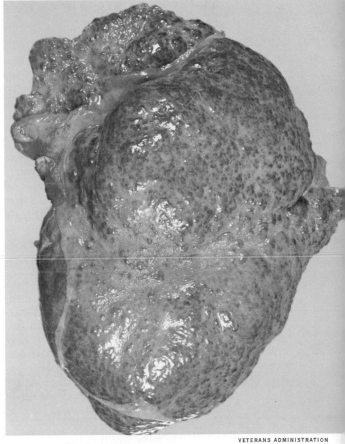

VETERANS ADMINISTRATION

Cirrhosis of the liver.

What to Do

1. If you suspect cirrhosis of the liver, consult a physician. His services will be necessary for an accurate diagnosis and, if the condition is present, in treating it.

2. The diet should be adequate and varied, but easily digestible and containing no flesh food, tea, coffee, or spices.

3. No alcoholic beverages are allowable.

4. Bed rest is advisable most of the time.

5. Blood transfusions may be necessary.

6. A low-salt diet or other medical management may control the collection of fluid in the abdomen and the lower limbs, but the fluid in the

abdomen may need to be removed by tapping.

FATTY LIVER.

Some cases of fatty liver do not cause symptoms definite enough to arouse a suspicion of the condition. In other cases—chiefly those in which the main cause is overindulgence in alcoholic beverages—there may be jaundice and a collection of fluid in the abdomen. Many of the symptoms are similar to those of portal cirrhosis of the liver, and they may be due to other causes. In fact, it is probable that factors which would lead to fibrous degeneration of the liver in one person would lead to fatty degeneration in another.

What to Do

1. If the condition is suspected, consult a physician to help determine the true nature of the illness.

2. If the physician decides that there is fatty degeneration of the liver, avoid all use of alcoholic beverages and take a diet similar to that recommended for a case of cirrhosis of the liver. (See previous item.)

LIVER ABSCESS.

Abscesses of the liver may occur when pus-producing germs have found their way into the bloodstream and caused general septic poisoning (pyemia), usually with abscesses in other parts of the body as well as the liver.

The outstanding symptoms are severe chills and a high fever followed by a drenching sweat which lowers the temperature. The victim is severely ill, and the outlook is grave. If only one abscess is present, it may be opened and drained; but the abscesses are usually multiple, which makes successful surgery impossible.

What to Do

The victim will usually already be under a physician's care on account of other manifestations of the infection. If a doctor is not actually present when symptoms suspicious of a liver abscess are noticed, consult one at once, as this is a very dangerous condition.

VIRAL HEPATITIS.

The term viral hepatitis is used to include two similar diseases caused by separate types of virus and typically transmitted by different means. These are designated as hepatitis type A and hepatitis type B.

1. *Hepatitis type A* (previously called *infectious hepatitis*). This type of hepatitis is more common among children and young adults than in older persons. The virus is usually transmitted by person-to-person contact, especially among those living under crowded conditions with poor hygiene. The virus can be transmitted by contaminated food or water. The symptoms of the illness begin from between two and six weeks after the virus was transmitted to the individual. The onset of symptoms is usually abrupt, and the duration of the illness is about six to eight weeks— shorter than the duration for hepatitis type B. Hepatitis type A is seldom associated with serious complications, there being a mortality rate of only about 0.1 percent. Hepatitis type A can be prevented or at least modified by the administration of immune serum globulin even after contacts have been made with persons ill with the disease. The protection afforded by the use of immune serum globulin lasts up to six months.

2. *Hepatitis type B* (previously called *serum hepatitis*). Hepatitis type B typically affects young adults, but it may affect older persons also. It seldom affects children. The virus for this type of hepatitis is usually transmitted by accidental injection by some contaminated instrument such as a hypodermic needle (as used in drug abuse), a tattooing needle, the instrument for piercing earlobes, or by blood transfusion. The "incubation period" (time lapse between transmission of the virus and the onset of

symptoms) is a long period of four to twenty weeks. The onset of the symptoms is usually gradual. The duration of the illness is three to four months. This is a more serious illness than that of hepatitis type A. Serious complications occur in 5 to 10 percent of cases, and these usually involve serious damage to the liver. The mortality rate for hepatitis type B is between 1 and 10 percent, usually not exceeding 2 percent. Hepatitis type B cannot be prevented by the administration of immune serum globulin. However, progress is being made by medical scientists in the development of a protective vaccine.

Course of the illness. For both types of viral hepatitis, the course of the illness may be described as having three phases: a prodromal phase, an icteric phase, and a recovery phase. In the prodromal phase the individual becomes ill with symptoms similar to those of influenza—malaise, loss of appetite, nausea, and fatigue. The prodromal phase is soon followed by the icteric phase in which there are evidences of temporary involvement of the liver, with the functions of the liver becoming abnormal. This evidence consists of jaundice (yellow coloring of the skin and whites of the eyes), dark-colored urine, and light-colored stools. The intensity of the jaundice reaches its maximum in seven to fourteen days, and thereafter it subsides progressively. During the phase of recovery, the symptoms and the jaundice gradually disappear. The patient is usually quite comfortable during this phase, but it is important that he not engage in any kind of strenuous activities lest there be a relapse of his illness.

What to Do

1. **Viral hepatitis should be taken seriously. If the patient is not already under the care of a physician, he should be as soon as the nature of the illness is recognized.**

2. **During the course of the illness the physician will arrange for re-** peated tests of the liver's function. The information provided by these tests will enable the physician to judge the seriousness of this particular case so that he can modify his treatment accordingly.

3. **Rest throughout the period of illness is the most important item in the treatment of viral hepatitis. The patient's strength and vitality should be definitely conserved.**

4. **The patient with viral hepatitis typically has a poor appetite. It is important, however, for adequate nourishment to be maintained throughout the period of his illness. In some cases, it is necessary to supplement his diet by the intravenous feeding of glucose.**

5. **Surgical procedures during the period of illness with viral hepatitis should be avoided as far as possible. The effects of an anesthetic can be damaging to the liver during this time when the liver's function is already reduced.**

6. **The condition of jaundice usually causes the skin to itch. This itching may be somewhat relieved by the use of frequent alkaline baths or by the application to the skin of calamine lotion.**

7. **It is important that the patient recovering from viral hepatitis be restrained from resuming his normal activities too soon.**

The Pancreas

ACUTE PANCREATITIS.

Acute pancreatitis is an inflammation of the pancreas usually resulting from the irritation or destruction of tissue in the organ by pancreatic juice which has been prevented from flowing out through the duct on its way to the intestine. It is rarely caused by infection.

The attack begins suddenly, with nausea, vomiting, and intense pain in the upper abdomen, usually radiating to the back. The victim will be prostrated and sweating profusely. Abdominal tenderness and distention will develop soon. The condition may resemble gallstone colic, intestinal obstruction, or perforated ulcer of the stomach or duodenum. Symptoms of shock frequently develop.

What to Do

There should be no delay in consulting a physician, because the condition is not only very distressing but very dangerous. It may need a physician's careful study to determine its true nature. Surgery may be needed, and, if so, it must be done early to be successful.

CANCER OF THE PANCREAS.
(See chapter 11 of this volume.)

CHRONIC PANCREATITIS.
Chronic inflammation of the pancreas may be caused by alcoholism, syphilis, tuberculosis, gallstones, pancreatic stones, cancer of the pancreas, or ulcer of the stomach or duodenum. The disease is characterized by increasing emaciation, general debility, fatty and foul-smelling stools, pain similar to that caused by gallstone colic or duodenal ulcer, and chronic indigestion that is made worse by eating fats or meats.

This condition tends to relapse again and again, with either symptom-free intervals or times with only mild symptoms between attacks. Each attack will be marked by a spell of nausea and vomiting, with upper abdominal pain radiating to the back, some fever, a rapid pulse, and abdominal tenderness. Since it is a companion or complication of any one of several other conditions, it may not be recognized as a separate condition; and its treatment is usually not separate from the treatment for some other condition.

What to Do

If chronic pancreatitis is suspected, have a physician study the case to find out its true nature. He will outline a proper diet and help in correcting such causative conditons as can be corrected. Do not attempt any course of home treatments.

DIABETES MELLITUS.
(See chapter 20 of this volume.)

Nutritional Diseases

It should be clear to everybody that too little food will result in starvation and that in most cases too much food will cause obesity, and also that both of these conditions are menaces to health. It is still a matter of argument as to whether or not obesity should be called a disease. In this book we shall consider it as such, because it paves the way for many other more serious diseases and because even without any other disease it often causes discomfort and reduces physical efficiency.

Nearly all nutritional diseases, however, are deficiency diseases—not necessarily from a limited total quantity of food, but from a shortage of certain food constituents, usually vitamins, sometimes minerals, occasionally proteins. On the other hand, a harmful excess of either minerals or vitamins, though uncommon, could cause nutritional disorders. For instance, large doses of vitamin D sometimes prescribed in medical treatment have in some cases seriously upset calcium metabolism in the body. Excessive vitamin A has also proved harmful.

Vitamin deficiency diseases are collectively called avitaminoses. Discussions of avitaminoses will comprise the bulk of this chapter, but a few other diseases with a nutritional basis will be included. Then, in the latter half of the chapter, problems and diseases of metabolism will be discussed, the term metabolism including the several processes by which the body assimilates nutrients.

Avitaminoses

VITAMIN A DEFICIENCY.

A mild deficiency of vitamin A tends to produce roughness and dryness of the skin. A greater degree of deficiency increases this tendency and causes damage to the epithelial tissues of the body, which become more susceptible to infection. In later stages, severe infections of the mouth, the genitourinary tract, the respiratory organs, and the eyes are likely to occur. The eye infection often develops into, or in connection with, a serious condition called xerophthalmia, which may lead to blindness. Another common effect on the eyes is a loss of ability to see in dim light, a condition called night blindness.

What to Do

1. Include more vitamin A in the diet. It may be convenient to take some oil rich in vitamin A, such as cod-liver oil or halibut-liver oil. Vitamin A is also available in purified form and may be taken as such.

2. It is best to consult a physician,

339

especially if eye symptoms are troublesome. He can advise as to what to take, how much, and how long to continue the treatment; and he can give, or arrange for giving, such special treatments as the eyes may need.

VITAMIN B DEFICIENCIES.

The so-called vitamin B complex consists of four separate vitamins: thiamine (vitamin B1), riboflavin (vitamin B2), niacin or nicotinic acid, and vitamin B12. Likewise, there are four separate nutritional problems in this area, each associated with a deficiency of one of these vitamins. There are two other B vitamins, folic acid and pyrodoxine, each with its associated nutritional problems.

A. *Thiamine (Vitamin B1) Deficiency.* The disease beriberi is the most common manifestation of serious thiamine deficiency. It is characterized by an inflammation and degeneration of nerve trunks, producing disturbances of both motion and sensation. There is loss of appetite. The patient becomes weak, especially in the legs. His muscles tend to waste away. Partial paralysis and a tendency to dropsy are common. The nerves controlling the heart action may be badly affected, and heart failure and sudden death may result.

Beriberi occurs most frequently among people whose diet consists mostly of polished rice, but anybody who lives chiefly on highly refined starchy or sugary foods may get it. It may develop in infants, especially those nursed by mothers who have the disease. If the disease is not far advanced, correction of diet usually will bring about rapid and complete recovery. If the neuritis has continued until the nerve trunks have degenerated, however, normal motion, sensation, and heart action can never be restored.

Wernicke's syndrome is also a condition caused by a deficiency of thiamine. It occurs most commonly among heavy users of alcohol. It is characterized by a clouded mental state, weakness of the muscles which move the eyes, unsteadiness, and deterioration of many of the nerves (peripheral neuritis).

What to Do

Correct the diet. No other remedy or treatment can do much good. Thiamine abounds in the outer layers of the grains of rice, wheat, and other cereals. Fresh milk, eggs, brewer's yeast, concentrated yeast extracts, and malt extract also contain generous amounts of thiamine. Fresh fruits and vegetables are helpful. Among flesh foods, liver is best.

B. *Riboflavin (Vitamin B2) Deficiency.* Riboflavin deficiency is likely to cause visual disturbances, eye pain in bright light, an overflow of tears, and redness of the eyes. Perhaps the commonest signs are wrinkling, moistness, and fissures of the skin at the angles of the mouth. The tongue tends to be unnaturally red. Loss of weight and vigor are common. B2 deficiency is often associated with B1 deficiency, giving a somewhat confusing picture. When either deficiency seems to be present, look for signs of the other.

What to Do

1. See that the diet contains adequate milk each day, and plenty of eggs and green vegetables.

2. In severe cases consult a physician. He will probably prescribe tablets of riboflavin, to be taken daily throughout the period of treatment.

Fresh fruits and vegetables, along with grains, nuts, and other natural foods, taken regularly and in moderate, balanced amounts, provide the surest safegaurd against nutritional diseases.

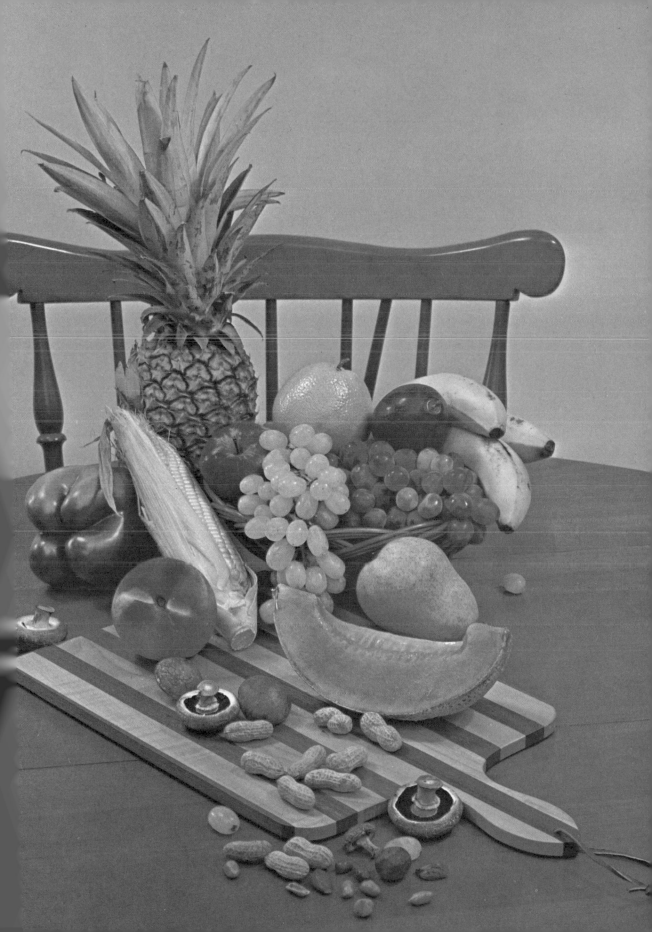

C. *Niacin Deficiency (Pellagra).*
One characteristic sign of pellagra is a peculiar skin eruption. The eruption looks much like a bad case of sunburn, with considerable cracking, crusting, and scaling, and occasionally some small blisters. It usually appears on the exposed areas of the skin, such as the backs of the hands and wrists, the face, and the neck, less frequently on the legs and ankles, and occasionally on the external genitals. The upper edge of the eruption usually has a well-defined border, giving rise to the descriptive term "glove-like" when it occurs on the hands and wrists. Exposure of the skin to sunlight is believed to stimulate the appearance of the eruption.

People with pellagra usually have capricious appetites and frequently digestive disturbances. Diarrhea is common. A victim's tongue usually looks abnormally smooth and deep red. Patients are often addicted to alcohol, and about one in fifty of them will probably eventually have mental disturbances severe enough to amount to true dementia. Many of them are troubled with such nervous symptoms as weakness, dizziness, insomnia, and disturbances of the sense of touch.

A correct diet will cure most cases of pellagra, but a pellagrin who continues to drink alcoholic liquor will be hard to cure. The cure is usually complete, except in those cases that have resulted in insanity; and even in them the mental condition is often much improved.

What to Do

1. In the acute stage of the disease there should be bed rest. The diet should consist of milk, vegetable purees, tomato juice, and softboiled or poached eggs. Yeast extract broths can be given with benefit.

2. If diarrhea is troublesome, give a teaspoonful of bismuth subcarbonate in water every three or four hours.

342

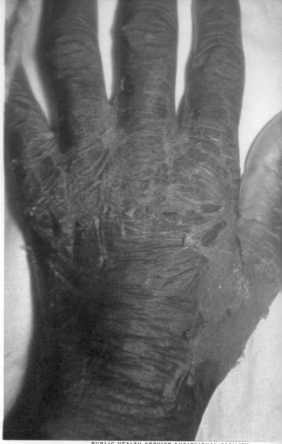

Pellagra characteristically causes eruptions on the skin similar in appearance to those caused by burns.

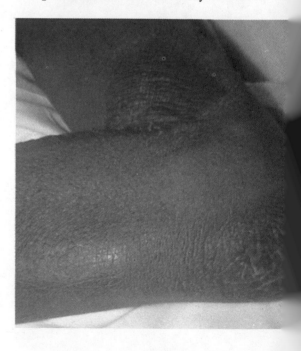

3. Lanolin to which 5 percent of boric acid powder has been added will help soothe the skin eruption.

4. When the acute stage of the disease is past, the chief remedy is still the diet. It should include a quart of milk a day and plenty of eggs and green leafy vegetables. Lean meat is allowable, but fat meat is valueless. The milk may be fresh, dried, canned, or buttermilk. Brewers' yeast or some concentrated yeast extract will prove helpful.

The following foods are all low in or almost devoid of niacin: corn and all products made from it, molasses, potatoes, carrots, yellow turnips, rice, ripe onions, most animal fats, cotton-seed oil, and gelatin. In parts of the country where people live wholly or chiefly on foods in this list, pellagra is common.

5. Alcoholic beverages should be left alone.

6. In severe cases the services of a physician are advisable. He will probably prescribe appropriate doses of niacinamide to be taken by mouth.

D. *Vitamin B*$_{12}$ *Deficiency.* When the body's tissues do not receive their necessary quota of Vitamin B$_{12}$, pernicious anemia (macrocytic anemia) develops. The deficiency is most frequently caused by a failure of absorption of this vitamin from the digestive organs. This condition is explained at greater length with recommendations for treatment in chapter 10 of this volume under "Blood Diseases, Anemia, B. Macrocytic Anemia."

E. *Folic Acid Deficiency (Megaloblastic Anemia of Infancy and of Pregnancy).* Folic acid, one of the group of B vitamins, is an important and widely distributed vitamin which occurs abundantly in many vegetables. Long-continued cooking of food is progressively destructive to folic acid.

Deficiency of folic acid occurs commonly among persons who are malnourished and produces a form of anemia very similar to pernicious anemia. (See the discussion of macrocytic anemias in chapter 10 of this volume.) The megaloblastic anemia resulting from a deficiency of folic acid is most likely to occur under conditions in which the body requirement for folic acid is greater than usual: in infancy and during pregnancy.

The megaloblastic anemia of infancy typically occurs between five and eleven months of age, a period of rapid growth. Infants who were born prematurely and those who have had repeated infections of the gastrointestinal organs are particularly susceptible. The condition may be easily confused with that caused by a deficiency of vitamin B$_{12}$. It is important to avoid such confusion, for the cure of this condition depends specifically on the administration of folic acid.

Megaloblastic anemia of pregnancy (pernicious anemia of pregnancy) appears in about one percent of pregnancies during the last three months, at a time when the personal requirements for folic acid are increased because of the rapid growth of the unborn child.

What to Do

The administration of tablets of folic acid, under a physician's direction, brings about a dramatic cure in almost all cases.

F. *Pyridoxine (Vitamin B*$_6$*) Deficiency.* Pyridoxine is another member of the vitamin B group. Symptoms of this deficiency are particularly important in infancy and early childhood, when they consist of convulsions. They develop in infants who have received formulas in which the milk or the cereal has been "over processed," prolonged processing having depleted the vitamin.

What to Do

There is an adequate quantity of pyridoxine in human milk, also in

343

cow's milk and in cereals if these latter are not overprocessed.

For the immediate treatment of convulsions due to a deficiency, an intramuscular injection of pyridoxine gives prompt relief. For infants who seem to be in danger of this deficiency, the physician will arrange for small doses of the vitamin to be added to the diet.

VITAMIN C DEFICIENCY (SCURVY).

A person with scurvy tends to become weak and anemic, to have spongy gums and loosening teeth, and to be subject to hemorrhages, especially about the joints and beneath the skin. The joint hemorrhages cause severe pain and sometimes lead to a mistaken diagnosis of arthritis or rheumatism. The spongy gums may bleed easily, become ulcerated, or become the seat of infection. In case the patient suffers a wound, the wound heals slowly.

A baby that is developing scurvy will be pale and stop gaining weight. The slightest bruise of its skin will result in a black-and-blue spot. Its gums will not make much trouble until the teeth begin to come through. The pain and swelling of the joints will likely cause the child to be irritable and to cry a great deal.

In scurvy, either in babies or in older people, correction of the diet brings about almost miraculous improvement. Pain may disappear within a day or two, and all other symptoms within a week or two. The same diet that will cure scurvy will prevent it. A person who takes a properly balanced diet will never have this disease.

What to Do

1. For the prevention of scurvy in a young child, give four ounces of orange juice per day or twelve ounces of tomato juice. Fruits and green vegetables should be added to the baby's diet as soon as the baby can take them.

2. For an older child or an adult, be sure there are plenty of green vegetables and fruit in the diet. Additional fruit juice may be helpful. Some very good sources of vitamin C are citrus fruits, strawberries, cantaloupes, tomatoes, green peppers, and raw cabbage (especially green cabbage).

3. For the treatment of a frank case of scurvy in either a child or an adult, the administration of ascorbic acid (vitamin C) by mouth may be used in the amounts prescribed by the physician.

VITAMIN D DEFICIENCY (OSTEOMALACIA, RICKETS).

Rickets develops almost exclusively among young children, though its effects may persist throughout life. Osteomalacia is a similar condition sometimes seen in adults. Rickets is most common between the ages of six months and eighteen months. It can be caused by a deficiency of calcium, phosphorus, or vitamin D in the diet. The vitamin D deficiency, however, is more common than the mineral deficiency. Calcium and phosphorus are the chief mineral elements in the framework of the body. Vitamin D is necessary for the work of building these elements into bones and teeth, and vitamin C helps it in this work.

The earliest symptoms of rickets are restlessness, irritability, and sweating of the head. Then the joints between bone and cartilage at the front end of the ribs begin to enlarge, forming two rows of hard nodules, one row beginning a short distance from each side of the upper end of the breastbone and running obliquely downward and sideways to the lower border of the ribs. These nodules can be easily seen in thin children with rickets, and they may be felt in those who appear to be well nourished.

The child's head gradually takes on a somewhat square shape. The fontanels, or "soft spots," in the top of the skull may remain open long after they should be closed. The bones that form the wrist joints, and often other joints, are softer and larger than they should be. The child with rickets is frequently bowlegged, though sometimes knock-kneed, and becomes even more so when he begins to walk. His abdomen may protrude markedly and his bowels be constipated. If his blood is tested, it will be found below normal in phosphorus or in calcium, but not necessarily in both. X rays of the joints of his limbs will show a characteristic lack of development near the ends of his long bones. Pelvic deformity due to rickets in a girl may persist until mature years, making normal childbirth difficult.

Since skeletal deformity resulting from advanced rickets is in so many cases an incurable condition, prevention is of prime importance. If it is not entirely prevented, but detected early, however, a satisfactory cure is not difficult. It is usually easy to obtain a diet containing sufficient calcium and phosphorus, especially if an ample quantity of milk is available. Milk is a good source of calcium, contains a considerable amount of phosphorus, and is a good source of vitamin D if whole milk is used, especially if the cows giving the milk spend a large part of their time out in the sunshine. Egg yolks also furnish good amounts of both phosphorus and vitamin D.

What to Do

1. Give a child who shows any signs of possible rickets at least a quart of whole milk a day. Milk fortified with vitamin D is now common.

2. From the age of five or six months onward, one egg yolk a day will be helpful.

3. Daily sunbaths are also helpful. (See discussion on this item in volume 3, chapter 20.) Exposure to sunlight, within reasonable limits, causes the skin to produce a certain amount of vitamin D.

4. Give the child cod-liver oil or some other good source of vitamin D. Begin at three or four weeks of age, giving half a teaspoonful twice a day, and increase gradually to one and a half teaspoonfuls twice a day at the age of three or four months and thereafter. A few drops of halibut-liver oil or of viosterol may be used instead of cod-liver oil, and this is better for babies who tend to be fat. It is well also to see that the baby's diet is not short of vitamin C. (See previous item.)

5. Properly graduated quartz-light treatments may take the place of sunbaths.

VITAMIN E DEFICIENCY.

Vitamin E is apparently conducive to health in several rather indefinite ways, but whether or not a deficiency of it will cause disease in human beings has not yet been conclusively proved. Furthermore, almost any otherwise well-balanced diet will contain sufficient vitamin E.

Two manifestations of rickets in a malnourished child are bowed legs and wrist joints larger than normal.

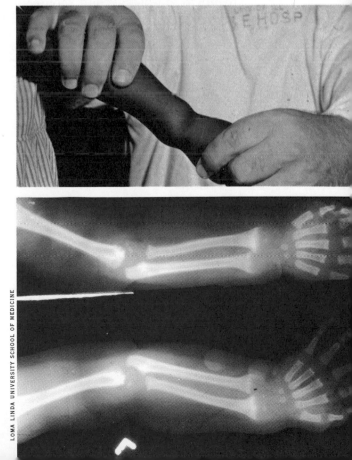

VITAMIN K DEFICIENCY.

Vitamin K occurs in sufficient abundance in most green leafy vegetables to make any serious deficiency of this vitamin rather uncommon. When an insufficient amount of it is eaten or absorbed, however, an increased tendency to hemorrhage develops; and laboratory studies have shown that this tendency is associated with a lessened amount of prothrombin in the blood. Hemorrhages due to this condition can often be prevented or checked by injections of vitamin K.

Vitamin K deficiency exists most commonly in newborn infants or in people with jaundice and whose intestinal absorption of digested food is poor. Attention to the diet is usually not enough to correct such a condition in people past infancy because dietary deficiency is rarely the sole cause. Ensuring that a prospective mother's diet contains an abundance of vitamin K is the best way to prevent a deficiency of this vitamin in her newborn baby. If her diet is inadequate in this respect, she should have injections of vitamin K during the last month or two of her pregnancy.

What to Do

If a newborn baby shows tendencies to hemorrhage, have a physician take charge of the case immediately. There may be other reasons for the tendency, but injections of vitamin K may prove to be the most helpful remedy.

MEGAVITAMIN THERAPY.

There has developed a popular sentiment regarding the use of vitamin preparations taken by mouth which applies the adage, If a little is good, more is better. But there is danger in following this sentiment.

A normally well-balanced diet contains all the vitamins that a person needs. It does no harm, however, to take one tablet a day of some reliable brand of a multivitamin preparation. Beyond this, the only justification for taking supplementary vitamin preparations is in the treatment of one of the vitamin deficiency diseases as mentioned in the preceding pages. The editor of the *Journal of the American Medical Association* quoted a recognized nutritionist as follows: "The use of massive-dose vitamin therapy appears to be without rational basis and may often be harmful." (JAMA, September 30, 1974, page 1850.)

Other Nutritional Diseases

NONTOXIC GOITER.

(See chapter 26 of this volume.)

NUTRITIONAL EDEMA (FAMINE EDEMA, WAR EDEMA).

Nutritional edema results from long-continued deprivation of protein that is biologically complete. It usually occurs in famine areas. The first step in its development is a general weight loss. Later there is water retention, which appears to check the loss of weight but leads to a pitting edema, appearing first in the legs but later spreading upward and sometimes involving the entire body.

A variety of nutritional edema fairly prevalent among babies and young children in parts of Africa, Asia, southern Europe, and Central and South America, where low protein foods are fed and milk is not available, has been called kwashiorkor. In this disease the liver is enlarged and the pancreatic tissue more or less degenerated. In addition to showing edema, the young victims do not grow well and are irritable and apathetic. Their appetite is poor, and they are troubled with vomiting and diarrhea. They are likely to have skin rashes, irregularity of pigmentation of skin and hair, and ulceration or inflammation about the mouth and eyes. If not treated early and properly, more than half of the victims of kwashiorkor die.

What to Do

Provide an abundant diet, otherwise well-balanced, but containing an abundance of protein, a considerable proportion of which should ordinarily come from nonvegetable sources. The amount needed to cure an adult who has developed nutritional edema is from 120 to 150 grams per day. For babies and young children, the most important dietary treatment is to give an

Having problems with overweight? There's hope. The solution generally lies in control of the appetite. This man lost 181 pounds in one year.

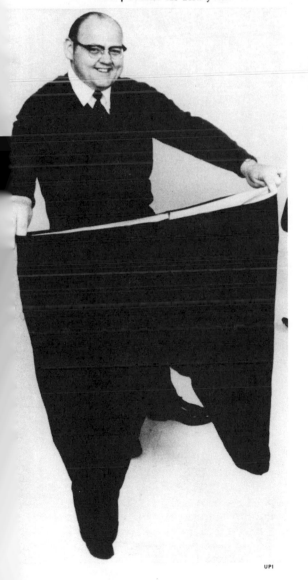

UPI

abundance of milk and eggs.

Since the disease usually attacks poor people, the expense of providing suitable dietary protein may be an obstacle to effective treatment. In some places a mixture of vegetable proteins has worked well. This should be easier where soybeans are grown or otherwise available, because soybeans are the best known vegetable source of complete protein.

OBESITY.

Obesity is nearly always due to overeating. There are a few cases—usually in childhood or early youth—in which glandular imbalance plays an important part. Obesity is objectionable chiefly because it is apparently a prelude to many cases of diabetes and heart disease. It makes arthritis of the hips and knees worse because of the abnormally great pressure it puts on the joints and articular cartilages. Different people may have other reasons for not wanting to be overweight, but very few have anything reasonable to say in its favor.

What to Do

1. If there is any question about the cause of the obesity, have a physician study the case.

2. If it is clear that overeating is the chief or only cause, reduce the weight to normal. (See volume 1, chapter 51.)

PERNICIOUS ANEMIA.
(See chapter 10 of this volume.)

SPRUE.
(See chapter 32 of this volume.)

Inborn Errors of Metabolism

A person's characteristics are determined in part by heredity and in part by environment. Heredity gives the individual his start in life and determines physical and mental traits which provide the gross outline of his body and of his personality. The influence of environment is then superimposed on that of heredity to fill in the details.

With respect to disease, there is considerable variation in the relative importance of heredity and environment. In some diseases the influence of heredity seems to be the main factor, with environment playing the minor role. In others environment plays the major role, with the influence of heredity serving only to make the person more or less susceptible to the disease. Under this subhead, "Inborn Errors of Metabolism," we deal with certain faults of metabolism caused essentially by unique heredity rather than by what may have happened to the person since his birth.

DISORDERS IN PIGMENT METABOLISM (PORPHYRIA).

The outstanding example here is the disease porphyria, in which there is a disturbance of the metabolic process by which the body uses the chemical substance known as porphyrin to help build its hemoglobin and some of its other pigments and enzymes. Heredity is blamed for most cases of porphyria. There are various forms of the disease, all resulting in an excess of porphyrin compounds in the urine.

In some forms of this disease there is a sensitivity of the skin to sunlight or to artificial ultraviolet light, with resulting skin lesions and abnormal pigmentation. In one form the patient shows symptoms of abdominal pain, vomiting, and constipation, together with paralysis of certain of the muscles. Acute attacks are usually brought on by the use of alcohol, by certain drugs, or by infections.

The treatment consists largely of avoiding alcohol and drugs and of protecting the skin from sunlight.

DISORDERS IN PROTEIN METABOLISM (PHENYLKETONURIA).

(See also *Phenylketonuria* in chapter 25 of this volume.)

Here the example is the disease phenylketonuria, the cause of which is hereditary. The laws of some states now require that tests be made on the blood of newborn infants as a means of detecting this disease in time to prevent its tragic complications. The problem occurs in about one child out of every 15,000.

The disease is caused by the lack of an enzyme necessary to the proper synthesis of tyrosine (one of the amino acids) within the body. As a result, phenylalanine (a precursor of tyrosine) accumulates within the body's tissues and fluids and flows over into the urine. The complications of the full-blown disease include damage to the patient's brain with resulting abnormal movements and mental retardation.

The treatment, which is quite effective, consists of arranging a diet which contains a minimum of phenylalanine. Obviously, a child with this disease must be under the care of a physician.

DISORDERS IN CARBOHYDRATE METABOLISM.

In this category there are two important hereditary diseases. First is galactosemia. In this disease the infant's body is unable to convert one form of carbohydrate into another (galactose to glucose) because of the absence of the necessary enzyme. An infant with this disease appears normal at birth but after a few days develops difficulty in feeding and begins to vomit. If the disease goes untreated, failure in growth and eventual death from malnutrition will result. Treatment is relatively simple, consisting merely of eliminating from the diet all galactose-containing foods. This means that milk and milk products are strictly forbidden. Even though the patient is still an infant, it will do very well on a properly designed diet which provides all the nutritional essentials by foods other than milk.

The second disease is glycogen storage disease. It is usually fatal within the first year or two of life, for it involves an inability to convert glucose to glycogen (two forms of carbohydrate) and vice versa, with the result that excesses of glycogen become deposited in various tissues of the body. Symptoms are fatigability and hypoglycemia (low blood sugar) with resulting shock and convulsions. In some cases the hypoglycemia can be combated by frequent feedings. If the patient survives the period of early childhood, his condition may gradually improve.

DISORDERS IN LIPID (FAT) METABOLISM.

In hereditary disorders of lipid metabolism some patients suffer from an increase in the amount of lipids in the body fluids and tissues, and others from a decrease. Perhaps the most notable disease in this group is essential hypercholesteremia (xanthomatosis). Here the amount of cholesterol is increased more than the other lipds that normally occur in the body, the amount in the blood serum being perhaps two or three times normal. Swellings produced by accumulations of cholesterol-laden cells (foam cells) occur in the skin (xanthomas); in the subcutaneous areas at pressure points such as knees, elbows, and buttocks; in the heart; and in certain tendons. Conditions such as arteriosclerosis and coronary artery disease, which are associated with an increase in cholesterol, are, of course, more frequent than usual in cases of essential hypercholesteremia.

These cases are benefited by instituting measures which tend to lower the concentration of cholesterol in the blood serum. Of first importance is a diet regimen which excludes the sources of saturated fatty acids such as meat, dairy products, eggs, and the common cooking fats. In their stead the patient may use vegetables and unsaturated fats such as corn oil. In extreme cases the physician may prescribe one of the cholesterol-lowering drugs.

DISORDERS IN KIDNEY TRANSPORT.

Among the numerous functions which the kidneys have to perform is the recovery from the "glomerular filtrate" of the chemical substances needed by the body's tissues.

As blood comes into the kidneys for renovation, the waste products to be eliminated from the body plus a great deal of water and such chemical molecules and radicals as glucose, carbonate, sodium, chloride, potassium, phosphate, calcium, and sulfate pass through the delicate membranes into the kidney tubules. All this makes up the so-called glomerular filtrate. But many of these chemicals cannot properly be spared, and so specialized cells which line the kidney tubules salvage what the body needs as the filtrate passes by.

In the hereditary disorders of kidney transport, the specialized cells of the kidney tubules are defective to the extent that they permit certain molecules or radicals to pass on through into the bladder.

A notable example of these diseases is called renal rickets. In this condition the cells of the kidney fail to recover as much phosphate as they should from the glomerular filtrate, with the result that the concentration of phosphate in the body's tissues and fluids falls to low levels. Symptoms similar to those of ordinary rickets develop. But even though the symptoms are similar, this disease typically does not respond to the administration of vitamin D as ordinary rickets does. The disease usually progresses to a fatal termination.

Diseases of Metabolism

In this group of diseases the metabolism (transport, synthesis, breakdown, or excretion) of some normal chemical constituent of the body occurs in an abnormal manner, and this abnormality of metabolism seems to be the primary cause of the illness. The various processes of metabolism are usually altered in other kinds of disease, but in these other instances the metabolic changes are the consequences of the disease rather than its cause.

CYSTIC FIBROSIS.

This is a serious disease of hereditary origin which affects that part of the pancreas which produces digestive enzymes, some of the salivary glands, the glands of the respiratory tract, and the sweat glands of the skin. The complications are (1) malnutrition because of the deficiency of the pancreatic digestive enzymes, (2) infections of the respiratory organs, and (3) a tendency to heat exhaustion because of the excessive loss of sodium chloride through the sweat. The disease typically begins in childhood, and many children with this disorder do not live to adulthood. With improved methods of treatment, the prospective length of life has increased.

What to Do

1. The recommended diet is high in calories, high in protein, and moderately low in fat.

2. Vitamin A in relative large doses is recommended.

3. Concentrates of pancreatic enzymes taken by mouth at mealtime serve to supplement the reduced output of the pancreas and help to allay the digestive symptoms and improve the patient's nutritional status.

4. The control of respiratory infections by the use of antibiotics and other medicinal agents is important.

GOUT.

Gout is mentioned here because its fundamental cause is a defect in metabolic processes with the result that deposits of uric acid occur in various parts of the body, notably in certain joints and in the kidneys. This causes a very distressing type of arthritis. Gout as a disease is discussed in chapter 14 of this volume.

DIABETES MELLITUS.

Of the two kinds of diabetes, diabetes mellitus and diabetes insipidus, diabetes mellitus is by far the most common. (For a discussion of diabetes insipidus, see chapter 26 in this volume.) When a person uses the term "diabetes" without qualification, he refers to diabetes mellitus.

This is a disorder of carbohydrate metabolism, with obvious hereditary background in about 50 percent of cases, characterized by the production of large quantities of urine and by excesses of glucose (sugar) in the blood and the urine.

It used to be assumed that the fundamental cause of diabetes mellitus is a deterioration of the islets of Langerhans in the pancreas, the cell groups which produce insulin. When the pancreases of persons who have died from diabetes mellitus are examined, in many cases there is an obvious deterioration of the islets of Langerhans. Strangely, however, in some cases no such deterioration can be detected. This observation together with other significant items of evidence has persuaded medical scientists that the disease is not always caused by difficulty in the pancreas itself. Other circumstances within the body's tissues can also interfere with the metabolism of carbohydrate. For this reason our discussion of diabetes mellitus is included here with diseases of metabolism rather than in the chapter on "Endocrine Gland Diseases."

Diabetes mellitus is not only a serious disease but a common one, occurring sometime during the lifetime of 4 percent of females and 2 percent of males in the United States. The onset may be at any age. Usually the disease first becomes apparent following some major demand on the body's resources such as severe injury, a serious infection, or a circumstance of emotional stress. The incidence of diabetes mellitus is higher in overweight persons than in people of normal weight.

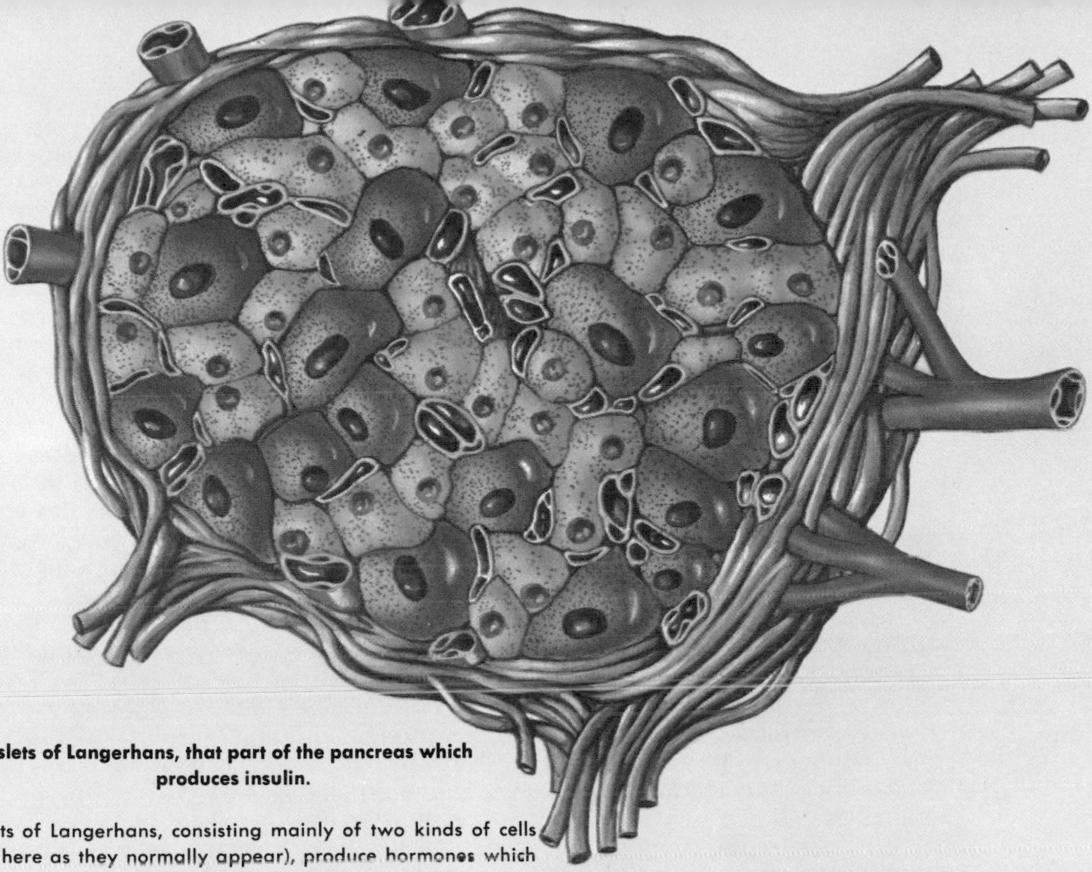

Islets of Langerhans, that part of the pancreas which produces insulin.

The islets of Langerhans, consisting mainly of two kinds of cells (shown here as they normally appear), produce hormones which regulate the body's use of sugar.

The cells of the islets of Langerhans as they appear when diseased and no longer able to perform their essential function.

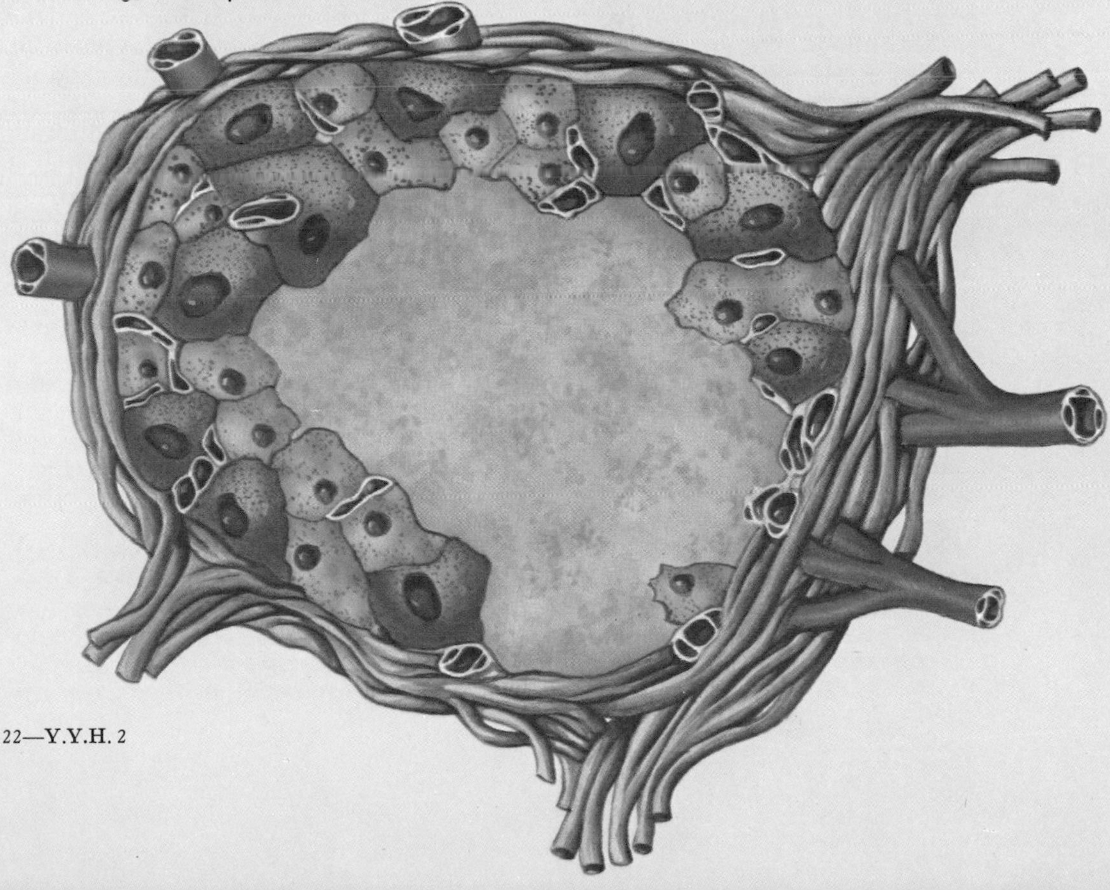

In diabetes mellitus there is an impairment in the storage of glucose by the liver and an interference with the process by which the body's cells are able to use glucose as their source of energy. A person suffering from this disease must therefore derive more of his energy from the metabolism of protein and fat than is normally the case.

Prior to the days of adequate treatment, the mortality rate for diabetes mellitus ran high. Even now for cases which begin in childhood it runs significantly higher than for those which begin in adult life. For a case in which the disease appeared first in adulthood, the life expectancy can be virtually as high as in a normal person, provided the treatment program is so carefully controlled at all times that the body processes proceed normally.

Symptoms the Patient Notices: When diabetes begins during childhood, the symptoms include excess production of urine, excessive thirst, a desire to void at night, bed-wetting, an increase in appetite in spite of a loss of body weight, weakness, and itching of the skin. For cases which begin during adulthood, the symptoms are excessive production of urine, increased thirst, weakness, and itching of the skin.

What the Physician Finds: When a physician examines a person with diabetes, he finds sugar in the urine, a higher than normal concentration of glucose in the blood, and evidence (revealed by a "glucose tolerance test") that the individual is not using up his blood sugar as quickly, following a meal, as in a normal case. These evidences all indicate that the body is unable to use glucose in a normal manner. In other words, glucose accumulates in the blood and is eliminated by the way of the urine instead of being used in the body for the production of energy.

A tragic feature of diabetes mellitus is that when it goes untreated serious complications develop, thus reducing the patient's life expectancy. One of these is a tendency to early degeneration of the body's arteries with arteriosclerosis developing throughout the body and with the coronary arteries of the heart being particularly involved. Abnormal conditions also tend to develop in the nervous system, such as peripheral neuritis, loss of the sense of vibration, and loss of normal control of the urinary bladder. Another complication of diabetes is kidney disease. A tendency to infection of the skin and other body tissues is much greater than normal. Also ever-present is the danger of a loss of consciousness.

Two situations representing opposite conditions may cause unconsciousness in a case of diabetes. The first develops gradually, when for some reason the glucose in the blood reaches high levels and is not offset by an adequate amount of insulin. This condition is called diabetic coma. The second may develop quite suddenly when, for some reason, the supply of glucose in the patient's blood and tissues reaches such a low level that the cells of his body run out of energy. This second condition is called hypoglycemic coma. It may develop when the diabetic patient has taken a larger dose of insulin (or of medication taken by mouth that has a similar effect) than he presently requires.

For the emergency treatment of these two conditions, see volume 3, chapter 18, "Handling Emergencies," under *Unconsciousness,* subsections B and C.

It is because of the lurking danger of coma that a diabetic patient is advised to carry a wallet card or wear a bracelet stating that he is a diabetic, and that if he is found to be acting strangely or if he becomes unconscious, his doctor or an ambulance should be called at once.

The card should also give the following information: patient's name, address, and telephone number; and physician's name, address, and telephone number.

Diet is essential in the control of

diabetes. Many cases, particularly those that develop during adulthood, can be handled satisfactorily without the use of insulin or other medicines, provided the patient follows a consistent dietary program. A suitable diet for a diabetic patient is relatively normal, with the exception that it does not include the more rapidly absorbed carbohydrates except in small amounts. The special feature in administering the diet is that all portions must be carefully measured so that the patient eats neither too much nor too little. In other words, the various food elements in his diet must be very carefully regulated. It is also very important that the diabetic patient avoid becoming or remaining overweight. It is when a diabetic patient becomes careless in following his diet, by eating more or less of some particular item, that he encounters difficulty.

The second important factor in the treatment of diabetes is the administration of insulin or of one of the "hypoglycemic agents." Insulin administered by hypodermic is the reliable means of controlling the level of blood sugar in diabetic patients. Great advances have been made in the preparation of insulin, and the physician may choose among various products available as he adapts the program of treatment to the particular needs of his patient. The so-called "hypoglycemic agents" are medications that are taken by mouth. In certain mild cases of diabetes in which the condition cannot be controlled by diet alone, these hypoglycemic agents may be used instead of administering insulin.

Once a case of diabetes has been diagnosed, it is well for the patient to spend several days in the hospital for his education in how to control his illness. Here he learns how to regulate his diet, how to test urine for sugar, and how to take his insulin or insulin substitutes as may be necessary. His ability to enjoy good health thereafter depends very definitely on his being consistent in following his treatment program. Also periodic checkups are necessary as a means of measuring his progress and of modifying the treatment program to fit changes in his condition.

Certain circumstances requiring special provisions may occur in the experience of a diabetic patient. During pregnancy, for instance, a diabetic patient requires closer supervision than usual. Infant mortality is higher in a poorly controlled diabetic mother. When a diabetic patient must have surgery, it is necessary for his treatment program to be altered accordingly and to be regulated very closely, day by day, throughout the period of his surgery and recovery. In case an infection develops in the skin or in any other of the body's tissues, the treatment program must be altered accordingly.

The diabetic patient must regulate the amount of his physical exercise almost as carefully as he regulates his diet. It is beneficial for him to have some physical exercise each day. Inasmuch as the amount of exercise changes his requirements for energy food, the possible consequences of his taking either too little or too much exercise during a given period may be just as serious as taking too little or too much food.

HYPOGLYCEMIA (LOW BLOOD SUGAR).

Hypoglycemia is the condition in which the amount of glucose (sugar) drops below the level of 50 mg. per 100 ml. of blood. Hypoglycemia is not a separate disease as such, for it may stem from any one of several causes.

The symptoms of hypoglycemia may follow two patterns, which can occur separately or in combination. First, certain symptoms relate to the nervous system and result from the brain's being deprived of sufficient glucose (energy food) to maintain the normal activity of its cells. These symptoms may include mental confusion and anxiety, hallucinations, aimless activity, convulsions, and eventual coma.

Second, other symptoms result from the body's automatic attempt to compensate for the lack of blood sugar by producing an emergency supply of epinephrine. These include sweating, pallor, chilliness, trembling, hunger, weakness, and palpitation.

The Causes of Hypoglycemia:

1. Hypoglycemia may result from an overdose of insulin. Insulin has the effect of accelerating the body's use of blood sugar. An overdose of insulin, therefore, reduces the amount of sugar in the blood. Hypoglycemia may also follow the excessive use of "hypoglycemic agents" (insulin substitutes).

2. A failure to eat the usual amount of food after taking insulin may cause hypoglycemia. In a diabetic patient, the amount of insulin must be carefully balanced against the amount of food the patient is expected to eat in order to maintain the level of blood sugar at its normal. When the patient does not eat this necessary amount of food after taking insulin, the effect is comparable to that of an overdose of insulin, with the result that the blood sugar is reduced.

3. Hypoglycemia may result from excessive exercise. If the body's sources for replenishing the available supply of blood sugar thus used up are not momentarily adequate, hypoglycemia will result. A person with diabetes mellitus is particularly susceptible in this instance.

4. Hypoglycemia may result from an overproduction of insulin within the body, as in the particular type of tumor of the pancreas in which the insulin-producing tissue becomes overactive.

5. It may develop in cases of liver disease in which the blood sugar is not stored or released by the liver in a normal manner.

6. Hypoglycemia may occur in connection with diseases of certain endocrine organs, as the adrenals and pituitary. Oddly, the "hypo" condition may occur early in the course of diabetes, before the usual "hyper" phase.

What to Do

1. The treatment of an acute attack of hypoglycemia will vary depending upon whether the patient is in the hospital or must be given emergency treatment elsewhere and on whether he is still able to swallow or has already lost consciousness. In the hospital the administration of glucagon by injection will usually produce a rapid elevation of the blood sugar level. Glucagon is a hormone which is normally produced in the pancreas and has the effect of counterbalancing the influence of insulin. The giving of glucagon may need to be followed by the intravenous injection of 10 to 25 mg. of glucose to replenish the body's supply. Subsequent treatment is determined by the results of laboratory tests indicating the level of the patient's blood sugar.

When the patient is not in the hospital but is still able to swallow, he should be given any sort of sweetened drink, such as orange juice, or its equivalent in candy or sugar. The symptoms of the immediate attack should improve within fifteen minutes. Then he should eat bread or other food containing starch and protein to provide the necessary source from which his tissues can produce additional glucose. When the patient is not able to swallow, he may be given sweetened fruit juice or a 5 percent solution of glucose by stomach tube. Prompt effort should be made to secure the services of a physician or to take the patient to the emergency room of a hospital.

2. For cases in which the cause of hypoglycemia may be organic disease of the pancreas or liver, a physician should study the case in order to determine the exact cause and arrange the treatment accordingly. Surgery or other definitive treatment may need to be carried out promptly.

3. For cases of functional hypoglycemia in which there is no actual disease of the liver or pancreas, an alteration in the patient's diet may correct the tendency to hypoglycemia. In such cases, the body's control mechanisms may have become unusually sensitive to the taking of carbohydrate food to the extent that insulin is produced in excessive amounts. A helpful procedure is to adopt a diet which is low in carbohydrate and high in protein and fat, thus enabling the individual to derive the necessary amount of calories for his energy needs without overstimulating his own production of insulin.

Intestinal Parasites

Animal parasites are commonly found in the human intestine, more often in children than in adults. Though especially common in countries with warm climates, this problem is not limited to such parts of the world. The parasites secure their food from the contents of the intestine in which they live, or from their victim's blood, which they usually obtain by attaching themselves to the intestinal wall. Most of them are either protozoans, roundworms, or tapeworms, though at least one of some importance is a fluke. Some of them are harmless, or at the worst do very little damage; others cause disease or distress; and a few are a grave menace to life, though usually not until the passage of considerable time.

Fluke or Trematode Infections

There are many flukes that can infect the human body but only one that spends any considerable time in the intestine. The disease which it causes is called fasciolopsiasis, and the name of the fluke is *Fasciolopsis buski*. The eggs of this fluke are passed out in the feces. They hatch out in water. Their first stage of development takes place in the bodies of snails. Then the partially developed parasites encyst upon water plants most commonly—

caltrops, water chestnuts, or water hyacinths. If these are eaten raw, the parasites mature in the eater's intestine. They usually attach themselves to the lining of the duodenum or the jejunum, causing inflammation and sometimes ulceration and bleeding. Diarrhea and abdominal pain are common. Later the stools become greenish-yellow and contain much undigested food. In severe infections, there is likely to be fluid in the abdomen, nausea, vomiting, and edema of the face, abdominal wall, and the lower extremities. These symptoms are suggestive that the infection is present, and would be meaningful if the person concerned had been eating any of the indicated foods; but a definite diagnosis depends upon finding the eggs in the stools. Death rarely results from the disease itself, except in children; but the victim is likely to become so weakened by it that some other disease easily overcomes him.

This disease is rare in the Western Hemisphere, but it is fairly common in the Orient.

What to Do

1. If the disease is suspected, have a stool examination to find the eggs of the parasite.

2. When the disease is known to be present, its treatment should preferably be supervised by a

356

physician. The accepted remedy is hexylresorcinol, available in 100-milligram pills. Recommended dosage for respective age groups is as follows:

Under six years of age, 1 pill for each year of age.

6 to 8 years of age, 6 pills.

8 to 12 years of age, 8 pills.

Over 12 years of age, 10 pills.

The evening before the drug is given, the patient should have a light supper and before retiring should take 1 tablespoonful of sodium sulfate in a half glass of water as a laxative. The next morning, the correct dose of hexylresorcinol should be taken on an empty stomach. Two hours after the pills are taken, another tablespoonful of sodium sulfate in a half glass of water should be taken. This completes one course of treatment. A second course, and perhaps a third course, of treatment is usually necessary, at four-day intervals.

3. As a preventive measure avoid eating raw caltrops, water chestnuts, or any other roots, plants, or "nuts" that might have Fasciolopsis buski cysts attached to them.

Protozoal Infections

Different kinds of protozoans may be found in the human intestine; but only two of them are important causes of disease. These are *Endamoeba histolytica* and *Balantidium coli*. Diseases caused by the former are much more common in warm climates than elsewhere, but it is not unusual to find cases in the United States and other countries in temperate zones. Most of these, however, are in people who have picked up their infection while living or traveling in tropical or subtropical regions or in areas where sanitation is poor.

AMEBIC DYSENTERY (AMEBIASIS).

Amebiasis, or infection with *Endamoeba histolytica*, is far more common than most people realize. Many are infected with this parasite without knowing it or being made noticeably ill by it. The parasite apparently always gains entrance to the body through the digestive tract, being carried in by contaminated foods or beverages.

When the parasites produce severe intestinal disease, the victim has diarrhea, cramps, and colicky pains; but these symptoms usually come on gradually rather than with a sudden onset. The stools contain pus, mucus, and blood, and may number twenty or more in a single day. Occasionally fever and a rapid pulse are present. In a majority of cases the diarrhea and other symptoms are mild, but more or less chronic, and tend to alternate between better and worse by spells. In some cases there may be only repeated spells of abdominal colic, with no diarrhea at all. The true nature of the condition can be proved, however, by finding the active amoebas or their cysts in the stools; and it is wise to suspect any case of recurring or chronic diarrhea as being amebic dysentery until proved otherwise, especially in warm climates.

Anybody infected with Endamoeba histolytica should have thorough and persistent treatment to rid his body of the parasites. A severe case may prove fatal. Even a mild infection—one so mild as to go unnoticed because of no definite intestinal symptoms—may cause a general impairment of health. Abscess of the liver is an occasional complication of amebiasis, but an amebic liver abscess may develop without there having been any previous detectable intestinal symptoms. The organisms are carried from the intestine to the liver through the portal circulation. As a rule, only one such liver abscess is present in a given case, but there may be more than one.

All of the effective remedies for amebiasis yet discovered are drugs that may harm the body if given improperly or in too large quantities. Emetine hydrochloride, carbarsone,

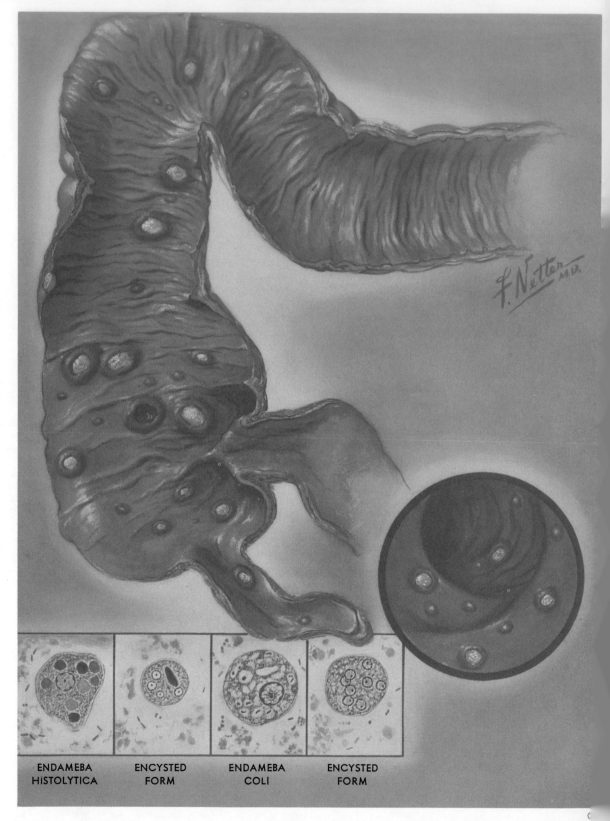

ENDAMEBA
HISTOLYTICA

ENCYSTED
FORM

ENDAMEBA
COLI

ENCYSTED
FORM

vioform, terramycin and certain other antibiotics, and several other remedies have been used with good results; but they should be given only under the supervision of a physician. The treatment should be continued not only until all symptoms have been brought under control, but until the organisms can no longer be found in the stools.

Prevention of infection is obviously important, and this includes prevention of the spread of infection from a known case to other people. The following preventive measures are recommended:

1. Protect all food, water, and other beverages from any chance of fecal or sewage contamination.

2. Carefully dispose of all human excreta.

3. Kill all flies, as far as possible, and take all practicable measures to prevent their breeding. All garbage should be kept in leakproof, covered containers. All animal fertilizer should be spread thinly on the ground or kept in tightly covered bins. All toilets or latrines should be carefully screened.

4. People living in places without fully adequate water sanitation should boil all drinking water, and after boiling store it in covered containers to prevent contamination.

5. Wherever human excreta are used to fertilize the soil, no vegetables or fruits should be eaten raw unless they are the type that can be peeled.

6. Food handlers should give careful attention to their personal habits. Fingernails should be kept trimmed and clean. Hands should always be washed with soap and water after defecation, and again immediately before beginning to handle food.

7. Before employing any person as a cook or other food handler, have his stools examined for the possible presence of amoebas or their cysts. Many people are unknowingly carrying these organisms. People who continue to be food handlers in areas where amebic dysentery is known to

occur should have annual stool examinations.

What to Do

1. If amebic infection is suspected, have a stool examination made to detect the presence of the causative organisms.

2. If the infection is found to be present, the infected person should stay under the supervision of a physician, since no home treatment or remedy is effective.

3. Have the victim's stools reexamined weekly until recovery seems to be complete, and yearly thereafter, since there is always considerable danger of relapse.

BACILLARY DYSENTERY.
(See chapter 28 of this volume.)

BALANTIDIAL DYSENTERY (BALANTIDIASIS).

Balantidial dysentery is in many respects similar to amebic dysentery, but less common and less severe, though more widespread geographically. A large proportion of the infected individuals are apparently healthy carriers of the parasite *Balantidium coli* and are never made ill by it. This is a common parasite of swine, and the infection is considerably more common among people who have contact with these animals than among people who do not. Liver abscesses are not produced as a complication of this infection, as is the case with amebiasis. Of the remedies that have proved valuable in cases of amebiasis, carbarsone is more effective than any of the others for balantidiasis; but some of the tetracycline antibiotics that have little or no effect on amoebas are of definite value against balantidia. For these reasons, the treatment of balantidiasis is less difficult than that for amebiasis.

What to Do

1. Follow the advice given under *Amebic Dysentery*.

2. Follow-up stool examinations are recommended, preferably yearly.

359

Roundworm Infections

COMMON ROUNDWORM INFECTION (ASCARIASIS).

Common roundworm infection is most prevalent in places with a warm, moist climate, but no part of the world is free from it. The worm is from six to fourteen inches (15 to 35 cm.) long, the female being larger than the male. It lives chiefly in the upper part of the small intestine, but may travel to other parts of the digestive tract. It may enter the stomach and be vomited up, or may find its way up into the throat, sometimes getting into the windpipe and the air passages, where it may cause strangulation or other serious injury. Only one or two may be present in the intestine, or possibly many.

The females produce large numbers of eggs, readily recognizable with the aid of a microscope. Several weeks' time is required for the embryo worms to develop in the eggs before they can infect humans. The eggs abound in places contaminated with fecal material. Children playing in contaminated dirt around houses or in gardens get the eggs on their hands, especially under their fingernails. Handling dogs or cats, or other pets that run about in contaminated places, may have the same result. Then when one eats with unwashed hands or uncleaned fingernails, or puts the fingers into the mouth, the eggs get into the mouth and go down to the stomach and into the intestine, where they hatch, liberating the tiny embryos. The embryos then burrow into the intestinal walls and migrate through the tissues to the lungs, from there making their way back to the intestine in much the same way that hookworm larvae do. (See following item.) In the intestine, the embryo worms develop into adults and live for a considerable period of time.

During the migration of the immature worms through the lungs, symptoms similar to those caused by the migration of hookworm larvae may be caused if the numbers of the parasites are considerable. The presence of these forms in the intestines, of children especially, may give rise to abdominal pain, fever, diarrhea, grinding of the teeth, restlessness, and sometimes convulsions; or their presence, especially if they are few in number, may cause no recognizable symptoms and may not even be suspected unless one of the worms is passed in the stool or unless a chance stool examination reveals the eggs. In regions known to be contaminated periodic examinations of the stools of children are recommended.

What to Do

1. The diagnosis of common roundworm infection should be confirmed by a laboratory examination of the stool specimen.

2. If a physician is available, arrange for him to order and supervise the treatment. Several effective remedies are now available, and it is best for the physician to choose the one best suited to the individual case.

3. At the time of writing, the remedy which is generally favored for the treatment of roundworm infection is piperazine. The dosage depends on the weight of the patient

Roundworm (actual size) and its ovum (enlarged 400 times).

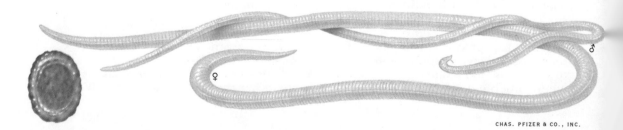

CHAS. PFIZER & CO., INC.

(see the table below). One dose per day is given on each of two consecutive days.

Patient's Weight In Kilograms	In Pounds	Daily Dose of Piperazine
14	30	1 gram
23	50	2 grams
46	100	3 grams
Over 46	Over 100	3.5 grams

4. One month after the course of treatment another stool examination should be made to determine whether the worm eggs are still present. If so, another course of treatment should be given.

HOOKWORM INFECTION (ANCYLOSTOMIASIS, GROUND ITCH).

Hookworms cause more cases of serious illness than do any other of the intestinal parasites. In many parts of the world, including some sections of the United States, hookworm disease is present in a considerable proportion of the population. In such localities, the average health and vigor of the people are below normal, their mental as well as physical efficiency being impaired.

Hookworms are small and slender, about half an inch (8 to 13 mm.) in length, the female being somewhat longer than the male. They live in the small intestine, where they attach themselves to the intestinal lining by means of their hooked mouths; and they feed by puncturing the blood vessels with their sharp teeth.

The female worms produce great numbers of eggs, which the human expels with his stools, and these hatch out after leaving the body. Contact with warm, moist soil favors the hatching of the eggs and the rapid development of the young embryos. When a skin surface, such as bare feet or hands, comes in contact with the moist earth containing these almost microscopic young worms, they rapidly penetrate the skin and enter the blood vessels. They are then car-

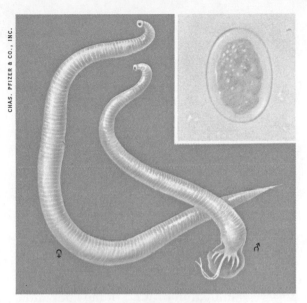

Hookworm (10 times actual size; ovum, 350 times).

ried by the bloodstream to the lungs.

The young hookworms enter the air passages in the lungs, make their way to the throat, and are then swallowed. In this roundabout way they finally reach the intestine, where they develop into fullgrown worms. If fewer than a hundred worms are present, symptoms are not likely to be noticeable. But the presence of five hundred or more will cause typical symptoms. In some of the most severe cases more than four thousand worms have been found in the intestines of a single individual.

The only way to be sure that a person is infected with hookworms is to find the eggs or the worms themselves in his bowel discharges, but in most cases there are characteristic signs and symptoms. The soiling of the skin of the hands or feet with contaminated earth, and the resulting penetration of the minute worms through the skin, cause itching and burning of the affected skin, followed by the formation of small papules and blisters, and later by crusting. This condition, commonly called ground itch, is also known as miner's itch, foot itch, toe itch, dew itch, or water itch. During the time when the immature parasites are passing through the lungs, there

361

may be spells of coughing, with sore throat and bloody sputum.

While the parasites are attaching themselves to the intestinal wall and growing to maturity, the characteristic symptoms are diarrhea, flatulence, and abdominal discomfort. Later, weakness, pallor, fatigability, weight loss, anemia, and difficulty of breathing become common. The symptoms are particularly noticeable in growing children in whom a definite slowing of mental development and body growth occurs. In some cases, especially where the number of worms is large, there may be swelling of the feet or of the entire body, and an accumulation of fluid in the abdominal cavity. A person with such severe symptoms cannot live long unless the worms are expelled.

The problem of preventing hookworm disease is one of great importance. Infected people must be helped to expel the worms from their intestines, and then be taught how to prevent further infection. Keeping the hands out of the soil and the wearing of shoes by people working in hookworm areas would help; but *it is of prime importance to make safe disposal of all human bowel discharges* so that the ground is not contaminated by them. Modern flush toilets or properly designed and constructed privies, if used as the sole depositories of fecal matter, would go far toward stamping out hookworm disease.

As a conclusion to the general discussion of hookworm infection, mention should be made of a peculiar condition called Larva migrans (creeping eruption). This is caused by the larvae of the dog and cat hookworm, which penetrate the human skin and migrate from place to place in it, usually without going deeper or traveling more than a few inches. The migration causes intense itching and a reddish eruption in the form of narrow, crooked, slightly elevated ridges. The eruption tends to persist for several months, but the migrating larvae finally die and are absorbed by the tissues. If they are numerous enough to be very troublesome, and especially if they are located near the skin surface, as is often true, a physician may use special methods to kill them. If they penetrate deeper, as sometimes happens, nothing can be done except to give symptomatic treatment while waiting for them to die.

What to Do

1. Tetrachloroethylene is among the most effective remedies, but it is dangerous to give it to alcoholic patients or to those with gastrointestinal disorders, severe constipation, any marked degree of anemia, or liver disease. It is difficult to be sure that none of the conditions warned against is present without tests and studies by a physician, and a physician should supervise the use of the drug. The physician may prefer some other remedy.

2. If no physician is available, piperazine may be used, administering it in the same way as recommended for a case of "Ascariasis." (See preceding item.)

PINWORM INFECTION (SEAT WORM INFECTION, OXYURIASIS, ENTEROBIASIS).

Pinworms live in the large intestine, especially in the rectum. They are usually present in large numbers, and females ready to lay eggs often crawl out through the anus and lay their eggs upon the surrounding skin. They cause much itching in this region, especially at night.

These worms are white in color and small in size. The female, much larger than the male, averages less than half an inch (8 to 13 mm.) long. She lays large numbers of eggs, and there is danger of the infection's being carried to other people, or of the child's reinfecting himself, through scratching about the itching anal region and later handling food or objects that he or other people will eat or handle, or by putting the fingers into the mouth. Underclothing and bedclothing easily become contaminated, and it has proved difficult to clear up the infection in one member of a family unless all the other members are treated at the same time.

When the eggs are swallowed, they hatch out in the duodenum and migrate downward. If the skin around the anus is not kept clean, the eggs may hatch out there and the immature worms migrate back through the anus into the rectum. Pinworm infection does not cause severe symptoms, aside from the itching, as a rule; but there may be vague gastrointestinal discomfort, restlessness, and insomnia.

What to Do

1. If a physician is available, arrange for him to order and supervise the treatment.

2. One of the preferred drugs for the treatment of pinworm infection is piperazine. Tablets of piperazine citrate or piperazine phosphate are usually available in either the 250 milligram or the 500 milligram sizes. The recommended doses depend on the weight of the patient as follows:

Patient's Weight in Pounds	Dose of Piperazine	Total Mgs. per Day
Under 15	250 mgs. (once daily)	250
16-30	250 (twice daily)	500
31-60	500 mgs. (twice daily)	1,000
Over 60	1,000 mgs. (twice daily)	2,000

3. For itching of the skin, apply 1 percent phenol in petrolatum or 1 percent yellow oxide of mercury ointment as needed.

4. Have any infected person wear tight-fitting shorts day and night, or use any other effective method to prevent him from scratching the anal region.

5. Change underclothing and bed linen daily, and use boiling as a

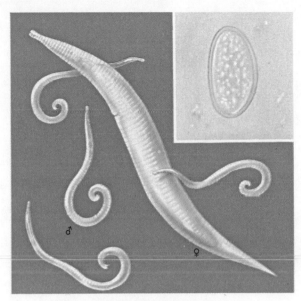

Pinworm (10 times actual size; ovum, 350 times).

part of the laundering procedure.

6. Scrub toilet seats with soap and water every day.

7. For greater safety, have all members of the family treated.

8. All members of the family should carefully wash their hands with soap and water after each bowel movement and before all meals; and their fingernails should be trimmed short and kept clean. They should all be warned to keep their fingers out of their mouths and not to scratch the skin in the anal region.

STRONGYLOIDIASIS (STRONGYLOIDES STERCORALIS [THREADWORM] INFECTION).

Strongyloides stercoralis infection is common in tropical and subtropical areas in all parts of the world, including the southeastern part of the United States. The larvae of this parasite usually enter the body and migrate through it in much the same way as do hookworm larvae. Some of them, however, may complete much of their development in the lungs or the air passages, giving rise to symptoms resembling those of bronchitis or bronchopneumonia. Infection of the intestines, which is the usual form, may produce no noticeable symptoms, though a watery diarrhea fairly often shows up, and occasional cases go on to ulceration.

The adult worms resemble hookworms in general appearance, but they are smaller. They are found in greater numbers in the duodenum than in any other part of the intestine. The anemia which they may cause is much less severe than that from hookworm infection. The eggs do not pass out in the stools as do the eggs of hookworms, but hatch while still in the intestine, and usually then the larvae pass out and contaminate the soil. Occasionally a few of the larvae do not pass out of the intestine, but perforate its walls, causing an unusually severe illness.

What to Do

1. Confirmation of the diagnosis of this infection depends, of course, on the finding of eggs and larvae in the feces.

2. The treatment should be under the direction of a physician.

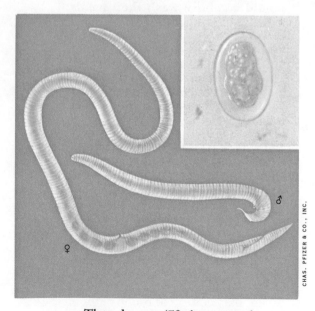

Threadworm (70 times actual size; ovum, 350 times).

TRICHINOSIS (TRICHINIASIS).

In contrast to other roundworms, trichinae live for only a comparatively short period in the intestines. Trichinosis is contracted by eating raw or insufficiently cooked flesh of animals containing the parasites in a dormant form. Nearly always the contaminated meat is the flesh of swine, though in a considerable number of reported cases it was bear meat, and apparently in a few cases other kinds of meat that had simply been chopped on the same block used to chop pork.

When infected meat is eaten, the embryo worms are liberated in the stomach and the intestine, where, in about three days, they grow to full size, most of them becoming rather deeply embedded in the intestinal mucous membrane. They do not lay eggs that pass out of the intestine, but produce great numbers of young worms, most of which burrow into the tissues and are carried throughout the body by the blood and lymph circulation. They finally become encysted and dormant in the muscle tissue as tiny coiled worms. They are not equally abundant in all muscles, but the diaphragm gets more than its proportionate share of them.

After infected meat is eaten, six or seven days are required for the full development of the first brood of young embryos, which are then ready to migrate in the body. The production of embryos continues for some time. Bowel symptoms, such as discomfort and diarrhea, may occur at the time of the multiplication of the worms in the intestine, and other and quite different symptoms develop while the young worms are migrating. These symptoms may be such as to arouse a suspicion of typhoid fever or rheumatism. They may be so severe that death results in some cases. Fever, chills, and abdominal and muscle pains are common. There is much muscle tenderness, with swelling of the muscles and the overlying skin during the period while the embryo worms are becoming encysted.

The small worms may lie dormant in the muscles as long as twenty years, but the symptoms of their presence largely disappear after the first few weeks or months.

Autopsy surgeons who have made a search for the encysted parasites in dead bodies have reported that in some parts of the world where pork consumption is high and where certain pork products are often eaten raw, more than 20 percent of the population is probably infected. The amount of illness caused by so much infection must be great. Many of the fevers, aches, and pains that people in such areas attribute to other causes are really due to their fondness for pork.

Of people with trichinosis severe enough to be recognized as such, probably one in twenty will die because of the infection, so it must be considered a very serious matter. Once the infection has taken place, there is no way to stop its progress, so prevention of infection is of vital importance. Those who do not eat flesh food, but especially pork, are safe; but others should remember that encysted trichinae embryos can be killed by thorough cooking of the meat containing them. It has also been proved that freezing the meat and keeping it frozen for several months will kill at least most of the parasites.

What to Do

1. If symptoms suspicious of trichinosis appear within three or four days after a person has eaten meat that might have been infected, the stomach and bowels should be thoroughly cleaned out, taking Epsom salts purgatives and copious enemas.

2. After the worms have begun to migrate through the tissues, no remedy or treatment can stop them; but a physician can use remedies that will at least partially relieve the symptoms.

3. Long-continued hot baths—temperature about 100° to 102° F. (38° to 30° C.) may help to relieve

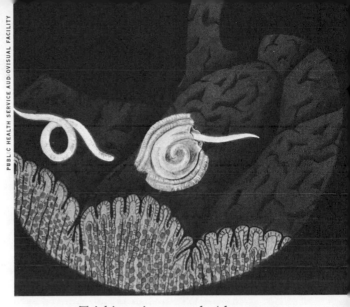

Trichinae in stomach (the worms shown much enlarged).

Trichinae encysted in muscle.

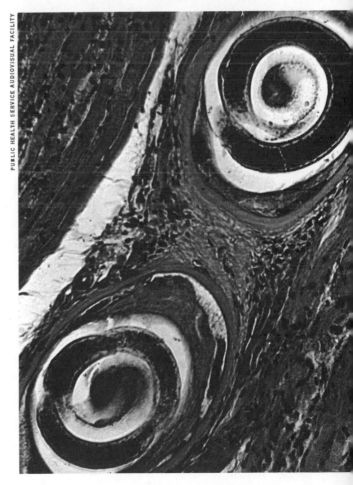

muscle pains; but cold compresses to the head must be given at the same time to prevent fainting, and the baths should not be continued long enough to produce profuse sweating. (See volume 3, chapter 20.)

WHIPWORM INFECTION (TRICHURIASIS).

Whipworms are about one and a half to two inches (35 to 50 mm.) long. They get their common name from their shape, looking like a whip with a slender lash and a thicker handle. The small end of the lash is the head of the worm. Sometimes as many as a thousand worms are found in a single individual's intestine. They live chiefly in the large intestine and rarely cause any symptoms. They produce large numbers of eggs of a characteristic appearance, being easily recognized under a microscope by a person who knows what they look like. The worms are usually detected by being passed in the stools from time to time. If present in great numbers, which is seldom true, they may cause some intestinal distress, diarrhea, and flatulence.

Whipworm eggs pass out of the intestine and hatch in the soil as a rule. They enter the body in larval form, but their manner of entry is similar to that of the eggs of the common roundworm.

What to Do

1. If whipworm infection is suspected, watch for the easily visible worms to be passed in the stools.

2. Arrange for a physician to supervise the treatment.

Tapeworm Infections

Ordinarily, a tapeworm has a double life history. The larva, after being hatched from the egg, is found in the flesh of some of the lower animals. Eating raw or insufficiently cooked flesh containing the larvae transfers them into the digestive tract of man, where they develop into their mature form.

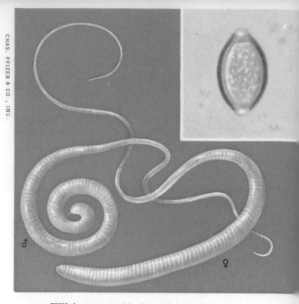

CHAS. PFIZER & CO., INC.

Whipworm (5 times actual size; ovum, 350 times).

All tapeworms are long, flat, and thin, with segmented bodies. The head is small and has sucking discs or hooklets or both, by which means it holds onto the intestinal wall. The old segments gradually drop from the back end as new segments are formed near the head. The segments that drop off and escape with the bowel movements often contain great numbers of eggs. These may later chance to be eaten by some lower animal along with its food. In the stomach and intestines of this animal, the eggs hatch into larvae, which migrate into the muscles or other parts of the animal's body and become encysted or dormant there, not developing further until the infected flesh of the animal is eaten by a human being or some other suitable host.

The varieties of tapeworms most commonly found in the human intestine are separately described below. The method of expelling them is the same for all varieties, and will be outlined following the descriptions.

BEEF TAPEWORM (TAENIA SAGINATA).

The head of the beef tapeworm has no hooklets. This may account for the comparative ease with which this worm is dislodged from its attachment to the intestinal wall when the proper remedy is used. Beef tapeworms may grow to a length of more than thirty feet (nearly 10 meters).

Eggs pass out in great numbers in the victim's bowel movements, but even more of them are discharged in the segments of the worm, which are frequently broken off from the back end of the worm. These separate segments seem to have an activity of their own, and often pass from the bowel at other times than when feces are passed. Anybody acquainted with the characteristic appearance of a tapeworm segment can easily tell the kind of worm from which it came.

The presence of the beef tapeworm sometimes causes diarrhea, hunger pains, and loss of weight. A greater than usual appetite may be the only noticeable symptom. All symptoms, however, are uncertain and are often absent. One can be sure of the parasite's presence only by discovering the segments of the worm as discharged from the bowel or by a microscopic examination of the stools to discover the tiny eggs.

DWARF TAPEWORM (HYMENOLEPIS NANA).

This is the smallest of the tapeworms whose adult forms infect man. It lives in the small intestine, sometimes in small numbers, but there may be as many as a thousand in one intestine. Individual worms grow to be from one to one and a half inches (25 to 35 mm.) long. This worm is found more often in children than in grown people, and the eggs can hatch out and grow to maturity without leaving the intestine. Infection comes generally from swallowing the eggs rather than from eating flesh containing the larval worms. This tapeworm may produce nervous symptoms and loss of appetite, but often it causes no symptoms at all. When it is present, there are many eggs in the bowel movements. These have a characteristic appearance, and are easily recognized by a trained observer with a microscope.

With Hymenolepis nana should be classed the rat tapeworm, Hymenolepis diminuta, and the dog tapeworm, Dipylidium caninum, which also infects cats. Both of these latter two worms are comparatively small. They do not often infect human beings, but they seem to be transmitted most commonly by the accidental swallowing of worms or insects containing the larval forms. The last of the three has reddish segments shaped like melon seeds, and it is somewhat larger than the other two.

FISH TAPEWORM (DIPHYLLOBOTHRIUM LATUM).

This is the largest of the tapeworms infecting man. It is not common in the United States. It may grow to a length of nearly forty feet (more than 10 meters). The segments may be half an inch (13 mm.) broad, and one worm may have three thousand or more segments. The egg of this worm must

Beef tapeworm. Note how segments break off the tail end.

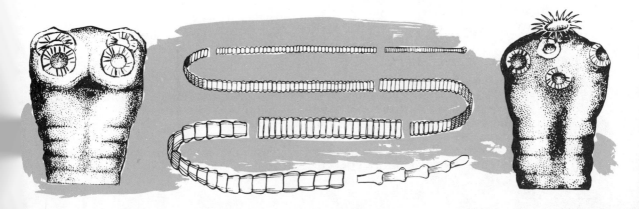

hatch out in the water, the larvae find entrance into the body of some fish, and the flesh of this fish be eaten by some person, if the person is to be infected with a fish tapeworm. Freshwater fishes are most often infected. Salting or smoking the flesh of the fish does not kill the larvae, but thorough cooking does. In some cases the fish tapeworm causes an anemia similar to pernicious anemia. Its presence may give rise to hunger pains, diarrhea, abdominal distress, and loss of weight.

PORK TAPEWORM (TAENIA SOLIUM).

In the United States the pork tapeworm is less common than the beef tapeworm; but this is not true everywhere. The muscles of the animal's body most often infected by the larvae are those of the neck, tongue, and shoulders. In many cases the infection produces no noticeable symptoms; but in some the infected person has digestive disturbances, hunger pains, and diarrhea alternating with constipation.

The pork tapeworm is comparatively difficult to expel, and may require repeated treatments. It sometimes grows to a length of about twenty feet (about 6 meters), and may live in the intestine for many years. In some cases people become infected with the larval form of this tapeworm from accidentally swallowing its eggs, but the larvae do not stay in the intestine. They burrow through the walls of the intestine and may infect almost any part of the body, including the brain, where their presence may cause symptoms similar to those of epilepsy or of brain tumor.

What to Do

Quinacrine hydrocholoride (atabrine) is the drug of choice. It is not recommended that it be used without a physician's supervision. A physician can arrange for proper safeguards and can best make the follow-up investigation needed to determine whether or not the treatment has been effective.

HYDATID DISEASE (ECHINOCOCCOSIS).

This is a tapeworm disease in one sense, but the adult worm does not infect the human intestine and the usual method of expelling the worm cannot be used, hence the discussion is kept separate from those concerning the worms that do infect the intestine and that can be thus expelled.

Echinococcosis is common in many sheep-raising regions. The adult tapeworm, Echinococcus granulosus, usually infects the intestines of dogs, foxes, wolves, et cetera, which animals become infected by eating the carcasses of sheep containing the larval worms. Infection of humans is with the larval form, and usually results from swallowing food accidentally contaminated with dog feces or from handling dogs and then putting the fingers into the mouth.

When a person thus swallows the eggs, they hatch out in the intestine. The young worms spend but a short time there, and then burrow into the tissues. Most of those that survive lodge in the liver, where they cause the formation of cysts filled with fluid and lined with a membrane that may produce large numbers of immature worm heads. Each of these heads could produce a mature worm if swallowed, but they would never be swallowed by any human under normal circumstances. Some of these cysts act like malignant tumors, so hydatid disease may become a severe malady. If this disease is to be prevented, care must be used in handling sheep dogs and in disposing of sheep carcasses.

What to Do

1. No medicine or home treatment is of any use.

2. If a cyst grows large enough to cause symptoms, or if it ruptures, consult a physician. An operation may be beneficial.

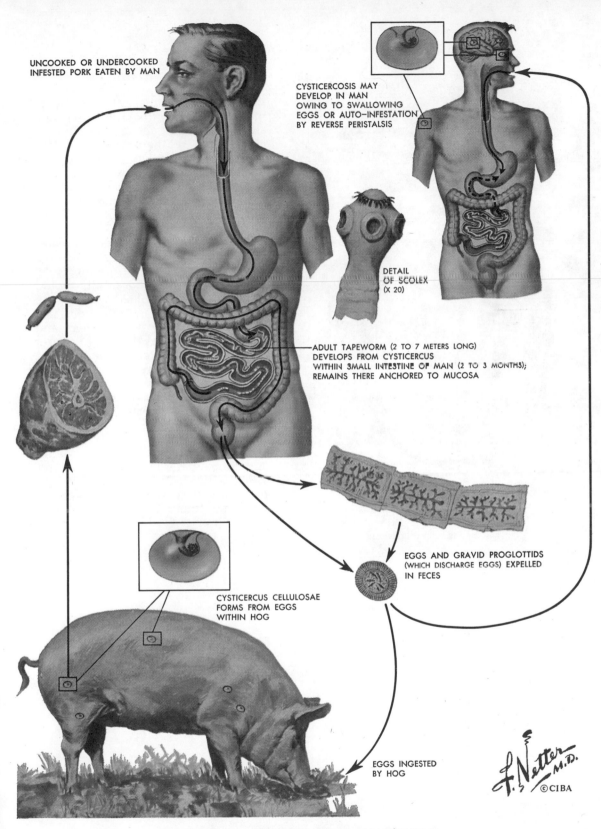

UNCOOKED OR UNDERCOOKED
INFESTED PORK EATEN BY MAN

CYSTICERCOSIS MAY
DEVELOP IN MAN
OWING TO SWALLOWING
EGGS OR AUTO-INFESTATION
BY REVERSE PERISTALSIS

DETAIL
OF SCOLEX
(X 20)

ADULT TAPEWORM (2 TO 7 METERS LONG)
DEVELOPS FROM CYSTICERCUS
WITHIN SMALL INTESTINE OF MAN (2 TO 3 MONTHS);
REMAINS THERE ANCHORED TO MUCOSA

EGGS AND GRAVID PROGLOTTIDS
(WHICH DISCHARGE EGGS) EXPELLED
IN FECES

CYSTICERCUS CELLULOSAE
FORMS FROM EGGS
WITHIN HOG

EGGS INGESTED
BY HOG

F. Netter M.D.
©CIBA

LIFE CYCLE OF THE PORK TAPEWORM

Conclusion

In the whole range of the diseases of man it is in the field of intestinal parasites that obedience to the rules of cleanliness and the laws of sanitation proves most effective in preventing disease. Adequate provision for the disposal of all human excreta and the use of proper toilets should become universal. Human excreta should not be used for fertilizing fields or gardens —at least in any way that creates a danger of contaminating food being grown for human consumption.

Neither children nor adults should go barefooted in places where the ground may be contaminated. They should keep their bodies clean and wash their hands thoroughly after defecating, before eating, and before handling food. Care is necessary in association with domestic animals, including especially dogs and cats. Children run the greatest risk of infection, because of their natural carelessness and because they come into such close contact with floors, the ground, and animal pets. They should be provided with clean places in which to play, and they should be taught to keep their fingers and all other objects except proper food and drink out of their mouths.

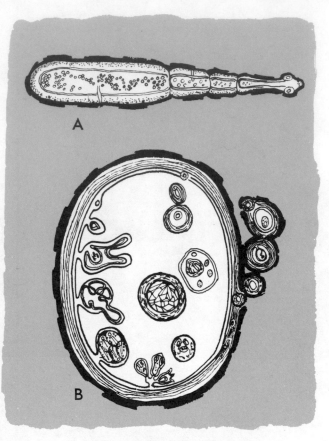

A. Echinococcus granulosus (magnified 23 times). B. Sectional view of a hydatid cyst.

Diseases of the Urinary System

The kidneys are the vital part of the urinary system. Blood flowing through the capillaries in the renal corpuscles carries excess water and certain other constituents. These are filtered out and collected by a funnel-like capsule, from which the filtrate flows into the kidney tubules. The cells lining these tubules are able to select part of the water and the materials still of use to the body, returning these materials in solution to the bloodstream. Waste materials in solution travel on down the tubules into the kidney pelvis, and from there through the ureter to be stored in the bladder. From time to time the bladder empties out of the body through the urethra. These waste materials in solution constitute the urine. A careful analysis of the urine will usually disclose whether or not a disease of the urinary system exists.

Diseases of the ureters and of the urethra are not common, except as they are affected by disease of the kidneys or the bladder. This fact makes the discussion of disease of the ureters and the urethra unnecessary in this chapter. The only important infection of the urethra which does not concern either the bladder or the kidneys is caused by the gonococcus, and this infection and its complications are dealt with in the discussion of gonorrhea in the chapter entitled "Venereal Infections." (See chapter 30 of this volume.) One of the common complications of neglected gonorrhea is urethral stricture, which is separately discussed in the following chapter on "Diseases of the Male Sex Organs."

BED-WETTING (ENURESIS).

Bed-wetting is really not a *disease*; it is a *symptom*. It is considered here, however, because it involves abnormal functioning of the urinary organs and because it is a problem in many families. At age two, about 40 percent of children wet their beds at night. By the age of four-and-a-half, about 12 percent are still bed-wetters, and by age eight, 7 percent of children are still troubled this way. Thus we see that the time of life at which a child develops control of his bladder-emptying function varies from one case to another. A few children do not gain this control until about age 12.

Pediatricians and urologists are not agreed on the exact reason behind a child's tardiness in developing control. This suggests that doubtless several factors cause the problem—one being responsible in one case and a different factor in another case. Some bed-wetting children sleep very soundly part of the time, and this may interfere with the development of the control pattern by which the brain

371

overrules the emptying reflex even during sleep. In some cases the capacity of the bladder does not increase as fast as does the growth of other parts of the body.

In an estimated 20 percent of cases of bed-wetting, an actual hindrance to the free flow of urine exists somewhere between the bladder and the outside. This may not seem to hinder the emptying of the child's bladder when he is awake, but it disturbs the functional balances sufficiently to cause bed-wetting at night. The hindrance may consist of simple folds in the membrane that lines the urethra (the tube that carries urine to the outside). It may consist of a narrow place (stricture) along the course of the urethra or of an unusually small opening at the external end of the urethra. Diabetes, when present, causes the person to drink more water and thus to have more urine to expel. Formerly it was thought that unsolved emotional problems of childhood were responsible for many cases of bed-wetting. It is now believed, however, that bedwetting of itself is not proof that a child is emotionally distraught.

What to Do

1. Abstain from punishing the child who wets the bed. He does not do this intentionally, for he is made uncomfortable by it. Be sympathetic and solicit his cooperation in overcoming the problem.

2. Establish a program to increase the capacity of the child's bladder. If the child can be encouraged to empty the bladder less frequently during the daytime, it will become stretched to accomodate the larger volume of urine, and this stimulates its growth. To start the program, a chart must be kept on which is recorded, day by day, the time of day each time the child goes to the toilet and the volume of urine that is passed each time. This requires that a measuring glass be used to measure the amount of urine at each voiding. After keeping the rec-

ord for a few days, the child is then encouraged to hold his urine as long as possible even after he receives the urge to void. He should be praised each time he holds his urine a little longer than usual and each time he voids a larger volume than usual.

Do not restrict the amount of water the child drinks during the day. At the start, it is well for him to drink very little water, if any, after his evening meal. He should not be criticized on the occasions when he still wets the bed. However, the occasions on which he wets the bed should become less frequent as the program procedes. He should be praised when he remains dry all night. This program of increasing the bladder's capacity may need to continue for as long as six months or more.

3. If the above program does not bring the desired results, then the child should be taken to a urologist (a physician who specializes in treating disorders of the urinary organs). After making a thorough examination, the urologist will advise on whether a simple surgical procedure (such as dilating the urethra) may be expected to relieve the bed-wetting problem.

4. Another method which the urologists sometimes use is the administration of the drug imipramine (Tofranil). The use of this drug may need to continue for several weeks and should be supervised by the physician.

Bladder Diseases

Diseases of the bladder usually have little to do with kidney function. The bladder is primarily a storage tank for urine and does not help to form it. This organ may be infected by germs that come down with the urine from an infected kidney, or by germs that make their way upward through the urethra. On the other hand, back pressure of urine which cannot escape freely from the bladder, or infection ascending from the bladder through the ureters to the kidneys, may cause kidney disease.

BLADDER FISTULAS.

Bladder fistulas are not very common. They usually consist of open tracts or canals that extend between the bladder and the rectum, the bladder and the vagina, or the bladder and the skin surface. If the fistula is of the first-mentioned type, urine may leak from the rectum or may be mixed with the stools, and the urine passed from the bladder nearly always contains bubbles of air or gas. Such urine has a foul odor, and sometimes contains small bits of fecal material. If of the second-mentioned type, there will be a leakage of urine from the vagina. If of the third-mentioned type, the leakage will be from some opening on the skin surface.

What to Do

If there is evidence of the existence of a bladder fistula, consult a surgeon, preferably a urologist. Only expert surgery can cure a bladder fistula.

BLADDER STONES (VESICAL CALCULI).

Stones in the bladder are common, but much more so in men than in women. Inflammation of the bladder, with a partial obstruction of the urethra, is believed to favor the formation and growth of stones, but an enlarged prostate gland can also cause such a partial obstruction. When it is known that such a partial obstruction has occurred, whatever the cause, periodic examinations for the detection of bladder stones are in order. These stones may be small or large—sometimes larger than a hen's egg. Some of them were originally kidney stones that came down the ureters to the bladder while still small, possibly causing much pain while doing so. Such passage, when it is known to have happened, constitutes an additional reason for periodic examina-

tions to detect possible bladder stones. The stones tend to become larger and larger in size as they remain in the bladder. Some cases of cancer of the bladder are caused by the irritation of stones that have been allowed to stay in the organ a long time.

It is a matter of importance to have bladder stones removed without delay. Bladder stones usually cause frequent and painful urination, but occasionally a stone of considerable size may become fixed in some pocket of the bladder wall and cause few or no symptoms. A small stone may be drawn into the urethra during urination, causing a sudden painful stoppage of the urine flow. When this happens a urologist should be consulted at once. The obstruction to urine may possibly be momentarily relieved in

Various types of bladder stones.

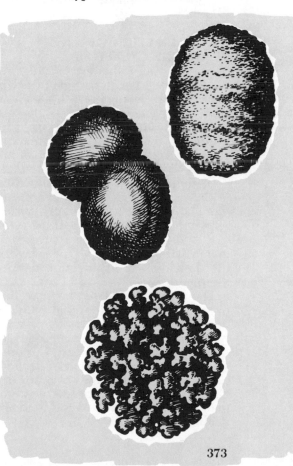

373

such a case by having the patient lie down while urinating into a small receptacle.

When there are stones in the bladder, a microscopic examination of the urine may reveal the presence of blood and/or pus. An X ray will show most bladder stones. By the use of a cystoscope a urologist can look into the bladder and see the size, shape, and number that may be present.

What to Do

1. If the presence of a bladder stone is suspected, consult a urologist without delay. Treatment may require surgery, but sometimes the stones can be crushed and the pieces washed out of the bladder by using a special instrument inserted through the urethra.

2. Temporary relief from pain may be obtained by taking a hot sitz bath or by sitting in an ordinary tub of hot water.

INFLAMMATION OF THE BLADDER (CYSTITIS).

In women, inflammation of the bladder often develops a day or two after sexual intercourse. In such a case, the bacteria that cause the inflammation have traveled up the urethra to the bladder. Inflammation can also occur as a complication of infection of the kidney.

In men, it may accompany infection of the kidney or it may follow an inflammation of the prostate. Any partial obstruction to the outflow of urine so that a residual amount of urine remains in the bladder at all times favors the development of infection within the bladder.

The symptoms relate mostly to the functions of the bladder and include burning on urination, a desire to void frequently, and a feeling of urgency to empty the bladder at once. General symptoms such as fever are usually caused by inflammations of other organs (as the kidneys or prostate) rather than by inflammation of the bladder itself.

The usual case of inflammation of the bladder responds readily to appropriate treatment. If the aggravating cause is an obstruction to the outflow of urine, as an enlarged prostate or a stricture of the urethra, such condition must be corrected. If the condition subsides and recurs repeatedly, there is some underlying cause which should be discovered and corrected.

What to Do

1. Antimicrobial drugs such as the sulfonamides are quite effective in clearing up an infection of the bladder. The choice of the particular drug and its mode of administration should be specified by the physician.

2. The person with inflammation of the bladder should drink ten glasses of water or fruit juice a day.

3. Hot fomentations over the lower part of the abdomen given three times a day or hot half baths help to make the patient more comfortable. (See volume 3, chapter 20.)

TUMORS OF THE BLADDER.

Cancer is probably the most common bladder tumor. It is often secondary to cancer of the prostate in men, and to cancer of the cervix or the body of the uterus in women. Noncancerous tumors of the bladder occasionally occur, however, among which the most important is the papilloma; but a papilloma may become cancerous in its later stages.

Tumors of the bladder may cause all of the symptoms of cystitis but not usually to a very severe degree. A papilloma may produce one symptom similar to that of a bladder stone. This tumor is treelike in form, and its branches wave about in the urine within the bladder. If the tumor is located near the bladder outlet, one of the branches may bend over it and produce a sudden stoppage of the urinary outflow. The outstanding symptom of a papilloma, however, is bloody urine, as is also true of other bladder tumors. The resulting bladder

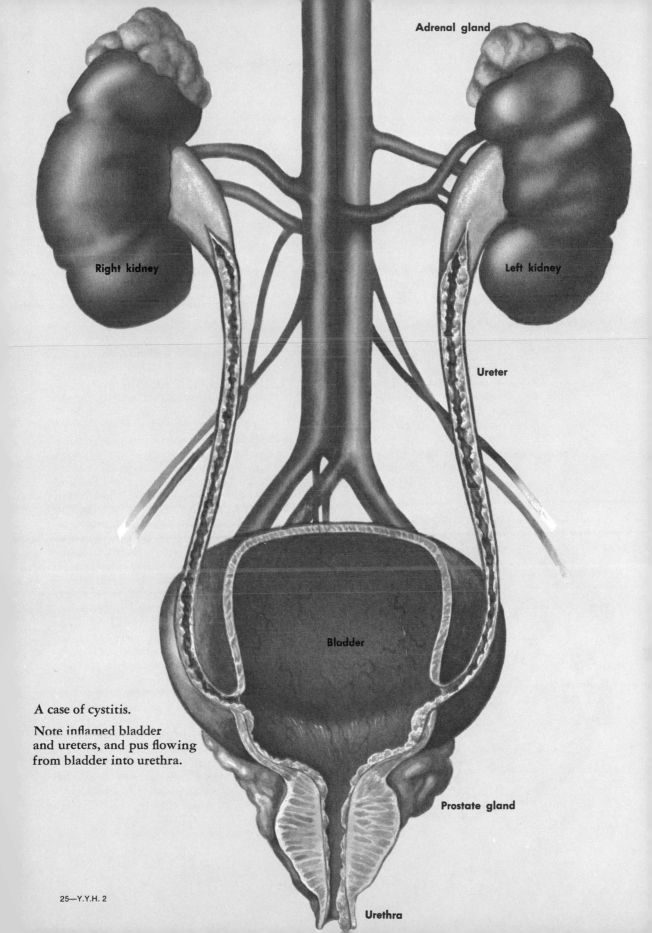

Adrenal gland

Right kidney

Left kidney

Ureter

Bladder

A case of cystitis.

Note inflamed bladder
and ureters, and pus flowing
from bladder into urethra.

Prostate gland

Urethra

hemorrhages may be profuse, even to the point of threatening life from loss of blood. An absolute diagnosis of the kind and seriousness of a bladder tumor demands the services of a urologist.

What to Do

If a bladder tumor is suspected, consult a urologist for diagnosis. If one is found, no treatment short of removal is satisfactory.

URINARY INCONTINENCE (INABILITY TO HOLD THE URINE).

In urinary incontinence, a most troublesome symptom, the patient loses normal control of the passage of urine. This loss occurs commonly when either the bladder or the urethra is involved with local infections (cystitis or urethritis). There is a sudden urgency to empty the bladder, and if the desire is not gratified urine may

Tumor of the bladder as observed through a cystoscope.

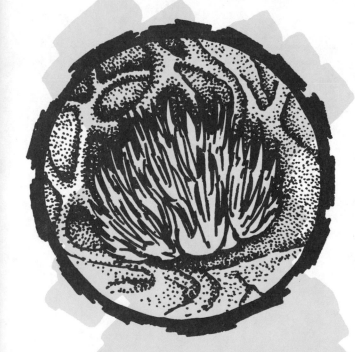

escape in spite of effort to retain it. The symptom occurs commonly in older men whose prostate gland has become enlarged. It occurs in women in whom tissue injuries sustained at the time of a difficult delivery for a child were not adequately restored by surgical procedures. In such cases, coughing, sneezing, laughing, or sudden lifting may cause the urine to leak.

Loss of urinary control occurs in cases in which the spinal cord or the nerves to the bladder have been damaged by disease or injury, compressed by a tumor, or severed.

What to Do

If urinary incontinence develops, consult a urologist.

URINARY RETENTION.

When there is partial obstruction to the outflow of urine, as from a stricture of the urethra, an enlargement of the prostate, a developing tumor within the bladder, or a growing bladder stone, the muscle in the wall of the bladder becomes stronger, at first, and forces the urine past the obstruction in a relatively normal manner. As the obstruction becomes more complete, a condition develops in which not all of the urine is emptied from the bladder at the time of voiding. That which remains in the bladder, called residual urine, reduces the bladder's effective capacity and makes it necessary for the person to void at more frequent intervals. Also, the presence of residual urine favors infection of the bladder lining, causing inflammation of the bladder (cystitis). Continued back pressure from an obstructed bladder causes damage to the kidneys.

As such a condition of obstruction progresses, there comes a time—often a sudden event—when the person can no longer empty his bladder at all. The bladder continues to fill, producing distention and considerable pain. This type of complete urinary retention constitutes an emergency.

What to Do

1. When complete urinary retention develops, consult a physician as soon as possible.

2. Do not eat or drink until relief is obtained.

3. Take a long-continued hot half bath, or sit in an ordinary tub of hot water. Two hours is not too long to stay in the bath if relief is not obtained sooner.

4. The physician will probably try to draw off the retained urine by means of a catheter, and such a procedure usually succeeds. Relief is only temporary, however, for catheterization is not a cure. Surgery may be necessary; and if so, the sooner it can be arranged, the better.

Kidney Diseases

FLOATING KIDNEY (NEPHROPTOSIS).

All kidneys are somewhat movable. Sometimes one is sufficiently so to make the organ easily felt through the abdominal wall. In most such cases, no symptoms are caused. Occasionally there is a disturbance of the circulation, causing some congestion and pain. In other occasional cases, the ureter may become kinked or otherwise partly or completely obstructed. The pain is usually a dull ache or dragging sensation, but sometimes it is acute and colicky, especially in the case of an obstructed ureter.

KIDNEY FAILURE AND UREMIA.

Some of the body's organs are more important to the individual's well-being than are others. Those essential to life are called vital organs. Others, like the spleen, the sex organs, and the gallbladder, perform important functions but can be removed should they become diseased, and their removal does not interfere too much with the functioning of other organs.

The kidneys belong to the vital organs—they are essential to life. A person will die after a few hours

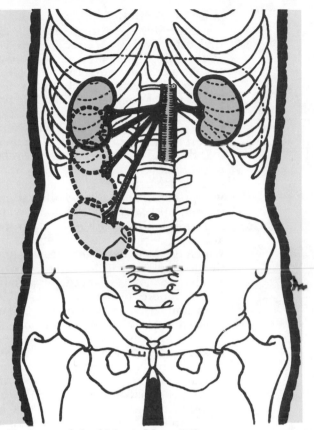

Prolapse of the kidney. Note different positions (dotted lines) a kidney can adopt in nephroptosis.

should the kidneys become totally inactive.

The function of the kidneys is to remove the waste products from the blood. Normally, they provide a wide margin of safety in that they contain much more functioning tissue than is necessary to keep the concentration of waste products in the blood well within safe limits. One kidney alone, if perfectly healthy, can care for the body's needs and still have functional capacity to spare.

Under certain conditions of disease, the working capacity of the kidneys is reduced. If this reduction is gradual, the elimination of wastes will still proceed normally for a time. Eventually a point is reached, however, beyond which the kidneys become un-

377

able to keep the concentration of waste products within safe limits. At first this inability occurs only under conditions of unusual demand, and at such times the concentration of the nitrogenous waste products in the blood increases above normal. If the accumulation of waste products becomes so great that toxic symptoms occur, the condition is called uremia.

If the damage to the kidneys is relatively sudden and severe, they may even cease to produce urine, and then we speak of acute kidney failure. Both uremia and acute kidney failure are life-threatening conditions. With the aid of modern laboratory methods by which the function of the kidneys and the concentration of the various waste products can be measured, physicians can evaluate a patient's condition from hour to hour. And by the use of the artificial kidney to eliminate the waste products from the blood and thus give the patient's own kidneys a new start in doing their work, the lives of many patients have been saved. Of course the final outcome of the illness depends upon whether the damage to the patient's own kidneys is permanent or whether his kidney tissue can resume normal functions after a period of rest.

NEPHRITIS.

The term "nephritis" covers a group of conditions in which both kidneys are involved in inflammatory or degenerative disease and in which some protein and some blood cells are found in the urine.

The normal kidney functions as a filtering device. Within the functioning units of the kidney there are actually pores of microscopic size. As the blood passes by these pores, a certain amount of water and many of the smaller molecules contained in the blood pass through these pores to become what is called "urinary filtrate." The pores are normally so small that the larger molecules (principally those of protein) and the blood cells cannot pass through.

In nephritis the kidney's filtering mechanism does not work properly and some of the large protein molecules (principally those of albumin) and some of the blood cells pass through the filter and eventually appear in the urine. The presence of the protein albumin in the urine is called albuminuria or proteinuria.

In many cases of nephritis there is edema (swelling of some of the body's tissues), elevated blood pressure, an accumulation of some of the nitrogenous waste products in the blood, and the presence of albumin in the urine (indicating that the kidneys are not functioning efficiently).

A. *Acute nephritis (acute glomerulonephritis).* Acute infectious diseases, such as smallpox, scarlet fever, typhoid fever, malaria, diphtheria, measles, and particularly sore throat caused by the streptococcus often cause an acute inflammation of the kidneys. Any pus infection may lead to this condition, but streptococcal infections are most frequently to blame. Phenol, potassium chlorate, and turpentine are among the drugs that can cause it. It may be a complication of pregnancy (in so-called "toxemia of pregnancy"). It occurs most frequently in children, and it is rare after middle age.

Contrary to common belief, a lame or painful back does not indicate kidney inflammation. One of the symptoms of acute imflammation of the kidneys is edema, although only the face and eyes may be puffy. Children afflicted with this disease may have convulsions, but convulsions in children are by no means always caused by nephritis. Headaches, nausea, and vomiting are other common symptoms. A severe headache may be the first warning of oncoming nephritis in a pregnant woman. There may be fever and great weakness. The changes in the urine are characteristic and important. It becomes scanty, highly-colored, turbid, and sometimes bloody. Albumin and pus are present in the urine, but these can be

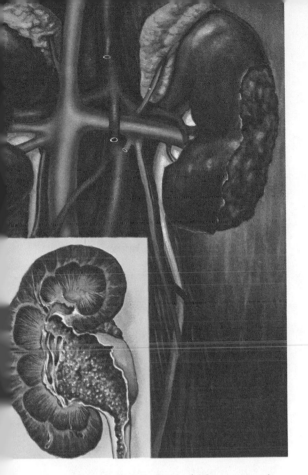

In nephritis both kidneys are involved. Lower left shows congestion inside the kidney.

detected and measured only by a physician or a trained laboratory worker.

Many people with acute nephritis can be completely cured; but, if it is neglected, it may gradually change into a chronic form, lasting over a period of several years before reaching a fatal termination. In other cases, death may come within a few days. Nephritis following or accompanying scarlet fever is especially dangerous.

What to Do

1. The patient should have bed rest and be kept warm. Care by a physician is important because there are many valuable treatments or remedies that can be given only by, or under the supervision of, a physician.

2. The diet should be planned carefully by the physician to comply with the patient's particular condition. Salt and protein may need to be restricted.

3. A warm bath may be given every day, but profuse perspiration should be avoided.

4. *No drugs* should be used other than what the physician orders.

5. As the acute stage of the disease subsides, more protein may be gradually added to the diet. Foods that can be added to good advantage are milk, cereals, and potatoes.

B. *Chronic Nephritis.* Chronic nephritis sometimes results from an acute nephritis that does not go on to recovery; but it more often develops gradually from a low-grade infection of long standing or from a low-grade irritation by chemical irritants taken or contacted over a considerable period of time. The damage done to the kidneys when toxemia develops in the course of pregnancy may be permanent, and may result in chronic nephritis.

A person with chronic nephritis may not realize that he has any serious kidney disease until it has progressed for several years. Accidental discovery of high blood pressure may be the first warning sign. Wastes are partly removed from the blood by the kidneys through a filtering process in the glomeruli, and blood pressure is necessary to make the kidney filters work. When the kidneys are damaged in the way characteristic of chronic nephritis, more pressure is required to force a given quantity of wastes through the filtering tissues. The high blood pressure, therefore, is at least partly the result of an attempt by the body to compensate for the kidney damage and to maintain the normal rate of waste disposal.

The kidney degeneration may have been progressing a long time before the characteristic headaches, loss of weight, weakness, shortness of breath, edema, and failing eyesight of

379

severe chronic nephritis appear. This is one of the reasons why a periodic urinalysis is advisable for everybody of middle age or past. The urinary symptoms, however, are not so characteristic as in acute nephritis. The quantity of urine passed may be above normal, causing frequent urination, especially at night.

Chronic nephritis may run a course of from two to twenty years, and its victim may die of some other disease before the kidney damage becomes severe enough to cause death. The final event may be uremia, stroke, coronary artery disease, or heart failure. Uremia is the condition that develops when the blood becomes overloaded with retained wastes, especially nitrogenous wastes, that the damaged kidneys have failed to throw off. Its accompanying symptoms are headache, weakness, loss of appetite, vomiting, emaciation, convulsions, and coma. In coma the victim becomes more and more stuperous, goes to sleep, and quietly passes away.

Stroke may be caused when a clot plugs a blood vessel in the brain or when such a blood vessel bursts. Coronary artery disease may be caused when a clot plugs one of the arteries that supply fresh blood to the wall of the heart. Heart failure may come on suddenly following some severe physical strain, but more often the heart gets tired from pumping blood under high pressure and fails gradually. Marked edema (swelling) of the feet, ankles, and legs, also asthma and great shortness of breath, may result from the weakening of the heart. The final stage of chronic nephritis may last a year or more. Treatment aims at prolonging life and increasing comfort. It cannot cure the disease, because the kidney tissue has been damaged beyond repair.

What to Do

1. It is advisable to have a physician in charge of the case all the time. The progress of the disease and the dangers accompanying it cannot be judged at all satisfactorily without repeated careful examinations and special laboratory tests. Hospital care may become advisable before the family realizes the need. If symptoms suspicious of uremia appear when the physician is not present, call him at once.

2. The victim should be protected from exposure to cold and all mental and physical strain.

3. A 30-minute tub bath at about 97° F. (36° C.) every evening just before retiring is beneficial.

4. Free water drinking is important unless there is edema, or swelling of the tissues under the skin.

5. The diet should consist chiefly of fruits and vegetables. Fruit juices and green leafy vegetables are especially good. Cases differ widely in their protein requirement, and it is wise to leave decision on this point to the physician.

6. Many cases are greatly benefited by the judicious use of an artificial kidney, a mechanical device for removing the nitrogenous waste products from the blood, such removal being either to reduce the load on the patient's own kidneys or to give them relief while healing takes place.

7. The procedure of kidney transplantation is becoming more and more successful. In this procedure, a healthy kidney from a live donor or from a person who has died from some other problem is surgically transplanted to the person whose kidneys are no longer functioning properly. The surgical procedure for kidney transplantation is now well perfected. There are still problems, however, in controlling the patient's immune mechanism so that the newly transplanted kidney can remain functional.

KIDNEY STONES (NEPHROLITHIASIS, RENAL CALCULI).

Kidney stones may be caused by some infection in the kidney such as

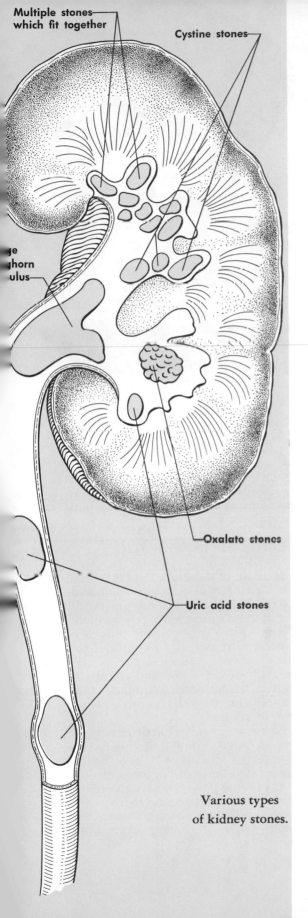

Multiple stones
which fit together

Cystine stones

e
horn
ulus

Oxalate stones

Uric acid stones

Various types
of kidney stones.

pyelitis; or they may result from stagnation of the urine in the kidney because of obstruction in its passage from kidney to the bladder. This obstruction may be caused by back pressure from an obstruction at the bladder outlet rather than by anything wrong in the bladder itself or in the ureter. Abnormalities in the metabolism of certain of the body's chemical substances may contribute to this condition. Notable among such metabolic disorders is gout, in which there is a considerable tendency to the formation of kidney stones. (See the discussion of *Gout* in chapter 14 of this volume.)

It is thought that improperly balanced diets or deficiencies of certain vitamins favor the formation and growth of kidney stones. The various chemical salts in the urine, especially the phosphates and the urates, may be precipitated and form the beginning of one or more stones. Such precipitation would be promoted by concentration of the urine such as may result from drinking too little water.

If the stones are small, they may pass down the ureters and be voided from the bladder without the person's knowledge. This is probably what happens to many kidney stones. If a stone remains in the pelvis of a kidney, it will steadily increase in size. A large stone may lie unsuspected in a kidney pelvis for years.

The symptoms of a stone in a kidney pelvis may be trifling. In fact, a kidney may be entirely destroyed before the victim has sufficient distress to persuade him to consult a physician. Usually, however, there is increased frequency of urination, especially associated with exertion or riding over rough roads. There may be vague pains and soreness through the upper back and side. If a ureter becomes blocked, there may be much pain, chills, and fever. If a stone starts to pass down through a ureter, it may cause sudden and excruciating pain, especially if it has sharp points or edges or if it is too large to pass down

381

the ureter easily. Such pain is often called renal colic. The urine in such cases will contain blood and possibly pus. The pain may be in the back, but more often it originates in the abdomen and radiates downward to the bladder, the groin, the inner aspect of the thigh, and the urethra. The pain may last from a few minutes to several hours or days, and it is one of the worst pains that humans ever have to bear, but it may stop as suddenly as it began.

There is a frequent desire to void urine during attacks of renal colic. In fact, the distress may be so closely confined to the bladder and its functions that the victim is deceived into thinking that the bladder is primarily at fault.

What to Do

1. Do not take any medicines with the idea of dissolving kidney stones.

2. To help relieve pain, apply heat, preferably fomentations if the pain is high in the back, or hot sitz baths if the pain is low in the back or the abdomen. (See volume 3, chapter 20.)

3. If satisfactory relief of pain is not promptly secured, consult a physician.

4. Drink plenty of water.

5. It is best to consult a physician, preferably a urologist, as soon as a suspicion of the presence of kidney stones is aroused. The treatment suggested in (2) above is preferably to be used only while waiting for a physician, or, if he approves it, as long as he suggests. Accurate diagnosis and proper treatment—sometimes including surgery—require the services of a physician.

NEPHROSCLEROSIS (ARTERIOLAR NEPHROSCLEROSIS).

A combination of high blood pressure and hardening of the small arteries of the kidneys is not an uncommon occurrence. Such a combination is likely to produce the characteristic symptoms of both hypertension and chronic glomerular nephritis. The treatment should combine the essential features of the treatments for both conditions.

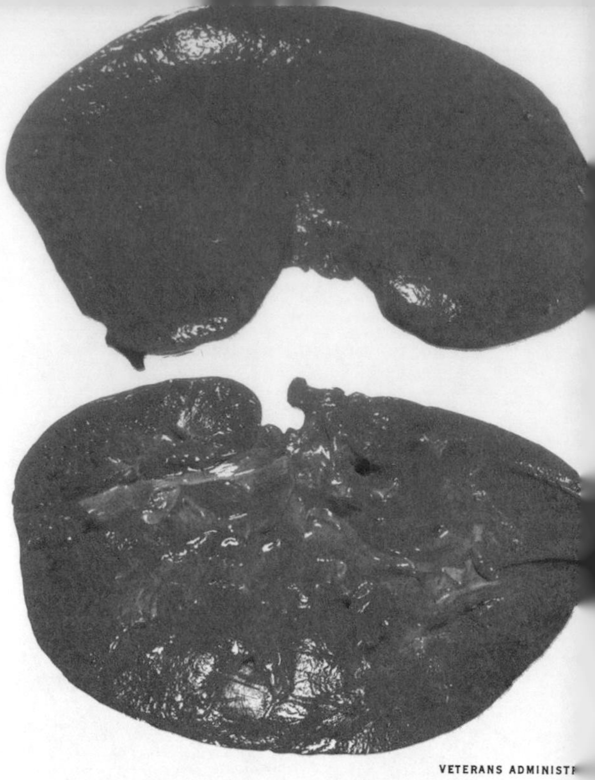

VETERANS ADMINIST

The human kidney as affected by nephritis, both external surface and interior being shown, this phase being between acute and chronic.

NEPHROSIS (NEPHROTIC SYNDROME).

Disease of the kidneys is responsible for this illness, which is characterized by pronounced edema (swelling of the tissues), protein (especially albumin) in the urine, and reduction of protein (principally albumin) in the blood serum. Children (especially between the ages of one and six) are affected much more frequently than adults, and boys have this disease more commonly.

The exact cause of the disease is not known, but it is sometimes associated with other diseases. It may be assumed that these or the prolonged effects of some poison, such as mercury, may cause damage to the kidneys and thus predispose to nephrosis. The nephrotic syndrome may occur as one stage in the course of nephritis.

In untreated cases the illness persists for many months, sometimes with periods of partial remission. In some such cases eventual spontaneous cure occurs, but in many some other disease of the kidneys develops or a severe infection of the tissues sets in. Tissues swollen with edema are particularly susceptible to infection.

Modern methods of treatment have greatly improved the possibility of eventual recovery. The use of corticosteroids brings about almost magic improvement in the majority of childhood cases and permits a fair proportion of adult cases to heal. The use of antibacterial drugs serves very well to control the infections that otherwise cause many deaths, but of themselves these drugs do not change the course of the kidney involvement.

What to Do

1. **A physician should supervise the treatment and the long-range care of the patient.**

2. **Bed rest is generally necessary to restrict the patient's activities.**

POLYCYSTIC DISEASE.

In some individuals, probably always happening during the developmental period before birth, segments of the kidney tubules fail to develop normally. These become blocked, forming closed sacs within which fluid accumulates. Such sacs are scattered throughout the kidney substance and are so numerous that they cannot be counted. As time goes on, they gradually increase in size, causing a steady enlargement of the kidney as a whole and progressive damage to its secreting tissue on account of increasing pressure. In some cases death occurs in early infancy. In others the enlargement is so gradual that symptoms leading to discovery of the condition may not show up before adulthood.

When the enlargement is sufficiently great, the kidney can be felt as an abnormal mass in the upper abdomen. Blood in the urine is a common finding. Symptoms and treatment are like those for *nephrosclerosis*. The condition is to some extent hereditary, nearly always involves both kidneys, and is incurable. Treatment can only afford temporary relief.

PYELITIS AND PYELONEPHRITIS.

The pelvis of the kidney is the enlarged upper end of the ureter, which is the tube that conveys the urine from the kidney to the bladder. Pyelitis, or inflammation of the kidney pelvis, may be caused by pus-producing bacteria. These bacteria may arrive through the bloodstream flowing through the kidney, or they may come upward through the ureter from an infected bladder. If the kidney substance is also involved, which is usually the case, the condition should be called pyelonephritis.

Infected tonsils, infected teeth, or other foci of infection are sometimes apparently the original source of the bacteria. One of the most common and persistent of the bacteria causing pyelitis or pyelonephritis is the colon bacillus, which always abounds in the large intestine. If not cleared out by thorough treatment, colon bacilli may remain in the pelvis of the kidney for years. These bacilli are often very resistant to treatment, and after apparent recovery recurrence of the infection is common.

A tendency to frequent voiding of urine may be the only symptom with mild infections. At other times the inflammation is so great that there is a constant painful desire to void. There may be severe chills, high fever, headache, nausea, vomiting, and extreme prostration for days at a time. There may be tenderness over the kidney region in the back. The distress, however, is often apparently confined to the bladder. In fact, many people have had bladder treatments for a long time, when the real trouble was in the kidneys.

If pyelitis becomes chronic, destruction or degeneration of the kidney tissue may progress until it becomes so extensive that surgical removal of the kidney is the only way to cure the disease. For this reason it is important to determine as early as possible whether one or both kidneys are involved and how far the infection has progressed. Obviously, if both kidneys are infected, the removal of either one cannot be considered, and suitable treatment must be started early enough to make surgical removal of a kidney unnecessary.

Pyelitis seldom proves fatal unless neglected, but a cure often requires expert and persistent treatment. In some cases the most effective treatment a specialist can give is dilation of the ureters so the kidneys can drain away the urine more easily.

What to Do

1. If the presence of pyelitis is suspected, it is important to obtain the services of a urologist promptly because it is necessary to have special examinations to detect it and special treatments to cure it.

2. Bed rest is essential as long as fever persists.

3. If the patient's temperature is not above 101° F. (38.3° C.), it may be helpful to give fomentations across the region of the back just above the hip bones (the flank). (See volume 3, chapter 20.)

4. Have the patient drink water freely to maintain a high urine output.

5. Sulfas or prolonged use of antibiotics are effective in many cases, and the physician in attendance will probably prescribe them.

6. Repeated urinalyses and cultures are always necessary, and they should be continued for some time after all symptoms have subsided— at least until the urine no longer shows the presence of bacteria.

TUBERCULOSIS OF THE KIDNEY. (See discussion of this item in chapter 29 of this volume.)

Tumors of the Kidney

Kidney tumors occasionally develop, most of them malignant. They may occur at any age. Even infants or young children may develop a rapidly growing fatal cancer of the kidney.

Bloody urine is usually the first and most persistent symptom noticed. The appearance of blood in the urine is an urgent indication that a physician should be consulted. If a kidney cancer is detected early, and if it is found that only one kidney is involved, surgical removal of the cancerous kidney may save life.

Diseases of the Male Sex Organs

EPIDIDYMITIS.

The epididymis is a small, soft-textured organ located in the scrotum next to the testis. It is composed chiefly of coils of the tube which carries the sperm cells (spermatozoa) from the testis into the abdominal cavity and through the prostate to the urethra. There is, of course, one epididymis on each side.

Epididymitis most commonly results from infection which makes its way from the prostate gland through the ductus deferens to the epididymis; and it is possible to have epididymitis on both sides. Neglected gonorrhea is a frequent cause, though not the only possible cause, of this condition. Any acute infection of the epididymis gives rise to swelling, pain, tenderness, and fever, which are made worse by physical activity.

What to Do

1. Have a physician determine the disease or infectious process causing the epididymitis, and have the condition properly treated according to his instructions.

2. Suggestions for home nursing care as outlined under *Orchitis* in this chapter may prove helpful.

GENITAL HERPES SIMPLEX.

(See also *Genital Herpes Simplex* in chapter 30 of this volume.)

That form of herpes simplex which affects the genital organs is caused by herpes simplex virus type II. This infection is acquired by sexual contact with a partner who already harbors this infection. It is manifested, in the male, by the appearance of clusters of small vesicles on the glans penis and occasionally along the shaft of the penis. If these vesicles rupture, they leave small, shallow ulcers.

As is true of other types of herpes simplex, so with genital herpes simplex, there is a so-called primary illness and the possibility of subsequent, recurrent manifestations. The lesions of primary genital herpes typically heal in three to six weeks. Those of the recurrent form of the illness usually heal within seven to ten days. Those of the secondary illness occur at the same sites as those of the primary illness.

What to Do

There is no effective cure for herpes simplex. The treatment is therefore symptomatic, with the intent of relieving the symptoms.

1. Should the small lesions on the skin of the penis become infected with ordinary bacteria, treatment with antibiotics is indicated. Antibiotics will have no effect on the infection caused by the virus, however.

2. If there is severe discomfort,

the use of some analgesic (pain relieving) medication may be indicated.

3. Compresses moistened with some antiseptic solution (such as benzalkonium 1:4000) may be applied for 15 to 30 minutes three or four times each day. This has the effect of reducing the risk of bacterial infection.

HYDROCELE.

Hydrocele is an accumulation of clear, watery, light-yellow-colored fluid in the membranous sac around the testis and epididymis. This condition may develop at any age. It is caused by some mild irritation in the lining of the sac. It may occur on both sides, but more often on only one side. Hydrocele sacs vary greatly in size. Some are so small as to be hardly noticeable. Some may be large enough to hold a quart or more of fluid. The tendency is to a gradual increase in size. A hydrocele causes little or no pain. It does not seem to injure the general health. The only problem that can arise is if the sac grows to a considerable size so as to cause inconvenience or discomfort.

By looking at a hydrocele sac with a light placed behind it, light is seen to pass quite readily through the clear fluid. This fact is often used to help distinguish hydrocele from some other kind of enlargement such as a tumor.

What to Do

1. If the hydrocele sac is small, no treatment is needed and none should be attempted.

2. A hydrocele sac large enough to cause discomfort calls for removal of the fluid by a physician. No home treatment is of any use.

IMPOTENCE

Impotence is the inability of a man to perform the sex act satisfactorily. It may consist of a weak erection, inability to gain an erection, loss of sex-

ual desire, premature ejaculation, or a loss of the normal sensation at the time of ejaculation. Most cases of impotence are caused by feelings of inferiority or by fear of the consequences of intercourse rather than by any actual disease or deformity of the sex organs. Impotence is a common development in older men, occurring even as early as the forties in some cases. Impotence occasionally occurs as a consequence of conditions involving excessive fatigue. It can be caused by diseases affecting the nervous system.

What to Do

1. Have no faith in remedies advertised as capable of restoring "lost manhood."

2. If impotence develops suddenly and independently of any unfavorable psychological influence, consult a physician.

3. Otherwise, for impotence developing in a man's prime of life, consultation with a psychiatrist offers the best prospect of cure.

4. Impotence developing gradually in the later years of life should be accepted philosophically as a part of the aging process.

ORCHITIS.

Orchitis is the name given to inflammation of a testis. It may be caused by injuries, by a tuberculous infection, or by a complication of other infections or infectious diseases, especially mumps. Orchitis is hard to distinguish from epididymitis, and the two conditions may be treated in the same way. In orchitis, the testis becomes swollen, painful, and very tender. The inflammation may involve one or both testes. When both are involved, it may be discovered later that the man concerned has been rendered sterile (incapable of becoming a father). This is especially likely to happen if he has not taken proper care of himself during the acute stage of the inflammation. The sterility in some cases is the result of damage to the testicle cells that produce the spermatozoa. In other cases it may be from scarring or stricture of the tubes through which the spermatozoa are discharged. Certain antibiotics are often helpful in controlling the infection causing orchitis, but these should not be taken without the prescription and supervision of a physician.

What to Do

1. Rest in bed until the acute symptoms subside.

2. Support the scrotum so that the weight of the testes will not hang on the cords.

3. Apply cold compresses continuously. (See volume 3, chapter 20.)

4. Keep the bowels open, preferably by proper diet, which should consist largely of fruit, vegetables, and skim milk. Drink water freely.

5. Avoid tobacco, liquor, tea, coffee, flesh foods, eggs, and all kinds of condiments.

6. Do not attempt to indulge in sexual intercourse until all painful inflammation has subsided.

7. If no definite improvement in the symptoms takes place within three days, consult a physician.

8. When the acute symptoms subside and bed rest is no longer necessary, wear a suspensory until there is no more tenderness in the affected organs.

PHIMOSIS.

Phimosis is the name given to an abnormal tightness of the foreskin. A cheesy mass, consisting of oily material, scales of dead skin, and dirt is likely to collect beneath such a foreskin and to set up irritation or even inflammation. An actual infection may develop which, if neglected, may heal by scar formation making it virtually impossible to retract the foreskin in a normal manner. Lack of cleanliness in the area beneath a tight-fitting foreskin, if allowed to persist for years, may even cause such irritation as favors the development of cancer.

What to Do

1. To prevent inflammation, retract the foreskin at the time of each bath and clean the area gently with soap. Do not leave the foreskin in a retracted position, but pull it back again over the tip of the penis.

2. In the case of an acute infection, consult a physician. He may have to resort to minor surgery to relieve the tightness and swelling of tissue.

3. After the acute inflammation has subsided, arrange for the removal of the tight foreskin by surgery (circumcision). See the discussion of *Circumcision* in volume 3, chapter 13.

PROSTATE, CANCER OF.

(See chapter 11 of this volume.)

PROSTATIC ENLARGEMENT (BENIGN PROSTATIC HYPERTROPHY).

Prostatic enlargement is generally a disease of elderly men. It is an overgrowth of tissue in the gland itself.

The prostate gland surrounds the neck of the bladder, and the first part of the urethra goes through it. An enlarged prostate causes trouble by pressing on the urethra and decreasing the size of the opening through it, or by forming a dam which holds back part of the urine in the bladder.

A man suffering from enlargement of the prostate will generally first notice that he has to get up oftener than usual to void urine at night. The stream will be small and slow to start. A long time may be required to empty the bladder, and toward the end of urination the urine may dribble instead of flowing freely.

Many men with enlargement of the prostate may have no further disturbance than the "nuisance" symptoms just mentioned. Again a case will get progressively worse until the patient is unable to empty the bladder and has to resort to a catheter to obtain relief. A bladder acutely distended with urine

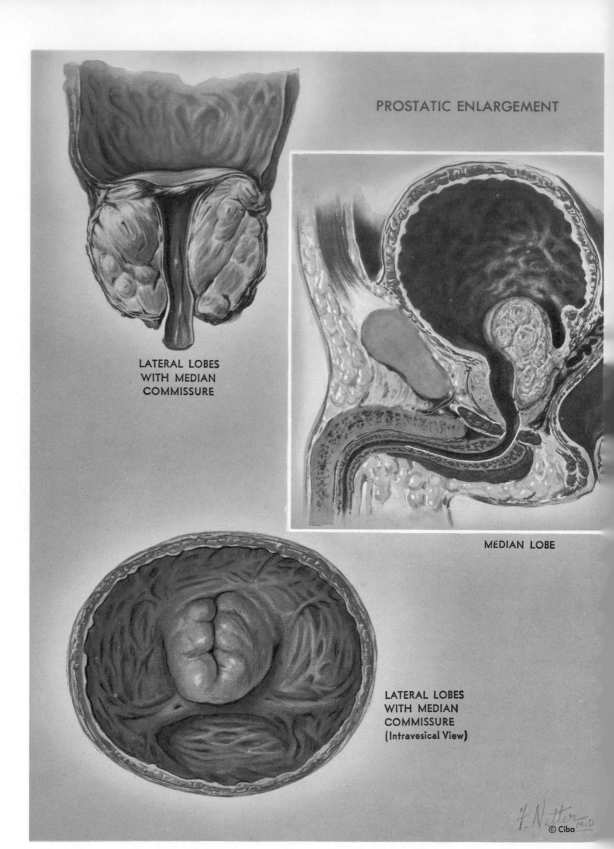

PROSTATIC ENLARGEMENT

LATERAL LOBES
WITH MEDIAN
COMMISSURE

MEDIAN LOBE

LATERAL LOBES
WITH MEDIAN
COMMISSURE
(Intravesical View)

is very distressing. After the urine has once begun to be drawn by catheter, the danger of infection of the bladder is very great; and all the symptoms and problems of cystitis are likely to result. (See chapter 22 of this volume.)

Enlargement of the prostate gland can be detected by a physician examining through the rectum. This sort of examination is also useful in detecting a possible cancer of the prostate. If a definite diagnosis cannot be made by this examination, use of a cystoscope may be necessary. This instrument is passed through the urethra into the bladder, making it possible for the physician to see the interior of this organ and judge as to what effect prostatic enlargement is having on the function of this organ.

Not all cases of prostatic enlargement require surgery with an external incision. In some cases it is possible to remove the gland by means of an instrument similar to a cystoscope passed through the urethral canal. The examining urologist's advice should be followed as to the type of operation most suitable in the individual case. After such an operation, the urethral opening sometimes has to be dilated one or more times, but this is a simple procedure and almost invariably succeeds.

What to Do

1. When symptoms suspicious of an enlarged prostate gland begin to be noticed, all spices, condiments, and other irritating substances should be eliminated from the diet to lessen the likelihood of irritating the bladder. Irritation promotes infection.

2. If it is known that the gland is already somewhat enlarged, it is wise to have an examination made by a physician two or three times a year to detect any increase in the danger of damming up the urine and creating back pressure from the bladder to the kidneys. A part of this examination should be the use of a catheter to draw off any urine

remaining in the bladder after voiding all that is possible in the natural way. This remainder is called residual urine.

3. When the enlargement becomes extensive enough to result in more than two ounces (60 cc.) of residual urine, when infection begins to result from the stagnant urine, or when the flow is temporarily stopped entirely, surgery may be needed; and it may be necessary to spend up to two weeks under the physician's care, preferably in a hospital, to prepare for the operation.

4. Hot half baths, and the avoidance of alcoholic liquor, of chilling, of getting the feet wet, of taking cold, or of holding the urine too long may aid in delaying the development of severe symptoms from prostatic enlargement, but the condition cannot be cured by home remedies or treatments.

PROSTATITIS (INFECTION OF THE PROSTATE).

Infection of the prostate gland may come through the bloodstream from some focus elsewhere in the body, but more often it comes from germs that pass upward through the urethra. On the other hand, a chronic infection in the prostate may in turn act as a focus of infection.

Sometimes the gland is acutely infected, or even abscessed. This causes frequency of urination, with pain and burning, both day and night; pain in the back, rectum, perineum, et cetera; blood or pus in the urine; a urethral discharge; chills and fever; and general prostration. With chronic infection, the chills and fever are not likely to be present, blood rarely shows in the urine, a urethral discharge is uncommon, and all the other symptoms are less severe; but there is likely to be a persistent feeling of fullness or discomfort in the region of the prostate gland.

A chronic congestion of the prostate, without infection, may result from sexual excitement, especially if not relieved by sexual intercourse; and it may produce a sensation of fullness in the external genitals, and sometimes generalized feelings of lassitude and nervousness. Under such circumstances, massage of the prostate, performed by a physician, usually relieves the symptoms.

What to Do

1. If symptoms give rise to a suspicion that an infection is present in the prostate, consult a physician. The prompt use of sulfas or antibiotics may quickly check the progress of the infection, remedies which, of course, a physician must prescribe.

2. Bed rest is advisable during the acute stage.

3. For relief of symptoms it is advisable to take a hot half bath daily, or twice a day if symptoms are severe. (See volume 3, chapter 20.)

4. Avoid alcoholic beverages, spices, condiments, and all irritating foods. The diet should consist largely of fruits and vegetables.

5. Drink plenty of water—at least two and a half quarts every day.

6. When the acute symptoms have subsided, or in a chronic case which had no acute stage, prostatic massage by a physician may be helpful.

SEMINAL EMISSIONS.

Once a boy reaches puberty (at about age twelve to fourteen), it is normal for his seminal fluid to overflow every week or two through the penis. This automatic discharge of seminal fluid is called a seminal emission, or "night loss." A married man may also experience such emissions if two weeks or more elapses between sexual intercourse.

The escape of seminal fluid in a seminal emission usually occurs during sleep and in connection with a dream about sexual matters, a perfectly normal process which should cause no concern. No attention should

be paid to charlatans or persons of abnormal sexual curiosity who may try to alarm a boy or young man by advising him on how to prevent seminal emissions.

STERILITY.

Sterility is the inability of a man to produce pregnancy in a normal woman. It may be because of abnormal or diseased testes that produce imperfect spermatozoa or none at all. Mumps can damage the testes in such a way as to render a man sterile. There may be an obstruction of the ductus deferens, which normally carries the sperm cells from the testes to the urethra. In some cases poor nutrition may be the cause. In others, too frequent sexual intercourse does not give the testes time to mature normal spermatozoa.

What to Do

1. See a physician and have an examination of the genital organs and an analysis of the sperm. Follow his instructions on treatment.

2. Avoid too frequent sexual intercourse.

3. Take a vitamin-rich and well-balanced diet, paying particular attention to vitamin E.

TESTICULAR TUMORS.

Tumors of the testes are not common, but it is important to detect them when present and to determine their nature. A firm, painless nodule or swelling in a testis may be a sign of a malignant growth, or of one which may eventually become malignant; and surgical removal may become advisable.

What to Do

If evidence of the possible presence of a tumor in a testis is noticed, consult a physician. He can make a definite diagnosis and possibly arrange for surgery. No time should be lost, for occasionally a tumor of high malignancy may develop in one of the testes.

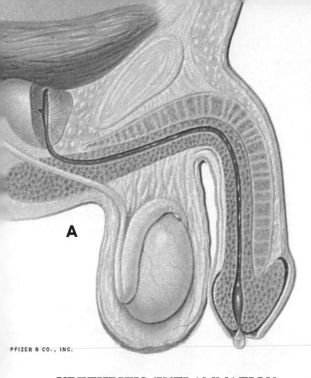

A. The male sex organs, showing inflammation of the urethra such as occurs in nonspecific urethritis. B. The inflammation sometimes extends into the epididymis and (C) also to the prostate.

URETHRITIS (INFLAMMATION OF THE URETHRA).

In urethritis the urethra (passage through which urine passes from the bladder to the outside) becomes intensely inflamed and a discharge escapes to the outside. The disease is listed here because it is more common in males. The most common cause is a gonorrheal infection. (See chapter 30 of this volume, on "Venereal Infections," under *Gonorrhea.*)

In some cases of urethritis it is not possible to identify any particular germ, and these are therefore called nonspecific urethritis. Even so there is usually pain in the urethra, at the tip of the penis, and in the testicles, and itching about the urethra.

What to Do

1. Consult a physician for the cause; then follow his recommended treatment, continuing it for a time even after symptoms disappear.
2. Abstain from sexual intercourse, from alcohol, and from coffee.

URETHRAL STRICTURE.

Urethral stricture is a narrowing or contracture of the urethra, the outlet tube of the bladder. It may result from accidental injury or from infection of the urethra, with scarring during the healing process. By far the most common cause is neglected gonorrhea. (See chapter 30 of this volume.)

What to Do

1. If because of a noticeable lessening of the size of the urinary stream a stricture is suspected, have a physician make an examination to determine the true nature of the condition.
2. If a urethral stricture is known or is found to be present, have a physician, preferably a urologist, gradually dilate it with special instruments.
3. If the condition has been neglected until no urine can pass, proceed as directed under *Urinary Retention.* (See under this item in chapter 22 of this volume.)

VARICOCELE.

Varicocele is a dilation or varicosity of the veins that carry blood from the testis and epididymis to the large veins of the abdomen. It is a common condition, most men having mild varicocele on the left side, especially during the years immediately following

391

puberty. The right side is much less frequently affected. The dilated veins feel somewhat like a bunch of earthworms at the side of the testicle and above it. Varicocele may sometimes cause a slight sensation of weight and mild, dragging pain; but it does not shorten life or cause a serious threat to health. A man with this condition should not allow himself to become frightened into using patent medicines to treat it—they cannot cure it.

What to Do

1. If the enlargement is not great, do nothing about it.

2. If the enlargement is large enough to give a sensation of weight and discomfort, wear a suspensory.

3. If the enlargement is extensive, which rarely happens, the condition can be cured by surgery. No other treatment is of any use.

Diseases of the Female Sex Organs

The female sex organs include the breasts, the ovaries, the oviducts, the uterus, the vagina, and the vulva. Their fundamental function is to help produce a new human being and nourish it until it can take other food than milk. In the production of such a new human being, no substitute has been found for either the ovaries or the uterus; however, the breasts all too often fail to do their duty, or they are discharged from the job without consideration of whether they should be or not.

Breast Diseases

ACUTE MASTITIS (INFLAMMATION OF THE BREAST).

The most common acute disorder of the breast is acute inflammation. It nearly always occurs during the early stages of the nursing period. Cracks or small injuries of the nipples usually precede the inflammation and prepare the way for the entrance of the disease germs which cause the trouble.

The inflammation occasionally affects only the nipples and the surrounding skin. In such cases careful cleansing of the nipples, with frequent applications of a saturated solution of boric acid, is all that is necessary. Boric acid solution, however, should not be applied to the nipples while the baby is being breast fed, unless thoroughly rinsed off with cooled boiled water after being applied.

When only the nipple or the nipple area is affected, the use of a nipple shield at the time of nursing is often helpful. Should tiny fissures (cracks) develop in the nipple, they can be painted with tincture of benzoin, which is readily available at the drugstore.

The inflammation is often more extensive, however, than described above, affecting deeper parts of the breast; and then it may not respond to simple treatment. It should be noted here that while we have been speaking of the breasts in the plural, an acute inflammation much more often affects only one breast rather than both of them.

The first signs and symptoms noticed when an infection begins to affect the deeper tissues of the breast are tenderness, pain, and swelling. There may be a chill, and the fever may be moderate or high, depending on the severity of the infection. In comparatively severe cases there will be a rapid pulse, with headache and other characteristic symptoms that usually accompany infection and fever.

Lower left, chronic cystic mastitis; center, cystic disease with single large cyst; right, benign tumor.

What to Do

1. When the first signs and symptoms of breast inflammation appear, consult a physician at once. The use of penicillin or some other antibiotic will usually prevent the formation of an abscess.

2. Take the baby off the breast so that the breast can be at rest.

3. There should be bed rest, but with toilet privileges.

4. Support the inflamed breast with a well-fitting brassiere or binder, which, however, should not be too tight.

5. The patient should be allowed to drink water freely, and as long as the fever lasts the diet should consist of soft and liquid foods only.

6. Cover the inflamed breast with a dry towel and lay an ice bag over the towel, keeping it in place for about two hours. The procedure should be repeated every three hours.

7. Do not try to pump milk out of the breast unless it becomes painfully engorged. If a physician is supervising the case, which will probably be true, he should give orders about the use of a breast pump.

8. If an abscess forms, the physician will take care of such surgical drainage as may be needed.

CANCER OF THE BREAST.

(See chapter 11 of this volume.)

CHRONIC CYSTIC MASTITIS.

This is the most common condition affecting the female breast, occurring, as it does, in about 5 percent of middle-aged women and, less frequently, in women of other ages. Usually both breasts are involved. In this condition, fluid-filled cavities of various sizes and in various numbers develop within the deeper breast tissues. These fluid-filled cavities (cysts) are often tender when compressed and are somewhat movable within the breast tissue.

Chronic cystic mastitis, of itself, is a benign condition. The importance of this condition, however, is that it produces lumps within the breast which feel very much like those which occur in a developing cancer. It is often impossible to tell, by simple examination, which condition, chronic cystic mastitis or cancer, is present. (See chapter 11 of volume 2 under "Common Locations for Cancer—Breast.")

What to Do

1. Have the lump or lumps examined by a physician as soon as possible. The only reliable way to detect or exclude cancer is to have a sample of the lump tissue removed

and studied under a microscope.

2. If cancer is found, arrange for surgery as soon as possible, since breast cancer begins to spread fairly early.

Miscellaneous Diseases of the Female Sex Organs

FEMALE GENITAL FISTULAS.

Accidents, infections, abscesses, malignancies, or tissue damage such as occurs infrequently at childbirth, may result in perforations or lacerations of various parts of the female genital tract; and fistulas of various sorts may be formed. There may be openings between the bladder and the uterus or the vagina, or between the urethra and the vagina, resulting in a dribbling of urine from the vaginal outlet. There may be an opening between the rectum and the vagina, with fecal material seeping into and out of the vagina. Other fistulas are rare.

What to Do

Arrange for surgical repair.

GENITAL HERPES SIMPLEX.

(See *Genital Herpes Simplex* in chapters 23 and 30 of this volume.)

Genital herpes simplex is a rather recent addition to the list of diseases that are acquired by sexual contact with an infected partner. This disease is caused by the herpes simplex virus type II which is a close relative of the virus that commonly causes skin eruptions at the border of the lips—so-called "cold sores."

Once this virus enters the tissues of a person's body, it tends to remain for the remainder of life. It causes two degrees of illness. The primary manifestation occurs at the time the virus is first acquired, and the symptoms during this primary illness are more severe than those occurring during the later, recurrent illnesses.

At the time of the primary infection, the individual feels ill with fever, loss of appetite, and general malaise. The lesions caused by the virus appear on the membranes of certain of the reproductive organs and on the skin areas of the genital region. These tiny vesicles may appear on the cervix of the uterus, on the lining of the vagina, on the vulva, on the perineum, and on the buttocks. Oftentimes the tiny vesicles break and form small superficial ulcers. Occasionally a single large ulcer may develop. These local lesions are often extremely painful.

In the primary illness the lesions of genital herpes simplex persist for a period of three to six weeks. In the recurrent attacks, which may occur unpredictably at later times, healing of the lesions usually occurs within seven to ten days.

There are two serious complications that may develop in connection with genital herpes simplex as it affects the female. One is the predisposing influence that this infection may have on cancer of the cervix of the uterus. Evidence now shows that cancer of the cervix occurs more frequently in women who have had an infection of herpes simplex.

The other serious complication is the possibility of transmitting this infection to the unborn child during pregnancy. This infection increases the risk of spontaneous abortion and also the risk that the child may be born prematurely. Even if the child is born at full term, there is a strong prospect that it will acquire the infection as it passes through the birth canal, and this infection is usually fatal for a newborn child. Many obstetricians, therefore, prefer to perform a cesarean operation for delivering the baby whose mother has genital herpes simplex.

What to Do

Inasmuch as genital herpes simplex is caused by a virus, there is no specific cure for the illness. The treatment program, therefore, is designed to ease the symptoms rather than to bring about a cure.

1. When the lesions of genital

herpes simplex are extremely painful, the discomfort can be relieved by the use of some analgesic (pain relieving medication).

2. The use of antiseptic compresses on the affected areas of membrane or skin will help to reduce the risk of an ordinary infection caused by bacteria. A suitable solution for such a compress is benzalkonium 1:4000. The antiseptic compress can be applied for 15 to 30 minutes to the affected area three or four times a day.

3. Should a secondary bacterial infection develop, it is then appropriate for antibiotics to be taken according to the doctor's directions.

4. The woman with genital herpes simplex should report to her doctor at regular intervals for examination and for his instructions relating to handling present conditions.

LEUKORRHEA.

Leukorrhea is not a disease, but it may be a symptom of some disease of the vagina, cervix, body of the uterus, oviducts, or some of the glands associated with the genital tract. It is a troublesome discharge of fluid containing pus or mucus or both. The discharge is usually white or whitish in color, which fact explains the word "leukorrhea." This word literally means "something white running or flowing down." Such a discharge is commonly present in chronic infections of the cervix, in gonorrhea, and in a host of other conditions, each of which may require its own specific treatment after careful study of its true nature by a physician.

A common and persistent form of leukorrhea results from an infection by a parasite called Trichomonas vaginalis. This infection affects the cervix and the membrane lining the vagina. It causes not only a discharge but a chronic inflammation with more or less itching and burning. Another parasitic infection which often causes intense itching and burning of the cervix and vaginal lining is that of Candida albicans, which produces a thick, white, cheesy vaginal discharge.

What to Do

Learn the cause of the discharge. It cannot be checked safely and permanently unless the cause is removed or corrected. Both detection and removal or correction usually require the aid of a physician. For each of the several causes of leukorrhea there is a specific treatment. It is especially important not to delay consulting a physician if the discharge between periods is at all blood-tinged.

PERINEAL LACERATIONS.

Some injury to the mother's pelvic outlet is unavoidable in childbirth. The tissues are more or less bruised, stretched, and torn. But with good obstetrical care the amount of laceration is usually so slight that it can be successfully repaired by a few stitches taken immediately after the delivery of the child. In spite of the best of care, however, bad lacerations, involving a large part of the pelvic floor, sometimes occur. The severity of the tear may not be apparent until a thorough examination is made a few weeks after delivery.

Unrepaired perineal lacerations may cause a feeling of heaviness in the pelvis, a sense of loss of support to the pelvic organs, pain in the ovaries, headache, general lassitude, physical debility, and nervousness. Constipation is common. The uterus is invariably in an abnormal position, pulling on some of the organs surrounding it and pressing on others. It may have sagged down to such an extent that the cervix protrudes from the vagina. Straining at stool causes the rectum to pouch into the vagina, producing what is called rectocele. Lack of proper support allows the bladder to pouch in on the front of the vagina, producing cystocele. This interferes with the proper emptying of the bladder, and

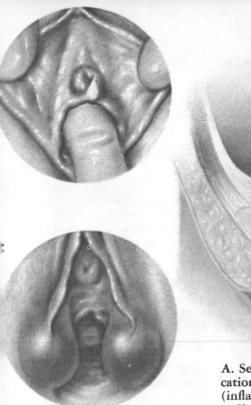

A. Sectional view of female sex organs, showing possible complications of nonspecific urethritis: urethritis, vaginitis, endometritis
(inflammation within the uterus), and salpingitis. B. Glands in
wall of urethra become involved in inflammation of urethritis.
C. Glands in wall of vulva frequently become inflamed as a
complication of urethritis.

cystitis may result. All these conditions taken together—and many of
them may exist at the same time—
result in a vast amount of discomfort
and ill health.

What to Do

If there are symptoms indicating
persistent results from cervical lacerations, have a physician, preferably a gynecologist, make a careful
examination. Have a perineal repair operation performed if he so
recommends. Surgical repair may
mean the difference between
chronic semi-invalidism and good
health.

STERILITY (INFERTILITY).

The inability of a woman to become
pregnant may be due to underdevelopment of some of the sex organs,
for which there is usually no cure,
though hormone injections may help
in some cases. It may also be caused
by constitutional conditions, or by
physical overwork, nervous tension,
endocrine disorders (especially ovarian), infections, tumors, cervical ero-
sions, or obstructions or strictures of
the oviducts. Before surgery or any
other extensive procedures are undertaken on behalf of the wife, consultation should be sought regarding sex
habits, and the husband's genital organs and semen should be examined.

What to Do

1. Consult a physician, preferably a gynecologist, to study the
cause of the trouble. He may be
able to detect it, and in some cases
to correct it.

2. Before going ahead with extensive corrective measures of the
wife's condition, have the husband
examined.

URETHRITIS (INFLAMMATION OF THE URETHRA).

Inflammation of the urethra is
commonly caused by a venereal infec-

tion. It can also be caused by other types of infection. In still other cases, no infectious agent can be demonstrated (non-specific urethritis). (For discussions of the symptoms and treatment, see the chapter on "Venereal Infections" under *Gonorrhea* and the chapter on "Diseases of the Male Sex Organs" under *Urethritis* in this volume.)

URETHRAL CARUNCLE.

Urethral caruncles are small tumors protruding from the urethral opening. They may be angiomas (blood-vessel tumors), small masses of granulation tissue growing from the membrane lining the urethra, or polyps. They are usually exceedingly sensitive and produce extreme pain on urination. A few of them become malignant.

What to Do

Do not attempt any home treatment. Consult a physician, preferably a urologist or a gynecologist, since surgery is the only effective remedy.

VAGINITIS.

(See *Leukorrhea* in this same subsection.)

VAGINAL (PUBO-COCCYGEAL) EXERCISES.

Many physicians are now recommending a simple exercise procedure to their women patients to strengthen the muscles and tone up the tissues of the perineum (in the region of the vagina). These exercises are especially beneficial (1) after childbirth, (2) in a case of urinary incontinence (dribbling of urine), (3) before surgery for the repair of old perineal lacerations, and (4) in a case in which sex relations are hindered because of the chronic relaxation of the perineal tissues.

The exercise is performed morning and evening (twice each day). It consists of voluntarily tensing the muscles at the outlet of the vagina as in the effort to prevent the flow of urine. The muscle tension is maintained for about six seconds and this is followed

by relaxation for six seconds. The 12-second sequence is repeated 12 to 24 times at each session (in the morning and again in the evening).

Ovarian Disorders

MENOPAUSE.

It is hardly proper to call the menopause a disease, because it comes naturally to every normal woman who lives out an average lifetime. But it is so often accompanied by various distressing symptoms that it is discussed here among the diseases of women's sex organs.

There is some logic, however, in considering it as an ovarian disorder. Menstruation begins as a result of the maturing of the ovaries, and it ends when their normal function ceases. The action of ovarian hormones has much to do with the changes in the lining of the uterus which produce the menstrual flow, and the use of ovarian hormones is often a useful remedy for the unpleasant symptoms of the menopause.

Menstrual periods normally come about once a month from puberty to the menopause, except during pregnancy or lactation. As the menopause, or change of life, approaches, there is often an irregularity of the flow—a missing of a period, or too frequent or too profuse flows. The menopause usually comes at about age forty-eight, but it may occur several years earlier or somewhat later.

At this time the pelvic organs begin to shrink in size, and the sex organs lose their reproductive power. As the menopause approaches, women often have hot flashes followed by chilliness. Some of them fail in general health, lose weight, and have a poor or capricious appetite. There may be reflex nervous symptoms—nausea, vomiting, and disturbances of the action of the heart or other organs. There may also be extreme weakness, depression, and even melancholia. All the symptoms that commonly plague women seem to crowd in during the menopause—headache, backache, digestive disturbances, fainting, constipation, diarrhea, soreness of the breasts, nervousness, et cetera.

The duration of the menopause varies greatly in different women. Some cease menstruating abruptly with no disturbing symptoms at all. On the average, the nervous and irregular menstrual symptoms last from a few months to a year or two. With some women the discomfort and nervous symptoms may persist for many years.

The menopause is a critical time in the life of a woman; and, before she reaches it, care should be taken to avoid disturbing influences as far as possible and to put the body into as good a condition of general health as can be attained. Much of the suffering that accompanies the change of life could be avoided by careful treatment of menstrual disorders before this time comes and by maintenance of good general health, both physical and mental.

What to Do

1. Light work, outdoor exercise, plenty of sleep, a wholesome diet, and tonic treatments such as daily cold mitten frictions could usually improve the general health and make the menopausal symptoms less severe. (See volume 3, chapter 20, for treatment procedures.)

2. Hormones taken under the direction of a physician are often helpful in relieving the headache, nervousness, and hot flashes characteristic of the menopause in many women. The physician may give the hormones by injection or prescribe them to be taken by mouth.

OVARIAN TUMORS.

Some tumors of the ovaries come as a result of abnormal developments in connection with the normal function of the ovaries. The ovaries normally produce the ova, or egg cells, any one of which, when fertilized by union with a male sperm, can develop into a child. Each of these ova lies in a separate sac in the ovary, and at a certain time in relation to each menstrual period one of them should normally escape when the sac containing it bursts. The little sacs (follicles) containing the ova sometimes fail to burst, however, and gradually become distended with fluid, forming troublesome ovarian cysts.

Cysts of other origin may also form in an ovary. Some of them can reach an immense size if not discovered and removed in time. These very large ovarian cysts, however, are rarely seen in places where the services of modern surgeons are available because they are discovered and removed before they reach such a large size. Cases are on record in the experience of missionary doctors where a woman weighed scarcely half as much after the removal of such an ovarian cyst as she did before it was removed.

One type of ovarian cyst is called a dermoid. This type is peculiar in that various body structures, such as bones, teeth, or hair, are found in the cysts. Solid tumors of the ovary also occur. Any tumor of the ovary may, as it becomes larger, produce pain and abdominal distention. All ovarian tumors that do not subside spontaneously within a short time should be surgically removed, as harmful or dangerous complications may occur if they are allowed to remain in the body and grow.

Some ovarian tumors are cancerous, or may become so, though the great majority are nonmalignant. The possibility of cancer, however, is another reason to have them removed.

What to Do

1. As soon as the presence of an ovarian tumor is suspected, consult a physician, preferably a gynecologist, and have him examine the condition to find out whether or not such a tumor is present.

2. If a tumor is found, arrange to have it surgically removed.

ECTOPIC PREGNANCY (TUBAL PREGNANCY).

(See *Tubal Pregnancy* in this list; also volume 3, chapter 15.)

Uterine Diseases

ABSENCE OF MENSTRUATION (AMENORRHEA).

Amenorrhea is a condition in which the menstrual flow fails to appear for one or more months during the time between puberty and the menopause. That which occurs during pregnancy or lactation is normal, of course, and needs no treatment. Fundamentally, amenorrhea may not indicate a disease of the uterus at all, the fault being elsewhere; but the uterus is the organ in which its manifestations appear.

It is a symptom, and not a disease. The condition occurs fairly often during the first few years after puberty. When it occurs in girls past the age of fifteen, it is most often because of overwork, excessive study, some infectious disease, heart disease, or merely emotional tension. As some women put on weight, they have a diminished flow; or the flow may entirely cease. This does not preclude pregnancy, though it makes it less likely.

Amenorrhea may be due to an obstruction in the cervical canal or to some malformation of the female organs. In rare cases the uterus remains in an infantile state; and, though hormone injections may help, as a rule no treatment does any good. Most cases of cervical obstruction and some cases of organ malformation can be corrected by surgery; but a cure of amenorrhea in the majority of cases must come from removal, correction, or treatment of the underlying cause by other than surgical methods.

What to Do

1. Give attention to the afflicted person's program of work or study, and to her general health habits. The way to cure her amenorrhea may thus become obvious. To change her work or study program may be difficult, but amenorrhea from these causes is not of itself a cause for alarm.

2. If the girl or woman is in run-down condition, correct the health habits. She should take an adequate amount of nourishing food. She should take at least an hour of moderate physical exercise in the open air every day. A cold mitten friction should be taken every day, except the days when the menstrual flow is due (or in progress). Alternate hot and cold applications every week would be helpful. (For a description of these treatments see volume 3, chapter 20.) She should get at least nine hours of sleep a night.

3. If the cause of the amenorrhea is not obvious, or if it is something that home treatments cannot cope with, consult a physician. Some causes of amenorrhea cannot be detected without study by a physician, and some of the most effective treatments for it must be professionally administered.

CANCER OF THE UTERUS.

(See chapter 11 of this volume.)

CERVICAL LACERATIONS.

Childbirth is always attended by some injury to the cervix (the outlet of the uterus). Small lacerations usually heal without trouble. Extensive lacerations, however, may cause much discomfort and ill health. Chronic inflammation of the membrane lining the uterus and a disagreeable discharge from the vagina are common complications of neglected cervical lacerations. Old, unrepaired, eroded lacerations predispose to cancer, a common and most serious disease of the cervix.

About six weeks after childbirth, every mother should return to her physician for a pelvic examination, at which time, if needed, treatment may be given to the cervix to prevent the development of possible chronic trouble. If this were done following every delivery of a child, and if the examination were repeated annually thereafter, most cases of cervical cancer could be prevented or detected at an early curable stage. Much suffering would thus be avoided and many lives saved.

What to Do

Follow the pelvic examination program outlined above, and have any abnormal conditions repaired without delay.

DISPLACEMENTS OF THE UTERUS.

The uterus is held in position by four pairs of ligaments, by the muscles and fascia below, and by the fat found in the tissues of the pelvis. The organ may be displaced backward, sideways, or downward.

Tumors of the uterus may drag or push it into various abnormal positions. Tumors located in any of the surrounding structures may displace it by pressure. Lastly, imperfect development of the supporting structures of the organ may result in displacement.

Displacement of the uterus.

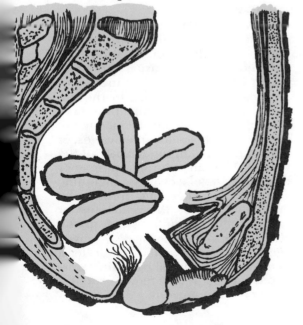

Only two types of uterine displacement may cause trouble. One is retroversion, or a backward tipping of the organ. This backward tipping may be accompanied by a sagging downward also. The most common position of the body of the uterus is forward and upward.

The other type of displacement is prolapse, or a settling downward of the organ, which is sometimes so extreme that the cervix protrudes from the vulva, and may drag down with it a part of the bladder and of the rectum. This condition is more common after the change of life than before. Loss of weight, weakening of the ligaments, and unrepaired lacerations are the chief causes of this downward sagging.

A displacement may be responsible for a woman's being unable to become pregnant; and, if she does conceive, abortion may result. With the backward position, the supporting ligaments may be stretched, causing congestion of the oviducts, ovaries, and uterus as they are pulled back into the hollow of the sacrum against the rectum. Other results are backache low over the sacrum, constipation, and menstrual pain. Most retroversions, however, are symptomless.

What to Do

1. If there is discomfort, and if displacement of the uterus is suspected, have a physician, preferably a gynecologist, make an examination to determine the true condition. If he finds the condition sufficiently serious, he may advise the insertion of tampons or pessaries into the vagina to help support the uterus. The doctor may recommend surgery.

2. If it is not necessary to have surgery or to use tampons or pessaries, and if the displacement is backward, as is usually the case, the following measures are recommended:

A. Avoid heavy lifting as far as possible, and do not stand any more than necessary while at work.

B. Build up the general health by taking moderate exercise, plenty of rest, a balanced diet, and hot half baths. (For a description of this latter treatment, see volume 3, chapter 20.)

C. If the displacement is due to a heavy uterus which has failed to return to its normal size after childbirth, a cold rubbing bath every day except during the menstrual period may help.

DYSMENORRHEA (PAINFUL OR DIFFICULT MENSTRUATION).

There are two forms of dysmenorrhea: the primary or congenital form in which no abnormality can be found in the pelvic organs, and the secondary or acquired form in which an examination reveals some abnormal condition as the cause of the pain. The acquired form may be the result of pelvic inflammation, tumors of the ovary or uterus, or obstruction to free uterine drainage. Obstruction may be caused by scar tissue following surgery or by a small tumor in some part of the uterine canal, most often in the cervix.

Many cases of dysmenorrhea can be partly or wholly relieved without the aid of a doctor, and it is recommended that the advice given below be tried before consulting one. Correct health habits will do much toward making the female organs function properly and without distress. It is remarkable what favorable results sometimes follow the correction of constipation. Taking cold, exposure to cold or wet, mental stress, late hours, and dissipation are common causes of pain at the menstrual periods, especially if they occur a short time before the flow begins; and one way to avoid such pain is obvious.

For the relief of pain, heat is the best local application. Heat or any other means of increasing the pelvic circulation will often help the flow to start; and, once the flow is well started, pain and other unpleasant sensations as a rule will gradually subside except in cases where obstruction is causing the trouble.

What to Do

1. Two days before the expected time for the flow to begin, reduce the amount of work done and increase the amount of rest. Take a warm tub bath or a warm half bath each evening for half an hour. (See volume 3, chapter 20.)

2. When the flow starts, go to bed and keep hot-water bottles to the feet and lower abdomen.

3. A hot saline enema will help both to clear the bowels and to relieve the pain. (See volume 3, chapter 19.)

4. Fomentations over the lower abdomen and lower part of the back often give relief from pain. (See volume 3, chapter 20.)

5. If distress persists after giving the above program a fair trial, consult a physician. He may find by examination that some obstruction is the cause of the trouble. If so, surgery may bring relief. If not, he may be able to give other useful advice, including the use of a mild analgesic.

ENDOMETRIOSIS.

Some comparatively young women, often sterile and troubled with irregular and painful menstruation, are afflicted with this unusual condition, which is characterized by masses or patches of tissue similar to the endometrium (the membrane lining the uterus). These may be attached to the lower part of the colon, the ovaries, or other structures in the vicinity of the uterus. When the uterine lining goes through its regular changes, including swelling and bleeding, during the menstrual cycle, these masses or patches of tissue do the same, giving rise to pain and hemorrhage. A physician can usually detect or at least guess at the condition by ordinary examination, but it may require surgical exploration to prove it.

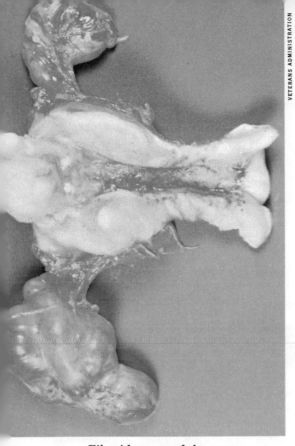

Fibroid tumor of the uterus.

What to Do

1. If irregular and painful periods are not known to have some other cause, a physician should study the case to detect possible endometriosis. The likelihood of it is greater if the woman concerned is sterile.

2. Medical treatment for suppressing of menstruation may relieve the distress, but the remedies used may have undesirable side effects.

3. Surgical removal of the abnormally placed tissue may be necessary.

FIBROID TUMORS OF THE UTERUS (FIBROMYOMAS).

Fibroid tumors of the uterus are composed partly of muscle tissue growing from and resembling the muscle in the walls of the organ. Tumors of this sort are rarely found elsewhere in the body. With this special muscle tissue are intermingled varying amounts of fibrous connective tissue. Fibroids are usually multiple—that is, several occur at the same time in the same organ. They vary much in size, from that of a pea to immense masses weighing two pounds or more. They are approximately spherical in shape, except when influenced by pressure, and are firm in consistency. Their cause is not known. They are hardly ever malignant.

When located in the lower part of the uterus, fibroid tumors are a source of danger during childbirth. If they are still lower down in the cervix or mouth of the uterus, they may press upon the bladder and the rectum. If located in the body of the uterus and close beneath its lining membrane, they usually cause profuse and prolonged menstruation, sometimes to the extent of menacing life from loss of blood. The discomfort and the hemorrhage tend to increase until the sufferer must remain in bed during the whole period of menstrual flow. There may be a feeling of weight in the pelvis, with backache; and, if the tumor is at all large, definite pressure symptoms may occur, such as irritation of the bladder, with a frequent sensation of need to urinate. The pressure sensations in the rectum are somewhat similar, but they are accompanied by chronic constipation. Pain does not come, as a rule, until the tumor has reached considerable size. Chronic anemia is common because of the abnormally profuse menstrual flow. Leukorrhea may be troublesome between the periods.

What to Do

1. If the tumor or tumors cause no symptoms, no treatment is needed. They should be watched for changes, however.

2. No medicine or home treatment is of any use.

3. When symptoms give rise to a suspicion of the presence of fibroid tumors, consult a physician, preferably a gynecologist. His examination will detect a tumor or tumors of

any considerable size. Surgical removal is the only cure; and if the tumors are large or numerous, it may be necessary to remove the entire body of the uterus.

HEMORRHAGE FROM THE UTERUS.

Excessive bleeding from the uterus most often occurs in connection with the menstrual periods, in which case it is called menorrhagia. Bleeding at other times is called metrorrhagia. The most frequent causes of uterine hemorrhage are the following:

1. Fibroid tumors, especially those located near the lining membrane of the uterus. (See above.)

2. Uterine polyps.

3. Cancer of the body of the uterus, of which either menorrhagia or metrorrhagia may be a complication.

4. Hyperplasia of the endometrium, a condition in which the membrane lining the uterine cavity is overgrown, thick and soft, and full of blood vessels.

5. Ovarian cysts. (See under subheading "Ovarian Tumors" in the previous subsection of this chapter.)

6. Retention of a portion of the placenta following childbirth.

7. General debility.

8. Endocrine gland imbalance.

9. Disordered circulation because of disease of the heart, liver, or lungs.

What to Do

1. For all sufferers from excessive menstrual flow, especially if they are debilitated, every possible effort should be made to build up the general health between periods, giving emphasis to moderate exercise, ample rest, and an abundant, nourishing, and easily digestible diet.

2. Between periods, a debilitated patient may benefit by a daily cold mitten friction. (See volume 3, chapter 20.)

3. More than the usual care is needed during and immediately after any childbirth so that the uterus will be restored to its normal size and not become a large, soft, and soggy organ.

4. It is important to determine the cause of the hemorrhage. A physician should study the case. Successful treatment will depend on dealing with the cause, and there is no single treatment that will succeed in all cases. Surgery or other treatments that can be given only by a physician may be needed.

5. Frequently the anemia produced by the excessive loss of blood requires special treatment.

PUERPERAL INFECTION.

The cause of puerperal infection is the entrance of disease germs, especially streptococci, into the exposed tissues of the cervical canal and the uterine cavity at the time of childbirth, miscarriage, or abortion. It is practically impossible to keep the vulva and vaginal tissues free from germs; therefore the introduction of instruments, fingers, or other objects into the birth canal or uterus, while sometimes necessary, is always accompanied by some danger of infection. Proper sanitary procedures during delivery, however, would prevent most cases of puerperal infection.

Such infections are always serious and may be fatal. The inflammation may extend from the uterus to the ovaries or to the tissues around the uterus, causing abscesses, and to the general peritoneum, resulting in peritonitis. In some cases the infection involves the large veins of the pelvis and the thighs, producing thrombophlebitis, or "milk leg."

A woman who has apparently been doing well after delivery, a miscarriage, or an abortion may have a rise of temperature, possibly preceded by a chill, on the third or fourth day. There may be no pain at all. The sudden rise in temperature in such a case indicates the strong possibility of puerperal infection and signals the urgent need for obtaining prompt professional care.

What to Do

1. If the symptoms give rise to a suspicion of puerperal infection, be sure that the woman concerned is under the care of a physician. Suitable sulfas or antibiotics given early will usually control the infection.

2. Do not use vaginal irrigations of any kind without a physician's orders, and he is not likely to order them.

3. Give the patient all the water she will drink.

4. As long as acute symptoms persist, keep an ice bag applied to the patient's lower abdomen twenty minutes out of each hour.

5. The diet should be abundant, but should consist only of soft and liquid foods as long as the fever persists.

6. When the acute symptoms have subsided, keep the patient out in the open air as much as possible.

Diseases of the Oviducts

INFLAMMATORY DISEASE OF THE OVIDUCTS (SALPINGITIS).

Inflammation of the female reproductive organs occurs in connection with three kinds of infection: that of gonorrhea (60 percent of cases), that produced by streptococcic and staphylococcic organisms (35 percent of cases), and that of tuberculosis (5 percent of cases). Although more than one of the pelvic organs and their surrounding tissues may be involved, it is usually the oviducts that are most seriously affected. Such an inflammatory involvement of the oviducts is called salpingitis.

The germs of gonorrhea gain access to the female reproductive organs by way of sexual intercourse with a partner already infected with this disease. The germs first cause an infection of the tissues in the vicinity of the vulva and the lower part of the cervix of the uterus. Then the infection follows the lining of the uterus upward and enters the oviducts, where it usually causes the greatest damage. It may continue through the oviducts to involve the peritoneum and the ovaries. This involvement of the oviducts may occur promptly after the initial gonorrheal infection or it may occur some time later—even years later. The lining membrane of the oviduct is virtually destroyed. There may be abscess formation. The oviduct is no longer capable of transmitting the ova, and permanent inability to become pregnant is a usual complication.

Infection by streptococcic or staphylococcic organisms usually begins as a puerperal infection (see discussion of puerperal infection under "Uterine Diseases" in the previous subsection of this chapter), in which these germs enter the tissues or the cervix of a uterus which has been unfortunately injured at the time of childbirth or miscarriage or, more commonly, in connection with an abortion. In this type of infection the germs find their way into the tissues which surround the uterus and are then carried by the veins and lymphatic vessels to the oviducts. The lining of the oviducts is not always destroyed in this type of infection, and thus in some cases it is still possible for the patient to become pregnant after the infection subsides.

Involvement of the oviducts by tuberculosis is always secondary to a tuberculous infection in some other part of the body, usually the lungs. The germs are carried to the oviducts by the blood. Early cases of tuberculous salpingitis may respond favorably to the administration of drugs now used for the treatment of tuberculosis in other parts of the body. Usually, however, it becomes necessary sooner or later to have the involved tissues removed by surgery.

Symptoms of salpingitis vary somewhat with the type of infection. In acute gonorrheal salpingitis the patient experiences severe pain in the lower abdomen with distension of the abdomen. There is nausea, vomiting,

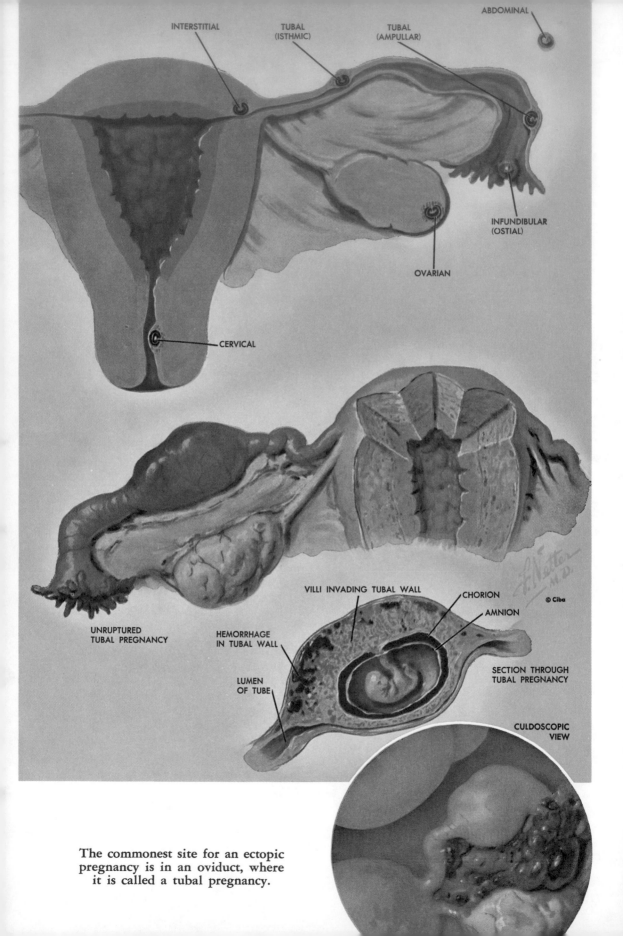

INTERSTITIAL

TUBAL (ISTHMIC)

TUBAL (AMPULLAR)

ABDOMINAL

INFUNDIBULAR (OSTIAL)

OVARIAN

CERVICAL

VILLI INVADING TUBAL WALL

CHORION

AMNION

HEMORRHAGE IN TUBAL WALL

SECTION THROUGH TUBAL PREGNANCY

UNRUPTURED TUBAL PREGNANCY

LUMEN OF TUBE

CULDOSCOPIC VIEW

The commonest site for an ectopic pregnancy is in an oviduct, where it is called a tubal pregnancy.

fever, and rapid pulse. In the septic type of salpingitis (that produced by streptococcus or staphylococcus organisms) the patient is weak with pelvic pain and possibly has chills along with the fever. In tuberculosis of the oviducts the symptoms are usually not as severe as in the other types, but pelvic pain is common and persistent, usually becoming worse at the time of menstruation. Sometimes there is excessive uterine bleeding. Often the complaint which brings the patient to the doctor is the inability to become pregnant.

What to Do

For the first two types of acute salpingitis the general program for the care of the patient is as follows:

1. Keep the patient in bed with the head of the bed raised eighteen or twenty inches higher than the foot (Fowler position).

2. Give the patient soft food including abundant fluid.

3. Take care to prevent the patient's becoming dehydrated. Dehydration may occur quickly on account of the vomiting.

4. Provide heat to the pelvic region. The best method is by hot sitz baths in which the patient sits in a specially designed tub of hot water while his knees and legs hang over the edge of the tub. (At home, use hot tub bath, with patient sitting up. See volume 3, chapter 20.) The temperature of the water should be gradually increased up to the patient's tolerance. The treatment should last about twenty minutes and may be given two or three times a day.

5. The physician in charge will doubtless prescribe a course of sulfonamides and antibiotics chosen to combat the specific infection.

6. When the acute phase has passed, the physician may recommend surgical removal of damaged tissues and organs.

For cases of tuberculous salpingitis, the first motive in caring for the patient is to combat the tuberculous infection, using the general principles of patient care mentioned in the chapter on tuberculosis (chapter 29 of this volume). If the case is taken early, the physician will doubtless prescribe drugs effective in combating tuberculosis. Even in a late case, these drugs are useful as a preparation for the surgical removal of the pelvic organs involved in the infection.

TUBAL PREGNANCY.

In an occasional case of early pregnancy the united sex cells fail to make their way into the uterus as is normally the case. In such event, the unborn child will begin its development wherever the united sex cells happen to lodge. This constitutes a so-called ectopic (misplaced) pregnancy. By far the commonest site for an ectopic pregnancy is within one of the oviducts, where it is called a tubal pregnancy.

The usual cause of a tubal pregnancy is that the oviduct is inflamed or so narrowed that the product of conception does not have room to pass through the remaining portion of the oviduct and on into the uterus.

The hazard of tubal pregnancy is that the tissues of the oviduct are not designed to stretch as much as are those of the uterus. Thus, after about three months of development, the fetus has grown to such proportions that it causes the oviduct to rupture, producing a serious hemorrhage for which prompt surgical treatment is the only satisfactory remedy. In the meantime, the unborn child perishes.

Introduction

Of all the organs and systems of the body, it is the brain and its associated structures in the nervous system that are of greatest importance to the normal functioning of the body and to the general welfare of the individual. Reasons for this top level importance are clear: (1) The activities of all other organs and tissues are controlled by nervous impulses received from the brain and spinal cord; (2) the brain is the coordinating agency for all nervous activity; and (3) the brain is the seat of consciousness and of all psychic functions related to consciousness.

When a portion of the nervous system is damaged by disease or injury, a corresponding deficit in function ensues, either in the part of the body normally controlled by the damaged structure or in the related activities of the brain. When demonstrable changes take place in some part of the brain, the spinal cord, or the nerves, we speak of "Nervous Disorders"—dealt with in the first part of this chapter. When there are no demonstrable changes in the tissues of the nervous system, even though the individual's brain functions abnormally, we speak of "Mental Disorders"—subject matter of the second part of this chapter.

Nervous and Mental Disorders

Nervous Disorders

PLEASE NOTE: It is urged that the following introductory pages be consulted before reading the discussions of individual diseases which follow. The basic understanding of the causes and manifestations of the nervous disorders thus acquired will enable the reader to place a better evaluation on the particular nervous disease in which he is interested.

General Considerations. The brain and spinal cord are composed of very fragile tissue. Both are protected by bones, the former by the skull and the latter by bony components of the vertebrae. In addition these organs are surrounded by durable fibrous coverings (the meninges), which provide further protection from injury. Thus, despite their delicate nature, these organs of the central nervous system fare very well under normal conditions. But once they are attacked by disease, once their supply of blood is curtailed, or once they receive a mechanical impact violent enough to injure their delicate tissues, their welfare is in jeopardy. And when a part of the nervous system is deranged, other parts of the body, or even the entire body, suffer also.

In the case of nervous disorders, home treatment is usually not appropriate. Furthermore, the outcome of most nervous disorders often depends upon whether the condition is recog-

nized early enough to allow adequate and appropriate care to be given in time to save the life or at least to minimize permanent damage.

When symptoms develop which indictate disease of the nervous system, a physician should be consulted promptly. Every physician is trained in the recognition and handling of the usual nervous disorders, but a specialist will be needed for those more complex.

Common Causes for Nervous Disorders

Many diseases and conditions involve the nervous system, some affecting only the organs of the nervous system but others, more general in nature, affecting additional parts of the body. The most common causes of nervous disorders are listed as follows:

A. *Developmental Defects.* When congenital faults of development affect the nervous system, the results to

409

the individual depend upon just what part of the nervous system is affected and on the degree of severity of the defect. Hydrocephalus—an enlargement of the head due to an increase of cerebrospinal fluid within the brain—is an example of developmental defects that may affect the central nervous system.

B. *Infections and Inflammatory Disorders.* These may affect the brain, spinal cord, or nerves just as they affect other tissues of the body. Two examples are encephalitis and meningitis.

C. *Toxic, Metabolic, and Nutritional Disorders.* These are conditions that often affect the entire body as well as the nervous system. Toxins produced by germs (as in tetanus, diphtheria, and botulism), absorption of certain heavy metals (such as lead), or the ingestion of certain chemical agents (such as alcohol), commonly cause damage to the brain and other tissues of the nervous system. Examples of metabolic disorders which affect the nervous system are phenylketonuria and diabetes. The nervous system is particularly susceptible to deficiencies in the diet, as when the B vitamins are insufficient.

D. *Trauma.* Although the organs of the nervous system are well protected by their bony coverings, falls or car accidents resulting in head or back injury may cause serious damage. In contusion, the delicate brain tissue is damaged by impact or by shearing stresses which pass through its substance causing varying degrees of disruption of the tissue. Hemorrhage into the brain or spinal cord may cause damage by disruption of the tissue and also by the pressure of the resulting blood clot. In some cases of injury the healing process involves the development of extensive scars which may irritate the delicate tissues of the brain so as to cause convulsions. In some injuries nerves are torn as they leave the brain to pass through the skull, or anywhere along their course to the structures they serve.

E. *Vascular Disorders.* The blood supply to the brain and spinal cord is very generous—necessarily so because the cells of these active tissues are critically dependent on a continuous supply of oxygen and nutrient materials, and on the removal of the products of brain metabolism. When the blood vessels of the body become diseased, the brain and spinal cord often suffer more quickly and more seriously than do other organs. Certain symptoms of senility are the result of a gradual diminution of the blood supply to the brain. When the blood supply to a particular part of the brain or spinal cord is shut off the resulting symptoms are related to the malfunction of this part. This is the usual background of a "stroke" in which a vessel becomes obstructed.

F. *Tumors.* Tumors of the brain and spinal cord are classed as "benign" if they do not invade the surrounding tissue, or "malignant" if they do invade the surrounding tissues. Even the benign tumors can cause serious symptoms and can threaten the patient's life by pressing against neighboring parts of the nervous system. In many cases of tumor of the brain or of the spinal cord early surgical removal of the tumor will remedy the situation. Brain surgeons have become very skillful in gaining access to most parts of the nervous system.

Common Symptoms Produced by Nervous Disorders

The human nervous system, consisting of brain, spinal cord, and the many nerves that reach out to all parts of the body, may be compared to a modern communications network. If there is a "break in the lines" at any point, the "territory" that is normally served by the broken "lines" will no longer be able to exchange messages with the headquarters. That is, if the nerve fibers that control a group of muscles are severed, these muscles will be paralyzed even though they may be at some distance from the actual site of the injury. Also, if some of

Traumata of the Brain

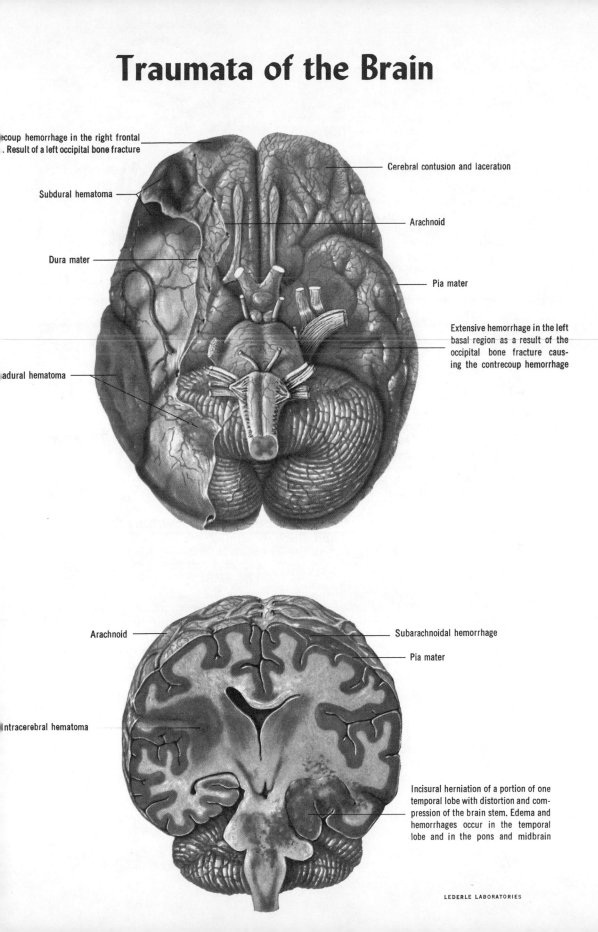

...coup hemorrhage in the right frontal... Result of a left occipital bone fracture

Subdural hematoma

Dura mater

...adural hematoma

Cerebral contusion and laceration

Arachnoid

Pia mater

Extensive hemorrhage in the left basal region as a result of the occipital bone fracture causing the contrecoup hemorrhage

Arachnoid

...ntracerebral hematoma

Subarachnoidal hemorrhage

Pia mater

Incisural herniation of a portion of one temporal lobe with distortion and compression of the brain stem. Edema and hemorrhages occur in the temporal lobe and in the pons and midbrain the fibers which normally bring sensations from a certain part of the body to the brain are severed, the particular sensations carried by these fibers can no longer reach the brain and thus loss of feeling in that particular part of the body will result. The loss of the ability to detect certain sensations that should come from a particular part of the body is called anesthesia.

The important symptoms of nervous disorders are more directly related to the particular part of the nervous system affected than to the specific cause of the disorder. Although a few areas of the brain can be affected without producing specific symptoms, most areas, when involved by disease or injury, cause interference in the control of muscles, in the functions concerned with sensations or with movement.

The common symptoms occurring in connection with nervous disorders are listed as follows:

A. *Abnormalities of Movement (of Muscle Action).* One of the functions of the nervous system is to control the activities of the muscles throughout the body. When those parts of the brain and spinal cord concerned with muscle activity become diseased or when the nerve connections between the central nervous system and the muscles are affected, the action of the muscles will be correspondingly altered and the particular type of these alterations will give a clue to the nature of the disease. The common kinds of abnormality of movement are:

1. Weakness. Weakness consists of a reduced power to use the muscles in the normal manner. For a discussion of the symptom of weakness, see volume 3, chapter 22, "List of Signs and Symptoms," under *Weakness.*

2. Paralysis. Paralysis, in contrast to weakness, involves a total inability of a muscle or muscle group to respond to voluntary commands rather than simply a reduced ability. The various kinds of paralysis and their general causes are considered in volume 3, chapter 22, "List of Signs and Symptoms," under *Paralysis.*

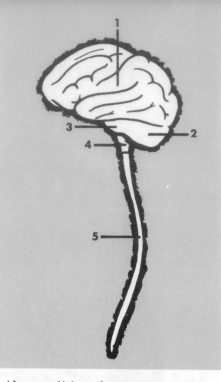

Abnormalities of movement correspond with impairment in specific areas of the brain or nervous system; such as (1) cerebrum; (2) cerebellum; (3) pons; (4) medulla oblongata; (5) spinal cord.

3. Spasticity and rigidity (stiffness). In conditions of health certain mechanisms cause the larger muscles of the body to remain firm, enabling a person to maintain his posture, for example without his having to give continuous thought to the movements of his body. When the person desires to use these same muscles in some rapid movement, the mechanism otherwise causing them to remain firm is automatically canceled out so that they can now move quickly. In certain diseases of the brain and spinal cord this ability to release the muscles from their contracted state is lost so that they remain firm even when the person desires to move them quickly. Spasticity may be seen in cases of stroke. Spasticity is somewhat different from paralysis because the muscles may still retain their power but lack their ability to respond quickly.

4. Involuntary (uncontrollable) movements. Certain disorders of the

412

nervous system, such as chorea and athetosis, cause spontaneous, purposeless movements involving certain muscles or muscle groups. For a more lengthy description see volume 3, chapter 22, "List of Signs and Symptoms," under *Movements, Abnormal.*

5. Gait disturbance. Walking is such a complex function that many types of disturbance of the nervous system may interfere with its normal progress. Gait may be altered by weakness, paralysis, spasticity, lack of coordination, disturbed sense of position, and even by hysteria.

6. Tetany. Tetany is a condition in which the muscles become abnormally responsive to stimulation. It occurs in the disease tetanus (see under *Tetanus* in chapter 28, "Infectious Diseases," in this volume), in conditions where the amount of calcium in the blood drops to low levels (as in hypoparathyroidism), or in conditions of alkalosis as when a person loses acid from the stomach by excessive vomiting or when a nervous person breathes too deeply with consequent loss of carbon dioxide from the body. Tetany also occurs in certain nervous disorders in which cells within the brain become abnormally responsive to the ordinary stimuli.

B. *Disturbances of Speech and Swallowing.* Both of these functions require a high degree of integration of muscle action. Disturbances of speech are particularly significant because they may indicate difficulty not only in the control of the muscles by the brain but in the intellectual processes. These disturbances are discussed in volume 3, chapter 22, "List of Signs and Symptoms," under the separate headings of *Speech Disturbances* and *Swallowing, Difficulty in.*

C. *Convulsions.* A convulsion usually consists of the abrupt occurrence of violent involuntary contractions of the muscles, often accompanied by loss of consciousness. For a discussion of the various causes of convulsions, particularly as these relate to disturbances in the brain, see the item on *Convulsions* in volume 3, chapter 22, "List of Signs and Symptoms."

D. *Disturbances of General Sensations.* By general sensations we refer to those that come from the skin, the membranes, and the muscles (pain, temperature, touch, position) as opposed to those which come from the organs of special sense (vision, hearing, equilibrium, taste, and smell).

When a given sensation is lost, such as of pain, temperature, or touch, we speak of "anesthesia," or else we speak of a loss of position sense. Oftentimes this loss of sensation is limited to some particular part of the body, and the physician interprets from this clue what part of the nervous system is affected. If irritation of the sensory nerve fibers causes abnormal sensations, such as the feeling of "pins and needles," we then speak of "paresthesia." If a normal sensory experience is exaggerated, we speak of "hyperesthesia."

E. *Headache.* Headache is perhaps mankind's most common symptom, occurring in many disorders of the nervous system. Its many causes and its possible involvements with other bodily ailments are summarized in volume 3, chapter 22, "List of Signs and Symptoms," under *Headache.*

F. *Dizziness.* Dizziness is a very uncomfortable symptom in which the individual receives a false sense of motion. There are several possible causes of this symptom, some being more mysterious than others. For a detailed discussion, see volume 3, chapter 22, "List of Signs and Symptoms," under the heading of *Dizziness.*

G. *Impairment of Vision.* Impairment or loss of vision should be taken seriously, and a physician who specializes in diseases of the eyes or of the nervous system should be consulted for an evaluation. Not all impairments of vision relate to the eyes themselves, for the difficulty may be in the pathways of nerve fibers that pass between the eyes and the brain or even in the tissues of the brain cortex.

Oftentimes defects of vision follow a significant pattern; for example, a restriction in the right side of what is seen by the right eye and in the left side of what is seen by the left eye (bitemporal hemianopsia, as in pituitary tumor). A person may not notice such a pattern of sight loss unless he checks the vision of each eye separately. For discussions on other impairments of vision, see in this volume, chapter 15, "Diseases of the Eye," and in volume 3, chapter 22, under *Eyes, Symptoms Pertaining to.*

H. *Unconsciousness.* The term "consciousness" is difficult to define, though the difference between the conscious and the unconscious state is easy enough to recognize. Perhaps the closest we can come to a definition of consciousness is to describe it as the normal functioning of a person's mental faculties to the extent that he is aware of his present circumstances and alert to what is going on around him.

Consciousness, in its broad sense, requires the normal functioning of the whole brain. Whatever interferes with a certain function of the brain interferes, to this extent, with the full experience of consciousness. Placed in the order of increasing impairment of consciousness, we may mention such terms as dullness, lethargy, stupor, and coma. A decrease in awareness of one's surroundings does not necessarily indicate a serious nervous disorder. It may only mean a temporary deficit in the blood supply to the brain, such as occurs in fainting, or the presence of toxins produced by germs causing some generalized disease. However, it may indicate a concussion or pressure produced by a tumor. Impairments of consciousness must therefore be evaluated by a physician. For further information see volume 3, chapter 22, under *Coma* and *Stupor.*

I. *Hallucinations and Delusions.* Hallucinations are false sensory experiences, the individual concerned seeming to hear, see, or smell something when, actually, his eyes, ears, or olfactory organs are not being stimulated in a manner to produce these sensations. Since some hallucinations are the result of abnormal stimulation of the brain areas where these sensations are ordinarily perceived, their occurrence justifies a study of the case by a physician or a specialist in nervous diseases.

Delusions are false beliefs to which an individual adheres in spite of evidence to the contrary. A person with delusions may confuse his identity with that of another, or he may draw conclusions that are false with respect to the information in hand. Delusions are more typical of mental disorders than of nervous disorders, but they may occur in either.

Consideration of the Individual Nervous Disorders

ABSCESS OF THE BRAIN.

An abscess of the brain is a localized infectious process with destruction of tissue. It is usually caused by the staphylococcus germ or sometimes by the streptococcus or the pneumococcus. The infection may be introduced at the time of a fracture or a penetrating wound of the skull or may spread from some neighboring area such as from an infection of the inner ear or an infection of the mastoid cells of the skull. In other cases the infection originates in the lungs or the heart and is brought to the brain by way of the bloodstream.

The symptoms of abscess of the brain vary considerably from case to case. In some cases the symptoms of brain abscess are generalized, relating more directly to the infectious process. These include chills, fever, loss of appetite, and a general feeling of illness. Other symptoms are caused by the irritation of the covering membranes (the meninges) and, possibly, of the brain cortex. These include stiffness of the neck and convulsions. Still other symptoms are caused by the disruption or compression of certain nerve fibers as the abscess enlarges.

In some cases, in fact, the only symptoms of an abscess of the brain may be those relating to the nervous system.

Abscess of the brain is always a serious condition and carries a mortality rate of up to 50 percent even with the best of care. It deserves prompt and adequate professional care. The treatment requires attention to the infection involved and to the need for surgical drainage of the fluid-filled abscess cavity.

AMYOTROPHIC LATERAL SCLEROSIS.

This is a rather rare, progressive disease which affects men more commonly than women and typically occurs above age forty. There is a degeneration of the nerve cells and fibers which supply the muscles of the body, with more and more cells and fibers being involved as the disease progresses. The average length of life after onset may be expected to be about three years.

Weakness and atrophy of muscles are the characteristic manifestations. The number of muscles thus involved gradually increases and various parts of the body may be affected, the most serious development being interference with breathing, swallowing, and chewing.

In spite of extensive studies, the cause of this disease is not yet known, nor has a satisfactory remedy been found. The patient should be encouraged to avoid fatigue; but he should remain as active as possible. Annual death rate in the United States from this disease is about one per 100,000 population.

ATAXIA.

A. *Cerebellar Ataxia.* This is a manifestation of disease of the cerebellum—that part of the brain located in the back part of the skull. Disease of the cerebellum from any cause may produce the main symptom of ataxia, failure of muscle coordination. There is no loss of muscle power as in paralysis but rather a series of back-and-forth groping movements when any precise action is undertaken. Writing and speaking are seriously handicapped. The development of ataxia indictes the need for professional care by a specialist in nervous disorders.

B. *Friedreich's Ataxia.* This hereditary disease is dominant in some families and recessive in others. It usually begins in childhood or youth and is characterized by unsteadiness and tremor. In addition to the lack of coordination of muscle movements, there is a paralysis of certain muscles and a lateral curvature of the spinal column.

No specific treatment is known. The disease progresses slowly, with death occurring, usually, at about the age of twenty.

BELL'S PALSY.

(See *Facial Paralysis* in this chapter.)

CEREBELLAR ATAXIA.

(See *Ataxia: A. Cerebellar Ataxia* above.)

CEREBRAL PALSY (LITTLE'S DISEASE).

The usual manifestation of this illness is an impairment of the control of the muscles (more commonly in the legs) coupled with spasticity (stiffness) and with awkward, jerking movements. The extent of the involvement and the severity of the manifestations will vary a great deal from case to case. There may be convulsions, impaired speech, and a degree of mental deficiency; but in many cases mentality remains quite normal. Some patients may be unjustly assumed to be mentally deficient because of their awkwardness and difficult speech.

The cause of cerebral palsy is not always clear. Either localized or diffuse damage to the brain which may have occurred prior to the time of birth or during the birth process, may cause it. Other possibilities include an inadequate supply of oxygen to the brain, mechanical injury, developmental defect, intrauterine encephalitis, and brain damage caused by some toxic agent. Sometimes the infant appears to be handicapped from the time of birth with vomiting, irritability, and difficulty in nursing. In many cases the manifestations of the disease are noted first when the child is about six months old, the evidences being a delay in the ability to sit up, crawl, and stand.

Many children with this affliction are capable of living relatively normal lives. The handling of a case centers around speech training, muscle reeducation, the wearing of braces, special tutoring in school, and vocational guidance.

CERVICAL RIB.

A small percentage of persons develop an extra rib on one or both sides, just above the usual first rib. This extra rib is in the lower part of the neck. Resulting symptoms, when they occur, are caused by a squeezing of nerves and blood vessels leading to the arm and lying between the extra rib and the scalenus anterior muscle. The symptoms are made worse when the arm is used for weight carrying or when it is raised for long periods above the head as in hanging up clothes or in washing walls. Usually the patient experiences no difficulty until adulthood. The symptoms consist of pain, tingling, numbness, and coolness in the forearm and hand, often on the side of the little finger. The muscles of the hand in this same area may atrophy.

This combination of symptoms is typical of several circumstances which cause damage to the roots of those nerves which supply the arm. Sometimes the symptoms occur when there is no extra rib, being caused by the pressure from other structures.

When the condition is not severe, the symptoms can be relieved by the avoidance of lifting with the involved arm and by care in supporting it by a pillow during sleep. For an overweight person, reducing often helps. In more severe cases, treatment requires surgery and usually involves the removal of the rib.

CHOREA.

Two principal diseases carry this name. As will be seen from the descriptions which follow, they differ greatly except that they present the common feature of purposeless, jerking, involuntary movements.

A. *Huntington's Chorea.* This hereditary disease is characterized by purposeless, jerking, involuntary movements and by progressive mental deterioration.

Symptoms usually appear about age thirty or forty. The purposeless movements and the mental deterioration usually appear concurrently, but in some cases one group of symptoms precedes the other. The purposeless movements consist of grimacing, lurching, and an unsteady, waltzing gait characteristic of drunkenness. As the disease progresses, the muscles become progressively weaker.

The mental symptoms vary from case to case, some patients being very cheerful and others suspicious, spiteful, and destructive. The intellectual faculties gradually deteriorate until the patient must be cared for in an institution. The disease usually progresses to death in about ten to fifteen years.

Many of the nerve cells throughout the brain and spinal cord show evidences of deterioration. The specific nature of the disease is not understood, but inasmuch as it runs in families as a dominant characteristic, it is advised that persons born into such families deliberately abstain from parenthood so as not to pass this disease on to children.

B. *Sydenham's Chorea (Saint Vitus's Dance).* Sydenham's chorea is a disorder of childhood characterized by rapid, involuntary, jerking movements which are irregular and purposeless. It occurs more commonly in females and is most frequently manifest between the ages of five and fifteen. As the illness begins, there is a clumsiness and a tendency to drop things. Presently the purposeless, involuntary movements begin and involve almost all muscles except those of the eyes. Purposeful movements can usually be executed but are performed in a jerky fashion. Coordination is poor, and a certain degree of weakness may develop. Chewing and swallowing may become difficult. Recovery usually occurs in six to ten weeks. In about one third of the cases, the illness recurs at some later time.

Although the exact cause of Sydenham's chorea is not known, a relationship to rheumatic fever and prior streptococcal infections seems probable. About half of all young patients with rheumatic fever develop chorea; and about three fourths of all chorea cases develop in persons who have had or are having rheumatic fever.

There is no specific treatment for Sydenham's chorea, but rheumatic fever should be looked for and treated when present. It is advised that a child ill with this disease should be kept quiet at home or in a hospital. Sedation may be necessary. As much attention should be given to his peace of mind as to his physical comfort. Certain procedures of hydrotherapy such as warm baths, fomentations, and continuous flowing baths may be helpful. (See volume 3, chapter 20.)

CONCUSSION.
(See *Head Injury* in this chapter.)

CONVULSIVE DISORDERS.
The cause of convulsions is not fully understood, but they are associated with a functional disturbance of the cortex of the brain such as can be demonstrated by the electroencephalogram (tracing of brain waves). Children are more prone to convulsions than are adults and may outgrow the tendency. In some instances, however, convulsions begin in later life.

A major ("grand mal") convulsion consists typically of the abrupt occurrence of violent, involuntary contractions of the body muscles, usually accompanied by loss of consciousness. The attack is often of short duration, but may recur.

Recurring convulsions are commonly called epilepsy. The duration and severity of the attacks may vary from case to case. In susceptible children diseases with high fever or ordinary breath holding (such as during a tantrum) may bring on convulsions. Convulsions may occur in persons with low blood sugar or low blood calcium. They may occur when the blood's reaction becomes more alkaline than normal as in continued deep breathing, persistent vomiting with loss of acid from the body, or the taking of too much alkali by mouth. They may occur when a confirmed alcoholic suddenly stops drinking or when a person addicted to barbiturates suddenly discontinues the drug.

Conditions that reduce the blood in certain parts of the brain or otherwise irritate it may cause convulsions: brain tumors, cerebral infections, brain injury, or diseases of the blood vessels within the brain.

Convulsions may occur in eclampsia, a serious complication of the latter period of pregnancy. They may also occur in cases of tetanus (lockjaw).

The occurrence of convulsions, especially in an adult who has not been known to have convulsions previously, should be considered a clue to some underlying disease. Therefore the services of a physician should be secured promptly. It will then be the physician's responsibility to discover the nature of the underlying condition and arrange suitable treatment. In the meantime, the patient should receive appropriate first-aid care, such as outlined in volume 3, chapter 18, "Handling Emergencies," under the item *Convulsions*.

DISK, HERNIATED.
(See *Spinal Injuries* in this chapter.)

ENCEPHALITIS.

Encephalitis is discussed in this volume in chapter 28, "Infectious Diseases," under the heading *Encephalitis, Epidemic*.

In the present connection, it is important to notice that certain nervous manifestations tend to appear after apparent recovery from the acute disease.

Among patients who recover from epidemic encephalitis some later develop residual nervous disorders which are often grouped under the term "chronic encephalitis." Some develop, after ten or more years, a form of parkinsonism. (See the item on *Parkinsonism* in this chapter.) Others develop disorders of the personality, including irritability and asocial types of behavior. Narcolepsy develops in some cases. (See the item on *Narcolepsy* in this chapter.) Some develop various abnormal movements of the muscles such as tics, grimaces, or tremors. Occasionally an oculogyric crisis occurs (uncontrollable turning of the eyes upward), which renders the patient helpless until it subsides, spontaneously or after rest.

EPILEPSY.

(See the item on *Convulsive Disorders* in this chapter.)

FACIAL PARALYSIS (BELL'S PALSY).

In facial paralysis the patient loses function of the muscles of facial expression on one side of the face. These muscles are supplied by the facial nerve. Although the basic cause often is not known, the paralysis results from a malfunction of this nerve. It is impossible for the patient to close the eye or wrinkle the forehead on the affected side of the face. The mouth droops on the involved side and is drawn to the opposite side when the person smiles.

Facial paralysis often causes undue alarm because of its being confused with the same types of paralysis in a stroke. However, in a stroke the

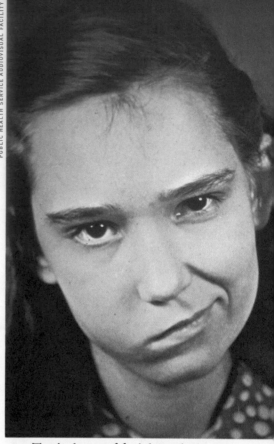

Typical case of facial paralysis.

weakness is mainly in the lower part of the face with little or no involvement of the muscles about the eye and forehead.

In favorable cases, improvement begins within two weeks. In other cases recovery may take several months, and in rare cases, the paralysis may be permanent.

What to Do

There is no specific remedy for facial paralysis, although some medicines prescribed by the doctor may hasten recovery. Because the eye on the affected side does not close securely during the course of the illness, it is important to protect the eye so that its membranes do not become injured and infected. A soothing solution designed for use in the eye should be dropped into the space behind the eyelids at least twice a day. A piece of Scotch tape placed across the affected eyelid serves to keep it closed during sleep. Heat and gentle massage to the muscles of the face on the paralyzed side will help to prevent their sagging by becoming stretched

FAMILIAL PERIODIC PARALYSIS.
(See *Paralysis, Familial Periodic* in this chapter.)

FRIEDREICH'S ATAXIA.
(See *Ataxia, B. Friedreich's Ataxia,* in this chapter.)

HEADACHE, MIGRAINE.
(See *Migraine* in this chapter.)

HEAD INJURIES.
A general description of head injury plus instructions on first aid for the victim of a head injury is given in volume 3, chapter 18, "Handling Emergencies," under the title *Head Injuries.*

The more common types of head injury are listed as follows:

A. *Skull Fracture.* Often the actual fracture of the skull is not serious in itself, but concurrent injury of the brain may be. Skull fracture may be complicated, however, by bleeding inside the skull, which can cause damaging pressure against the brain. Also when a fragment of the skull is depressed, the surgeon must relieve the pressure against the underlying brain tissue by elevating that portion of the bone. A compound skull fracture is often complicated by endriven fragments of bone. These may permit the entrance of infection into the tissues of the brain. It is desirable to enlist the services of a neurosurgeon in such a case. In some extensive skull fractures, the cerebrospinal fluid, which is watery in appearance, may escape from the nose or from one or both of the ears. For the emergency care of skull fracture, see the item on *Fractures: Fractures of the Skull* in volume 3, chapter 18, "Handling Emergencies."

B. *Concussion.* In concussion there has been sufficient shock to the brain

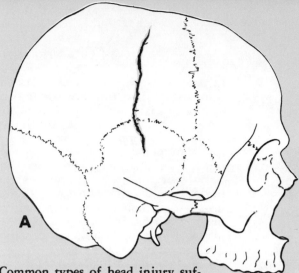

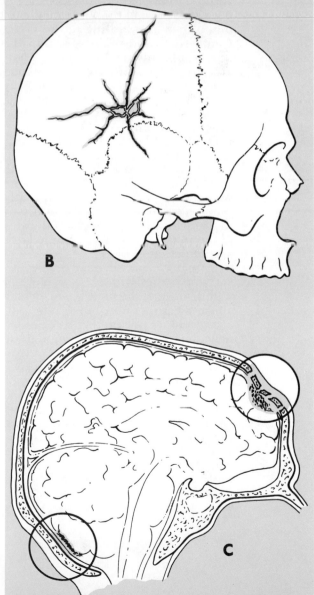

Common types of head injury suffered in accidents: A. Fracture. B. Compound fracture. C. Cerebral contusion and laceration.

to produce some impairment of consciousness. The duration of unconsciousness is a rough measure of the severity of the damage to the brain. Often concussion is associated with a loss of memory for events just preceding the head injury (retroactive amnesia). In minor head injuries the period of unconsciousness seldom lasts more than a few minutes. In major injuries, the unconsciousness may last for several hours or possibly even several days.

C. *Cerebral Contusion and Laceration.* In severe head injuries the surface of the brain may become bruised and/or torn. There may be hemorrhage into the brain substance or into the space around the brain, and generally there is swelling of the brain. Confined as the brain is within the bony skull, this swelling poses a hazard. In severe injuries with these complications surgical intervention may be necessary in order to control the hemorrhage or to relieve the increased pressure within the skull.

D. *Hemorrhage.* Hemorrhage into the brain substance often occurs in connection with a severe injury in which the brain is damaged (see the preceding paragraph). Frequently bleeding into the brain tissue occurs in many locations throughout the area of the injury without any single large accumulation of blood.

In many cases of head injury, associated either with skull fracture or with tearing of the membranes which surround the brain, bleeding will occur and an accumulation of blood may develop either between these membranes or between these membranes and the skull. Oftentimes such an accumulation of blood develops slowly. As time passes and the blood clot degenerates, it absorbs fluid and swells. The swelling produces such pressure against the brain as may endanger the patient's life. This critical complication of hemorrhage inside the skull may develop several days or even several weeks after the original head injury. The only satisfactory remedy is to remove the blood clot through a surgical opening.

It is important that the person who has suffered a severe head injury be observed carefully during his period of recovery. In case there is a secondary lapse of consciousness, impaired speech, or dragging or weakness of a limb, such a condition should be reported promptly to the physician, for once the pressure produced by a blood clot becomes great enough to interfere with consciousness, the relief of the pressure must be accomplished quickly if the patient's life is to be saved.

E. *Damage to the Cranial Nerves.* In some cases of skull fracture, particularly those involving the base of the skull, there may be damage to certain of the cranial nerves at the site where they leave the skull. The nerve most commonly damaged is the olfactory nerve, which conveys impulses for the sense of smell. Other nerves, such as the optic nerve or the auditory nerve, may also be damaged.

Aftereffects of Head Injuries. In many cases of head injury certain symptoms follow which are collectively called the "postconcussion syndrome." This group of symptoms, which may persist for some time after the injury, includes headache, dizziness, difficulty in concentrating, and certain alterations in the personality. The severity of the symptoms may not correlate with the severity of the injury. In favorable cases in which the individual receives adequate medical care, the symptoms gradually disappear. In other less fortunate cases the symptoms interfere with the patient's return to normal life, causing prolonged disability.

Another possible complication of severe head injury is the later development of recurring convulsions. These are presumably caused by the irritation of the brain by scar formation. Such convulsions are usually treated by the use of anticonvulsant drugs. In an occasional case, surgery is indicated.

HERPES ZOSTER.

For a description of this disease, see chapter 28, "Infectious Diseases," under the heading *Herpes Zoster*, also chapter 12, "Skin Diseases," under *Shingles*, both in this volume.

The disease is self-limited, usually terminating after several days. In the meantime, the treatment consists essentially of relieving the intense pain by appropriate medication and of preventing secondary infection of the skin lesions. Occasionally, in elderly individuals, the pain persists even after the lesions have healed (postherpetic neuralgia).

HUNTINGTON'S CHOREA.

(See *Chorea, A. Huntington's Chorea* in this chapter.)

HYDROCEPHALUS.

Hydrocephalus is a condition in which the head enlarges because of an excessive accumulation of cerebrospinal fluid inside the skull. Cerebrospinal fluid is a watery fluid most of which is produced within the internal spaces of the brain (ventricles). It circulates slowly throughout the brain spaces and throughout the space between the exterior of the brain and the membranes which enclose it and the spinal cord. Normally the cerebrospinal fluid is absorbed at the same rate it is produced; but in hydrocephalus, there is either an overproduction of cerebrospinal fluid, a reduction of absorption of the same, or most frequently a blocking of its normal flow. Thus the amount of fluid gradually increases, producing pressure within the skull.

Many cases of hydrocephalus are congenital. In such a case the infant's head becomes enlarged and portions of the brain atrophy because of the increased pressure. Usually, the enlargement of the infant's head is not noticeable until several weeks or months after birth. If the condition is not successfully treated, death may be expected within months or a few years.

PUBLIC HEALTH SERVICE AUDIOVISUAL FACILITY

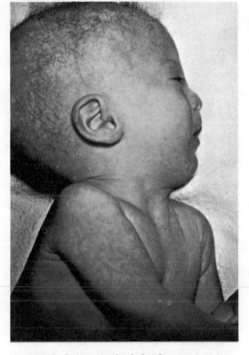

Case of congenital hydrocephalus.

By certain surgical procedures the excess cerebrospinal fluid can be drained away through an implanted plastic tube which empties into a vein, a body cavity, or the heart itself. The opinion of a neurosurgeon should be obtained regarding the advisability of such treatment.

INJURY.

(See *Head Injuries* and *Spinal Injuries* in this chapter.)

KORSAKOFF'S SYNDROME.

Korsakoff's syndrome consists of a defect of mental function characterized by confusion of thinking, defective memory for recent events, and a tendency to confabulate—invent answers to questions whose real answer the patient does not know. The memory defect is so severe that the patient may not remember things which happened a few minutes previously. Familiar faces and surroundings are forgotten, so that the afflicted person does not know where he is or the time of day or the day of the week.

This aggravates his mental confusion and causes him to be anxious.

Korsakoff's syndrome typically occurs in persons who are long-time users of alcohol. It is presumed to be the result of a deficiency of the B vitamins niacin and thiamine.

Korsakoff's syndrome occasionally occurs in persons who have not used alcohol but who have suffered brain damage from head injuries or other injuries to the brain. The syndrome is sometimes associated with polyneuritis. (See under *Neuritis* in this chapter.)

What to Do

Appropriate treatment usually brings about some improvement, but complete recovery is seldom realized. The treatment consists of withdrawing alcohol and of administering large doses (20 to 50 mg.) of thiamine chloride (vitamin B₁) daily for a week or more. Some physicians prefer to use the total vitamin B complex in this condition rather than just the vitamin B₁. This should be followed by the administering of smaller doses of thiamine chloride or by having the patient drink powdered yeast in iced milk three times a day. It should be made certain that the patient does not resume the use of alcohol—not even small amounts.

LITTLE'S DISEASE.
(See *Cerebral Palsy* in this chapter.)

MENIERE'S DISEASE.
(See *Meniere's Disease* in chapter 16 of this volume.)

MENINGITIS, ACUTE.
(See chapter 28, "Infectious Diseases," in this volume, under the heading *Meningitis*.)

MENINGITIS, TUBERCULOUS.
Tuberculous meningitis develops secondarily to a tuberculous infection in some other part of the body—usually the lungs. It may develop in a patient totally unaware of any such infection.

The disease occurs most frequently in children between one and five years of age, but it may occur at any age.

The onset of the infection of the meninges (the coverings of the brain) is usually gradual with symptoms of irritability, drowsiness, headache, loss of appetite, vomiting, and a mild fever. The drowsiness may progress to stupor, and convulsions may develop. Certain of the cranial nerves may be affected, with resulting difficulties in vision and hearing. Without treatment, tuberculous meningitis usually leads to death within about three months.

The patient should be under the care of a physician well informed on the intensive treatments of tuberculosis. Most important is specific drug therapy, but the patient's general nutritional needs must be met adequately, even to the extent of using artifical feedings as may be indicated. Treatment must be continued for many weeks.

MENINGITIS CAUSED BY FUNGOUS INFECTIONS.
Several kinds of fungous infections may involve the meninges. Examples of fungous infections which may cause meningitis are actinomycosis, cryptococcosis, candidiasis, coccidioidomycosis, blastomycosis, and histoplasmosis.

The symptoms are often those of a subacute meningitis. In other cases the onset of symptoms is sudden, and the disease progresses rapidly to a fatal outcome. The symptoms are headache, dizziness, vomiting, and usually stiffness of the neck.

Drugs which are fairly effective are available for the treatment of most of these fungous infections, but before beginning treatment the physician must identify the fungus which is causing the infection. This requires hospitalization and extensive laboratory procedures.

MIGRAINE.

Migraine is a functional disorder in which the afflicted person experiences distressing symptoms in recurring episodes, with the attacks coming at intervals of a few days to as long as a month or more. The outstanding symptom is a severe headache which is often limited to just one side of the head. The attack is usually preceded by certain unusual sensations, such as the seeing of bright or colored lights, which a person soon learns by experience indicate the onset of another attack. During the attack there is often severe nausea and vomiting. The attack lasts for several hours, ends spontaneously, and leaves the person rather exhausted.

Migraine may begin at any age, sometimes in childhood, and, once established, may continue for many years.

More than half of the persons who have migraine belong to a family in which migraine has occurred in other relatives—grandparents, parents, and brothers and sisters. Migraine occurs somewhat more frequently among women than among men. In women, migraine attacks frequently are related to menstruation. The attacks may lessen or disappear during the period of the menopause. They may increase or decrease during pregnancy.

Persons who have migraine are usually perfectionists who drive themselves relentlessly toward reaching some goal. Possibly the reason migraine tends to run in families is that persons in the same family have similar personality characteristics.

What to Do

1. The first consideration in dealing with the problem of migraine is to evaluate the individual's personality by helping him to discover what factors provide him with stress and unsolved tensions. There may be certain circumstances that tend to bring on an attack of migraine. In other cases, however, the attacks seem to occur at somewhat regular intervals regardless of the immediate circumstances. These persons need to learn to be more at ease—at their job, at home, and in pursuing their ambitions. In order to relieve the migraine attacks, it may be necessary to change to a job that is more enjoyable. It may mean facing up to some family problem that bothers the sufferer. It may mean finding some form of enjoyable recreation that provides physical activity to counterbalance the mental strain under which the individual finds himself. It may mean a reevaluation of religious philosophy. It may involve radical altering of life-style.

2. Certain kinds of medication are quite effective in relieving the symptoms of a migraine attack. These should be used only under a doctor's supervision. The primary emphasis, however, should be on finding the basic cause of the tendency to migrain attacks rather than on relieving the symtoms when the attacks occur.

MINIMAL BRAIN DYSFUNCTION SYNDROME. (MBD, HYPERACTIVE CHILD, HYPERKINETIC CHILD.)

This designation refers not to a specific disease, but to a group of behavior abnormalities affecting children in which a child of near normal intelligence may have one or more of the following characteristics: hyperactivity, listlessness, impulsiveness, aggressiveness, low tolerance for stress, short attention span, difficulty in learning to read or write, difficulties in muscle coordination. This group includes the "problem children" that are perplexing to the parents and the teachers alike.

Oftentimes there is some unusual circumstance in the child's past history which, presumably, may have caused his handicap. There may have been a difficult labor at his birth. He may have been a premature infant.

423

His mother may have had complications during her pregnancy or at the time of his birth. He may possibly have had an attack of mild encephalitis which was considered to be only "flu."

In such cases, there may or may not be some structural changes in the brain tissue. The electroencephalogram (brain wave tracing) may be perfectly normal or may show only slight variations from normal.

What to Do

The treatment of a case of minimal brain dysfunction syndrome involves cooperation between parents, teacher, and physician. The parents need to establish and maintain an atmosphere at home in which the child feels comfortable, and yet one in which he is not treated as being different or abnormal.

The teacher's role in dealing with children who have minimal brain dysfunction syndromes is one that requires patience and ingenuity. When facilities at school make it possible, children with this difficulty should have their schoolwork adapted to their particular problems so that they receive special tutoring and considerable encouragement as they make rather tedious progress. Some of the larger schools provide special classes conducted by teachers who have had particular training in the handling of such cases.

Obviously there is no magic cure for the problem of minimal brain dysfunction syndrome. In most cases, the problem will resolve itself spontaneously as the child matures. There may be mild evidences of the former problems that have carried over into adulthood. For the most part, however, children with this problem can make satisfactory adjustments to adult life. The drugs that have been used in an effort to aid the children in this category have varied all the

way from tranquilizing drugs to stimulating drugs. Surprisingly, it is the drugs with the effect of stimulating the brain function that seem to have accomplished the best results even though the child is described as being hyperactive. Presumably the beneficial effect of stimulating drugs is to make the child more alert with a longer attention span, and thus more susceptible to the learning process. In some cases, a combination of stimulating drugs and tranquilizers has given good results. More important, however, is the combined patient efforts of parents and teachers as they encourage such a child to react favorably to his environment.

MONGOLISM.

Mongolism is a serious congenital condition characterized by mental retardation (intelligence quotient between 20 and 50), stunted growth, small skull, coarse and scanty hair, flat face, depressed bridge of the nose, short and thick hands and feet, and a laxity of the ligaments. Mongolism is so named because there is a lateral upward slope to the eyes somewhat similar to that of the Asiatic races. Mongolism occurs about once in 600 births and accounts for nearly 10 percent of feeblemindedness. Mongolism is usually associated with the defect in the chromosomes which is designated as "trisomy 21." By this it is meant that the chromosomes designated as "pair 21" produce three individual chromosomes rather than the usual two, giving a total of forty-seven chromosomes in each cell of the body rather than the normal forty-six.

Because of the congenital nature of mongolism, it is understandable that no cure for it exists. The problem of caring for a child with this abnormality centers around training him to do as much as it is possible for him to do and sheltering him from life's competitions. Some cases are best cared for by relatives, whereas others would fare better if placed in an institution.

MULTIPLE SCLEROSIS.

This slowly progressive disease involves various parts of the central nervous system and presents numerous symptoms which tend to come and go only to return again in greater severity. The symptoms usually begin between ages twenty and forty, men and women being affected about equally. In some cases the progression of the disease is so slow that the patient lives out a normal life-span and dies of some other cause. In other cases the disease progresses to a fatal outcome in five to ten years. Early in the course of the disease the patient will appear to be perfectly normal during the periods of remission.

A tremendous amount of research is being carried forward in the hope of discovering the basic cause of multiple sclerosis. At the time of writing the evidence points to a virus as a probable cause. The lesions of multiple sclerosis which interrupt the nerve pathways are characterized by a loss of the usual insulating material (myelin) which covers the nerve fibers.

The symptoms vary a great deal from case to case and from time to time in the same case. The mental symptoms may include lack of judgment, inattention, and frequently, unwarranted optimism, but occasionally depression. There is often a reduced emotional control. In some cases there are convulsions; in some, abnormal or reduced sensations; and in others, spasticity or weakness in certain parts of the body. Some patients have difficulty in talking. In many cases there are episodes of double vision or partial blindness. Scanning speech is a common symptom as are also tremors and impaired coordination.

What to Do

As yet no cure is known for multiple sclerosis. Effort should be made, therefore, to help the patient live as nearly a normal life as possible, consistent with his physical and mental condition. He should use moderation in all he does and avoid fatigue. Physical therapy measures are useful. Among the benefits from physical therapy is the preventing of deformities of those parts of the body that may be weakened or paralyzed.

MUSCULAR ATROPHY.

Another name for this disease is "familial progressive spinal muscular atrophy of childhood"—a rare disease with many characteristics of a recessive hereditary disorder. In some family lines, however, it is transmitted as an incomplete dominant trait. The onset of symptoms is usually within the first year of life. Although the child is mentally alert and able to smile and recognize his family members, he does not learn to sit up and stand as a normal child does. He has poor control of his head and there is difficulty in swallowing. Eventually he develops difficulty in breathing. Inability to contract the muscles becomes progressively worse, and death usually occurs in about five years.

For purposes of comparison with other diseases it should be mentioned that the difficulty here is in the nervous control of the muscles, not in the muscle tissue itself. There appears to be a reduction in the number of nerve cells which normally activate the muscles and also a loss of the insulating layer (myelin) on the nerve fibers that serve the muscles.

There is no satisfactory treatment for this disease. Physical therapy procedures may be of some help.

MUSCULAR DYSTROPHY.

This is an inherited disease characterized by a progressive degeneration of muscle fibers with resulting weakness. It is to be differentiated from muscular atrophy because, in this disease, the primary difficulty is with the muscle tissue rather than with the nerves which control the muscle.

For a more detailed discussion see *Muscular Dystrophy* in chapter 13 of this volume.

MYASTHENIA GRAVIS.

Myasthenia gravis is a rare disease characterized by the development of muscular weakness which fluctuates from time to time and which especially affects the muscles about the eyes and face. The muscles of swallowing and those of the limbs are also affected in most cases. The disease may begin at any age, but most commonly in the second or third decade, beginning earlier in women than in men. The muscles fatigue quickly on use, the first few excursions being nearly normal but the muscle power fading with continued use.

Some cases progress rapidly to a fatal termination, with death being caused by failure of the respiratory muscles. In others the patient lives on for years.

The immediate cause of myasthenia gravis is an alteration in the chemical activity at the junction between the nerve fibers and the muscle fibers. Patients with this disease respond miraculously for a short period following the administration of one of the anticholinesterase compounds such as neostigmine or pyridostigmine. The use of such a drug does not cure the disease or even retard its progress, but it does make life easier for the sufferer. Such drugs must be taken under the supervision of a physician, for there is danger of overdose resulting in more severe weakness and other complications. Abnormalities of the thymus, including tumors, are frequently associated with this condition.

MYOTONIA.

In myotonia, of which there are several types, there is difficulty in relaxing the muscles after they have once contracted. Repeated use of the same muscles seems to "warm them up" so that their function becomes virtually normal. Many cases of this unique disorder seem to have hereditary backgrounds. Some forms of myotonia appear early in life, others later. In some cases the difficulty is aggravated by prolonged rest, by exposure to low temperatures, and by emotional excitement.

There is no satisfactory treatment for myotonia, but in many cases the disease does not shorten life. Many victims of the disease learn to live quite normally in spite of their handicap.

NARCOLEPSY.

Narcolepsy is a syndrome (group of symptoms) characterized by (1) the tendency to fall asleep spontaneously, even during the daytime and in spite of adequate sleep at night, (2) the occurrence of unusual dreams, (3) sleep paralysis in which the individual is unable to move his muscles for about the first minute on awakening, and (4) the sudden occurrence of muscle weakness so severe that the patient falls even though he does not lose consciousness. This sudden muscle weakness is called cataplexy and usually comes in response to some surprising emotional experience such as mirth, anger, or fear.

The symptoms develop most commonly during the second decade of life. Narcolepsy is relatively uncommon, but it occurs four times as frequently in men as in women. It does not interfere with the usual life-span except as it introduces an element of hazard because of the tendency to go to sleep even while otherwise occupied—as while driving a car.

Treatment consists of the carefully supervised use of drugs which tend to keep the individual awake.

NEURALGIA.

Neuralgia is generally considered to be a symptom rather than a disease. It consists of a series of attacks of acute pain in the area supplied by some particular nerve, usually one of the cranial nerves located in the face or neck region. In neuralgia, in contrast to neuritis, no demonstrable change occurs in the structure of the nerve involved. Formerly, certain painful conditions such as sciatica were placed under the heading of neuralgia. Now it is recognized that sciatica is usually caused by a compression of one or more nerve roots by the herniation of an intervertebral disk. (See under *Spinal Injuries* in this chapter.) The usual examples of true neuralgia are trigeminal neuralgia, glossopharyngeal neuralgia, and causalgia.

A. *Trigeminal Neuralgia (Tic Douloureux).* The trigeminal nerve is the sensory nerve to the face and consists of three branches, one supplying the skin of the forehead and eye, one supplying the skin of the side of the face between the eye and the mouth, and the third supplying the skin of the side of the jaw, the lower lip, and the chin. One or more of these branches may be involved in trigeminal neuralgia.

Trigeminal neuralgia may occur at any time in adult life but usually begins about age 50. It is somewhat more common in women than in men.

The pain is a lightninglike stab which occurs in paroxysms and usually lasts a moment or two. In the early stages it may not recur for days. As the disease advances, the intervals between paroxysms may become shorter. The pain of trigeminal neuralgia is usually so intense that the patient writhes in agony. In most cases there is some activity of the face or mouth which seems to trigger the attack— touching or washing of the face, exposure to cold, talking, eating, or drinking.

Trigeminal neuralgia is a most difficult illness to treat satisfactorily. The use of medication is usually given a good trial before recourse to the other, more drastic measures. Dilantin, a drug ordinarily used for epilepsy, may give relief. However, the newest effective drug for relieving the symptoms of trigeminal neuralgia is carbamazepine (Tegretol). This drug is said to be effective in at least two thirds of the cases of trigeminal neuralgia, but the problem is that in some cases it produces serious side

effects including skin rash, dizziness, ataxia, and damage to the blood-forming tissues of the body. It should be used, of course, only under the supervision of a physician, and he will want to arrange for frequently repeated blood tests and liver function studies in order to check on the possibility of serious side effects.

The use of narcotic pain-killing drugs should be avoided because they give little relief and because of the great danger of addiction. One of the more drastic measures that is sometimes used for the treatment of trigeminal neuralgia, in cases in which the use of medications is not effective, is injection of alcohol into the involved nerve. This may cause temporary cessation of the pain, lasting for 18 months, more or less. Surgical procedures for destroying the sensory portion of the trigeminal nerve have been more permanently successful in many cases. It is advised that the patient with trigeminal neuralgia consult a specialist in neurology.

B. *Glossopharyngeal Neuralgia.* In this type of neuralgia there are paroxysms of pain which involve the back of the tongue, one tonsil, one side of the throat, and the middle ear on the same side. The symptom usually makes its first appearance after age forty and, strangely, affects males more commonly than females. The attack is often brought on by chewing, swallowing, talking, or yawning. The attack of pain is brief, lasting only a few minutes but being so severe that the patient sometimes faints.

The use of drugs in the treatment of glossopharyngeal neuralgia is seldom completely satisfactory. Indiscriminate use of narcotics leads to addiction. Surgical treatment by severing or removing the involved nerve offers the best prospect of relief.

C. *Causalgia.* Causalgia, though not a typical example of neuralgia, is included here because of the element of excruciating pain. This symptom follows injury to a nerve such as the median nerve in the arm or the sciatic nerve in the hip, thigh, or leg. The persistent burning pain is easily aggravated by almost any stimulus such as exposure of the involved area to the air, a sudden noise, some startling experience, or mere emotional excitation.

It is believed that injury to the sympathetic nerve fibers contained in the injured nerve is responsible for this unusual symptom. In some cases relief has been obtained by surgical severing of the sympathetic nerve fibers which supply this part of the body. A person with causalgia should consult a specialist in neurology.

NEURITIS.

Neuritis is a condition in which degenerative changes occur in one or more nerves as a result of mechanical damage to the nerve, metabolic disturbance, or toxic insult. When a single nerve is involved, we speak of mononeuritis; when more than one or many nerves are involved, we speak of polyneuritis.

Because most of the body's nerves contain a variety of fibers, the symptoms appearing in neuritis correspond to the various types of nerve fibers injured. In the usual case there will be symptoms resulting from damage to the sensory fibers. These include various kinds of discomfort, described as sharp pains, burning sensations, sensations of tingling, the feeling of "pins and needles," and numbness.

Involvement of the motor fibers in a nerve produces weakness of the muscles which may progress to complete paralysis with eventual atrophy of the muscles. Involvement of the autonomic nerve fibers may produce an increase in skin temperature in the involved area, sweating, and skin lesions. In other cases there may be paleness and dryness of the skin. The various types of neuritis will now be discussed.

A. *Mechanical Damage to the Nerve.* This may occur in connection with penetrating injuries, crushing injuries, or fractures of bones in which nerves are damaged. It may be caused by long-continued pressure against a nerve, as when an intoxicated person sleeps in a chair with his arm over the back. What the patient notices is a distortion of nerve functions such as occurs commonly when a person's leg or arm "goes to sleep" on account of sustained local pressure.

B. *Metabolic Disturbance of the Nerve Tissue.* In these generalized conditions the damage is usually to many nerves, and therefore we speak of polyneuritis. It occurs in conditions or diseases in which there is not a sufficient amount of thiamine (vitamin B_1) in the diet. Polyneuritis of this kind develops in such diseases as beriberi and pellagra, and in alcoholism. The chronic alcoholic derives much of his energy from calories contained in the alcohol and thus does not eat sufficient food to provide the required nutritional elements, including thiamine. Other metabolic diseases, such as diabetes, may also cause polyneuritis.

C. *Toxic Insults to the Nerves.* Here we include the toxic conditions that result from diseases such as diphtheria, in which neuritis may develop because the toxin from the germs damages certain nerves. Also, there are many chemicals and heavy metals which injure nerve tissue. These include alcohol, carbon tetrachloride, and benzine among the chemicals, and lead, arsenic, mercury, and bismuth among the heavy metals. Persons exposed to these substances in excess are prone to develop symptoms of polyneuritis.

Treatment of neuritis consists of discovering and removing the cause of the damage to the nerves. Once the cause is removed, recovery may be prompt in mild cases. In severe cases, however, in which damage to the nerves has been inflicted over a long period, the normal function of the nerve may never be completely restored. A good diet and high intake of vitamins may hasten recovery.

PALSY.

(See *Cerebral Palsy* and *Facial Paralysis* in this chapter.)

PARALYSIS AGITANS.

(See *Parkinsonism* in this chapter.)

PARALYSIS, FAMILIAL PERIODIC.

Familial periodic paralysis is a rare hereditary disease characterized by recurring attacks of profound weakness of the muscles of the trunk and extremities. Usually the muscles of breathing and those of the face remain normal. The individual attack lasts somewhere between two and twenty-four hours. Attacks may occur every day or as infrequently as once a year. The disease usually begins during the first or second decade of life, persists for a few years, and then improves over the next few years, with attacks becoming less frequent and less severe. Interestingly, attacks usually occur after a period of rest or after a meal consisting largely of carbohydrate food. Oftentimes a person will suffer an attack upon awakening in the morning. In most cases attacks are associated with a reduction in the concentration of potassium in the blood serum.

Usually persons with this disease live out an average life-span, but occasionally death occurs because of involvement of the muscles of breathing.

In most cases the attack of paralysis can be relieved by the administration by mouth of potassium chloride. This is not advisable for all cases, however, because in some reduction in the concentration of potassium in the blood serum is not the problem. Noting this diversity, some scientists believe that the fundamental difficulty is in the body's metabolism of sodium rather than in the handling of potassium. In fact, when the amount of sodium in the diet is reduced appreciably, attacks of paralysis do not occur.

The handling of a case of familial periodic paralysis should be under the direction of a physician.

PARESIS (GENERAL PARESIS).

(See *Syphilis of the Nervous System* in this chapter.)

PARKINSONISM (PARALYSIS AGITANS).

Parkinsonism is a chronic, progressive disorder, usually occurring in middle-aged or elderly persons. It is characterized by slowness of movement, rigidity of the muscles, involuntary tremor, and progressive weakness.

The usual case of parkinsonism begins gradually and is without known cause. The rate of progress of the disease will vary from case to case. Usually the patient becomes gradually incapacitated over a period of several years. Parkinsonism occurring earlier in life may be a sequel to encephalitis or to some circumstance in which the cells of the brain were deprived of their supply of oxygen for at least five to ten minutes and were thus permanently damaged. Such a circumstance may develop in connection with carbon monoxide poisoning, asphyxia, or head injury.

The victim of parkinsonism presents a characteristic appearance. The muscles of his face become immobile, and blinking of the eyes becomes infrequent so that he appears to stare and seems unable to register his emotions. In advanced cases, saliva may drool from a corner of the mouth. The patient leans forward as he walks, moves with short, shuffling steps, and may break into a run, trying to keep from falling forward. At times he may even fall backward. Typically his arms are flexed at the elbows, and he carries his hands near his abdomen. There may be tremors in various parts of his body, but the most characteristic one involves a repetitive movement by which the tips of the fingers brush past the ball of his thumb—the so-called "pill-rolling movement." The tremors are worse when the patient is tired or when he becomes excited.

Although weakness of the muscles develops gradually in parkinsonism,

429

there is a rigidity which interferes with rapid movement of any part of the body. Speech becomes hampered both in volume of sound and in clarity of enunciation. Intellectual capacity is retained quite well until the terminal phase of the disorder.

Inasmuch as there is no cure for parkinsonism, the care of a patient with this disorder centers around keeping him active as long as possible, maintaining his morale by cheerful surroundings, and using such drugs as may minimize his tremors and reduce the rigidity of his muscles. Various surgical procedures have been tried which aim to destroy those parts of the brain in which the tremors and the spasticity are activated.

Recently, however, the surgical treatment of parkinsonism has been largely superseded by the use of the drug levodopa ("L-dopa"). In about two thirds of cases of parkinsonism the symptoms are very materially improved by the use of levodopa. There is even some evidence that the use of levodopa retards the progression of the disease and thus lengthens the patient's life-span.

In quite a number of cases the use of levodopa is accompanied by unpleasant side effects such as nausea, vomiting, and, occasionally, transient mental disturbances. The control of the side effects requires cooperation between the patient and his physician. Variations in the dosage of the levodopa, altering the daily pattern of administering the levodopa, or using supplementary drugs will usually reduce the severity of the side effects satisfactorily.

PHENYLKETONURIA (PKU).

Phenylketonuria is perhaps the best known of several hereditary metabolic diseases. The disease, striking about one child in every 15,000, is caused by the lack of an enzyme necessary to the proper synthesis of tyrosine (one of the amino acids). As a result of this metabolic defect, phenylalanine (a precursor of tyrosine) accumulates in the body's tissues and fluids, and is excreted by way of the urine. From the standpoint of our present consideration of nervous disorders, the importance of phenylketonuria is that children with this disease display awkward gait, tremors, and continuous purposeless movements of the hands. Epileptic seizures occur in about one fourth of the cases.

The mental deficiency of phenylketonuria develops gradually, beginning soon after birth. If the infant so affected is placed on a special diet at once—a diet which contains only a minimum of phenylalanine—he may not develop mental deficiency or other neurological manifestations. Of course, it is not easy to determine in the case of a young infant whether or not he is becoming mentally retarded and is possibly afflicted with phenylketonuria. The only way to be sure is to make tests of the urine. Some states require that these examinations be carried out on all newborn infants as a means of detecting the occasional one who would benefit by treatment for phenylketonuria and thus be spared the tragedy of becoming mentally deficient. The special diet must be adapted by the physician to the needs of the individual case.

POLIOMYELITIS.

(See under *Poliomyelitis* in chapter 28, "Infectious Diseases," in this volume.)

POLYNEURITIS.

(See under *Neuritis* in this chapter.)

POSTEROLATERAL SCLEROSIS (COMBINED SYSTEM DISEASE).

Posterolateral sclerosis is a serious involvement of the nervous system associated with pernicious anemia or other macrocytic anemias. The deficiency of vitamin B_{12}, the cause of pernicious anemia, has its effect on the tissues of the nervous system, causing a degeneration of areas of the spinal cord. The degeneration interferes with the normal transmission of nervous impulses. (For a more complete discussion of pernicious anemia as a disease, see in this volume, chapter 10, "Blood-vessel and Blood Diseases," under the heading *Macrocytic Anemias.*)

Sometimes it is the symptoms of posterolateral sclerosis that first call the physician's attention to the possibility of pernicious anemia in a given case. The first symptoms usually consist of tingling and numbness in the skin of the toes and soles of the feet. Soon the same sensations develop in the fingers. If the disease still goes unrecognized and untreated, these sensations spread to the feet and legs and, possibly, to the thighs and lower parts of the body. The tingling and numbness of the fingers usually spreads to include the hands; but it seldom involves the arms, particularly the upper arms.

Next is noticed an unsteadiness and stiffness in gait, which may be accompanied by weakness of the muscles of the legs. The patient tends to stumble, especially when walking in the dark. As the weakness progresses, the knees may give way unexpectedly. The hands become clumsy.

In severe cases there is an involvement of the brain with certain psychic symptoms including loss of recent memory, ideas of persecution, and even stupor and coma. Commonly, vision is impaired with a developing blindness at the center of the visual field.

In untreated cases of pernicious anemia the symptoms of posterolateral sclerosis become progressively worse.

When treatment is begun early, at least by the time unsteadiness in gait is first noticed, there is a good prospect that the sypmtoms will disappear and, if treatment is continued consistently for the remainder of life, that the victim of this disease can live out a normal life-span. If treatment is long delayed, however, the damage to the tissues of the spinal cord becomes so serious that normal conditions can probably never be reestablished. Even in such cases, however, treatment may bring about a significant improvement.

Since posterolateral sclerosis is part of pernicious anemia, the treatment is one and the same. It consists of the administration, by intramuscular injection, of vitamin B_{12}. A case of pernicious anemia with posterolateral sclerosis should, of course, remain under the continuing supervision of a physician.

RABIES.
(See under *Rabies* in chapter 28, "Infectious Diseases," in this volume.)

RIB.
(See *Cervical Rib* in this chapter.)

SAINT VITUS'S DANCE.
(See the discussion of Sydenham's chorea under *Chorea* in this chapter.)

SCLEROSIS.
(See *Amyotrophic Lateral Sclerosis, Posterolateral Sclerosis* and *Multiple Sclerosis* in this chapter.)

SCIATICA.
Sciatica is a term used to describe pain in the distribution of the sciatic nerve. This nerve derives its fibers from the spinal cord in the lower part of the back and passes through the buttock and thigh into the leg. The usual cause of sciatic pain is pressure produced by a herniated intervertebral disk. See the discussion of *Herniated Intervertebral Disk* under "Spinal Injuries" in this chapter.

SHINGLES.
(See under *Herpes Zoster* in this volume in chapter 28, "Infectious Diseases," and in chapter 12, "Skin Diseases.")

SPINA BIFIDA.
Spina bifida is a malformation of the vertebral column which, in the more

serious cases may be accompanied by involvement of the spinal cord and the spinal nerves. It usually occurs in the lower part of the back and affects one or more vertebrae. It is commonly associated with other congenital defects such as clubfoot or hydrocephalus. In the least severe cases there are no symptoms relating to the nervous system; a clue to such a defect may be a dimple in the skin at the site of the deformity, a discoloration of the overlying skin, or a tuft of hair in this area. The deformity of the vertebrae can be discerned of course, by X-ray examination.

In the moderately severe cases in which some of the nerve roots are involved, the infant may have difficulty in learning to walk and may have a clumsy gait. In the very severe cases there may be a weakness and wasting of the muscles of the legs and feet in addition to some diminution of the skin sensations in the areas of the buttocks and adjacent portions of the thighs. In these more severe cases there is usually a surface protrusion of the membranes that normally cover the spinal cord, the protrusion appearing in the midline at the lower part of the back. This protruding sac of soft tissue may in some cases include portions of the large nerve roots, and occasionally even the spinal cord.

In these cases an opening may be eroded in this protruding soft tissue through which cerebrospinal fluid may escape. There is then grave danger, of course, of an infection of the meninges with resulting meningitis.

The immediate treatment for cases of spina bifida that have symptoms is reparative surgery. However, surgery will not restore functions of the nervous system already deficient. Furthermore, hydrocephalus sometimes develops as a complication after surgery.

The care of the patient includes a carefully planned program of rehabilitation aimed to make it possible for the child, as he grows up, to live a reasonably normal life.

SPINAL INJURIES.

By spinal injuries we refer to those accidents that damage the vertebral column and may at the same time injure the spinal cord and/or some of the spinal nerves. The reason spinal injuries may affect the spinal cord or the spinal nerves is the very close anatomical relationship which exists between the vertebral column and the spinal cord with its emerging spinal nerves.

The vertebral column consists essentially of the bodies of the vertebrae plus their bony processes which extend to the sides and backward from the vertebral bodies. These bony processes form a complete arch behind each of the vertebral bodies. It is within the spinal canal formed by these arches that the delicate spinal cord (a downward continuation from the brain) is located. The spinal nerves originate from the spinal cord and then pass outward on the right and on the left between the bony processes.

The greatest danger to the spinal cord occurs when the vertebrae are crushed or sharply bent on one another so that they pinch or crush the spinal cord, or when one vertebra is displaced in its relation to its neighbor so that the spinal cord is sheared. The spinal nerves which emerge between the bony processes of the vertebrae may be compressed or damaged by injuries which bring pressure against them. There are four principal types of spinal injuries as indicated in the following descriptions:

A. *Herniated Intervertebral Disks.* The intervertebral disks are composed of fibrocartilage, a dense connective tissue, and are interposed between the vertebral bodies to provide for cushioning and also to permit a certain amount of flexibility. Each of these intervertebral disks is composed of a softer central part, the nucleus pulposus, and a surrounding ring of the dense tissue designated as the anulus fibrosus.

Injuries to the intervertebral disks

constitute the most common type of spinal injury. When a disk is injured, the nucleus pulposus often herniates through the damaged part of the anulus fibrosus and brings pressure against an adjacent nerve root, causing discomfort and often some loss of function.

Herniation of an intervertebral disk occurs most commonly in the lumbar region of the lower back. The second most common site is in the lower part of the neck. The usual cause of damage to a disk in the lumbar region is lifting while in a stooping or twisted position. At the time of this first injury the patient will usually suffer pain for a few days, experiencing a "catch in the back" or a "crick in the neck." The discomfort is caused by torn ligaments or strained muscles. It may be some time later, possibly after several incidents of discomfort, that the nucleus pulposus at the center of the intervertebral disk actually squeezes out and brings pressure against the adjacent nerve root, causing the typical pain that radiates throughout the course of the nerve thus compressed.

The discomfort associated with a herniated disk located in the lower back usually consists of severe aching pain in the buttock and the back and side of the thigh and leg. Often numbness and tingling is felt in the same area. The pain is often aggravated by coughing or sneezing or by straining at stool. It may be made worse by twisting, stooping, or lifting. Certain muscles in the thigh, leg, or foot may become weak. There may or may not be pain in the lower part of the back.

When the damaged intervertebral disk is in the lower part of the neck, the pain involves the shoulder, the arm, the forearm, and the hand, the latter either on the thumb side or on the little finger side. Again there will be numbness and tingling in these areas with a weakness of certain muscles—particularly the triceps muscle in the back of the arm.

Treatment for cases of herniated intervertebral disk falls into two categories: conservative and surgical. Conservative treatment consists of bed rest for several days or a few weeks in order to eliminate the mechanical pressure which has caused the intervertebral disk to collapse and bulge. In cases where the damaged disk is in the lower back, the patient's bed should be very firm so as to keep the structures of the vertebral column in the most favorable position. A relatively unyielding mattress should be used, and this should be laid on plywood or other firm foundation.

For cases in which the injury is in the neck, it is often advisable to provide traction. This is arranged by attaching a weight by a rope that runs over a pully at the head of the bed so as to exert a continuous pull on a closely fitting head harness. As the patient improves, he may be allowed out of bed during the daytime provided he wears a supporting collar. The traction is usually continued at night for a longer time.

Surgical treatment for herniated intervertebral disk involves removing the nucleus pulposus pressing against the nerve root and, in some cases, inserting a bone graft to stabilize the spinal column at the site of difficulty.

B. *Sprains.* A sprain of the vertebral column involves a stretching of the spinal ligaments which hold the vertebrae in place. Inasmuch as the cervical portion (in the neck) of the vertebral column is most flexible, this is the part most commonly sprained. It is this type of injury, occurring in the neck, that is called "whiplash." It occurs as a result of direct violence or of excessive muscle pull as when the head is suddenly thrown backward in an automobile accident.

In a sprain, the vertebrae are usually not displaced; therefore seldom does a sprain injure the spinal cord. Symptoms consist of pain on moving the neck, of local tenderness, and of stiffness.

Occasionally a person who has sustained this type of sprain becomes

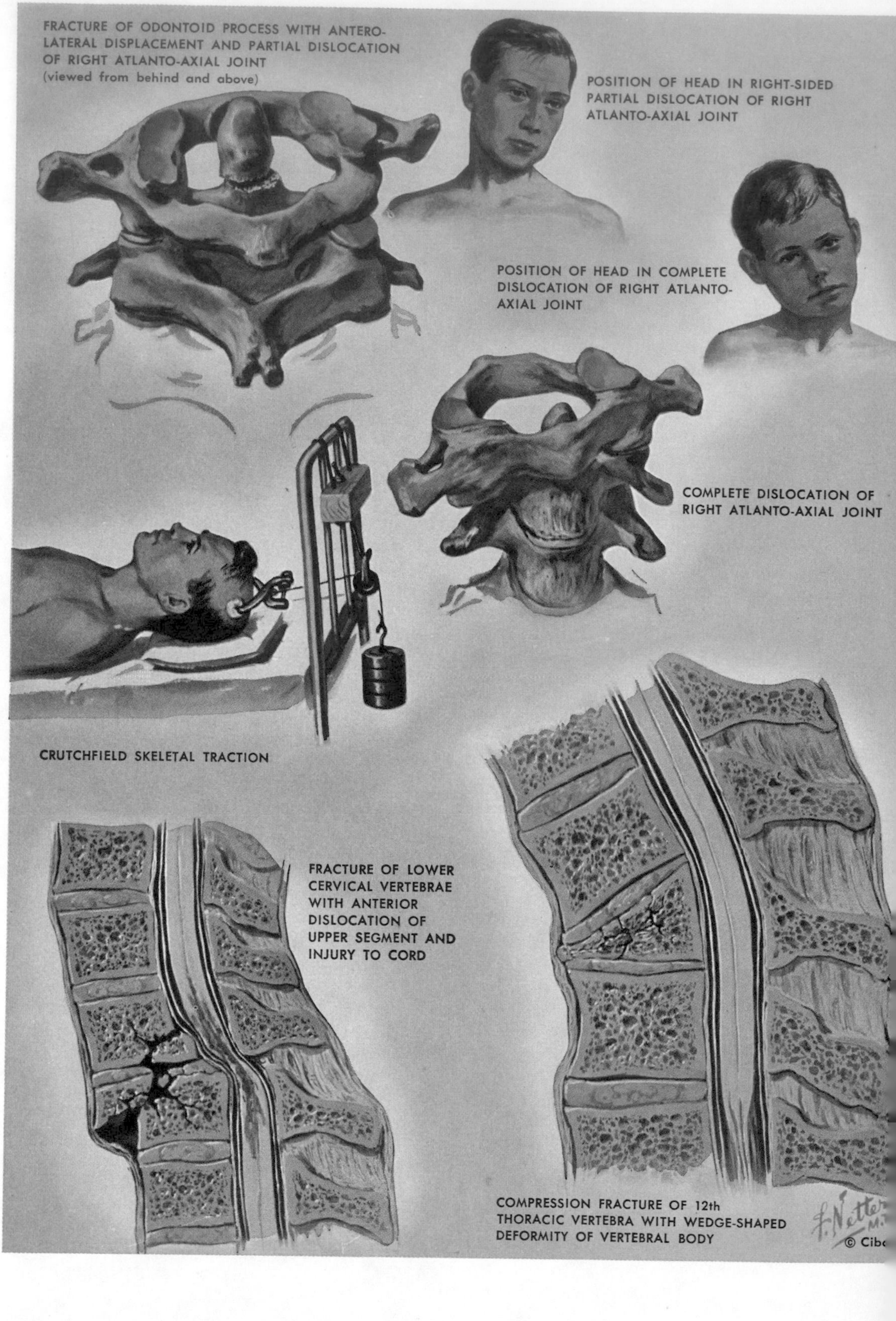

FRACTURE OF ODONTOID PROCESS WITH ANTERO-
LATERAL DISPLACEMENT AND PARTIAL DISLOCATION
OF RIGHT ATLANTO-AXIAL JOINT
(viewed from behind and above)

POSITION OF HEAD IN RIGHT-SIDED
PARTIAL DISLOCATION OF RIGHT
ATLANTO-AXIAL JOINT

POSITION OF HEAD IN COMPLETE
DISLOCATION OF RIGHT ATLANTO-
AXIAL JOINT

COMPLETE DISLOCATION OF
RIGHT ATLANTO-AXIAL JOINT

CRUTCHFIELD SKELETAL TRACTION

FRACTURE OF LOWER
CERVICAL VERTEBRAE
WITH ANTERIOR
DISLOCATION OF
UPPER SEGMENT AND
INJURY TO CORD

COMPRESSION FRACTURE OF 12th
THORACIC VERTEBRA WITH WEDGE-SHAPED
DEFORMITY OF VERTEBRAL BODY

F. Netter
M.D.

© Ciba

self-centered in his desire for sympathy or compensation. This attitude tends to prolong the symptoms even beyond the time required for the tissues to heal. Most physicians therefore advise these patients to return to their normal way of life within a reasonable period of time, encouraging them to ignore their continuing symptoms.

C. *Dislocations.* In a dislocation of the vertebral column an actual displacement of one vertebra in its relation to another takes place. Dislocations are often associated with fractures, torn ligaments, and injuries to the intervertebral disks. Because of the displacement, there is great danger of injury to the spinal cord.

Dislocations may be caused by diving into shallow water or by falling on the head, shoulder, or even in a standing-up position. A heavy blow such as causes the vertebral column to bend sharply in any direction may cause a dislocation. Symptoms consist of local pain, tenderness, and a deformity of the bony structures such as can be observed by X ray or by careful digital examination.

In any case of dislocation of the vertebrae, great care must be taken in handling the patient lest damage be done to the spinal cord. Even a slight movement of the patient's body might cause the displaced vertebra to compress the spinal cord, with resulting permanent damage.

Immediate care of the case requires the same precautions as when the back is broken. If the patient must be transported, great care should be taken to avoid body or neck movement. (See volume 3, chapter 18, "Handling Emergencies," under *Fracture of the Back* and *Fracture of the Neck.*) Usual hospital treatment for such a patient includes traction of the head so that if the parts of the vertebral column which are injured shift their position, they will do so in the direction of their normal position rather than in a direction that might press on the spinal cord.

D. *Fractures.* Fractures of the vertebrae are somewhat more common in the middle and lower back. Sometimes they consist merely of the compression of a vertebral body without its being displaced. As mentioned above under dislocations, fractures may well be associated with damage to the intervertebral disk or to the ligaments that normally hold the vertebral bodies in place. Fractures are usually the result of a fall with forceful bending or of a direct blow on the back or of the intense pressures produced by sudden strong muscle action as in a convulsion.

If there is no displacement of the bony structures so as to endanger the spinal cord or the nerve roots, fractures are not so serious to the patient's total welfare as are dislocations. Symptoms of a fracture consist of local pain, tenderness, and muscle spasm. Treatment consists, usually, of the use of casts and braces to support the patient's back during the period of healing. For instruction on the first-aid handling of persons with fractures of the vertebral column, see in volume 3, chapter 18, "Handling Emergencies," under *Fracture of the Back* and *Fracture of the Neck.*

STROKE.

A stroke, commonly called apoplectic stroke or a stroke of paralysis, is caused by severe damage to some part of the brain resulting from a hemorrhage or an interruption of the blood supply. The exact symptoms in a particular case are determined by the specific part of the brain that has been damaged. For a detailed discussion of the various causes of stroke and for instruction on the immediate care of a stroke victim, see chapter 10, "Blood-vessel and Blood Diseases," under the heading of *Stroke,* in this volume. The paralysis that commonly occurs in connection with a stroke is discussed in volume 3, chapter 22, "List of Signs and Symptoms," under the heading of *Paralysis From Cerebral Vascular Accident.*

Not all strokes result from something that happens to the blood vessels inside the skull. Sometimes an obstruction to the flow of blood develops in vessels in the neck—vessels which normally carry blood to the brain. Thus the brain is deprived of its usual blood supply just as effectively as when the mishap occurs inside the skull. Usually certain warning signs indicate that the brain is not receiving a sufficient amount of blood. There may be "transient strokes" in which the symptoms last only a few minutes. It can then be determined by an X-ray study of the vessels (arteriography) whether the difficulty is caused by a narrowing of the vessels in the neck. If so, the lumens of these vessels may be enlarged by a surgical procedure (end-arterectomy).

SYDENHAM'S CHOREA.

(See *Chorea, Sydenham's* in this chapter.)

SYPHILIS OF THE NERVOUS SYSTEM.

Syphilis is produced by a spiral-shaped germ, the Treponema pallidum. It is classed as one of the social diseases and is usually transmitted by sexual contact. As explained in chapter 30, "Venereal Infections," in this volume, it affects many organs and tissues of the body. In the present chapter we are concerned with its involvement of the nervous system.

Antibiotic drugs have brought about a marvelous improvement in the treatment of syphilis. When adequately used early in the course of the disease, they will prevent most of the serious complications from developing. Syphilis could doubtless be stamped out within a few months or years if all who have the disease, throughout the world, would submit to adequate treatment. The facts that syphilis is transmitted by sexual contacts, however, and that syphilis patients are reticent to admit their social indiscretions, make it difficult for physicians and health agencies to conduct a successful campaign against the disease.

Involvement of the nervous system is one of the later manifestations of syphilis, occurring typically in the so-called third stage of the disease. The germs of syphilis seem to remain quiescent in the tissues of the nervous system for many months or even several years after they have entered these tissues. Then, for some unknown reason, they begin to produce damage so disastrous that even intensive treatment may not restore the patient completely to his previous condition.

A person need not remain in uncertainty as to whether he needs treatment for a syphilitic infection. Blood tests for syphilis are now available at any doctor's office, at any venereal-disease clinic, and at any public-health headquarters. More than this, it is possible, by drawing a sample of the cerebrospinal fluid, to determine whether or not the germs of syphilis have entered the nervous system. If they have, the need for intensive treatment adapted to this complication is most urgent even though no symptoms of the involvement of the brain or spinal cord have yet appeared.

Syphilis affects the brain and spinal cord in several ways. It may produce a unique type of meningitis or it may involve, primarily, the blood vessels of these organs. It may produce degenerative changes which seriously affect the intellect or cause a destruction of certain of the nerve pathways. In the present consideration we will discuss only the two most important manifestations of syphilis of the nervous system: (A) general paresis and (B) tabes dorsalis.

A. *General Paresis of the Insane.* This is a serious late complication of syphilis, typically developing several years after the individual's first syphilitic infection. It is serious because it destroys the intellect and progressively limits the victim's usual activities, bringing death, on the average, about three years after the first appearance of symptoms. Fortunately, general paresis of the insane is seldom seen now because most cases of syphilis receive adequate treatment in their earlier stages.

The general symptoms of this disorder include headache, ataxia (unsteadiness of gait and station), slurred speech, tremor of the fingers and tongue, and mental deterioration.

Personality-wise there is a progressive impairment of the individual's efficiency both in family life and in business. He begins to use poor judgment and is prone to make serious mistakes such as unnecessarily incurring debt or spending money for things not needed. There is a progressive failure in memory and a tendency to tell untruths. The individual becomes disoriented so that he no longer knows the time of day or the day of the week or month and is confused as to his whereabouts and the identity of himself and those he contacts. This leads to a dreamlike state. A person with this condition commonly has delusions, imagining himself to be somebody great. The emotions of joy and sorrow may alternate suddenly and without adequate justification. There is a rapid deterioration of moral and ethical standards. As the disease continues, the victim becomes apathetic and finally completely demented.

Intensive treatment with antibiotic drugs may at least partially arrest the progress of general paresis; but, inasmuch as the disease involves a degeneration of nerve cells and nerve fibers, treatment cannot always be expected to restore the individual to his normal state. Because of such reasons it is urged that any syphilitic infection be treated intensively early in its course.

B. *Tabes Dorsalis (Locomotor Ataxia).* In this manifestation of syphilis it is primarily the spinal cord and the nerve roots that are affected. Fortunately this disease is much less common now than it was before adequate treatment for syphilis be-

came available. Tabes dorsalis tends to develop from five to twenty years after the primary syphilitic infection.

In the usual case, the first symptom is an aching pain in the legs, often confused with rheumatism. The pain becomes progressively worse until it is described as lightninglike. These pains come in bouts, usually occurring at least once during each twenty-four hours, the severity usually being more intense at night than during the day. In some cases the patient receives the impression of a tight girdle about his abdomen. In others agonizing pains (so-called tabetic crises) develop in certain organs of the body. These excruciating pains occur most commonly in relation to the stomach. They may last for several days, the pain being either continuous or intermittent. Any attempt to drink or eat causes vomiting. The pain may disappear as suddenly as it begins, only to recur at a later time.

Various neuralgias, involving nerves here and there throughout the body, may develop as a part of tabes dorsalis. There may be numbness and a feeling of coldness in various skin areas. Often the patient reports a sensation as though he were walking on cotton. Certain areas of the skin may be less sensitive than normal, approaching a complete loss of sensation. The sense of position suffers greatly in most cases so that the individual becomes unaware of the position of his feet or legs except as he watches these and observes their movement and position. With walking thus made difficult, the victim typically uses a cane and watches each step he takes. When he stands, he stands with his feet wide apart so as to brace himself because of his unsteadiness. There is often a loss of tone in the muscles of his extremities so that they move in a flail-like manner. His strength and energy become progressively poor.

In well-established tabes dorsalis, as well as in general paresis of the insane, the deteriorated nerve fibers cannot be restored even by intensive treatment. Once the damage has been done, repair is impossible. Again it should be emphasized that any syphilitic infection should be treated intensively as soon as possible after the infection has been acquired. (See chapter 30, "Venereal Infections," in this volume.)

SYRINGOMYELIA.

This is an unusual disease in which a cavity develops in the central portion of the spinal cord, causing a progressive destruction of the adjacent nerve fibers. The cause of the disease is unknown, but some evidence indicates that it harks back to a congenital fault of development. Exact symptoms depend upon which part of the spinal cord happens to be involved, whether a part in the neck or lower down. The first symptoms often appear between ages ten and thirty. The disease is slowly progressive but may remain stationary for several years. Some patients live as long as forty years after the disease begins.

At first the patient notices loss of certain sensations for pain and temperature in the particular part of the body (usually the arms and trunk) related to the location of the cavity within the spinal cord. The sense of touch remains normal. This loss of sensation for pain and temperature is usually brought to the patient's attention when he observes that he suffers no pain in the involved part of his body from minor injuries or even a burn.

Another early evidence of the disease is progressive weakness and atrophy of certain of the small muscles, usually those in the hands.

There is no satisfactory treatment for syringomyelia. The patient should be encouraged to remain active as long as feasible. In view of the danger of burns of the skin, now that the natural protective influence of pain and temperature has been lost, appropriate means to prevent injury to the victim should be employed. Reasonable measures should be taken to help the patient retain an attitude of cheerfulness in spite of his handicap. In some cases surgery may provide partial relief of symptoms and may retard the progress of the disease.

TABES DORSALIS.

(See *Syphilis of the Nervous System* in this chapter.)

TIC DOULOUREUX.

(See *Neuralgia: A. Trigeminal Neuralgia* in this chapter.)

TORTICOLLIS.

(See under *Neck, Stiffness of* in volume 3, chapter 22, "List of Signs and Symptoms.")

TRAUMA.

(See *Head Injuries* and *Spinal Injuries* in this chapter.)

TRIGEMINAL NEURALGIA.

(See *Neuralgia: A. Trigeminal Neuralgia* in this chapter.)

TUMORS.

A. *Tumors of the Brain.* There are various kinds of brain tumors. Some grow slowly, others rapidly. All kinds are hazardous because their increase in size brings pressure against the delicate tissues of the brain. Some invade the brain tissue itself, causing destruction of the nerve cells and fibers as they do so. Others remain within a fibrous capsule and inflict damage by the pressure which their growth produces. Those which grow rapidly and invade the nervous tissue are usually the most dangerous and threaten the patient's life within the shortest period of time. Tumors of the brain occur at any time of life but are most common in early adulthood and middle age.

Based on the possibility of cure, tumors of the brain may be classed as either benign or malignant. Benign tumors are curable if they can be safely removed by surgery. An example of a benign tumor is the meningioma which develops in the membranes surrounding the brain.

Malignant tumors are seldom curable because of their tendency to grow rapidly, to invade the tissues, and to recur after removal. These may be subdivided into primary and second-ary tumors. Primary brain tumors originate withing the skull. An example of a primary malignant tumor is the astrocytoma which consists of cancer cells that have developed from cells which normally support the nerve cells of the brain. Secondary malignant tumors are those which spread usually by the bloodstream from a tumor in some other part of the body such as the lung or the breast. Small portions of such a tumor are carried by the blood to the brain where they become secondarily implanted.

Symptoms of tumors of the brain are of two types: (1) those that result from the pressure which the tumor produces, and (2) those caused by the destruction of nerve cells and nerve fibers. A tumor located in one part of the brain will produce a different group of symptoms from one located in some other part, even though the size of the two tumors may be the same.

Headache is sometimes the first symptom of a brain tumor. Inasmuch as headache is commonly produced by other causes, this symptom is not diagnostic except as it may persist unnaturally. Unexplained nausea and vomiting are also symptoms which occur commonly in brain tumor. In some cases weakness, awkwardness, and/or convulsive seizures develop. In other cases there may be drowsiness, changes in personality, strange conduct, and impaired thinking.

Treatment for tumors of the brain, always of course under the direction of a neurosurgeon, is either surgical removal, radiation therapy, and/or chemotherapy.

B. *Tumors of the Spinal Cord.* These are much less frequent than tumors of the brain, but are classified in about the same manner. Symptoms depend on the location of the tumor and upon the particular groups of nerve fibers or of nerve cells destroyed or compressed as the tumor grows. There may be weakness of certain muscles, also changes in the sensations relating to certain parts of the skin area—either abnormal sensations or the loss of sensation. Early surgical removal of a tumor of the spinal cord usually offers the best possibility of a favorable result. Even then the outcome will depend upon how much tissue of the spinal cord has already been destroyed. In certain cases of tumor of the spinal cord, radiation therapy is preferable to surgery.

WERNICKE'S SYNDROME.

This combination of symptoms is somewhat similar to Korsakoff's syndrome, described earlier in the chapter, in that it is the result of a vitamin deficiency which usually occurs in chronic alcoholics. A rather clear evidence that it is due to a vitamin deficiency and not to the alcohol, as such, is that it has occurred among war prison inmates who were fed a vitamin-deficient diet consisting mostly of carbohydrate food. In this syndrome certain nerve cells located near the center of the brain deteriorate. The particular groups of cells involved will vary from case to case and thus the symptoms of the illness vary somewhat when comparing one case with another.

The usual symptoms include double vision, ataxia, neuritis, and mental changes such as apathy, disorientation, and forgetfulness. In some cases there are hallucinations similar to those occurring in delirium tremens.

What to Do

The success of treatment depends upon how early in the course of the disease the treatment program is begun. Without treatment, the disease proves fatal.

The treatment consists of the injection of 100 mg of thiamine each day for one week. Afterwards, 50 mg of the vitamin are administered by mouth for as long as is necessary

for the relief of the symptoms. It is desirable for other components of the vitamin B complex to be given to the patient at the same time.

WRYNECK.
(See *Neck, Stiffness of* in volume 3, chapter 22, "List of Signs and Symptoms.")

Mental Disorders

The first portion of this chapter discusses disorders in which organs of the nervous system are affected to the extent that the patient's general health is impaired or certain of his normal abilities may be diminished or destroyed. In this final portion of the chapter, devoted to mental disorders, we deal with abnormalities of the personality usually not based on disease as such but on the individual's unfavorable adjustment to life. We now consider psychological problems rather than neurological problems. Physicians specializing in such disorders are psychiatrists.

Psychoneuroses

In the psychoneuroses the affected individual reacts in an abnormal manner to certain conflicting circumstances in his life but still retains his mental capacities to the extent that he can think normally and, for the most part, exercise normal judgment. The person with a psychoneurosis often realizes that his reactions under some circumstances differ from those of other people. The psychoneuroses are not forms of insanity but, rather, personality disorders in which the behavior and the emotional responses are abnormal. The several classic types of the psychoneuroses will now be described, followed at the end with a paragraph on treatment.

THE ANXIETY REACTION.

In this type of emotional illness there are attacks of an unsettled state of mind characterized by apprehension, nervous tension, physical and mental fatigue, and panic. Attacks occurring at night may be associated with nightmares. The attack is often accompanied by physical symptoms of tremor, sweating, vomiting, diarrhea, and urinary urgency. There may be an overpowering dread of some imminent disaster. The attack may vary in duration from a few minutes to longer periods. Usually the problem relates to some intolerable situation in the patient's present or immediate past experience.

THE DISSOCIATIVE REACTION.

This is similar to the anxiety reaction except that it is more intense. In this instance, the individual actually loses control of certain of his mental functions so that he experiences extreme stupor or loses his memory or conducts himself automatically without being aware of his actions or resorts to aimless running.

THE CONVERSION REACTION (HYSTERIA).

In the conversion reaction the individual subconsciously converts energy pent up as a result of intense anxiety or frustration into some abnormal form of behavior or into some form of supposed illness which tends to protect the individual from the unbearable situation. This is an unhealthy solution to life's problems. The conversion reaction is a great imitator of many symptoms of disease,

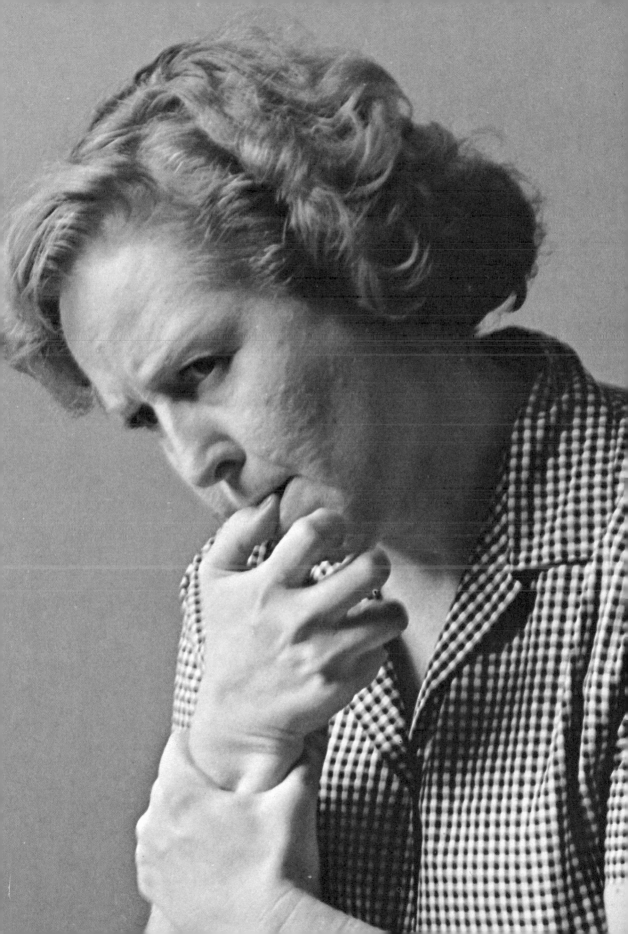

such as paralysis, anesthesia, blindness, or loss of consciousness. Oftentimes the physician's skill is taxed to tell the difference between the conversion reaction and actual disease.

THE PHOBIC REACTION (PHOBIAS).

In the phobic reaction the individual manifests an unreasonable, unjustified anxiety regarding some particular situation. Consciously he recognizes that no actual danger is involved, but he finds himself unable to control his intense fear, even so. Phobias may be directed toward high places, closed spaces, elevators, dirt, the danger of contamination, cancer, or certain animals. Phobias represent a carry-over of some unresolved conflict. It is assumed that the phobia becomes symbolic of this conflict to the extent that the individual puts the true conflict out of consciousness by focusing on the phobia.

THE DEPRESSIVE REACTION.

In this type of psychoneurosis the individual becomes downcast, pessimistic, unhappy. He feels that he is personally inadequate. He lacks energy and becomes disinterested in most of the activities about him. Crying for insufficient cause is a cardinal evidence of depression. The depressive reaction may be accompanied by certain symptoms relating to the body's functions such as loss of appetite, constipation, headache, and sleeplessness. The condition is often associated with anxiety. The attitude of discouragement may become so profound that the individual may contemplate suicide and may even make an attempt in this direction. Proper precautions should be taken so that such a patient is not left alone.

THE OBSESSIVE-COMPULSIVE REACTION.

An obsession consists of an almost uncontrollable urge to follow the same line of thought over and over. Often the thought is unwelcome but,

try as he may, the individual finds it nearly impossible to banish it from his thinking. A compulsion consists of an unreasonable urge to perform some act even though the act is entirely unnecessary and may even be unreasonable in nature. A person may become obsessed with the thought that he is carrying a germ which could infect other members of his family and even cause their death. As a result he may develop the compulsion to wash his hands frequently, particularly at certain times such as before eating, after shaking hands, or at fifteen-minute intervals. Mild degrees of the obsessive-compulsive reaction may occur in persons who live normally. This tendency may become manifest in the immaculate housekeeper or in the accountant who is meticulously accurate.

A person may develop the obsession that he is changing in appearance, and this may prompt the compulsion that forces him to look in the mirror repeatedly for evidences of such change. A person with an obsession may be constantly troubled by obscene thoughts out of harmony with his standards of conduct. A religious person may be obsessed by doubts regarding the foundation of his beliefs. A person may develop the compulsion that he must remove his clothes in a certain routine. This may become so troublesome that if anything interferes with the routine, he will have to put his clothes on again and start the routine all over. A person with a compulsion may feel that he is forced to touch all power poles as he passes them on the sidewalk.

The obsessive-compulsive reaction is supposed to be a subconscious form of penance associated with guilt and self-condemnation. The individual who develops these obsessions and compulsions is not consciously aware of the background of his reactions.

Treatment of the Psychoneuroses. A person with a psychoneurosis will frequently gain benefit from a series of conversations with a

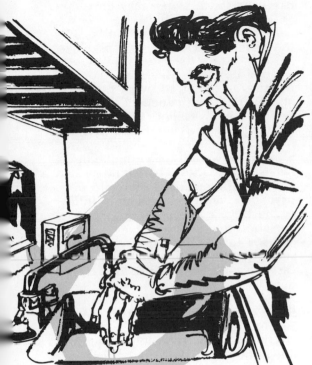

An obsessive fear of germs leading to frequent hand washing can be a part of a psychoneurotic pattern.

psychiatrist intended to help him recognize the relationship between his present symptoms and the unsolved problems which lie at their foundation. The patterns of thinking and acting are usually so firmly established that a mere explanation of the cause of the symptoms will not enable the individual to overcome them. The patient has to have time to reorient his thinking to the extent of accepting the fact of his unfavorable circumstances and planning ways of being realistic rather than hiding behind excuses or dodging the real issues.

The physician can often aid the patient during his period of reorientation by prescribing one of the modern tranquilizers to relieve anxiety or by using one of the antidepressant drugs to help the patient rise above his periods of depression.

Psychotic Disorders

The psychotic disorders include several forms of mental derangement any one of which constitutes "insanity" in the usual meaning of the word. When a person becomes ill with a psychosis, he loses control of his thinking and acting to the extent that his behavior no longer is in harmony with accepted standards or consistent with the realities of his situation in life. Efforts to persuade him that his thinking is confused or that his actions are not acceptable do not change his abnormal patterns.

The person with a psychosis is no longer able to carry his share of responsibility in the family or in the community. He may be irrational and irresponsible and, for his own good, may have to be required to comply with regulations that others consider best rather than being allowed to follow his own dictates.

Fundamental causes of the psychoses are still debated. Most psychiatrists feel that hereditary factors sometimes make one person less able than others to adjust successfully to life's demands and that such an individual's personality may disintegrate under stresses in life that require greater adjustments than the patient is capable of making. Others, however, believe that the psychoses are caused by some yet undiscovered abnormality of the chemical processes that occur within the nerve cells of the brain.

In some instances persons with a psychotic disorder become difficult to manage. For a discussion of this problem, see volume 3, chapter 18, "Handling Emergencies," the item entitled *Insanity, Handling of a Disturbed Person.*

For a discussion of some of the common manifestations of the psychoses, that may be encountered, consult volume 3, chapter 22, "List of Signs and Symptoms," under the headings of *Delirium, Mental Deficiency,* and *Mental Disorders.*

443

THE AFFECTIVE PSYCHOSIS (MANIC-DEPRESSIVE PSYCHOSIS).

This form of psychosis is characterized by an exaggerated mood with only a minor involvement, if any, of the ability to think. The affective psychosis tends to occur in attacks, between which the individual may be entirely normal.

The disturbances of mood may be in either direction, that of mania and elation or that of depression and melancholy. In one attack, mania may predominate; in another, depression. In some patients, the mood in each attack shifts toward mania; in others, toward depression. In still other cases, there may be a shift from mania to depression or vice versa in the same attack.

The first attack of affective psychosis typically occurs in young adulthood. It is assumed that heredity plays an important role in setting the stage for the development of this illness. Without adequate treatment, the typical attack of affective psychosis may last up to a year or more. With modern methods of treatment, the time is usually shortened.

In the manic phase of the illness, the patient tends to become more and more excited. There are tireless overactivities and feelings of elation. Judgment and insight are usually poor, and the patient may act in a mischievous manner to the extent of tearing his clothing, disarranging his room, and engaging in mild vandalism. Commonly he sings and shouts and even displays occasional delusions of grandeur. He may become easily annoyed with those who try to restrain or control him. He talks a great deal but not on sensible topics.

In the depressed phase the patient is downhearted and fearful and experiences feelings of inadequacy. He sleeps poorly, and all physical activity is accomplished with great effort. He typically develops delusions of self-condemnation in which he believes, "I am not worth anything." There may be attempts at suicide. In extreme cases a state of stupor may develop.

Treatment of the affective psychosis consists of four parts: (1) arranging for the professional services of a psychiatrist, (2) placing the patient in suitable surroundings, (3) using shock therapy or drugs to hasten recovery from the attack, and (4) influencing the patient by kind conversation to avoid the foolish business schemes which he is prone to develop and to look forward to recovery and to the resumption of his usual activities. There is no essential loss of mentality in the affective psychosis, and the patient is influenced by his surroundings and conversation to a greater extent than he appears to be. He may even understand quite well that he is ill. Most cases respond favorably to kind treatment.

SCHIZOPHRENIA (DEMENTIA PRAECOX).

Schizophrenia is the most serious one of the group of mental disorders. Although recovery occurs in some cases in response to modern methods of treatment, many cases become chronic and progressively incapacitating. The usual chronic nature of the illness can be emphasized by noting that less than 20 percent of the first admissions to public mental hospitals are for schizophrenia whereas about 60 percent of all who remain permanently in these hospitals are victims of this disease.

In schizophrenia the patient loses his ability to distinguish clearly between fantasy and reality. Both his ability to think and his emotional responses become confused.

It is generally assumed that some particular hereditary predisposition makes certain people susceptible to a breakdown of personality structure once they are subjected to difficult situations. Some persons living perfectly normal lives have traits of personality that resemble, in mild degree, the victim of schizophrenia. Presumably such persons would become ill with this type of mental disorder

444

should they become seriously distressed because of problems in their environment for which they could not find adequate solutions. The fact that some people respond more favorably than others to treatment suggests that the hereditary predisposition is more pronounced in some individuals than in others.

Schizophrenia may develop at any age, but it is less frequent in childhood and after age fifty than it is in young adulthood. The disease often begins insidiously. As the victim begins to withdraw from reality, he appears to others to be preoccupied. His conversations may assume an odd pattern, but the individual experiences no concern even when this is brought to his attention.

As the disease progresses, delusions, hallucinations, and odd mannerisms develop. In his delusions, the patient with schizophrenia often hears persons saying unkind things about him. He seems to live in a world apart and may spend time staring at himself in the mirror or smiling or laughing to himself. His emotional responses are often inappropriate.

Treatment for schizophrenia has been modified a great deal in recent years. The use of drugs particularly adapted for psychotic disorders has now largely replaced the previous use of shock therapy. The use of psychotherapy and maintenance of a friendly, understanding attitude by workers in the hospital where the schizophrenic is placed contribute greatly to the success of the drug therapy. Although many cases do not recover completely, a large proportion respond well enough to be able to live relatively normal lives outside the hospital.

PARANOIA.

Paranoia is not a clear-cut disease independent of those just described. It is a type of response seen in persons who may have schizophrenia or who may have affective psychosis. It is characterized by delusions in which the individual attempts to bolster his self-esteem by assuming that people are plotting against him. He craves recognition; but, having failed to obtain the acclaim he desires, he develops false explanations which indicate that he has failed in life only because of the plottings and jealousies of others.

Paranoia may have its roots in childhood because of experiences that deprived the individual of the degree of social acceptance which most children receive. In these early stages disappointment in life could have been overcome had the individual become successful in his chosen enterprises. Success in these would have brought about the recognition he desired. In persons who have found life to be disappointing, however, it is easy for the early childhood experiences of sullenness and hatred to become exaggerated to the extent that a psychosis develops.

The delusions of paranoia often lead the patient to imagine himself as being some important or great person—a king, a queen, or an inventor.

The paranoid may become dangerous because of the possibility that he may do bodily harm to those he feels are plotting against him. Many patients will respond favorably, however, to the kindness and sympathy of some person whom they feel they can trust. It is such a person who may be able to bring about improvement in a case of paranoia as he tactfully persuades the patient to accept reasonable interpretations of his circumstances. Successful treatment of paranoia consists more of sympathetic relationships than of any specific therapy.

Organic Brain Syndromes

Many conditions of poor general health exert an influence on the functioning of the brain and may be responsible for symptoms similar to those produced by specific brain disease or by genuine psychotic disorders. The fundamental fault is with the systemic disease that has adversely affected the brain and only secondarily with the person's way of thinking or reacting to life's realities.

Many forms of illness cause temporary mental confusion which we commonly designate as delirium. Arteriosclerosis, as it affects the vessels of the brain, is frequently the cause of mental confusion and excitement with deterioration of the intellectual capacities. Tumors of the brain, general paresis of the insane (a complication of syphilis), chronic alcoholism, and other toxic conditions may also have such adverse effects.

Treatment of the organic brain syndrome obviously consists of removing the cause of the problem if such removal is possible.

Endocrine Gland Diseases

Many of the body's glands discharge their products through tubes called ducts. Other glands have no such outlets. Instead, their secretions are discharged into the blood and carried by it to parts of the body far distant from the glands themselves. For this reason these ductless glands are sometimes called endocrine glands, or glands of internal secretion; and the substances which they secrete are correspondingly called hormones.

The secretions of the endocrine glands are also called hormones because of the way they act. This name comes from a word which means "an agent or messenger to stir up activity." Hormones help to stimulate or control growth and many other activities of the body which are carried on without our consciousness or thought. The circulation of the blood is partly regulated by them. Changes in the cells which enable food to be absorbed and wastes to be prepared for excretion are brought about largely by hormone action. Whether a child will grow up to be intelligent or stupid in mind, and healthy or sickly in body, depends to a great extent on the influence of the secretions of his endocrine glands.

The most important endocrine glands are the adrenals, the islets of the pancreas, the parathyroids, the pituitary, the sex glands, and the thyroid.

The endocrine glands and their hormones are described in detail in volume 3, chapter 12, "The Glands." Some of the data given there are also mentioned here to help explain disorders that result from abnormalities of the glands. In many cases what might be spoken of as a disease of one endocrine gland also concerns the action of other glands. The fault is usually either an underproduction or an overproduction of one or more hormones, and in most cases the so-called disease cannot be detected as easily or treated in as simple a way as can diseases of many of the other organs of the body. For these reasons most of the discussions in this chapter will be quite general; and only in exceptional cases will a disease be given individual discussion with definite suggestions as to what to do.

Adrenal Disorders

The adrenal glands are shaped somewhat like caps, one resting on the upper end of each kidney. Each gland has an inner core called the medulla and an outer layer called the cortex. The secretion of the medulla, epinephrine (adrenaline), has something to do with the heart muscle and with the small muscles in the blood-vessel walls so that it keeps the pressure of the circulating blood high enough to

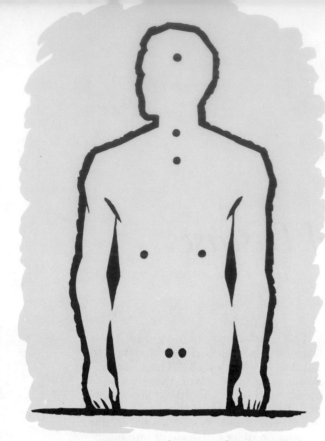

Location of main endocrine glands.

The secretion of the adrenal cortex, a mixture of thirty or more related compounds called steroids, is quite different from epinephrine. One of the compounds, aldosterone, helps to control sodium, potassium, and water distribution in the body. Cortisone and hydrocortisone help to regulate protein, carbohydrate, and fat metabolism in the body and to control inflammatory and immune reactions. Still another, androsterone (like the male sex hormone, testosterone) is a masculinizing hormone, but present in both males and females.

A close relation exists between the cortical hormones of the adrenals and the adrenocorticotrophic hormone (ACTH) of the front part of the pituitary gland. If the pituitary is removed, the adrenal cortex will largely waste away. When both of these glands work in harmony, they do much to ensure normal secondary sex characteristics, and they have a beneficial effect on

Adrenal gland rests on kidney.

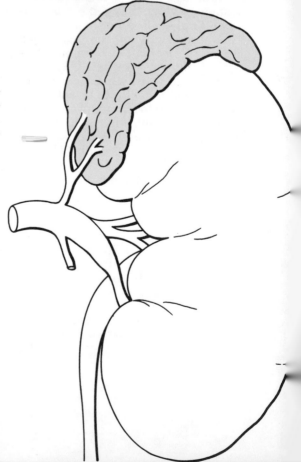

meet all needs. It also stimulates the sympathetic nerves and tends to raise the level of blood sugar, in this latter respect having an effect opposite to that of insulin.

If a person takes certain poisons, the first noticeable result is an increased pulse rate and heart action because of the irritating or stimulating effect of the poison on the adrenals and the consequent increased production of epinephrine. This in turn quickens those activities responsible for the oxidation and excretion of the poison. Fear, rage, and pain also stimulate epinephrine production. This is a wise provision of the Creator. Such emotions or conditions are likely to demand sudden and vigorous muscle action, and the muscles need a quickly available supply of energy fuel for the emergency. It has been proved that epinephrine is able to bring about the liberation of the sugar that the liver cells have stored, thus making it quickly available for use as muscle fuel.

448

tissue nutrition and general body vigor.

Increased adrenal activity may be caused by tumor growths within the glands or by a general increase in glandular activity. Tumors may develop in either the cortex or the medulla. A noteworthy tumor that develops in the medulla of the adrenal is the pheochromocytoma. It is important because it eventually causes death if allowed to persist; but, when taken in time, it can be cured by surgical removal. The pheochromocytoma produces an excess of the same hormones as are normally produced in the adrenal medulla. Its cardinal effect is to produce excessively high blood pressure. Of course, this is only one of the many things that may cause high blood pressure.

Although not all tumors developing in the cortex of the adrenal glands make hormones, those that do cause symptoms the nature of which is determined by the type of hormone produced. Those which make androsterone betray their presence by their effects on the sex characteristics. In early childhood, they tend to hasten the changes characteristic of adulthood, particularly male adulthood. In mature years they accentuate masculinity in both men and women.

In those conditions in which the cortex of the adrenal gland produces excess quantities of cortisone and hydrocortisone over long periods of time a condition known as Cushing's syndrome develops. This is characterized by general weakness; fragility of the bones; a tendency to diabetes; a peculiar kind of obesity affecting the face, neck and trunk; and high blood pressure.

ADDISON'S DISEASE.

Addison's disease is the name given to a serious condition caused by deficiency of the cortexes of the adrenal glands. The damage to the glands results from some wasting degeneration or destructive lesion such as that caused by tuberculosis. In adrenal insufficiency of this type, the person concerned suffers from chronic fatigue, exhaustion, low blood pressure, and usually a loss of sodium chloride and water from the blood and tissues. He has poor appetite and frequent attacks of nausea, vomiting, and diarrhea.

Rational treatment includes the giving of salt, cortisone, and an abundance of water, with prompt attention to any aggravating condition, such as an infection. This disease is often accompanied by many and varied complications, and it demands expert study and medical guidance; but, while the malady was once a hopeless condition, it is no longer so. Given good medical supervision and intelligent cooperation on the part of the afflicted person, an active and comparatively normal life is now possible for most victims of Addison's disease. It is fortunate, however, that there are not many of them.

The symptoms of Addison's disease do not develop until about 90 percent of the tissue of the cortex of the adrenal glands has been incapacitated. There are some intermediate cases of adrenal cortical insufficiency in which the cortexes of the adrenal glands are still producing part of their quota of steroid hormones. These cases, once recognized, should receive the same kind of carefully regulated treatment as for full-blown cases of Addison's disease.

The physician's task of evaluating a case of Addison's disease is made more difficult if it happens that the patient has received steroid medications within the recent year. In such case, the patient should, by all means, mention to his doctor the taking of such medications.

Pancreatic Islet Cell Disease

In the pancreas are found numerous groups or "islands" of cells that are smaller than the cells which secrete pancreatic juice. The "islet" cells secrete a hormone called insulin, which helps control carbohydrate metabolism in the body. Sometimes these cells degenerate, resulting in a shortage of insulin and a consequent decrease in the body's ability to utilize carbohydrates, as in the disease diabetes mellitus. This is not the only factor, however, which may interfere with the body's use of carbohydrates.

DIABETES MELLITUS.

Diabetes mellitus as a disease is considered in chapter 20, "Nutritional Diseases," in this volume.

Parathyroid Diseases

Normally there are four parathyroid glands, each about the size of a navy bean, two located behind each lateral lobe of the thyroid gland. The parathyroid glands produce a hormone which controls the amounts of calcium and phosphorus which circulate in the blood serum. The principal diseases are (1) hypoparathyroidism (in which an insufficient amount of hormone is produced) and (2) hyperparathyroidism (in which an excess of the hormone is produced).

HYPOPARATHYROIDISM.

In this disorder the amount of calcium in the blood serum is low, the amount of phosphorus, high. When it begins in childhood, a stunting of growth takes place, with malformation of the teeth and a deficiency in mental development. In the acute phase of the disorder there are cramps of the muscles (especially the abdominal muscles), difficult breathing, sensitivity to light, and convulsions. When the condition becomes chronic, there is a tendency to the formation of cataracts of the eyes and permanent brain damage.

Cases of hypoparathyroidism that develop spontaneously are rare. The usual circumstance that causes hypoparathyroidism is the removal of the parathyroid glands when thyroid surgery is performed. Persons who have had thyroid surgery should therefore be alert to the possibility of the presence of hypoparathyroidism.

What to Do

Originally the treatment for this disorder was very unsatisfactory with most cases terminating fatally. Now that doctors better understand the body's chemical processes and controls, cases respond favorably to a carefully regulated program of therapy. This requires the administration of salts of calcium (by vein in acute cases) and of a special type of vitamin D preparation. Dairy products should be avoided because of their high content of phosphorus. Frequent laboratory checkups must be made to keep track of the patient's response to the treatment and thus to avoid recurrence of the symptoms.

HYPERPARATHYROIDISM.

Hyperparathyroidism occurs more commonly than hypoparathyroidism. It is characterized by a high level of calcium in the blood serum and in the urine. This may be responsible for the development of kidney stones (because of the large amount of calcium being eliminated through the kidneys) and for fatal damage to the kidneys by deposits of calcium within their tissues. There also occurs a rarefaction of the bones as observed by X ray on account of the withdrawal of calcium salts. The symptoms include excessive thirst, excessive urination, pains in the back and in various bones and joints, and loss of appetite even with nausea and vomiting.

Usually, the cause of hyperparathyroidism is the development of some kind of tumor within one or more of the parathyroid glands. Increased function of the parathyroid glands can also develop in association with chronic kidney disease and in rickets. Certain malignant tumors in other parts of the body apparently may produce a hormone with function similar to that of the parathyroid hormone even to the extent of producing symptoms of hyperparathyroidism.

When hyperparathyroidism is caused by the development of a tumor within the parathyroid glands, surgical removal of the involved tissue is necessary.

Pituitary Diseases

The pituitary gland is located in a saddle-shaped bony pocket just below the central part of the brain. It is made up of two principal parts, though both parts taken together do not make a mass larger than the end of a finger. It is remarkable how much activity can take place within such a small space. The anterior lobe of the gland is the largest part, and looks like gland tissue. The posterior lobe looks like

Gigantism stems from an excess of the growth-promoting hormone.

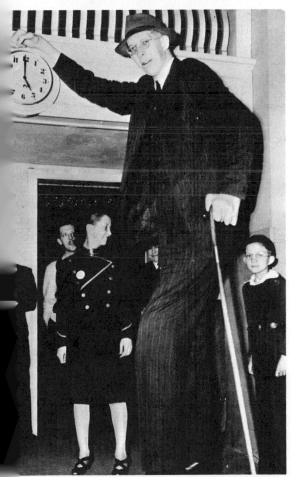

UNITED PRESS INTERNATIONAL

Intermediate lobule

Infundibular stem

Posterior lobule

Anterior lobule

The vital pituitary gland is located at the base of the brain deep inside the head. The diagram shows its main parts.

nerve tissue. The middle part serves chiefly to attach the gland to the brain.

The various hormones produced by the pituitary gland together with their normal functions are discussed and summarized by a chart in volume 3, chapter 12, "The Glands."

ACROMEGALY AND GIGANTISM.

In these diseases there is an overproduction of the growth-promoting hormone elaborated by cells in the anterior lobe of the pituitary. The overproduction usually results from the development of a tumor of the pituitary gland, the cells of which manufacture an excess of this hormone. The tumor may be either slow-growing or fast-growing. If the overproduction occurs during childhood, gigantism results with adult height ranging from six and a half feet upward. If the overproduction of hormone begins after adult growth has been attained, acromegaly is the result. In acromegaly

451

there is no apparent further increase in height but a gradual enlargement of hands and feet with an exaggeration of facial features, with the jaw, lips, nose, and ridges above the eyes becoming prominent.

The only satisfactory treatment of acromegaly and gigantism requires the destruction of the overactive tumor. The case therefore deserves the supervision of highly trained specialists who will decide on the treatment best suited for the individual case. Radiation treatment or some form of surgery are the usual methods of therapy.

CUSHING'S SYNDROME.

This disease, mentioned earlier in the chapter under *Adrenal Disorders,* is mentioned again here because it sometimes results from an overproduction in the pituitary of the adrenocorticotrophic hormone (ACTH), which, in turn, stimulates the adrenal gland to produce an excess of the adrenal corticoids. The symptoms of Cushing's syndrome may also be produced, and commonly so, by the taking of excessive doses of adrenal cortical steroids (cortisone).

It is a rare disease, more common among females. The usual symptoms are obesity (involving the face and trunk), muscular weakness, excessive growth of hair on the face and chest, atrophic changes in the skin, elevation of blood pressure, suppression of menstruation in women and decrease of sex desire in men, a thinning of bone structure. Often diabetes mellitus will develop as a result of the disease.

Prospect for recovery from this disease is poor. If a tumor, either of the pituitary or of the adrenal gland, is known to exist, surgical or radiation treatment may be helpful.

PITUITARY DWARFISM.

There are several kinds of dwarfism, but here we speak of the kind caused primarily by a decrease in production of the growth-promoting hormone elaborated by the anterior lobe of the pituitary gland. In this kind, the body's proportions are relatively normal. Dwarfs of this type have become famous circus performers. Some also have become wealthy. Often the sexual development is retarded.

To be effective, the treatment of pituitary dwarfism must be begun early in childhood. It consists of administering pituitary growth-promoting hormone of human origin (that of animal origin is not effective). Understandably, the medication is very expensive. Cases of dwarfism should be treated by specialists at a medical center.

HYPOPITUITARISM (SIMMONDS' DISEASE).

Here we refer to a condition in which all the secreting cells of the anterior lobe of the pituitary fail to produce their respective hormones. In view of the close relationship between the pituitary and the other endocrine glands, these other glands are affected also. In the mildest form of the disease, there is atrophy of the sex organs with a reduction in axillary and pubic hair and a tendency to premature aging. In more severe cases, there is also weakness, low blood pressure, low blood sugar, low body temperature, and loss of appetite.

The treatment of this condition requires the use of many hormone preparations under the direction, of course, of a specialist in endocrinology.

DIABETES INSIPIDUS.

Diabetes insipidus is a rare chronic disorder in which large quantities of dilute urine are produced. It is accompanied, of course, by a desire to drink large quantities of water. The urine in this disorder does not contain glucose (sugar) as is the case in diabetes mellitus, (For a discussion of diabetes mellitus, see chapter 20 of this volume.) The fundamental difficulty is a failure of the posterior lobe of the pituitary to produce the normal amount of the antidiuretic hormone (ADH), which acts on the cells of the kidney tubules in such a way as to favor the resorption of water from the kidney tubules.

The treatment of diabetes insipidus requires the careful planning and supervision of a highly qualified specialist.

Sex Gland Endocrine Disorders

The sex glands are important glands of internal secretion, and their hormones have much to do with the physical and mental changes that distinguish males from females as children grow up. As with the other glands of internal secretion, the sex glands constitute a part of the endocrine gland system. Diseases or disorders of these glands are, therefore, so intimately involved with disorders of other glands of internal secretion that it is difficult to classify them as separate diseases

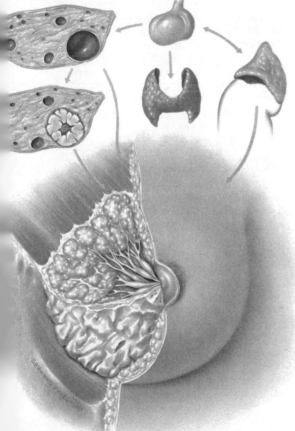

PFIZER & CO., INC.

with definite remedies for each disease.

The fundamental sex glands are the testes and the ovaries. The function of the internal secretion of the testes is simple, having to do chiefly with the development of male secondary sex characteristics, a work which it shares with the secretions of the adrenals and the pituitary. The internal secretions of the ovaries help to control menstruation, the female procreative functions in general, and many sympathetic nervous system activities associated with puberty, menstruation, and the change of life. Various disturbances of menstruation, such as too-frequent menstruation and profuse or prolonged menses, may be caused by an increase or a decrease in the amount of one or more of the female sex hormones produced by the ovaries.

The fundamental sex organs may be absent or atrophied in either the male or the female. Their vitality may be destroyed by local disease or too much exposure to radiation of any kind. If either condition dates from before puberty, it greatly influences the disposition, the sex impulses, and certain body characteristics that distinguish men from women. In the case of either sex, however, while typical secondary sex characteristics are lacking, intelligence is normal, the bones of the limbs tend to grow somewhat longer than otherwise, and the pituitary gland becomes overactive. These conditions, due to absence or devitalization of the sex glands, cannot be cured; but they are not fatal and do not prevent their victims from living useful lives.

Sexual development too early in life may be caused by tumors of the sex glands or the adrenals. They may cause all the signs and symptoms of puberty to occur at an early age. Such tumors have in some cases been removed with great benefit, but it is always a question whether or not successful surgery is possible.

A great mass of popular opinion,

453

Interrelationship between the endocrine glands and the growth and development of the breast.

much of it little better than superstition, has collected around the outward manifestations of the differences between the sexes. The mannish woman and the feminine man have to labor under greater handicaps than they should. As a matter of fact, it is hard to say exactly what is normal in either case; and there is more or less masculinity in most women, and more or less femininity in most men. Those whose build or appearance does not measure up to their masculine or feminine ideal should not worry unduly about the fact.

Disorders of the ovarian functions and their treatment deserve special attention.

Surgical removal of the ovaries late in a woman's life, or even before the natural menopause, may have little influence on her temperament or her sex impulses. Menstruation, if present, ceases, of course; and the disturbances of the "change," such as hot flashes and nervousness, may be comparable to those occurring in the natural change of life.

Some of the symptoms usually attributed to "the change of life" (the menopause), rather than being caused by actual disturbances of the endocrine organs, are of psychological origin. Here we refer to feelings of being left out, to attitudes of personal worthlessness when the children leave home, and to fears that one's feminine appeal has declined. Such symptoms may occur in a woman who feels uncertain regarding her status in the family when she reaches the late forties and early fifties, whether or not her ovaries have been previously removed by surgery.

The symptoms of the menopause such as hot flashes, nervousness, and rheumatic pains can often be wholly or partly relieved by the proper use of hormones. This applies both in cases in which the menopause is brought on prematurely by the surgical removal of the ovaries and in cases in which nature follows its usual course at the age of forty-five to fifty.

Teen-age girls and young women who suffer from painful menstruation can often be benefited by the carefully supervised administration of hormone preparations.

The ovarian functions are intimately associated with those of the thyroid and the pituitary, and in normal health the actions of the three are well balanced. Since the ovarian function is greatly altered at the change of life, pituitary and thyroid function must be adjusted in order to restore the balance. It is this intimate association that makes what seems to be an ovarian disorder such a complex problem. A woman experiencing symptoms which seem to indicate trouble with her ovaries should consult a physician, preferably one with experience in women's diseases, and this physician may wish to call an endocrinologist for consultation.

Thyroid Diseases

The thyroid gland consists of two lobes, one lying on each side of the upper part of the trachea, and an isthmus connecting the lobes and extending across in front of the trachea immediately below the Adam's apple. Considerable interaction takes place between the thyroid gland and the adrenal glands, the anterior lobe of the pituitary, and the female sex glands.

The thyroid gland produces three hormones: thyroxine, triiodothyronine, and thyrocalcitonin. Thyroxine is the principal hormone and the one to which we will give attention here. The effects of the three thyroid hormones are summarized in chapter 12 of volume 3 under "The Thyroid Gland."

An enlarged thyroid gland is called a goiter, whatever the cause of the enlargement. In some goiters an excess of thyroxine is produced, and in others a reduced amount. An overabundance of thyroxine causes a speeding up of many body activities. More than the normal amount of oxygen is used by the body's cells. The relative activity of the thyroid gland can be deter-

Goiter

(an enlarged

thyroid gland).

mined by a laboratory procedure in which the thyroid hormones in the blood are measured.

NONTOXIC GOITER.

In this condition the thyroid gland enlarges, but it does not produce more than the normal amount of its hormones. In fact, in some cases of nontoxic goiter there may even be a deficit of hormone production.

The basic cause of the nontoxic goiter is some interference with the mechanism for producing thyroxine. Because thyroxine is now in short supply, the thyroid gland enlarges (under the overruling stimulation of the pituitary gland) in an effort to compensate for the deficiency. Factors which may provoke this condition are (1) a shortage of iodine, one of the constituents of thyroxine; (2) the excessive use of one of the thyroid-depressing drugs; and (3) inherited defects of the body's enzyme system.

In former decades nontoxic goiter was much more common than now because iodine was in short supply in certain geographic areas. This deficiency has been corrected by the widespread use of iodized salt.

What to Do

The essential treatment for nontoxic goiter is the administration of thyroxine as a medication. This compensates for the reduced amount of the hormone produced by the thyroid gland and thus removes the stimulus for the gland to function beyond its normal capacity.

HYPERTHYROIDISM.

Hyperthyroidism, as the term implies, is a condition in which the thyroid gland is more active than normal. The condition is usually due to overproduction of both of the hormones thyroxine and triiodothyronine. There are several manifestations of hyperthyroidism. We will discuss the two most common ones: (1) thyrotoxicosis (Graves's disease) and (2) toxic nodular goiter.

A. *Thyrotoxicosis (Graves's disease, exophthalmic goiter).* Thyrotoxicosis is more common in women than in men in the ratio of three to one. It may occur at any age but is most frequent between the ages of ten and fifty. The predisposition to the disease often runs in families. The basic cause is now assumed to be a disturbance in the body's immune system.

The symptoms of thyrotoxicosis may develop suddenly or gradually. The sudden onsets often follow some injury, a severe infection, or some psychic upset. The usual symptoms are nervousness, intolerance for heat, rapid heartbeat, weight loss, tiredness, increased appetite, excessive thirst, difficult breathing, weakness of the muscles, fine tremor, frequent urination, and diarrhea. A goiter (enlargement of the thyroid gland) is usually obvious, although in a few cases the thyroid may remain normal in size. A prominent symptom in about 70

455

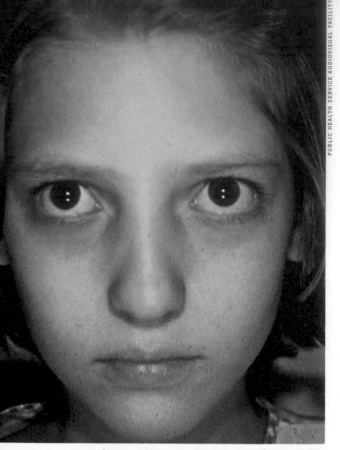

Abnormally prominent eyes characterize thyrotoxicosis (Graves's disease).

percent of the cases is a "staring expression" of the eyes so that the eyes may even appear to bulge. It is this appearance of the eyes that prompted the term "exophthalmic goiter" (goiter with protruding eyes).

What to Do

1. **Every person with thyrotoxicosis should be under the care of a physician. The excess production of thyroid hormones causes all tissues of the body to function beyond their normal rate, as though they were operating under a condition of perpetual emergency. The outlook for untreated cases is unfavorable, the eventual death being caused by problems of nutrition or by heart failure.**

2. **There are certain "antithyroid" drugs which have the effect of suppressing the excess activity of the thyroid gland. Inasmuch as these** often produce unfavorable side effects, they must be used only under careful professional supervision.

3. **The administration of radioactive iodine is now being used very successfully in many clinics. The thyroid gland absorbs and retains the iodine which, because of its radioactivity (it emits beta rays), destroys many of the overactive cells in the gland. Even this form of treatment has its complications, however, for in about 40 percent of cases the gland eventually fails to produce as much of its hormones as the body requires. Thus the condition of hyperthyroidism regresses into that of hypothyroidism.**

4. **Surgical removal of part of the hyperactive thyroid gland is still being used for cases in which other methods of treatment are inadequate.**

B. *Toxic Nodular Goiter.* Although an excess of thyroid hormones is produced in this type of goiter, as in thyrotoxicosis, it has a different background of origin. Toxic nodular goiter usually occurs as a late complication of nontoxic goiter. In such a case isolated areas of tissue within the thyroid gland become unresponsive to the body's normal checks and balances and proceed to produce excesses of hormones.

Toxic nodular goiter usually develops later in life than does thyrotoxicosis. The symptoms always come on more slowly and are not so extreme. Bulging of the eyes (exophthalmos) does not occur. In neglected cases damage to the heart may develop.

What to Do

The treatment for toxic nodular goiter is similar to that for thyrotoxicosis. The response to the use of radioactive iodine is usually good. For those cases in which radioactive iodine does not bring

456

relief, the surgical removal of the affected "nodules" of thyroid tissue is indicated.

THYROID MALIGNANCY (CANCER OF THE THYROID).

Although still a relatively rare disease, cancer of the thyroid has shown a marked increase in recent years. Some instances occur in persons who have had a goiter for many years. Others seem to occur independent of any previous thyroid disease. It is important, however, for a person with goiter to report promptly to his doctor should he notice a sudden enlargement or pain in an existing goiter or should he suddenly develop difficulty in swallowing, a cough, difficulty in breathing, or a change in the quality of his voice.

The use of radioactive iodine in the treatment of goiters seems not to predispose to cancer of the thyroid. However, cancer of the thyroid is more common in persons who, during childhood, received X-ray treatments to the tonsils or any other tissue within the neck. A person with such a history should inform his physician.

What to Do

1. The treatment of thyroid malignancy is surgical removal of part or all of the thyroid gland.

2. Following surgery some clinics use radioactive iodine in the hope that this will seek out and destroy any remaining islands of malignant thyroid tissue or of malignant tissue that has migrated (metastasized) to some other part of the body.

3. After removal of part or all of the thyroid gland it is often advisable for the patient to take appropriate doses of thyroxine for the remainder of his life in order to restore the amount of thyroid hormone which his body requires.

THYROIDITIS.

Thyroiditis is an unfortunate name for a small group of conditions which involve the thyroid gland; the members of the group seem not to be related to each other.

A. *Acute Thyroiditis*. This is a rare condition in which the thyroid gland becomes inflamed because of the invasion of bacteria. In this case the term "thyroiditis" is justified because of the presence of acute inflammation. The infection reaches the thyroid from surrounding tissues of the neck or because a cyst of the thyroid has become infected. The patient suffers from fever and pain in the neck and notices an enlargement in the area of the thyroid gland.

What to Do

The treatment of acute thyroiditis consists of eradicating the infection by the use of antibiotic medications as prescribed by a physician.

B. *Subacute Thyroiditis*. In this inflammatory condition there is a painful enlargement of the thyroid gland which persists over a period of weeks or months. It is caused, presumably, by a virus. In mild cases the illness subsides spontaneously after days or a few weeks. In the severe cases, if untreated, there may be remissions and relapses over a period of one or two years.

What to Do

The severe cases respond favorably to the administration of a corticosteroid medication which should be tapered off within a period of one month. Such medication, of course, should be under the direct supervision of a physician.

C. *Chronic Thyroiditis*. This is really not an inflammatory condition at all, in spite of the implication of the term "thyroiditis." The term embraces a small group of chronic diseases in which the thyroid becomes enlarged to various degrees and in which the functioning tissue of the thyroid is gradually replaced by connective tissue and, sometimes in part, by lymphocytes.

Hashimoto's thyroiditis is the outstanding member of the group. This disease is twenty times more frequent in women than in men. Its usual occurrence is between the ages of thirty and fifty. Typically it results in a reduction of the normal function of the thyroid gland. Patients complain of fatigue. The thyroid gland may be two or three times its normal size and is of firm consistency.

What to Do

The treatment consists of administering thyroid hormone (thyroxine) to make up for what the gland is no longer producing on its own.

HYPOTHYROIDISM.

Hypothyroidism is a condition in which the thyroid gland secretes less than the normal amount of thyroxine or a poor quality of it; however, rather surprisingly, the gland may in some cases be considerably enlarged. The most extreme cases of hypothyroidism are the congenital or childhood type, known as cretinism, and the later-developing type, myxedema.

A. *Cretinism.* Cretinism usually starts because of thyroid deficiency in the mother, but the child also develops this deficiency. Children with this condition do not grow so rapidly or so symmetrically as they should. Their minds are slow in development. No abnormality may be seen at birth, but within a few weeks the skin begins to thicken and the cry becomes hoarse. The tongue becomes large and the facial expression piglike. The teeth are late in developing. If not treated, cretins become and remain deformed, feeble-minded dwarfs, for whom little improvement is possible after the usual growing years are past.

Now that adequate treatment is available for cretinism, it is urgent that the condition be recognized in early infancy and treatment be begun promptly.

What to Do

Whenever there is question regarding an infant's progress in development a physician who specializes in such matters (either a pediatrician or an endocrinologist) should be consulted.

The treatment for cretinism consists essentially of the administering of thyroxine to make up the deficiency in what the child's own thyroid gland is producing.

B. *Myxedema.* In myxedema the production of thyroxine is below normal, oxidation in the body is decreased, and all the chemical activities of the body are slowed down. The heartbeat and the breathing become slower, and the heart action becomes weaker. The heart may become dilated. Perspiration is scanty, and susceptibility to infection is greater. The temperature is below normal. The patient feels chilly and asks for more clothing, especially bedclothing. A peculiar type of tissue swelling follows, which may occur in any or all of the body tissues. It changes the skin, causing it to become puffy, rough, and thickened. The hair becomes dry and falls out easily. The nails are brittle and cracked. The body as a whole appears fat and soggy. The voice often sounds hoarse and harsh, hearing is impaired, and the victim appears mentally dull.

Myxedema is, typically, a disease of adults and occurs whenever the production of thyroid hormones is greatly reduced. Myxedema may occur in a case in which there has been intensive treatment for hyperthyroidism. In such an instance, the treatment has caused the production of thyroid hormones to be reduced below the normal level. This does not necessarily mean that the treatment of the hyperthyroidism was faulty. The treatment may have been the means of saving the patient's life. In such a case, in which the thyroid gland is no longer producing as much hormone as it should, it is relatively easy for the physician to arrange to make up the deficiency by prescribing thyroxine medication.

What to Do

▌The doctor can confirm the suspicion of hypothyroidism by order- ing the laboratory test to determine the amount of thyroxine present in the patient's blood. In addition, he may want to order other laboratory studies.

The treatment of myxedema consists of administering thyroxine medication.

Lymphoid Tissue Diseases

The human body contains several organs or masses composed of lymphoid tissue. This tissue is made up mostly of cells called lymphocytes. About one third of the total number of circulating white cells in the bloodstream are lymphocytes. There is a constant interchange between these circulating cells and the lymphocytes of the lymphoid tissues. Some of the lymphoid organs are the spleen, a large solid structure in the upper left side of the abdominal cavity; the thymus, in the chest cavity, just behind the upper part of the breastbone; and the lymph nodes, of which there are five or six hundred scattered in different parts of the body. These latter vary in size but are all small, most not larger than a small bean. There are many in the sides of the neck, the armpits, the groin, the central part of the chest cavity, and the abdominal cavity.

Other important collections of lymphoid tissue are the Peyer's patches in the lower part of the small intestine; the tonsils, situated on the sidewalls of the throat near the back part of the tongue; the adenoids, also called the pharyngeal tonsils, on the upper part of the rear wall of the throat; and the appendix, attached to the large intestine near the place where the small intestine joins it.

In recent years the lymphoid tissue system has been found to have extremely important and complex responsibilities in the normal day-to-day function of the human body. The body's tissue fluid (lymph) moves slowly through lymph channels which are separate from the blood vessels except that they finally empty into blood vessels. The lymph, as it moves along, passes through lymph nodes which act as guardians to keep foreign particles, disease germs, and cancer cells from entering the bloodstream. Also the lymphoid tissue system is quickly mobilized to produce antibodies (killer proteins) which help to control viral, bacterial, fungal, and some parasitic infections. Lymphoid tissue helps the body reject poisons and injurious proteins. It probably regulates the healing process. Malfunctions of this system are presumably responsible for diseases such as allergies and certain ailments of the joints, skin, lung, and kidney in the so-called autoimmune category. It is the body's lymphoid tissue that causes transplanted tissues and organs to be rejected. Since the lymphoid tissue system is widely scattered throughout the body, the physical removal of part of it, if diseased (i.e. spleen, lymph nodes), appears not to have any major deleterious effect on the body. Certain chemicals however can paralyze or destroy the entire lymphoid tissue system.

Diseases associated with the

thymus, also inflammations of the tonsils, adenoids, and appendix, are discussed elsewhere in this volume. Inflammation of the Peyer's patches occurs almost solely as a feature of typhoid fever. The spleen is involved in several different diseases, but it is seldom if ever the seat of a disease by itself. Virtually every infection or infectious disease that attacks the human body involves the lymph nodes but usually only secondarily. In this chapter we shall consider in detail only (1) Hodgkin's disease, in which the lymph nodes are primarily affected, and (2) swelling of the lymph nodes, which occurs almost every time they are involved in any other disease. Involvement of the lymph nodes occurs sooner or later in most cancers, as well as with infections by disease germs or viruses.

HODGKIN'S DISEASE.

Hodgkin's disease, a serious, chronic, progressive disease, has a higher incidence among men and boys than among women and girls. Typically it begins in young adulthood. If not treated, Hodgkin's disease causes death in about two years. The precise cause is not known. It is assumed to be a form of cancer which in early stages involves the lymphoid tissue.

The first evidences may appear gradually. The lymph nodes enlarge progressively. Those located where they can be felt are firm and elastic to the touch. Early they remain freely movable and do not mat together. Troublesome itching may accompany early node enlargement, and episodes of night sweats are common. Later the victim has spells of moderate fever, is weak, loses weight, and becomes pale and anemic. The symptoms and signs of this disease, however, are so nearly like those of some other diseases that about the only sure way to detect its presence is for a physician to arrange for the removal and microscopic examination of one of the enlarged lymph nodes.

Many distressing conditions may develop in the course of Hodgkin's disease. While the lymph nodes in the neck are usually the first to be affected, and while the swollen nodes are not painful, those in the interior of the body often press upon various organs and structures and interfere with their functions.

Many highly specialized tests have been developed which properly determine the extent of the disease. This knowledge when properly applied allows for the intelligent choice of proper treatment for each patient.

Modern methods for the treatment of Hodgkin's disease require the judicious and skillful use of adequate radiation therapy and/or the administration of specially selected and combined anticancer medicines. Because these treatments are potentially dangerous, they must be given under the direction of specially skilled physicians. When such treatment is properly administered, the ten-year relapse-free rate of survival for patients with mild to moderately advanced Hodgkin's disease (stages I, II, and III) is over 50 percent. Even with advanced disease (stage IV) the patient's chance of a ten-year relapse-free survival is now over 30 percent and is improving steadily as physicians become increasingly skilled.

What to Do

When it is noticed that the lymph nodes in the neck, in the axilla, or in the inguinal region enlarge without the evidences of infection in these areas, the findings should be reported to a physician. The enlargement of the lymph nodes in the early stages of Hodgkin's disease may be on one side of the body only. There are other conditions, of course, in which enlargement of the lymph nodes may occur. However, it is important in any such case to determine the cause for the enlargement.

The physician will make the necessary examination in order to determine the exact cause of this enlargement of the lymph nodes. If it is discovered that this is a beginning case of Hodgkin's disease, the patient should be referred to the nearest major medical center where the modern methods of treating the disease are available.

SWELLING OF THE LYMPH NODES.

Nearly all the disease conditions affecting the lymph nodes produce an enlargement which can easily be seen and felt if the affected nodes are situated near the body surface. These swellings are more likely to be painful and tender if they are caused by inflammation or if they develop rapidly.

A sore throat, a sore mouth, a bad cold, infected tonsils, or disease of the middle ear is usually accompanied by swollen and tender lymph nodes on the sides of the neck and underneath the jaws. An infected hand or a sore on a hand or an arm is likely to be accompanied by swelling of the nodes in the corresponding armpit. Sores on the scalp often lead to swollen nodes behind the ears and on the back of the neck. Infections of the feet or legs frequently cause swelling of the nodes in the groin. These swellings usually subside with the disappearance of the conditions which occasioned them, but meanwhile some of them may require medical or surgical treatment on their own account.

In various acute infectious diseases, including scarlet fever, smallpox, and typhoid fever, many of the lymph nodes throughout the body are inflamed and swollen. Bubonic plague gets its common name from the fact that, in most cases, the lymph nodes throughout the body, but often most noticeably those in the groin, are inflamed, and pus forms in them. Such inflamed lymph nodes are called buboes. Uninformed or ignorant people sometimes call them "blue balls."

A peculiar disease known as glandular fever or infectious mononucleosis causes many of the lymph nodes throughout the body, but especially those in the neck to be swollen and tender. This disease may last from a few days to three or four weeks, but is seldom a menace to life. It is probably caused by a virus. It is characterized by fever, sore throat, and general weakness in addition to the swollen lymph nodes; and the spleen is often enlarged and the liver often inflamed. Occasionally there is a skin rash. The most distinctive sign, however, is the presence in the blood of a special form of protein produced by the body as a reaction against the virus infection. The test to detect this protein is called a "Mono Spot Test." This is the simplest of several tests now used by medical laboratories to determine if the infectious mononucleosis is present. Sometimes weakness may persist for two or three months after all other symptoms have subsided.

Tuberculosis frequently involves the lymph nodes of the body. In most cases of tuberculosis in which the nodes seem to be affected more than any other tissues, children are the victims; and the nodes eventually heal, but with calcium deposits in many of them, especially those in the chest. Tuberculous nodes may break down and form pus, however. Lancing such a node is not likely to do much good, but sometimes it is advisable to remove the entire node.

Syphilis always involves the lymph nodes. Accompanying the primary sore on the genitals, there is painless swelling of the nodes in the groin. Later, in the second stage of the disease, the nodes throughout the body become hard and feel as if they were enlarged; but during this stage they neither become painful nor have pus in them.

As mentioned earlier in this chapter, there is an important connection between cancer and the lymph nodes. Enlargement of the nodes because of cancer is different from that from many other causes. It comes from the transference of cancer cells to the nodes from the original sites and the development of cancer in the nodes themselves. An outstanding example of this process occurs in the armpits, cells being carried there from cancer in the breast. Other nodes frequently involved are those under the jaws and on the neck, to which cells are carried from cancer of the lips, mouth, or tongue. In the treatment of cancer anywhere it is as important to detect any lymph nodes that may be involved and to remove them as it is to detect and remove the original tumor. Otherwise no real cure is possible, and improvement is only temporary, because the cancer has spread to a new site in the nodes.

What to Do

1. Try to learn the cause of the swelling, securing the aid of a physician if needed.

2. If the swollen lymph nodes are painful and tender, and if they are located in an accessible place near the body surface, apply hot fomentations over them three times a day. (See volume 3, chapter 20, "Simple Home Treatments.")

3. Keep the patient under a physician's care, if possible, so that any pus formation may be promptly detected, and the node or nodes may be lanced and drained without delay if such treatment should be needed.

Infectious Diseases

Infectious diseases are those caused by entry into the body of one of the infectious agents commonly called germs. These agents subdivide into four groups:

1. Plantlike organisms, among which are bacteria, yeasts, and molds.

2. Organisms of animal origin consisting principally of protozoa (organisms such as those causing amebic dysentery and malaria) and worms which invade the body's tissues or cavities.

3. The rickettsiae, small organisms usually carried by arthropods and capable of producing such diseases as typhus fever and Rocky Mountain spotted fever.

4. Viruses, the causative agents of many infectious diseases such as chicken pox, influenza, German measles, mumps, poliomyelitis, and rabies.

Many diseases caused by infectious agents are not discussed in the present chapter, being considered rather under "Skin Diseases," "Diseases of the Respiratory Organs," "Intestinal Parasites," "Tuberculosis," "Venereal Infections," and "Warm-climate Ailments" in this volume.

When an infectious disease can be transmitted from person to person it is called contagious or communicable. Most of the common contagious diseases are described in the present chapter. Many of these are spoken of as "childhood diseases" because children are affected more frequently than adults.

An immunity is developed against many of these diseases once a person has had them. Thanks to current methods of immunization, it is possible also for a person to be made immune in many cases without ever contracting the disease. See chapter 3 of this volume for a discussion of immunity.

Home Care for Contagious Diseases

The procedure for general care of a patient at home is discussed in volume 3, chapter 19. But with contagious diseases special measures must be taken to minimize spread, some requiring greater precautions than others. Specifics will be discussed as we take up the various diseases in the chapter; but first let us note a few general principles on caring for a person with a contagious disease at home:

One particular room should be set apart as the sickroom, and the patient should remain in this room until the doctor indicates that the patient has passed the time when the illness is "catching."

The sickroom, usually a bedroom, should be kept attractive in appearance. It is not necessary to remove drapes, pictures, and desirable articles of furniture except as these make the room too crowded or interfere with the care of the patient. It must be remembered that one of the factors in recovery is a happy state of mind. The room should be kept in such condition, therefore, as to make it cheerful and homelike.

If there is a choice, the room selected for the sickroom should be as close as possible to the bathroom.

The windows of the sickroom should be screened so as to prevent the entrance of insects, which in some diseases serve as carriers of germs.

Certain materials and utensils necessary for the care of the patient, though they be articles commonly used in the home, will now have to be kept in the sickroom until the patient recovers. These should be kept neatly on a small bedside table or chair.

Special care should be taken in the daily cleaning of the sickroom to avoid raising dust that might carry germs to other parts of the house. The floor should be damp-dusted or mopped rather than swept with a broom. The use of a good vacuum cleaner is reasonably safe.

First Steps in Protection. Germs are easily carried by "droplet infection." They ride as passengers on tiny droplets of moisture expelled from a person's mouth during a sneeze or vigorous cough. For this reason all persons are advised to cover the mouth and nose with a handkerchief at the time of sneezing or coughing, a precaution doubly important for the patient with a contagious disease. The nurse or family member in attendance should instruct the patient to cover all sneezes and coughs; he should also try to remain out of the path of the current of air coming from the patient's nose and mouth. If the patient does not cooperate by covering his mouth and

A cheerful atmosphere in the sickroom aids in recovery from disease.

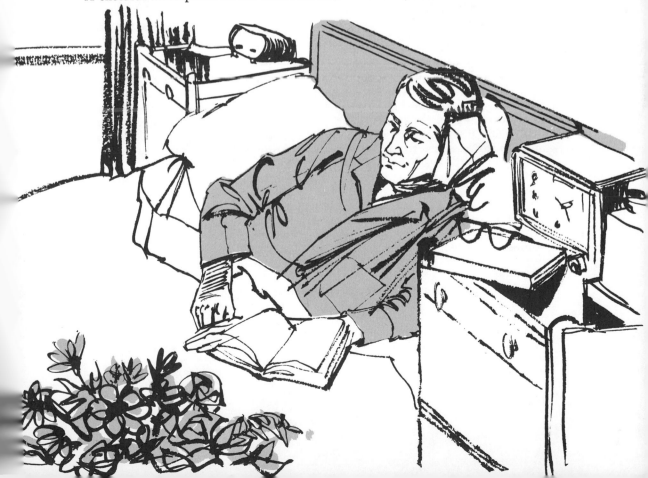

nose when sneezing, it may even be advisable for the attendant to wear a surgical mask while caring for the patient.

Germs can also be carried by the patient's sputum, by discharges from his nose and open wounds, and by the urine and feces. More will be said about these matters in the paragraph dealing with the disposal of wastes.

Hand Washing and Nail Care. In the routine care of a patient, it is the attendant's hands which become contaminated first. Without proper cleansing, the hands readily carry germs from the patient to objects about the room and to other parts of the house. Anyone caring for a sick person should develop the firm habit of not touching his own face and hair.

Hands should be carefully washed after each contact with a person suffering from an infectious disease, preferably with warm running water and plenty of soap. Time should be taken to work the suds in between the fingers and high onto the wrists. Fingernails should be given careful attention by cleaning beneath them with an orange stick or other blunt instrument while the hands are being washed. Paper towels are preferable for drying because they are disposable. When frequent washings irritate the skin of the hands, a mild hand lotion may be applied after each washing.

Wearing a Gown. It is easy for the attendant's clothes to become contaminated while waiting on a patient. Without precaution, this may lead to the spread of the infection to other persons. The usual method of precaution is for the attendant to wear a covering garment (gown) whenever he comes in contact with the patient or the patient's bedclothing. It is not necessary, of course, to put on a gown simply to hand the patient a book or a drink of water.

The gown need not be the same type as worn in a hospital. It should have long sleeves, however, and should fully cover the attendant. A housecoat or long smock is quite suit-

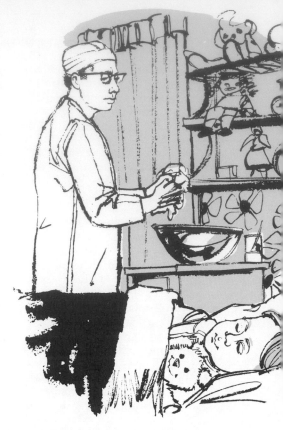

able. It should be left hanging near the door in the patient's room when the attendant leaves so as to be easily available when he returns. The attendant should wash his hands, of course, each time after the gown is removed. In case only a short-sleeved gown is available, the hands and forearms, up to the elbows, need to be washed thoroughly.

Care of the Patient's Dishes. All food remaining on the patient's dishes should be discarded at once. If the method of disposal requires that the garbage be placed in a garbage can, it is best to place the leftovers from the patient's dishes in a paper or plastic sack and close this tightly before placing it in the garbage can. This precaution prevents flies and other insects from making contact with the germs that the food fragments may carry.

Dishes from the patient's room should be washed separately either in an automatic dishwasher or by hand, with abundant soap or detergent.

After the usual washing, they should be stacked in a position that permits them to drain and then rinsed with boiling water, following which they should merely drain dry rather than being dried by a dish towel. After they are dry, they may be safely returned to the dish cupboard along with other household dishes. Many people prefer to save time and effort by using disposable plastic or paper dishes so that these can be discarded after use.

Disposal of Wastes. For discharges from the patient's nose, mouth, or infected wounds, the safest method of disposal is to collect them in paper tissue and to keep the accumulation in a tightly closed paper or plastic sack to be taken out later and burned.

Urine and feces from the patient can be safely flushed down the toilet, provided the home has a properly functioning septic tank or is connected to a city sewer system in which the sewage is scientifically treated rather than being merely discharged into a stream or a lake. Under other circumstances, the patient's urine and feces should be chemically treated with a disinfectant before being emptied. For this, they may be placed in a covered container of at least two gallons capacity and mixed with a 5 percent solution of a phenol or cresol type of disinfectant. Such disinfectants are available at the drugstore, and a 5 percent solution is prepared by mixing one part of the disinfectant as it comes from the drugstore with nineteen parts of water. The urine and feces should remain in contact with the disinfectant solution for an hour before being finally emptied. Care should be used to keep the bottle of phenol or cresol disinfectant out of the reach of children, for it is poisonous.

The Patient's Laundry. The patient's laundry, including bedclothing, bed linen, and towels, should be washed as soon as possible after removal from the sickroom. It should be washed separately from other laundry, but may be washed in the washing machine or by whatever other method is usual. The water used should be steaming hot, and abundant soap or detergent should be used. Pieces of laundry that are heavily contaminated by the patient's discharges should be boiled for five minutes before being washed in the usual manner. If the household wash is sent to a commercial laundry, that from the patient's room should be packaged separately and this package plainly labeled to warn that it contains contaminated articles.

Mental Hygiene for the Patient. It must be constantly recognized that a patient has emotional as well as physical needs. Attendants should maintain a cheerful attitude and do what is reasonably possible to make the surroundings pleasant. As conditions permit and as the doctor approves, the patient should be allowed to engage in pleasant, trivial activities, even while still in bed. These will help to occupy his mind and will improve his morale.

Returning the Sickroom to General Use. Even after a patient with a contagious disease has recovered, the germs associated with his illness may linger in the sickroom. Thus, certain precautions should be taken before the sickroom is returned to general use. Woodwork, the bare portion of the floor, and furniture should be washed with soap and water and the room aired for several hours. Articles such as toys and hot water bottles should be washed and placed in the sunshine to dry. Bed clothing, rugs, drapes, and other articles which are not easily washable should be aired in sunlight for six hours or more. Utensils which have been used in the sickroom should be washed carefully with soap and water and, if they will not be damaged by the heat, placed in actively boiling water for at least five minutes. The thermometer which has been used to take the patient's temperature should be washed with soap and cool water, soaked in alcohol (rubbing alcohol is suitable) for thirty minutes, rinsed, and dried.

The Infectious Diseases

The following pages in this chapter contain discussions of the various infectious diseases. The items are arranged in alphabetical order. In cases where the principal description of the disease is in another chapter cross-reference is made to this location.

ACTINOMYCOSIS.

This noncontagious disease occurs in all parts of the world, most commonly in young male adults. It is caused by a fungus. When the fungus is breathed in, it affects the lungs. Otherwise it enters through some break in the skin or mucous membrane. It typically causes draining sinuses and abscesses in the face, neck, chest, and abdomen. Usually the infection is acquired while one is working in proximity to cattle.

What to Do

Actinomycosis is a serious disease which carried a high percentage of fatality before antibiotics became available for use in treatment. In many of the more serious cases appropriate surgery must be combined with the use of penicillin or other antibiotic drug. Of course all cases of actinomycosis must be under the supervision of a physician.

ADENOVIRUS INFECTIONS.

The adenoviruses are a group responsible for causing a small percentage of the cases of "common cold." In some epidemics of the common cold among military recruits, one of the adenoviruses has been responsible for most of the cases.

There is no specific treatment for adenovirus infections. Bed rest and suitable symptomatic treatment tend to shorten the course of the illness and reduce the possibility of complications.

AMEBIASIS.

(See chapter 21 in this volume under "Amebic Dysentery.")

ANTHRAX (MALIGNANT PUSTULE; WOOLSORTER'S DISEASE).

Anthrax is acquired by contact with animals. Though not common, it is dangerous when it occurs. The germs of anthrax (anthrax bacillus) occur commonly as spores (the latent form) which adhere to the skin or hair of animals and may remain potentially dangerous for a long time.

Human infection may occur when people handle animals, their hides, or their hair. The spores usually enter through a break in the skin. In a small number of cases the spores are inhaled into the lungs. In another small group of cases the spores are introduced into the body by eating contaminated meat.

The form of the disease which results when the spores are taken into the lungs or into the organs of digestion is much more serious and progresses more rapidly than the form in which the spores enter through a break in the skin. Even in the latter, the infection may spread throughout the body with fatal results in about 20 percent of the cases.

In a typical case of anthrax involving the skin, a small, red, slightly

Typical case of anthrax.

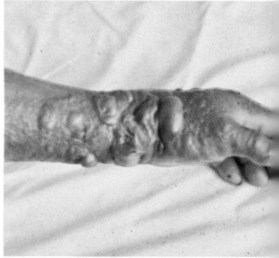

raised spot appears at the site where the spores entered. The lesion increases rapidly in size to form a flattened blister, which becomes a dark-colored ulcer around which the tissue is swollen. There may be itching but very little pain. It is usually this dark-colored ulcer surrounded by swollen tissue which attracts attention to the infection.

The type of anthrax which forms a skin ulcer and remains localized usually responds favorably to the use of an appropriate antibiotic.

ATHLETE'S FOOT.
(See chapter 12, "Skin Diseases," in this volume.)

BLASTOMYCOSIS.
Blastomycosis occurs occasionally in the central and southeastern parts of the United States. The organism which causes it is a yeastlike fungus, the spores of which are carried by the air and breathed into the lungs. The disease is not transmitted from person to person and therefore is not classified as contagious. It affects the lungs, the skin, and, sometimes, the bones.

Care of a patient with blastomycosis should be under the direct supervision of a physician. The essential feature of the treatment is the administration of some antibiotic drug which is particularly effective against fungous infections.

BOTULISM.
(See *Poisoning: Food Poisoning* in volume 3, chapter 18, "Handling Emergencies.")

BRUCELLOSIS.
(See in this chapter under *Undulant Fever*.)

CAT-SCRATCH DISEASE.
This mild, noncontagious illness affects children more commonly than adults and usually follows a scratch or bite inflicted by the family cat. Occasionally scratches by animals other than cats, or even a puncturing thorn, have been the means of introducing the causative agent, probably a virus, into the body.

In the usual case a scabbed ulcer of the skin develops at the site where the scratch occurred. This may disappear at the end of two or three weeks. In the meantime an enlargement of the lymph nodes has usually developed in the affected part of the body—axilla, groin, or neck. General symptoms of loss of appetite, weakness, and nausea may also develop.

What to Do
The disease is not serious, and recovery occurs spontaneously within a few weeks. There is no specific remedy for the disease. Making the patient comfortable and treating symptoms as they develop are the accepted procedure for patient care.

CHICKEN POX (VARICELLA).
This extremely contagious disease, occurring in all parts of the world, is caused by a virus and appears most commonly in children under eight years of age. It is characterized by general symptoms of mild illness and by a skin rash in which there are crops of lesions which pass through the sequence of macules (red spots), papules (small pimples), vesicles (small blisters), and crusts.

Chicken pox usually begins ten to sixteen days after contact with someone who has the disease. At the onset there is usually a slight fever, a feeling of chilliness, aching in the back and extremities, and vomiting. The older the patient, the more severe the symptoms are likely to be. The skin rash makes its appearance about one day after the symptoms begin. The skin lesions appear in "crops" which usually develop first on the scalp and face and eventually become most numerous on the chest and upper back.

The skin lesions pass through four distinct stages. First is the small macule—an area of mild redness. Sec-

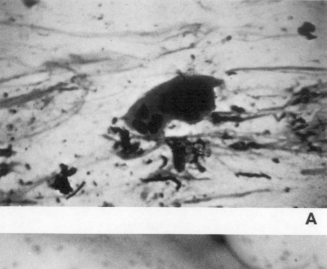

A

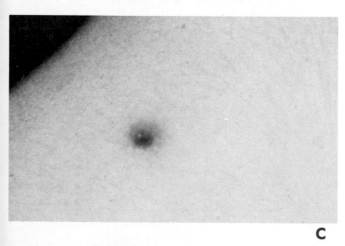

B

A. Greatly enlarged view of multi-nucleated giant cell as affected by chicken pox virus. B. Red papules on the skin. C. Small crusted blister.

ond, the macules develop into red papules, which are slightly elevated and resemble fleabites or mosquito bites. Third, the papules become small water blisters (vesicles), each surrounded by a tiny red zone. Fourth, if the vesicle does not become infected by ordinary germs, there develops a crust which soon breaks away, leaving no permanent scar.

With the skin lesions developing in crops, there may be present at one time on any given area red spots of different sizes, blisters, and scabs. The recovery from chicken pox is usually uneventful and rapid, once the skin rash disappears. In occasional cases, complications occur involving various organs of the body. The most common complication is that the itching skin lesions become infected by ordinary germs.

Relationship Between Chicken Pox and Herpes Zoster. Chicken pox and herpes zoster (shingles) are caused by the same virus, and in some instances a person who has come in contact with a case of chicken pox has developed herpes zoster. It is supposed that the particular form the disease takes, whether it be chicken pox or herpes zoster, depends on whether the individual has some immunity to the virus, herpes zoster developing in those who have a partial immunity. Herpes zoster is a very uncomfortable illness in which the virus affects one or more of the nerve roots and the skin area served by this particular nerve. The involved area is typically limited to one side of the body and consists of a band of skin in which there is severe pain.

Although chicken pox is highly contagious, it is not considered serious. Children of school age who have chicken pox should be kept home until all the skin lesions have developed crusts and have become brown in color. If there happens to be another child in the family who is not in good health and who has not had chicken pox, it is best to keep such a child away from the patient in the

C

hope that the feeble child will not catch the disease. But generally it is considered best for a child to have chicken pox and thus develop his own immunity before he reaches school age.

As yet there is no satisfactory way of preventing chicken pox by vaccination.

What to Do

The itching of the skin is the most troublesome symptom during the usual course of chicken pox. This may be relieved somewhat by sponging the affected areas with a strong solution of baking soda. Calamine lotion may also help to relieve the itching.

It is very important to guard against infecting the skin lesions. The patient's fingernails should be clipped short and kept clean, and his hands should be washed at frequent intervals. If an infection develops in skin lesions which have been scratched, the physician's attention should be called to this. He may find it advisable to use antibiotics for the control of such an infection.

As the lesions progress to the crusting stage, gentle application of olive oil to the skin surface will have a soothing effect.

CHOLERA.

(See chapter 32, "Warm-climate Ailments," in this volume.)

COCCIDIOIDOMYCOSIS (COCCIDIOIDAL GRANULOMA, VALLEY FEVER).

This highly infectious, noncontagious disease is caused by a fungus, the spores of which can be inhaled with the dust in areas in which the soil is infected. The disease occurs in the southwestern United States and in parts of South America. It is most frequent between ages twenty-five and fifty-five and occurs more commonly in men than in women. There are two forms of the disease: (1) primary pulmonary coccidioidomycosis and (2) disseminated coccidioidomycosis.

In the primary pulmonary type symptoms develop from one to four weeks after the spores are carried to the lungs. They are similar to those of influenza and may even suggest a mild form of pneumonia. With appropriate treatment, prospects of recovery are excellent in this type of the disease.

In the disseminated form of the disease, the fungous organisms which cause the illness are carried by the blood from the lungs to various parts of the body. Often there develop burrowing abscesses and draining sinuses in the skin and even in the bones. Sometimes the meninges which cover the brain are involved. There may be involvement of other organs as well. In this form of the disease, the mortality rate runs as high as 60 percent.

What to Do

The patient with coccidioidomycosis should be under the care of a physician. At the time of writing, the most effective treatment consists of the administration of amphotericin B, an antifungal drug. Inasmuch as the disease is not contagious, nursing care consists of the usual means of providing patient comfort. All discharges from the body however, particularly the sputum and the discharges from openings in the skin, should be handled in the manner outlined at the beginning of the chapter, for these discharges will probably contain the fungous organism which causes the disease.

THE COMMON COLD.

The common cold is an infection of the upper air passages by any one of a group of thirty-eight or more types of virus. There are also more than 100 additional viruses that can cause the same symptoms as in the common cold. Easily transmitted from person to person by infected droplets of mois-

471

ture floating in the air or by contaminated dust, it is properly classed as a contagious disease. The symptoms develop from one to two days after exposure. A person who harbors the infection is able to transmit it to other persons a few hours before his own symptoms begin and for as long as five days after the symptoms have appeared.

Exposure to cold or to wind, extreme fatigue, loss of sleep, or other causes of reduced vitality seem to make a person more susceptible to the common cold.

Inasmuch as the common cold may be caused by any one or more of such a large number of different viruses, protection by immunization is practically impossible. Even after having had an attack of the common cold, a person becomes immune for the time being only to the particular virus or viruses which caused his recent illness. He is still vulnerable to other viruses in the group. There is therefore no effective means of prevention except by the relative advantage of maintaining good general health and vigor and by avoiding excesses of fatigue and exposure.

Symptoms of the common cold usually begin with a roughness or irritation in the throat. This is followed quickly by sneezing and by the discharge of watery fluid from the nose. In most cases there are systemic symptoms such as mild chilliness, general aching in various muscles and body tissues, and a feeling of indisposition.

Among possible complications are infection of the middle ear (otitis media), infection of the nasal sinuses, bronchitis, and even pneumonia. The irritated tissues of the upper respiratory tract become vulnerable to invasion by common bacteria always present in the air passages, and these cause the complications.

What to Do

1. **For infants and children and for all sufferers from the common cold who have fever, rest until the**

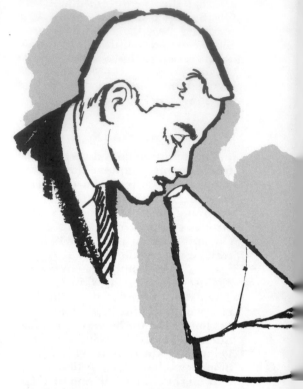

Steam inhalations may relieve discomfort from a common cold.

symptoms subside is recommended. Even for the adult patient who does not develop fever, avoidance of fatigue and exposure is recommended.

2. **As a courtesy to other people, anyone suffering from a common cold should cover his face with a handkerchief when he sneezes or coughs and should avoid close proximity to other people while his symptoms persist.**

3. **The use of antibiotic drugs is not effective in relieving the common cold. Antibiotics are useful only in the treatment of the complications that may develop as a result of invasion by bacteria.**

4. **The use of nose drops and of steam inhalations may make the patient more comfortable.**

5. **The use of a heating compress**

472

to the throat or to the chest, particularly during the night, will help to relieve the symptoms and hasten recovery from the common cold. (See volume 3, chapter 20, "Simple Home Treatments.")

CRYPTOCOCCOSIS (TORULOSIS).

Cryptococcosis is produced by a fungus. It occurs occasionally in all parts of the world and most frequently affects adults between forty and sixty years of age, with males having the disease twice as frequently as females. The most serious cases are those in which the central nervous system and its coverings are affected. The disease may also involve the lungs, the skin, the bones, and other organs.

The means by which the fungus enters the human body is not known for sure, but some evidence suggests that the lungs are involved first even in those cases in which the central nervous system seems to be principally affected. This type of fungus has been found in the excreta of pigeons, but it seems that the birds from which such excreta come are not ill with the disease. Cryptococcosis is not considered to be contagious, the disease apparently not being transmittable directly from person to person or from animals to humans.

In that form of the disease which affects the central nervous system, the mortality rate is very high.

What to Do

1. The use of some of the newer antibiotics has greatly improved the prospects of recovery in all forms of cryptococcosis. The use of these must be supervised, of course, by a physician.

2. In some cases surgical removal of the lesions is advisable.

DIPHTHERIA.

This very serious, acute, and highly contagious disease is caused by the diphtheria bacillus. Children be-

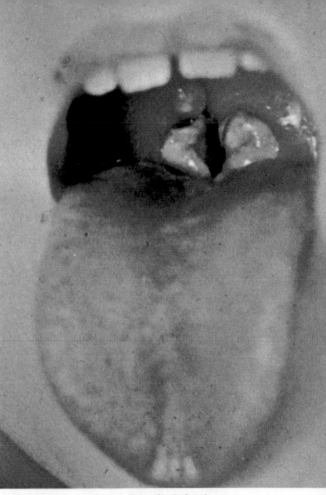

Appearance of throat in diphtheria.

tween the ages of one and ten are especially susceptible, but the disease also attacks older persons. The diphtheria bacillus does not survive long when not in contact with human tissues. The germs are usually carried by infected secretions from the nose or throat of a person who harbors these germs. Most commonly they are introduced into the body of the susceptible person through the mouth or nose either by inhalation of contaminated droplets of moisture, by contact with contaminated fingers or with a soiled handkerchief or towel, or by the use of contaminated food or milk.

The time between exposure to the diphtheria infection and the beginning of the illness is about the shortest of any of the diseases caused by bacteria, the incubation period being one to five days.

473

Diphtheria has been in existence for many centuries, having been described even before the time of Christ. It has been a dread disease, often occurring in epidemics and causing hundreds of thousands of deaths. Even after surviving the illness, many a person suffers permanent handicap from damage to the heart or the kidneys, or from paralysis of certain of the muscles.

The first encouraging chapter in the diphtheria story began in 1890 when Von Behring developed an effective antitoxin which, when administered early enough during the illness, prevented the usual complications of the disease. The next improvement in the handling of the disease came in 1923 with the development of diphtheria toxoid which, when administered to a susceptible person, stimulates the development of immunity and thus keeps him from acquiring the disease. As of the present time, immunization against diphtheria is part of the routine for protecting children against the various contagious diseases. It is on this account that the disease is relatively rare in the United States. When it does occur, it is usually in persons who have not been immunized.

Usually the bacillus invades the membranes of the upper air passages (pharynx, larynx, and trachea). The membranes are seriously damaged, and there develops a unique structure, called a pseudomembrane, which coats over the infected areas. The pseudomembrane becomes thick and constitutes the first threat to the patient's life because, as it loosens from the underlying tissues, it may obstruct the passage of air and cause death by asphyxiation. In serious cases where the passageway through the larynx is obstructed, life is sometimes saved by the surgical procedure known as tracheotomy, in which an opening from the outside into the trachea is made in the lower part of the neck.

Once the diphtheria bacillus is entrenched in the upper air passages, it produces a very potent toxin which circulates throughout the body by way of the blood. Except for the danger of asphyxiation as mentioned above, it is the effect of this toxin that accounts for the high death rate in diphtheria. It is this toxin that causes damage to the heart, to the kidneys, and to the nerves. Damage to the heart and to the kidneys accounts for the greatest number of deaths. The nerve damage often causes temporary paralysis of muscle more commonly in the area of the throat and face but, occasionally, in other parts of the body.

In rare instances the diphtheria bacillus affects other parts of the body rather than the upper air passages. The eyes, the ears, or a skin wound may be the site of infection.

The symptoms in the usual early case of diphtheria include a mild sore throat, and elevation of body temperature, difficulty in breathing and swallowing, and the beginning evidences of damage by the toxin produced by the diphtheria germ. The circulation of this toxin through the body causes severe prostration. In some cases there is a tremendous enlargement of the lymph nodes in the neck.

What to Do

1. It is urgent that a patient with diphtheria be under the direct supervision of a physician. Once the diagnosis is confirmed, he will want to administer adequate doses of antitoxin to prevent the complications which may threaten the patient's life. Antitoxin itself does not kill the diphtheria germs but only neutralizes the toxin which they produce. The doctor may therefore want to administer an antibiotic, such as penicillin, in order to kill the diphtheria germs.

2. Inasmuch as diphtheria is highly contagious, the nursing care of a diphtheria patient should include all of the precautions mentioned earlier in this chapter.

3. The patient should be kept absolutely quiet in bed for at least two

weeks—longer in serious cases, particularly when the heart has been affected.

4. During the acute phase of the illness, there must be constant monitoring of the patient's breathing so as to make sure that this does not become obstructed by the pseudomembrane which develops in the air passages.

5. Inasmuch as it is difficult for the diphtheria patient to swallow, the taking of food and fluid becomes a major problem. It may be necessary to administer fluid by vein to keep the patient from becoming dehydrated. Also, it may be advisable to give nourishment by artificial means, as the doctor orders.

6. The pain of the swollen lymph nodes in the neck may be somewhat relieved by applying an ice collar for fifteen minutes out of the hour. This can be prepared by placing chipped ice inside a narrow plastic bag and covering the same with a hand towel.

7. Mouth and throat irrigations with warm salt solution (1 teaspoonful of salt to a pint of water) may relieve some of the discomfort of the sore throat.

8. Because of the possibility of damage to the heart, the diphtheria patient should be very deliberate about resuming his normal activities after the acute phase of the illness is past. Physical activity, even normal play for a child, if resumed too quickly, may cause death on account of the damage to the heart muscle.

9. The recovering patient should not be permitted to mingle with people until after two successive laboratory examinations have indicated that the diphtheria germs are no longer present in his tissues.

DYSENTERY, AMEBIC.

(See the discussion in chapter 21, "Intestinal Parasites," in this volume.)

DYSENTERY, BACILLARY.

Bacillary dysentery is a disease of the bowel caused by germs belonging to the Shigella group of bacilli. It is characterized by frequent stools (up to one hundred or more a day) which contain mucus, blood, and pus. There are abdominal cramps, a general feeling of illness, and fever. The disease occurs in all parts of the world, particularly in the tropics.

Bacillary dysentery occurs frequently where families live in overcrowded quarters in which the sanitation is not satisfactory. It affects young children more commonly than older people. It is a contagious disease, the responsible germs being carried from person to person usually by food which has lacked refrigeration and which has been contaminated by contact with germ-laden soil or with flies that have carried the germs from human excrement.

The symptoms begin within one to four days after the germs have been taken into the patient's mouth. The onset of symptoms is often sudden, particularly with children. There is fever, loss of appetite, drowsiness, a desire to vomit, abdominal pain, and the frequent passage of stools which soon contain mucus, blood, and pus.

The greatest danger to life in the case of a young child is caused by the loss of fluid from the body (dehydration). Also, as the illness persists, the lack of nutrition becomes serious.

What to Do

Four important considerations in caring for a patient with bacillary dysentery are the restoration of water and chemical salts that have been lost from his body by the diarrhea, the overcoming of the infection by the use of drugs which kill the organisms causing the infection, the providing of adequate nourishment, and the prevention of the spread of the infection to other persons.

1. The restoration of fluid and

chemical salts is accomplished by intravenous injections of solutions made up to meet the patient's present needs. These are administered, preferably, in a hospital and, necessarily, under the direction of a physician.

2. Drugs are available which assist the body in combating this disease and in minimizing the usual complications.

3. The problem of nutrition becomes a major concern in the case of an infant. As soon as the vomiting and diarrhea have ceased, the infant can be fed appropriate solutions for restoring fluid and providing nourishment at hourly intervals. As recovery occurs, the usual formula can be added to these solutions. For older children, a high-protein, low-residue diet supplemented by vitamins is indicated.

4. The general principles for preventing the spread of bacillary dysentery require adequate sanitation, the safeguarding of food supplies (refrigeration and avoiding contamination), effective disposal of sewage, and proper methods to exterminate flies and to keep even an occasional fly from entering the house.

The nursing care of the patient should conform to the routines mentioned earlier in the chapter for the care of contagious disease cases.

ENCEPHALITIS, EPIDEMIC.

Encephalitis is a condition characterized by an inflammation of the brain tissue. In the epidemic type, sometimes called sleeping sickness, the causative agent is probably a virus. The disease has been known in various parts of the world for many years. It typically affects persons between the ages of ten and forty-five years. The virus is probably carried from one person to another by the minute droplets of moisture discharged by a sneeze or by way of contact with articles which have been soiled by the discharges from a patient's nose or throat. The symptoms of epidemic encephalitis are similar to those of influenza except that in this case there is a greater tendency to stiff neck and to lethargy (sleepiness). There is often a disturbance in the action of the muscles in the form of coarse tremors and, sometimes, purposeless movements or weakness.

It is common for persons who have had epidemic encephalitis to develop symptoms after their apparent recovery from the acute attack. Sometimes these late symptoms develop several years later resulting in invalidism, change of personality, or the symptoms of parkinsonism. (See chapter 25, "Nervous and Mental Disorders," in this volume.)

Epidemic encephalitis is a serious disease with a fatality rate between 10 and 30 percent. As yet, there is no specific treatment.

In recent years special kinds of encephalitis have been recognized, such as the "Saint Louis type," the "Eastern type," and the "Western equine type." Manifestations of these types usually occur in epidemics. There is some evidence that the virus causing these types of encephalitis may be carried to human beings by insects, including mosquitos.

Forms of encephalitis may also occur as a complication in chicken pox, measles, mumps, or smallpox, but the seriousness of these cases of encephalitis is not as great as that of epidemic encephalitis.

What to Do

1. Inasmuch as the virus causing epidemic encephalitis can be carried from person to person, great care should be used in disposing of the discharges from the nose and throat of patients with this disease. Linens and other articles soiled by these discharges must be sterilized or destroyed.

2. The patient with encephalitis should be protected from undue

noise or excitment of any kind.

3. Because of the possible difficulty in swallowing, it is important to make sure that the patient receives sufficient fluid and that his nutrition is not neglected. If there is a question on this, the doctor should be consulted on the proper way to administer fluid and nourishment, if necessary, by vein. For the patient who is able to swallow, abundant fluid by mouth and semisolid food are recommended.

ENTEROVIRUS INFECTIONS.

Many types of viruses commonly inhabit the digestive tract of human beings. Ordinarily they do not cause symptoms. The diseases that they may cause occur more commonly in the summer months than at other times of year. The common members of this group of viruses are the polioviruses, the Coxsackie viruses, and the ECHO viruses. For a full discussion of poliomyelitis, the disease caused by the polioviruses, see *Poliomyelitis* in this chapter.

The other diseases caused by viruses of this group may vary all the way from a very mild illness which is hardly recognizable to serious illnesses causing aseptic meningitis, paralysis, and even death.

No specific remedies are known. Treatment and patient care consist of efforts to relieve the symptoms.

EPIDEMIC NAUSEA AND VOMITING ("INTESTINAL FLU").

During recent years there have been repeated reports of epidemic waves of what first seemed to be bacterial food poisoning, but which later proved to be unrelated to food or drink. Typically, epidemics of this disease sweep through a community in two to four waves about two or three days apart, the second wave usually being the most extensive. A considerable proportion of the pupils in a school, for instance, will be absent, complaining of symptoms quite similar to those of food poisoning. Two or

three days later most of them will be back in school, though decidedly weak for a day or two more. Even in the milder cases, nausea will appear as a prominent symptom.

The general features of this disease suggest that it is caused by a virus transmitted through the air from a person ill with the disease. The disease runs a short course. No effective treatment is known.

ERYSIPELAS.
(See chapter 12, "Skin Diseases," in this volume.)

EXANTHEM SUBITUM (ROSEOLA INFANTUM).

This acute disease affecting infants and young children (six months to three years of age) is presumably caused by a virus and is characterized by high fever which lasts three or four days and ends by crisis (abrupt disappearance of the fever). At the time the fever drops, a mild skin rash starts on the trunk, spreads to the arms and neck, and involves the face and legs only slightly. The rash lasts for a few hours, or at the most one or two days, and then fades, leaving the skin in normal condition. The outstanding characteristic of the disease is the absence of symptoms or physical disturbances other than those mentioned above. During the phase of high fever, convulsions occur in some cases. There is no known method for shortening the disease or for preventing it. When the body temperature rises above 104° or 105° F., it is desirable to bring it down by the use of cool sponges or alcohol rubs.

FLU.
(See *Influenza* in this chapter. For Intestinal Flu refer to the discussion in this chapter on *Epidemic Nausea and Vomiting*.)

FOOD POISONING.
(See *Poisoning: Food Poisoning* in volume 3 chapter 18, "Handling Emergencies.")

GERMAN MEASLES (RUBELLA).

PUBLIC HEALTH SERVICE AUDIOVISUAL FACI.

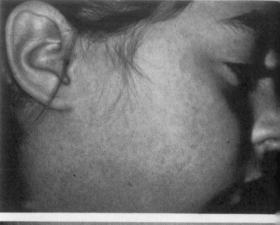

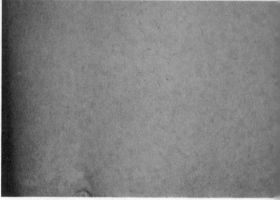

German measles is caused by a virus—a virus different from any other of the viruses, even that causing ordinary measles. The symptoms, which usually begin between seven and fourteen days after exposure, vary a great deal from case to case and are usually mild. The first symptoms may be a cold with cough and sore throat; or there may be headache, a feeling of general illness, aching of the muscles with fever, and an enlargement of the lymph nodes, especially those behind the ears. The skin rash usually appears within twenty-four hours of the first symptoms. It consists of a faint redness of the skin (easily confused with the rash of scarlet fever) which is blotchy in arrangement like that of ordinary measles. It usually appears first on the face and neck and spreads rapidly to the trunk and extremities, sometimes leaving one area before it appears at the next. The red areas fade under mild pressure. The rash usually lasts two or three days. In some cases no rash appears.

German measles may appear anytime after the first six months of life. It is especially common in young adults. The virus is transmitted from one person to another by personal contact and seems to enter the body through the membranes of the respiratory passages.

German measles is usually a mild disease and rarely causes any complications. However, as mentioned below in the case of expectant mothers, the unborn child may suffer deformity.

The tragedy of German measles is that it may interfere with the development of an unborn child when an expectant mother becomes ill with this disease during the first three months of her pregnancy. About 90 percent of the children born to mothers who have had German measles during these first three months are perfectly normal, but the disease is so prevalent that the 10 percent of children who are deformed on this account constitute quite a large number.

The rash of rubella appears on the face and neck first, spreading then to the trunk and extremities.

As a result of German measles occurring during the first three months of pregnancy there may be death of the unborn child, or retardation in its mental or physical development. Blindness, deafness, and defects of the heart are common deformities that occur under these circumstances. Even though German measles constitutes a definite hazard to the unborn child, the illness which a prospective mother suffers is no more severe than that occurring under other circumstances. Because the disease occurring under ordinary circumstances is so mild, it has even been proposed that girls should be deliberately exposed before they approach adulthood so that, by having the disease, they will develop an immunity which will prevent them from being susceptible when they later become pregnant.

What to Do

1. There is no specific treatment for German measles. The care of the patient consists of making him as comfortable as possible.

2. The patient should be kept at home and isolated from other persons until after the skin rash has completely disappeared. In cases associated with fever, the patient should be kept in bed until the temperature becomes normal.

3. When the lymph nodes at the back of the neck become particularly painful, an ice bag applied over the area for a few minutes out of each hour may give considerable relief.

4. A vaccine for German measles became available in 1969 after years of research. Immunization by this means should be carried out for all children and young adults who have not yet had the disease. Because of the possibility that the vaccine might cause an unborn child to be deformed, it should be determined that a young woman is not pregnant before giving the vaccine to her.

5. In the case of an expectant mother who has been exposed to German measles, a physician should be consulted at once and his recommendations followed carefully.

GLANDULAR FEVER.

(See *Mononucleosis* in this chapter.)

HERPES SIMPLEX.

The various manifestations of herpes simplex are due to the presence of the herpes simplex virus. The illness occurring when the virus first enters the tissues of a susceptible person is called primary herpes simplex. The manifestations occurring sub-

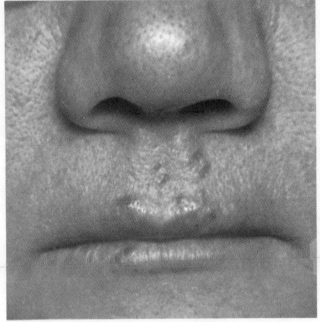

PUBLIC HEALTH SERVICE AUDIOVISUAL FACILITY

Herpes simplex, the common cold sore or fever blister.

sequently, from time to time, are caused by a reactivation of the virus which has remained latent in this person's tissues since the time it first entered. These are called recurrent herpes simplex.

A. *Primary Herpes Simplex.* Primary herpes simplex may be localized or generalized. If localized, the characteristic small blisters may appear on the mouth and gums, on the tissues of one of the eyes (even involving the cornea), on the delicate tissues of the genitals, or at the site of some injury to the skin. The disease may produce no symptoms and may thus pass unnoticed. Antibodies are produced, however, as a result of this first infection, and it is because of these that the subsequent manifestations of the disease are different from those of the first infection.

In infants who are infected at or soon after birth, primary herpes simplex may cause a very serious, commonly fatal illness. In such cases a multitude of small blisters appear on

479

the skin and mucous membranes. (See *Genital Herpes Simplex* in chapters 23 and 30 of this volume.)

Recurrent Herpes Simplex. The condition which may cause a reactivation of the virus which has remained latent in the tissues of a person's body are several. For the lesions which occur on the lips or around the face, an overexposure to sunlight or a stretching of the tissues around the mouth such as may occur when a dentist repairs a tooth may be a sufficient stimulus to cause reactivation of this infection. For herpes simplex lesions in other parts of the body, undue emotional stress or some systemic disease which reduces the individual's general resistance may cause a reactivation of the herpes simplex.

Cold Sore. The manifestation of herpes simplex which occurs on the lips and exposed portions of the face are caused by herpes simplex virus type I. The "cold sores" or "fever blisters" that commonly appear on the lips or around the mouth first consist of small vesicles which develop on a slightly inflamed base. Within a few days these form a yellowish crust and usually disappear within about ten days.

As mentioned above, herpes simplex becomes a serious disease when it affects a newborn infant. In such a case, the care of the infant must be carefully supervised by a physician. In some cases herpes simplex affects the tissues of the eye. In these, the services of a physician who specializes in diseases of the eye should be secured.

What to Do

Inasmuch as herpes simplex is caused by a virus, there is no specific medication that will bring about a cure. For fever blisters and cold sores, the use of some drying lotion or spirits of camphor may be of some help. In any case in which the lesions become secondarily infected with ordinary germs, they should be treated as any other infection, probably by the use of antibiotics as directed by the physician.

Persons who are subject to recurrent attacks of cold sores on the lips and face will do well to protect the skin of this area by the use of some anti-sunburn ointment or "sun screen" preparation.

Genital Herpes Simplex. Herpes simplex infections involving the genital organs are caused by herpes simplex virus type II. This type of infection has become quite frequent in recent years and is classed as one of the venereal diseases. (See *Genital Herpes Simplex* in chapters 23 and 30 of this volume.)

HERPES ZOSTER (SHINGLES).

Herpes zoster consists of a virus infection which involves one or more of the nerve structures that transmit sensations from a particular skin area. The involved area is typically limited to a small part of the skin on one side of the body, neck, or head. This area of skin becomes very painful, and tiny water-filled blisters develop in the area. Herpes zoster is caused by the same virus as causes chicken pox. For further discussion, see the item *Chicken Pox* in this chapter and also the discussion of *Shingles (Herpes Zoster)* in chapter 12, "Skin Diseases," in this volume.

HISTOPLASMOSIS.

This disease is caused by a specific fungus, the ordinary habitat of which is the soil, principally such as is adjacent to chicken houses and pigeon lofts. No proof exists that the disease can be transmitted from animal to man or from person to person. The infection is probably introduced into the body by inhaling the spores. The infection starts in the lungs and may be spread from the lungs to other parts of the body. This disease occurs most commonly in the Mississippi Valley. About 30 percent of those affected are children. A striking feature is that the disease may be so mild as to pass unnoticed or it may be so severe as to prove fatal.

Primary Acute Form. In this form the lungs are principally involved, thus causing symptoms of lung disease: cough, shortness of breath, chest pain on breathing, hoarseness, and blood spitting. The patient feels ill, loses weight, and may have muscle pains, chills, and fever. With this form of the disease, the patient usually recovers rapidly.

Disseminated Form. In this form the infection spreads from the lungs to other parts of the body, and the particular symptoms depend upon which organs of the body are involved. There are generalized symptoms of anemia, loss of weight, enlargement of the lymph glands, enlargement of the liver, and fever. Except for the benefit of the newer methods of treatment, this form of the disease carries a mortality of about 80 percent.

Chronic Cavitary Form. It is not known for certain whether this form of the disease is caused by a new infection or whether it is an aftermath of one of the other forms of the disease. It mimics tuberculosis quite closely and can be easily confused with it. Cavities form in the lung tissue. There is cough, weight loss, difficult breathing, chest pain, blood spitting, and a lowgrade fever just as in tuberculosis.

What to Do

The primary acute form of histoplasmosis is usually a rather harmless disease from which the patient recovers rapidly. All that is necessary in caring for such a patient is to contribute to his general comfort.

In the more serious forms of the disease, the outcome has become much more favorable since the availability of amphotericin B, which is an antifungal antibiotic drug. This preparation is injected into the patient's vein and the treatment program must be carefully supervised by a physician.

HYDROPHOBIA.
(See *Rabies* in this chapter.)

IMPETIGO.
(See chapter 12, "Skin Diseases," in this volume.)

INFANTILE PARALYSIS.
(See *Poliomyelitis* in this chapter.)

INFECTIOUS MONONUCLEOSIS.
(See *Mononucleosis* in this chapter.)

INFLUENZA.
(For intestinal flu see *Epidemic Nausea and Vomiting* in this chapter.)

Influenza is a very contagious disease of short duration caused by either A, B, or C types of influenza virus. The disease causes an initial sense of chilliness, followed by fever, general weakness, various aches and pains including headache and pain in the muscles, loss of appetite, and inflammation of the membranes of the nose and pharynx.

Once the vitality of the membranes of the nose and pharynx has been weakened by the influenza virus, it is common for bacteria (not viruses) which are always present in the mouth and pharynx to invade tissues and produce complications such as sinusitis, ear infection, and bacterial pneumonia. The most serious of these complications, and the usual cause of any death that follows influenza, is bacterial pneumonia. (See under *Pneumonia* in chapter 17 of this volume.)

Except for the development of complications, relatively early recovery from influenza is the rule. The patient usually remains somewhat weak for several days after the other symptoms have disappeared.

Vaccines are now available for the prevention of influenza. Inasmuch as any one of the three types of influenza virus may cause the disease, effective vaccines must provide immunity against all three types of the virus. The

Photograph of influenza virus
(Imai strain) showing magnification of
166,400 times.

resulting immunity lasts only about a year, so it is recommended that booster doses be administered early each autumn. Vaccination against influenza is especially recommended for pregnant women, for older people, and for persons with chronic diseases. It should be made clear that the protection provided by influenza vaccine does not protect against other types of respiratory infection.

What to Do

At the time of this writing, progress is under way in the development of certain antiviral drugs which, it is hoped, will be effective in the treatment of influenza.

For the uncomplicated case, the plan for care consists simply of making the patient as comfortable as possible. Should secondary in-

fections and their resulting complications develop or threaten, it is urgent to arrange for the services of a physician.

1. Rest in bed for the duration of the symptoms helps the patient to conserve his strength and hastens his recovery. As symptoms subside, return to activity should be gradual so as to avoid fatigue.

2. An ice bag applied intermittently to the forehead helps to relieve headache.

3. For cough, steam inhalations three times a day are helpful.

4. A simple diet, including a great deal of fruit juice and other liquids, is indicated as long as symptoms persist.

5. The drug amantadine gives promise of aiding in the prevention and, possibly, in the treatment of influenza type A.

LAVA MIGRANS.

(See the discussion of *Hookworm Infection* under the heading of *Roundworm Infections* in chapter 21, "Intestinal Parasites," in this volume.)

LOCKJAW.

(See under *Tetanus* in this chapter.)

MEASLES (RUBEOLA).

Measles is one of the most contagious of the common diseases of childhood. It is most easily transmitted from person to person in its earliest stages before the symptoms become full-blown. The virus which causes measles is conveyed by invisible droplets of moisture discharged from a patient's mouth or nose when coughing or sneezing.

The symptoms of the disease first appear about seven to fourteen days following exposure to the measles virus. The patient begins to sneeze, his nose runs, and his eyes water and become sensitive to bright light. He feels tired, is sleepless and restless, develops a fever, and has a hoarse, dry cough. There may be pain and sore-

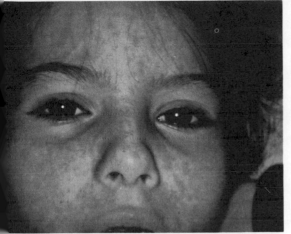

The pink spots of measles appear first on the head, spreading next to the trunk and limbs.

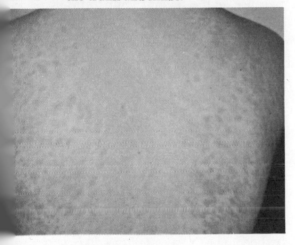

ness in the chest. It is during this early stage before the skin rash appears that measles may be confused with an ordinary respiratory infection or with bronchitis.

The skin rash first appears about three to five days after the onset of the symptoms mentioned above. It consists of well-defined pink spots which are first seen behind the ears, on the neck, at the roots of the hair, or on the forehead. Later the rash appears on the trunk and limbs. These pink spots tend to become darker as time passes, becoming almost purple before they disappear. As these spots increase in number, they tend to run together to form irregular blotches. Even in those cases in which the rash is profuse, small patches of natural-appearing skin may be seen among the blotches. Often the rash on the face begins to fade before it is fully developed on the legs. Fine, silvery scales are shed from the skin surface at about the time the rash disappears.

The severity of measles may vary a great deal from case to case. In the severe cases there may be high fever, delirium, cracked tongue, rapid pulse, and even unconsciousness.

A possible complication of measles is encephalitis, which is caused by the invasion of the measles virus into the brain tissues. Other possible complications are the result of a lowered resistance to other germs. The hazard of measles is really not in the disease itself; for, without complications, recovery is quite prompt. The serious complications include pneumonia, middle-ear infection, damage to the heart, and the exacerbation of latent tuberculosis.

Measles can be effectively prevented by the use of the presently available measles vaccines. The protective antibodies which develop in response to the use of vaccines are believed to provide protection for many years, possibly for life. It is therefore advisable that persons, particularly children, who have never had measles should be vaccinated.

Once a susceptible person has been exposed to measles, it is possible for him to receive such treatment as will make the disease less severe or will even prevent it altogether. This consists of the administration of gamma globulin. The protection conferred by such a procedure is short-lived and lasts only a very few weeks.

What to Do

The care of a patient with measles is directed primarily toward the prevention of complications. Secondarily it is intended to make the patient as comfortable as possible during his illness.

1. The patient should remain quietly in bed until after the skin rash disappears. Following this time he should be protected for at least two weeks from sudden changes of temperature or from other conditions that might make him susceptible to infections.

2. During the illness, the patient's eyes should not be exposed to strong light. It is not necessary that the room be completely darkened, but only that the light be subdued.

3. Increasing the humidity of the room or arranging for steam inhalations may reduce the patient's tendency to cough.

4. The diet should be simple and easily digested and should include an abundant intake of fluid.

5. Itching of the skin may be at least partially relieved by the application of phenolated calamine lotion applied to the skin several times a day. This is available at most drug counters.

6. Antibacterial drugs (sulfonamides or antibiotics) are indicated only as a means of preventing or controlling certain of the complications that may develop. The physician's judgment will indicate when these are needed.

MEASLES, GERMAN.

(See *German Measles* in this chapter.)

MENINGITIS.

Meningitis is an acute inflammation of the meninges (the covering membranes of the brain and spinal cord). The inflammation may be caused by various germs: viruses, bacteria, fungi, or yeasts. Except for the infection of the meninges that develops from a nearby brain abscess or that occurs in contaminated, penetrating head injuries, the infection is usually brought to the meninges from some other part of the body—the middle ear, the nasal sinuses, the tonsils, the lungs, or the valves of the heart.

Meningitis is always serious, regardless of its cause. The usual evidences of meningitis are fever with severe headache, pain and stiffness in the neck and back, accompanied with changes in the patient's pattern of thinking and acting. These changes typically range all the way from slight irritability to deep coma.

The common forms of meningitis are meningococcic, tuberculous, influenzal, pneumococcal, streptococcal, staphylococcal, syphilitic, and purulent meningitis of the newborn (usually caused by the E. coli bacillus). Of these, meningococcic meningitis is selected for a more complete description (see the following item) because, of the several acute forms, it alone is communicable.

MENINGITIS, MENINGOCOCCIC (EPIDEMIC MENINGITIS, SPOTTED FEVER).

Meningococcic meningitis is a very common complication of meningococcic disease. The infection is caused by the germ called meningococcus. It is spread from person to person by the droplets of moisture violently exhaled at the time of a sneeze or cough. The germs, once taken into the body, establish an infection in the region of the pharynx. While the infection resides here, the victim may easily become a "carrier" of the disease. From the infection in the pharynx, the germs may be carried by the bloodstream to other parts of the body. It is by this route that the meninges commonly become involved by the meningococcic infection.

The disease is endemic in all parts of the world, but from time to time it flares up as an epidemic. Notable epidemics occurred in 1917, 1929, 1936, and 1943. About 45 percent of the cases of meningococcic meningitis occur in children under fifteen years of age.

During that phase of the disease in which the infection is being carried by the blood, groups of the germs congregate in various parts of the skin and membranes, where they cause purple-colored irregular blotches. It is because of this occurrence that the disease is often called spotted fever.

The symptoms of meningococcic meningitis develop rapidly and consist of a severe headache, irritability, forceful vomiting, chills with high fever and rapid pulse, convulsions (especially in infants), rigidity of the muscles (especially those of the neck and back), pain on flexing the neck, and delirium progressing to stupor and coma.

Before the availability of modern antibacterial agents the fatality rate for meningococcic meningitis was about 75 percent. With modern methods of treatment the figure has dropped to 10 percent or less.

What to Do

1. When symptoms such as the above develop, a physician should be alerted at once. The success of treatment in cases of meningococcic meningitis depends upon early recognition of the disease and prompt, adequate treatment.

2. Appropriate antibiotic drugs will be administered intensively under a physician's direction. He will usually find it necessary to perform a spinal puncture as a means of assisting in the diagnosis and, later, of checking on the patient's progress.

3. Appropriate nursing care is an important part of the treatment and should follow general procedures useful in caring for other serious infectious diseases. Precautions mentioned in the first part of this chapter should be used to prevent the spread of the infection to other persons.

4. The patient should receive adequate fluid, as indicated by an output of urine of at least one liter (one quart) per day.

5. An ample easily digested, nour-

ishing diet should be provided.

6. It may be necessary (on the doctor's order) to administer fluid and nourishment by vein.

MONONUCLEOSIS.

Mononucleosis, also called infectious mononucleosis and formerly called glandular fever, is an acute infectious disease which continues for a variable period between one week and three months. It occurs most commonly between the ages of fifteen and thirty. The specific cause, still unknown, is assumed to be a virus. Usually the disease occurs sporadically, but occasionally it spreads as an epidemic where young people have close association as in schools and colleges. The disease is probably transferred from person to person by way of the air that is exhaled and breathed.

Fever and enlargement of the lymph nodes throughout the body are the outstanding characteristics of mononucleosis. Sore throat, weak-

A symptom of mononucleosis is enlargement of the lymph nodes.

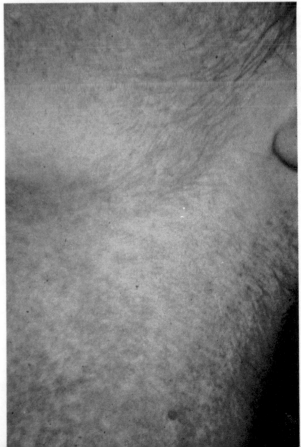

PUBLIC HEALTH SERVICE AUDIOVISUAL FACILITY

ness, muscle pains, and loss of appetite are accompanying symptoms. The spleen and liver frequently become enlarged. One of the serious complications of the disease is caused by rupture of an enlarged spleen.

Because the symptoms may be vague and somewhat variable, a precise diagnosis requires a laboratory examination of the blood and the blood serum.

What to Do

Since the exact cause of mononucleosis is not known, there is no specific treatment. Bed rest with good nursing care, making sure that the patient drinks an adequate amount of fluid, constitutes the basis for treatment. Should complications develop, the services of a physician are imperative.

MUMPS.

This contagious disease is characterized by enlargement of one or more of the salivary glands. It is caused by a virus, in the usual case occurring during childhood. Complete recovery takes place in a few days. Complications frequently develop, however, most commonly in patients older than twelve years.

The symptoms—chilliness, headache, lack of appetite, and moderate fever—begin between two and four weeks after contact with a person who has the disease and usually appear a few hours before the salivary glands become painful. It is usually the parotid gland, situated just in front of the ear, that is primarily affected. Any one or more of the several salivary glands, however, may be involved. Pain in the involved gland is induced by external pressure on the gland, by swallowing, or, particularly, by taking sour substances into the mouth. The swelling of the salivary glands usually lasts from three to six days.

The most common serious complication of mumps is an involvement of the sex glands, either of the testes (orchitis) or of the ovaries.

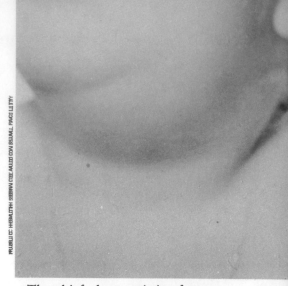

The chief characteristic of mumps is a swelling of the salivary glands.

In about 25 percent of the cases of mumps among older boys and men, at least one of the testes is affected. The affected testis becomes swollen and very painful. In some cases the organ later atrophies, thus being rendered incapable of producing male sex cells; but unless both testes are thus involved, a man is still capable of fatherhood. Even when one or both testes atrophy, the male sex hormones are produced in normal fashion. The comparable involvement of the ovaries in women is not so common or so serious as is the involvement of the testes in men.

About 10 percent of all cases of mumps develop some degree of encephalitis with severe headache, drowsiness, and vomiting. Usually this complication clears up spontaneously.

Another occasional complication of mumps is pancreatitis, in which severe nausea, vomiting, and abdominal pain develop. Even with this unpleasant and rather serious development, spontaneous recovery usually ensues within a week.

What to Do

There is no specific treatment for mumps. Unless complications develop, it is considered to be one of the less harmful contagious diseases. A child with mumps should be kept at home and out of school until all swelling of his salivary glands has disappeared. Effort should be made to keep him away from other children or from grown people who have not had the disease. Persons older than twelve years who have mumps should remain in bed until their fever has disappeared. The nursing care for mumps may be summarized as follows:

1. The patient should be protected against chilling throughout the period of his illness. This is especially important for patients above twelve years of age.

2. Swollen salivary glands may be less painful if either a hot water bottle or an ice bag is placed over the swollen area for a few minutes out of each hour. The choice of heat or cold depends on which makes a patient more comfortable.

3. The patient should receive a light diet of food which is easily swallowed.

4. The patient is made more comfortable by rinsing the mouth every two or three hours with a warm salt solution (one level teaspoonful of salt to a pint of water).

5. In cases in which the testes become involved, the patient should be kept at absolute bed rest and the scrotum should be supported by a large tuft of cotton or by an adhesive tape bridge placed between the thighs so as to support the weight of the swollen scrotum. The periodic application of an icebag to the scrotum may provide some relief.

6. When the pancreas becomes involved, it is usually advisable to feed the patient by vein rather than by mouth. This must be under the direction of a physician.

7. In all cases of mumps in which complications develop, a physician should be in charge of the case.

8. A mumps vaccine is available for purposes of immunization.

NAUSEA.
(See *Epidemic Nausea and Vomiting* in this chapter.)

ORNITHOSIS.
(See *Psittacosis* in this chapter.)

PARATYPHOID FEVER.
(See *Typhoid Fever* in this chapter.)

PARROT FEVER.
(See *Psittacosis* in this chapter.)

PERTUSSIS.
(See *Whooping Cough* in this chapter.)

PLAGUE.
(See *Plague* in chapter 32, "Warm Climate Ailments," in this volume.)

POLIOMYELITIS (INFANTILE PARALYSIS).
Poliomyelitis is an acute infection caused by a virus which most commonly (80 to 90 percent of cases) produces a mild illness lasting one to three days but which sometimes produces a major illness resulting in serious damage to certain of the nerve cells controlling the muscles of the body and which therefore often produces paralysis of the corresponding muscles.

Symptoms of the minor type of illness include headache, slight fever, sore throat, and possibly vomiting. In this minor form the illness does not seem to involve the central nervous system.

In the less frequent major type of illness symptoms include severe headache, stiffness of the neck and back, and deep muscle pain, with a developing weakness of certain muscles—these symptoms associated with fever. In these cases, in which the nervous system is involved, slightly more than 50 percent recover without permanent paralysis of the muscles; about 25 percent have minor muscle weaknesses for the remainder of life; the remainder (slightly less than 25 percent) carry severe disabil-

487

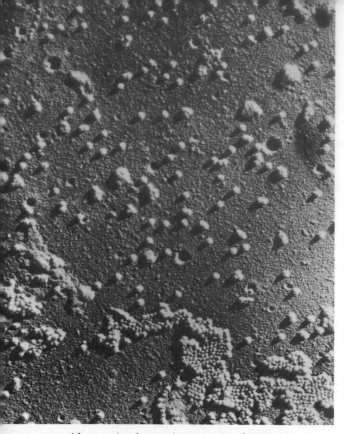

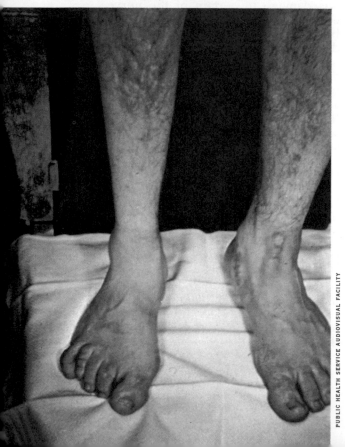

Above: A photomicrograph of one type of polio virus, enlarged 77,000 times actual size. Below: Atrophy of leg from polio.

ity for life because of permanent paralysis of important muscles. In these severe cases the greatest danger is the possibility of failure of the breathing mechanism. It is for these that the use of mechanical respirators (iron lungs) may be lifesaving.

Prevention. Thanks to the availability of effective vaccines, beginning in 1955, poliomyelitis is now a preventable disease. The more recently developed type of vaccine (live attenuated vaccine) is administered by mouth and is so effective in preventing poliomyelitis that there is no longer any excuse for persons having this dread disease. The occasional case of poliomyelitis indicates a disregard for the program of vaccination as advocated by all physicians and all health-promoting agencies. For details on the plan of immunization for poliomyelitis see chapter 3, "Immunizations," in this volume.

What to Do

Treatment for the minor type of poliomyelitis consists essentially of bed rest for several days, an adequate intake of fluid, and the use of simple remedies to combat the symptoms. There is no specific treatment for the disease, once a person becomes ill.

For the major type of poliomyelitis with involvement of the central nervous system, there must be absolute rest in bed. It is in this form of the disease that fomentations ("Kenny packs"), applied to the areas where the muscles are painful, are most beneficial. These should be applied for about twenty minutes, several times each day. (See volume 3, chapter 20, "Simple Home Treatments.") Of course these major cases must be carefully supervised by a physician, who will be alert to the need for a mechanical respirator should the patient's breathing begin to fail.

All persons who have had contact with a poliomyelitis patient, unless

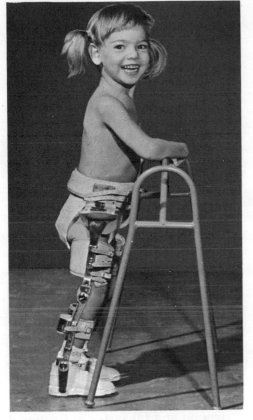

Braces help to compensate for muscle weakness resulting from polio.

it is known that they are already immune to the disease, should be immunized at once by the use of the live oral polio virus vaccine.

PSITTACOSIS (ORNITHOSIS, PARROT FEVER).

This disease is caused by a virus which primarily infects birds. When transmitted to humans, it produces an atypical form of pneumonia. The onset of the disease is rapid, with chills, fever, pain in the muscles, a dry cough, and loss of energy. The disease is rare among children but common among those who handle pets and among poultry workers. The symptoms—including headache, loss of appetite, vomiting, and possibly delirium or stupor, in addition to those mentioned above—typically appear one to two weeks after the individual has been in contact with the infected bird. The virus is carried by dust particles and can thus be inhaled by anyone who comes into near contact with an infected bird.

What to Do

Inasmuch as some cases of this disease become serious, the care of a patient with psittacosis should be directed by a physician. Certain antibiotic drugs give excellent results in controlling the disease.

It is preferable to have the patient in a hospital. If he is cared for at home, the treatment is similar to that for pneumonia, involving strict bed rest, the use of oxygen inhalations as indicated, and the use of simple remedies for the relief of other symptoms. The use of fomentations to the chest, morning and evening, is helpful. (See volume 3, chapter 20, "Simple Home Treatments.")

Q FEVER.

In this acute illness the symptoms develop two or three weeks after exposure to the germ which causes the disease. It usually ends spontaneously after two or more weeks of illness. There is usually an abrupt onset of symptoms—high, irregular fever, headache, pain behind the eyes, with cough and chest pain developing at about the end of the first week of illness.

The disease occurs in persons who have contact with animals, particularly cattle, sheep, and goats.

What to Do

The tetracycline drugs are remarkably effective in the treatment of Q fever. These must be administered under the direction of a physician.

Other than this, patients with Q fever should rest in bed but may have bathroom privileges. Cool sponges or alcohol rubs may help in controlling the fever if the temperature tends to run excessivly high. Easily digested soft or liquid diets are recommended.

RABBIT FEVER.

(See *Tularemia* in this chapter.)

RABIES (HYDROPHOBIA).

Rabies is a serious disease which typically follows the bite of a "mad dog" and ends fatally if not treated. It is caused by a virus capable of invading the brain of many of the mammals, especially the carnivores. Once the virus enters the body through a break in the skin, it travels by way of the nerves to the brain and then to the salivary glands so that the saliva of an animal or person ill with this disease can convey the virus to another animal or person.

The disease occurs quite commonly among wild animals such as skunks, foxes, raccoons, and coyotes; and from these the infection is easily transmitted to the domestic dog, which is the usual agent for infecting man. Healthy bats may also serve as carriers of the disease.

Because of the involvement of the brain, a dog with rabies behaves in a furious manner and because of its own discomfort bites other animals or humans even without provocation. The wound caused by the bite becomes infected because the dog's saliva is laden with the virus. The infection may be transmitted even though the dog does not bite, if circumstances permit its infected saliva to come in contact with an open wound or a break in the skin or mucous membrane of the susceptible animal or person.

In the human, symptoms of the disease may develop anytime between ten days and one year after exposure. The average is thirty to fifty days. This period of time is shorter when the wound through which the virus enters is in the region of the neck, face, or head. Once the symptoms of the disease begin, the infection invariably progresses to a fatal outcome. It is therefore imperative that treatment be given as soon as possible after exposure to the virus. If there is early and adequate treatment, the symptoms will not develop.

The symptoms in man start with mental depression, fever, and a growing restlessness which progresses to a stage of excitement. As the salivary glands become involved, there is excessive production of saliva accompanied by painful spasms of the muscles of the larynx and pharynx. These spasms are triggered by minor activities such as the attempt to take a drink of water. It is for fear of causing another of the painful spasms that the patient now refuses to drink. Death occurs within about five days after the symptoms begin.

What to Do in Case of Exposure

Treatment of the person who has been exposed to rabies, either by the bite of an animal which is possibly rabid or by such contact with the animal's saliva as may have permitted the virus to enter the tissues through some break in the skin or membranes, consists of two phases: (1) local treatment of the wound and (2) systemic treatment to provide immunization. In the meantime, the animal in question should be kept alive if at all possible and under the observation of a veterinarian for a period of at least five days, preferably seven to ten days. Only by such observation can it be determined for sure whether the animal is actually ill with rabies. If it is clear at the end of the observation period that the animal does not have rabies, the systemic treatment of the person who has been bitten may then be discontinued.

The local treatment of the wound requires a thorough cleansing with large amounts of soap and water. After such treatment, it is recommended that the wound be left open, without suturing. It is also recommended that antirabies serum be injected into the tissues surrounding the wound.

The decision regarding the use of antirabies vaccine must rest with the physician who cares for the per-

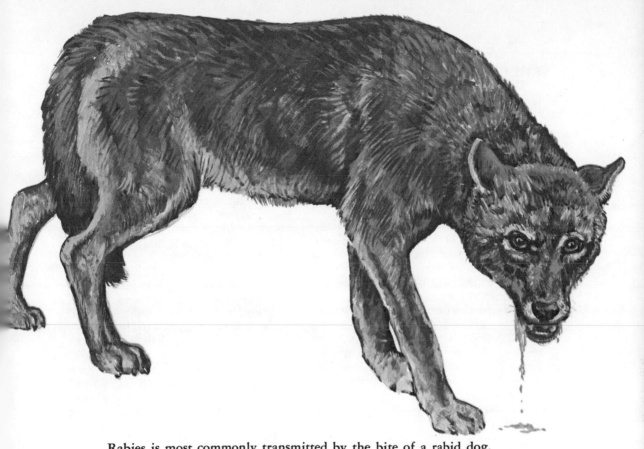

Rabies is most commonly transmitted by the bite of a rabid dog.

son who has been exposed. The general rule is that the series of vaccine injections should be started immediately under any one of three conditions: (1) when it is known that the biting animal has rabies; (2) when the animal is not available for examination but it is known that there has been rabies in the area; and (3) when the bite was inflicted by some wild animal, including bats.

When it is possible to keep the biting animal in captivity and under the observation of a veterinarian, the program of vaccination may be discontinued at the end of five to ten days if at that time the animal is judged to be normal.

RELAPSING FEVER.

This acute infectious disease is caused by spirochetes belonging to the species Borrelia. The disease occurs commonly in animals, especially rodents, and is conveyed from animal to human by ticks. It may be transmitted from person to person by infected lice. The disease is characterized by recurring periods of fever, each lasting a few days. The interval of time between the attacks is usually one to two weeks. There are from two to ten attacks in the series, with the attacks becoming less severe as the patient's immunity improves. A mild skin rash, followed by rose-colored spots, commonly occurs during the attacks. Jaundice commonly develops late in the course of an attack.

What to Do

Specific treatment for relapsing fever is the administration of appropriate antibiotics. Other than this, rest in bed and good nursing care are important. The patient should receive adequate fluids each day with an easily digested, nourishing type of diet.

491

RHEUMATIC FEVER.

This is a serious disease characterized by fever, pain, and inflammatory involvements of various of the body's tissues. Fortunately the incidence of the disease has been declining in recent years—presumably as a result of generally improved living conditions. Rheumatic heart disease is the most serious complication of rheumatic fever.

Rheumatic fever occurs as an aftermath of an infection caused by group A beta hemolytic streptococci—an infection such as tonsillitis, streptococcal sore throat, or scarlet fever. Rheumatic fever as such is not caused directly by the presence in the tissues of these germs, but seems to be caused by a mysterious hypersensitivity to the germs or to their products. Rheumatic fever can be prevented by prompt and adequate treatment of persons who have streptococcal infections, using the appropriate form of penicillin or of a related antibiotic preparation.

There are many cases of sore throat, for example, that are not caused by the streptococcus. In order to determine for sure whether a given infection is the kind that may lead to rheumatic fever, it is necessary for the physician to take a sample of mucus from the affected area. He will have this sample cultured and examined in a medical laboratory.

In some cases of rheumatic fever or its complication of rheumatic heart disease, there is no knowledge of a previous streptococcal infection. It is presumed, however, that even in such cases there must have been a streptococcal infection with such mild symptoms that it went unrecognized.

A person who has once had rheumatic fever is prone to have another attack of the disease. It is of vital importance, then, to arrange antibiotic treatment for such a person whenever he has a streptococcal infection. The cause of rheumatic fever and that of Sydenham's chorea (Saint Vitus's dance) are related. Some persons afflicted with rheumatic fever have chorea at one time or another. Frequently chorea is followed by the same serious complications (such as rheumatic heart disease) as follow rheumatic fever.

The course of an attack of rheumatic fever runs somewhat as follows: While recovering from a streptococcal infection (such as tonsillitis, streptococcal sore throat, or scarlet fever) a child develops fever and certain of his larger joints become painful, hot, red, swollen, and tender. The involvement of the joints may move from certain joints to others. There is loss of appetite, general sweating, and possibly redness of the skin. Sometimes painful nodules appear just under the skin. Pain over the heart with irregularities of the heartbeat may accompany the development of "rheumatic heart" with its consequent deformity of the heart valves. The lungs may also become involved, as indicated by symptoms of cough and difficult breathing.

The course of an attack of rheumatic fever varies a great deal from case to case. In most cases the attack is over within twelve weeks. In some it is much shorter, and in others, longer.

What to Do

1. The person with rheumatic fever deserves the careful supervision of a physician.

2. In the acute phase, the physician will first want to make sure that the original infection with streptococci is eradicated. He will therefore probably give intensive treatment with penicillin.

3. Bed rest with nursing care is important in the early phases of the attack. Usually the physician will allow the patient to leave his bed to go to the bathroom after his temperature remains below 100° F. (37.8° C.). The rate at which physical activity can be gradually resumed will depend on the physician's appraisal of the patient's progress.

4. Salicylate drugs are usually administered to reduce the involve-

ment of the joints and to provide comfort from pain. The usual doses are large and require the physician's supervision.

5. Complications such as rheumatic heart disease require special treatment as they arise.

6. It is very important that steps be taken to prevent a recurrence of rheumatic fever. At the time of writing it is considered essential that continuous antibiotic treatment be used after an attack so as to prevent the possibility of another infection by the hemolytic streptococcus.

7. Proper steps must be taken to prevent the child who has had rheumatic fever from developing the concept that he is an invalid. His schoolwork should be continued as soon as the acute phase of the illness is over, even with arrangements for a teacher to come to his home while he is still under treatment. Pampering should be minimized, and the child's preparation for the responsibilities of adulthood should be encouraged.

RICKETTSIALPOX.

This mild disease runs its course in about two weeks. It is caused by an organism similar to that causing Rocky Mountain spotted fever. It is transmitted from mice to humans by mites. About ten to twenty days after the mite has penetrated the skin, a single initial skin lesion develops at the site of the infection. This initial lesion becomes red and elevated, spreads to about half an inch in diameter, and eventually develops a blister at the center. A few days later the patient suddenly experiences chilly sensations, sweats, headache, loss of appetite, pains in the muscles, and fever which remits each morning. These symptoms continue for about a week. A generalized skin rash, similar in appearance to that of chickenpox, usually develops either during the period of fever or immediately thereafter. This rash continues for about a week.

The treatment consists of good nursing care plus the administration by the physician of appropriate antibiotic drugs.

ROCKY MOUNTAIN SPOTTED FEVER.

This disease was at first supposed to be limited to the Rocky Mountain area but it is now known to occur throughout most of the United States as well as in Canada, Mexico, Colombia, and Brazil. It is caused by a tiny rickettsial organism which is introduced into the body by the bite of an infected tick.

The illness comes on suddenly three to eight days after a tick bite. There are chills, sweats, fever, headache, eye discomfort from bright light, pain in the skeletal tissues, sore throat, and vomiting. The breathing and heartbeat become rapid. A skin rash usually appears between the third and fifth days of the illness, beginning on the ankles and wrists and

Skin rash characteristic of Rocky Mountain spotted fever.

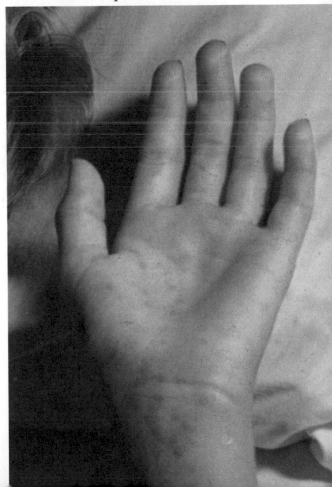

spreading to the limbs and trunk. This rash first consists of small rose-colored spots that blanch under pressure. As time progresses, the spots darken in color and refuse to blanch on pressure. In some cases there is an associated obstruction of the tiny blood vessels in the skin, which accounts for bluish to purplish blotches which in severe cases give rise to local areas of skin destruction. In severe cases of illness there are certain nervous symptoms consisting of sleeplessness, restlessness, delirium, and possibly stupor or coma.

Without specific treatment, the disease runs its course in about three weeks. In fatal cases, death may occur about two weeks after the onset. Formerly, mortality rates in this disease were alarmingly high. Now that effective drugs are available, the mortality rate is as low as 3 percent, the deaths usually occurring in those who receive the treatment late in the course of the disease.

A vaccine is now available which produces immunity to Rocky Mountain spotted fever. Immunization by this means is recommended for those who live in areas where the disease is prevalent.

What to Do

1. Antibiotics are effective remedies and serve to shorten the course of this disease. They must be administered, of course, under the direction of a physician.

2. Nursing care is directed toward making the patient comfortable and conserving his strength.

ROSEOLA INFANTUM.
(See *Exanthem Subitum* in this chapter.)

RUBELLA.
(See *German Measles* in this chapter.)

RUBEOLA.
(See *Measles* in this chapter.)

SCARLET FEVER (SCARLATINA).

Scarlet fever is an acute infectious disease in which the symptoms appear from one to ten days after contact with a "carrier" or with a case during the communicable stage of the disease. The various phases of the disease last for a total of about three weeks after symptoms first appear. The disease is characterized by fever, extremely sore throat, vomiting, headache, a coated tongue, and a skin rash which makes its appearance about two days after the onset of the other symptoms.

It used to be assumed that scarlet fever is a separate disease entity. It is now recognized as one of the possible manifestations of infection by "group A" of the germs called hemolytic streptococci. Other diseases caused by group A hemolytic streptococci include streptococcal sore throat and erysipelas.

The principal site of infection in scarlet fever is the soft tissues of the pharynx. It is here that the toxins are produced that may cause serious damage in various organs of the body.

Germs of scarlet fever are carried from person to person by the air or by the small droplets of moisture emitted through a person's nose or mouth. A person with this disease may transmit it to others beginning about a day before his symptoms appear, continuing through the course of the disease, and extending as long as a month or more after recovery. Certain persons become "carriers" of the infection even though they have never been ill with the disease. It is said that more cases of scarlet fever develop after contact with carriers than after contact with actual cases of scarlet fever.

The skin rash of scarlet fever appears first on the upper chest and back, later on the lower back, upper extremities, abdomen, and lower extremities. Often the rash does not appear on the face, but the face is flushed and there is a pale area around the mouth. Typically, the tiny elevations of the skin rest on a background of redness which fades on pressure. The tiny elevations are about the size of goose pimples, and these remain after the red color of the skin has become pale. In some cases numerous tiny blisters develop. In most cases the skin begins to peel as the rash fades. In contrast to the peeling of some other diseases, the sections of skin which become loose in scarlet fever are relatively large, particularly so on the palms and soles.

Typically in scarlet fever the lymph nodes of the neck become greatly enlarged. Occasionally abscesses develop in these nodes. Complications which may occur in untreated young children include sinusitis, middle-ear infection, mastoiditis, and impetigo. Other serious complications are arthritis, meningitis, damage to the tissue of the heart, and damage to the kidneys.

Fortunately the severity of the average case of scarlet fever has declined in most countries during recent years. The fatality rate for the disease is now less than 1 percent.

What to Do

1. **Penicillin is the antibiotic drug of choice in the treatment of scarlet fever. It does not neutralize the toxin that has been produced by the infection in the pharynx, but it does eliminate the causative germs and thus reduces the danger of complications and hastens recovery.**

2. **In children who have been exposed to scarlet fever and in whom it is desirable to prevent the disease because they are not vigorous, the proper and prompt administration of penicillin can keep the disease from developing.**

3. **Nursing care of the scarlet fever patient should provide rest in bed, adequate fluids, and an easily digested, nourishing diet.**

4. **For excessively high fever, tepid sponge baths or alcohol rubs may be helpful. (See volume 3, chapter 19, "Home Care for the Sick.")**

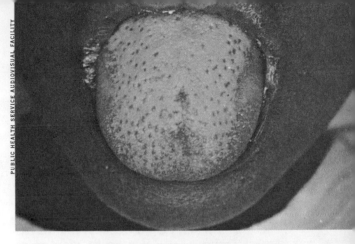

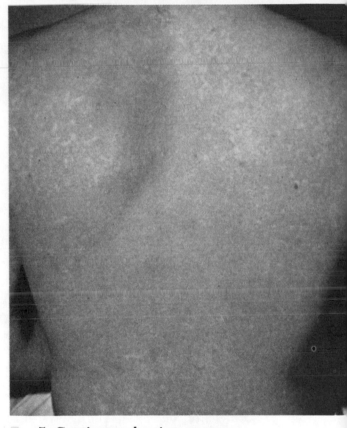

A coated tongue and a skin rash help to identify scarlet fever.

5. **Continuous heating compresses to the neck are helpful in allaying the discomfort of severe sore throat. (See volume 3, chapter 20, "Simple Home Treatments.")**

6. **Cleanliness of the mouth may be promoted by using a salt-water mouth rinse (1 level teaspoonful of salt to a pint of water).**

7. **Frequent examinations by the**

495

physician should be made so as to detect early any complications involving the heart or kidneys. When such develop, they must be treated as separate illnesses.

8. At the time scaling of the skin occurs, it is helpful to rub the skin with olive oil.

9. It is recommended that the recovering patient remain in bed a few days even after symptoms disappear and that he be slow in returning to full activity—this as a means of minimizing the damage that may have been done to the tissues of his heart or kidneys.

SEPTIC SORE THROAT.
(See *Streptococcal Sore Throat* in this chapter.)

SHINGLES.
(See *Herpes Zoster* in this chapter.)

SMALLPOX (VARIOLA).

Smallpox is an acute, highly communicable disease caused by a virus and characterized by suddenly developing symptoms of severe illness and a progressive skin rash followed, after recovery, by blemished and pitted skin.

Prior to the widespread use of vaccination, smallpox was very common, usually contracted during childhood. Thousands of people died in the severe epidemics, and those who recovered were usually disfigured for life by scars left from the skin lesions.

As of the present, smallpox is all but completely conquered. Only a very few cases have been reported in the last few years, and these in remote areas of the world. The conquest of smallpox is one of the great triumphs of modern medical science.

Vaccination against smallpox is no longer recommended in the United States. In the unforeseen event that a susceptible person should become exposed to smallpox, immediate vaccination should be effective in preventing the disease.

Before starting on international

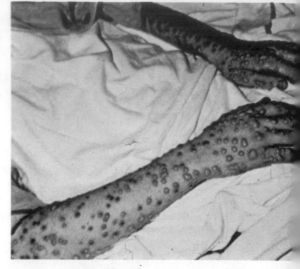

PUBLIC HEALTH SERVICE AUDIOVISUAL F

Smallpox in the vesicle stage.

travel, one should check to see which countries still require a certificate of vaccination for smallpox.

The virus that causes smallpox is present in the skin lesions, in the dry crusts and scales that follow the skin lesions, and in the droplets of moisture expelled through the mouth when coughing. Probably the virus can even be transmitted by the air which the patient exhales—especially during the early stages of the disease.

Twelve to fourteen days elapse after exposure before the symptoms of smallpox appear. At first there are three or four days of a mild general illness such as may occur in influenza. Then the symptoms become suddenly worse and include a severe chill, intense headache, pain in the back and limbs, loss of appetite, vomiting, fever, and sometimes convulsions. When the skin rash appears, about the third day after the onset of severe symptoms, the fever drops and the patient may feel reasonably well. It is at this time that great danger of exposing other persons prevails. As the skin eruption continues to develop, the patient's temperature rises for the second time and may now become quite high.

At first the skin rash of smallpox consists of small, dark-red, elevated lesions which appear on the forehead, neck, and wrists. These feel like small shot embedded in the skin. They gradually fill with clear serum, forming small blisters. The blisters, or vesicles as they are called, soon become depressed at their centers. After about a week the fluid within the vesicles becomes cloudy, and the lesions are now called pustules. Within another few days the pustules begin to dry and crusts are formed. A few days later the crusts loosen and fall off, leaving scars which may be permanent.

In a mild case of smallpox there may be only a few pustules, mainly on the forehead, neck, and wrists. In the average case many hundreds of lesions develop, chiefly on those parts of the body which face forward and including the palms and soles. In very severe cases bleeding may occur into the vesicles and pustules. It is in these severe cases with large numbers of skin lesions and in which skin hemorrhages occur, that there is grave danger of death.

A mild case of smallpox may be mistaken for chicken pox. The comparisons in the accompanying table should be helpful in differentiating the two diseases.

What to Do

A smallpox patient should be placed in a hospital where care is provided for communicable-disease cases. If the patient must be cared for at home, the following instructions apply:

Smallpox	Chicken Pox
1. Headache, backache, and fever begin four or five days before the skin eruption appears.	1. Few or no symptoms occur prior to the skin eruption.
2. Lesions appear all in one crop; at any given time the lesions on a given area of skin will be in the same stage of development.	2. Lesions come out in successive crops—papules, vesicles, and crusts all being present at the same time on a given skin area.
3. Papules are hard and deep-seated, feeling like small shot.	3. Papules are not hard and not deep-seated.
4. It is difficult to press all the fluid out of a vesicle.	4. It is easy to break open a vesicle and press out all of its fluid.
5. Lesions are located chiefly on the exposed skin areas—face, hands, feet, forearms, and legs.	5. Lesions are located chiefly on areas covered by the clothing such as the chest and back.
6. The smallpox patient is extremely ill in proportion to the severity of his skin eruption.	6. The skin eruption may be very profuse without making the patient feel severely ill.

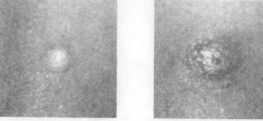

Day 1   Day 4

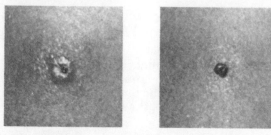

Day 7   Day 14

The technique of vaccination developed by Dr. Edward Jenner in the eighteenth century has made smallpox a rare disease. Illustration shows how site of the vaccination appears progressively on the first day, the fourth day, the seventh day, and the fourteenth day.

1. Follow carefully the directions for preventing the spread of a contagious disease as given at the beginning of this chapter.

2. The patient should be kept in a separate room with no visitors allowed until all the crusts have fallen away from his skin lesions.

3. There is no drug that appears to be useful in treating smallpox or in protecting those who have been exposed to the disease. Many physicians will order one of the antimicrobial drugs in order to prevent the development of secondary infections starting when the skin lesions break.

4. When the illness is severe, it is important to make sure that the patient drinks sufficient fluid and that he receives adequate nourishment even though he has no desire for food. It is sometimes necessary for the physician to arrange for fluid and even for food to be administered by vein or by stomach tube. Otherwise the diet should consist mostly of milk, cereal, gruels, and fruit juices.

5. Excessively high fever may be controlled by sponging the patient's skin with lukewarm water or by the use of alcohol rubs, or by other measures prescribed by the doctor.

6. As the skin lesions begin to form crusts, the itching may be relieved somewhat by the use of carbolated vaseline.

STAPHYLOCOCCAL INFECTIONS.

Prior to the introduction of the antibiotic drugs, staphylococcal infections were considered less serious than those caused by the streptococcus. It is the staphylococcus that is usually involved in infections of the skin such as boils and in infections that produce abcesses. Now that antibiotic drugs have come into general use, infections caused by the streptococcus are under reasonably good control. It has developed, however, that staphylococcal germs are not so readily controlled by the antibiotic drugs. Furthermore, certain strains of the staphylococcus (the so-called "resistant strains") do not respond well to the usual types of antibiotic drugs.

Staphylococcal infections prove to be most serious in the very young or the very old and in those whose resistance has been reduced by illness. The danger of staphylococcal infections is greatest in newborn infants, nursing mothers, persons ill with influenza, those with such chronic lung diseases as emphysema, those with long-standing skin disorders, persons recovering from surgery, and persons with extensive burns.

In their usual manifestations, staphylococcal infections may cause abscesses, pneumonia, or bacteremia (blood-stream infection).

Prevention. Because some staphylococcal infections are life-threatening and because their treatment is so difficult, emphasis is placed on preventing them in preference to treating them after they occur. Particularly in hospitals, both in nurseries and in the facilities for surgery, great care is used to avoid the transfer of staphylococcal germs to someone who may be susceptible. Precautions involve the use of all possible methods of preventing contamination.

In the hospital nursery sterile gowns and masks must be worn by the persons who take care of the infants. The hands of the attendants must be washed with soap and rinsed with disinfectant solution. Any infant with an infection is isolated to prevent spread of the infection to others. Any materials or body discharges that may possibly carry staphylococcal germs are handled strictly in accordance with hospital techniques. Similarly in the handling of surgical patients, all precautions are taken to prevent the entrance of staphylococcal germs into the tissues of susceptible patients.

Staphylococcal germs (shown here highly magnified).

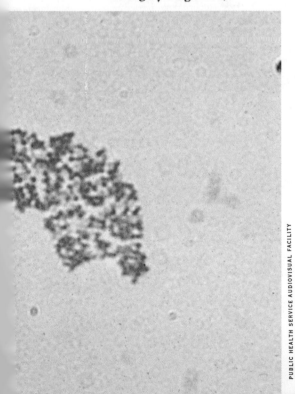

PUBLIC HEALTH SERVICE AUDIOVISUAL FACILITY

When a patient with such an infection is cared for at home, the patient should not only be isolated from other persons who may be susceptible but his bedding, personal linen, and all body excretions must be handled in the strictest possible manner to prevent further contamination.

What to Do

As mentioned above, the older antibiotic preparations usually do not prove effective in combating staphylococcal infections. Fortunately, several of the newer antibiotics are quite useful. The physician in charge of a case will use his best judgment in selecting the particular antibiotics effective against the type of staphylococcal germ involved.

Abscesses that develop in the course of the infection must be surgically drained. Careful attention must be given to make sure that the patient receives an adequate amount of easily digested food during each twenty-four-hour period. High fever is best controlled by the use of tepid sponge baths or by alcohol rubs.

STREPTOCOCCAL SORE THROAT (SEPTIC SORE THROAT).

This severe sore throat is caused by a strain of hemolytic streptococcus very similar to that which causes scarlet fever. In fact, there is very little difference between streptococcal sore throat and scarlet fever as far as the disease processes are concerned, there being in both a serious infection in the tissues of the pharynx. But in scarlet fever there is in addition a skin rash caused by the effect of the toxin on the capillaries of the skin.

Streptococcal sore throat occurs both as isolated cases and in epidemic form. Epidemics of this disease are usually the result of a streptococcal contamination of milk or milk products. Spread of the disease from person to person is usually by contamination of articles of food and drink by

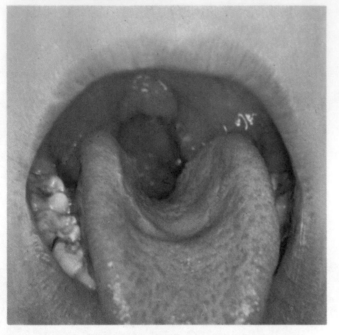

Typical case of sore throat.

germs derived from the throat of someone ill with the disease.

The potent toxin produced in the infected tissues of the pharynx makes the patient very weak. The possible complications of streptococcal sore throat include arthritis, persistent infection of the lymph nodes in the neck, middle-ear infection, occasional infection of the lining of the heart, and damage to the delicate tissues of the kidneys.

What to Do

1. As with other infections caused by the streptococcus, that of streptococcal sore throat is quite amenable to treatment by antibiotic drugs. Properly selected and administered, these reduce the severity of the illness and shorten its duration.

2. Nursing care of a patient with streptococcal sore throat should include the usual precautions for preventing the spread of the infection, as detailed in the early part of this chapter. Discharges from the mouth and nose are laden with the streptococcus germs and should be handled appropriately and destroyed.

3. In the adult, soreness of the throat may be relieved by using a gargle containing ten grains of aspirin to half a glass of warm water. In the child, the amount of aspirin in the gargle should be proportionately less.

4. The painful lymph nodes in the neck are best treated by the use of either hot or cold applications, depending upon which makes the patient more comfortable. Cold can be applied by the use of an "ice collar" for about ten minutes out of each half hour. Heat can be applied by the use of hot packs.

5. It must be made certain that the patient drinks a sufficient quantity of fluid to enable him to produce copious quantities of urine. This "forcing of fluids" reduces the danger of damage to the kidneys. Remember that the patient is tempted to refuse fluid because his sore throat makes it difficult to swallow. If it is impossible for him to take enough fluid by mouth, a physician's instructions should be obtained relative to administering fluid by vein.

TETANUS (LOCKJAW).

In tetanus there is a persistent spasm of the voluntary muscles plus convulsions.

The disease is caused by a specific germ which forms spores and grows best where there is very little oxygen. The spores are abundant in garden and barnyard soil, in the dust along the roadside or in playgrounds, and especially in soil or dust where there is horse manure. When the spores find their way into a deep wound, particularly a puncture wound where they have no access to the air, they grow and produce their toxin. It is the toxin which gives rise to the serious symptoms characteristic of this life-threatening disease.

Symptoms usually appear within five to ten days after the injury. The original wound may have begun to heal by this time. There develops a stiffness of the muscles of the face, noted when the patient attempts to open or close his mouth. The victim becomes restless and worried. The stiffness spreads to other muscles of his body. His face becomes contorted, and he responds so sensitively to slight noises or any sudden contact with his skin that all the muscles of his body may suddenly contract. Pain becomes intense, and there is high fever with sweating, exhaustion, and retention of urine. The illness usually ends fatally unless early adequate treatment is given. One of the pathetic features of the disease is that the victim remains conscious, in spite of his suffering, right up to the time of death.

Fortunately, this disease is not very common. But it is so dangerous to life and causes such great suffering that every reasonable means should be used to prevent it. It is urgently recommended that every young child be vaccinated with tetanus toxoid and that booster doses of the toxoid be given every two or three years. Whenever the kind of injury is sustained that may cause an infection with the spores of tetanus, a booster dose of toxoid should be administered to bring the victim's immunity up to maximum potential for protection.

What to Do

When any person not adequately protected by vaccination against tetanus sustains an injury in which tetanus spores may possibly be implanted in the wound, a physician's services should be obtained without delay. He will want to clean the wound in such a way as to eliminate the injured tissue and thus reduce the production of the toxin should infection occur.

In addition to cleaning the wound, the physician will probably administer a special tetanus antitoxic serum which confers protection for a few days. This should be given, of course, before there is opportunity for symptoms to develop.

For a person so unfortunate as to develop the actual symptoms of tetanus, hospital care should be arranged at once.

TORULOSIS.
(See *Cryptococcosis* in this chapter.)

TULAREMIA (RABBIT FEVER).
Severe symptoms consisting of headache, chills, vomiting, fever, and prostration develop two to four days after the specific germ has entered the tissues. A day or two after the onset of symptoms a single elevated lesion de-

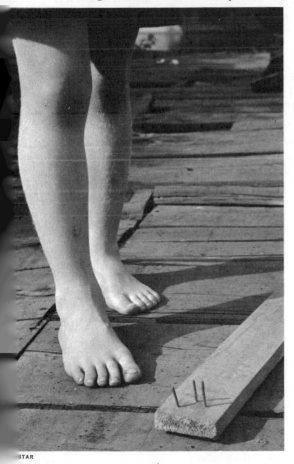

Puncture wounds give tetanus germs access to the body.

STAR

501

velops at the site of infection. This later ulcerates. There may be more than one such lesion if the mouth or eye is involved. The lymph nodes in the vicinity of the ulcer or ulcers soon become enlarged and form abscesses. By the fifth day of the illness a persisting high fever develops and, in many cases, an involvement of the lungs similar to pneumonia occurs. The spleen often becomes enlarged. In untreated cases, the temperature remains high for three or four weeks before it gradually declines.

The germs which cause tularemia enter the body through a break in the skin or by contact with the internal membranes. Although the germs occur widely in nature, most cases are traceable to a contact with infected wild rabbits. It is possible to acquire the disease through bites of insects or by eating the flesh of infected animals in which cooking has been inadequate, or by drinking contaminated water. Cases in which the lungs become involved are particularly serious and, without adequate treatment, may end fatally.

Prevention. Prevention of tularemia requires the exercise of great caution in the handling of wild rabbits and other rodents. The germs may be present not only in the tissues of the animal but in its fur. The flesh of wild birds and game should be cooked thoroughly before it is eaten. Drinking water of questionable purity should be adequately disinfected before use.

What to Do

1. **Streptomycin is the antibiotic of choice in the treatment of tularemia.**

2. **The patient should be kept in bed, should receive a generous diet of easily digested food, and should drink adequate amounts of fluid.**

3. **Application of an ice bag for about ten minutes out of each half hour to the areas which are ulcerated or in which there are swollen lymph nodes brings some comfort.**

4. **When one or both eyes are affected, special treatment and medication should be prescribed by the physician.**

TYPHOID FEVER (INCLUDING PARATYPHOID FEVERS).

A. *Typhoid Fever.* A specific germ, the typhoid bacillus, causes this acute, generalized, infectious disease. The body's lymphatic tissues are primarily affected. Symptoms include fever, a relatively slow heart rate, and, commonly, a rose-colored skin eruption. There is usually an enlargement of the spleen.

The germs of this disease enter the body through food or drink contaminated by bowel or kidney discharge from a typhoid fever patient or a "carrier." One agent which transfers the germs to food is the common housefly.

The symptoms begin one to four weeks after the germs enter the body. The onset is usually gradual with a tired feeling and general weakness. There may be headache and nosebleed. The fever rises higher each day until by the end of the first week it may reach 104° F. (40° C.)—higher in the evening than in the morning. The appetite is poor, the tongue is coated, and the teeth and lips are covered with a brownish deposit.

Diarrhea is common, especially at first; but there may be constipation instead. The stools have a very offensive odor. The abdomen is distended and tender to pressure. After seven to ten days, small, rose-colored spots may appear on the skin, most abundant over the abdomen but sometimes on the chest and back also. Near the beginning of the third week of illness, the fever usually begins to fall gradually.

During the early part of the disease the face is flushed and the eyes are bright; but by the second week the expression becomes listless and dull. Cough is fairly common, especially early. As a rule, the skin is dry; but sweating may occur late in the course of the disease.

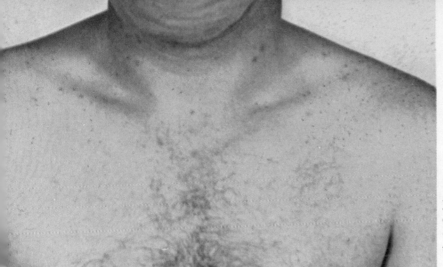

Rose-colored spots
on the chest
commonly characterize
typhoid fever.

The symptoms and the severity of typhoid fever vary greatly. The onset may be with convulsions, severe headache, and delirium.

Many serious complications may develop, the most common being intestinal hemorrhage and intestinal perforation. When these occur, they usually come during the third week of the illness. The occurrence of intestinal hemorrhage is indicated by a sudden drop in temperature, a weak and rapid pulse, and a dark discharge from the bowel. Intestinal perforation is indicated by sudden pain in the abdomen (often on the right side), a rapid drop in temperature, a spread of the abdominal pain to include the entire abdomen, and a weak but rapid pulse.

In some cases of typhoid fever the symptoms are so mild that the patient feels it unnecessary for him to go to bed or to consult a physician. Even in these mild cases, however, there is danger of intestinal hemorrhage. It is the mild cases that create the greatest danger of transmitting the infection to susceptible persons, the reason being that the mildly ill person may be careless about the proper disposal of discharges from the bowel and bladder.

Persons in reasonably good health but whose bodies still harbor the typhoid bacillus to the extent that it is present in their bowel or bladder discharges are called "carriers." A person who has a very mild attack of typhoid fever is just as likely to become a carrier as one who has a severe attack. It is in the effort to eliminate the carriers of this disease that the public-health departments insist on laboratory tests being made after a person recovers from this disease. If the germs are still present in the body discharges, a course of treatment with the proper antibiotic drugs will usually remedy the situation. One of the reasons that food handlers are required to have periodic examinations is to detect typhoid carriers. Many cases of the disease are traceable to food inadvertently contaminated by food handlers who are carriers of this infection.

In communities with poor sanitation, water is the most frequent means of transmitting typhoid fever. Food, especially milk, is the next most frequent offender. In urban areas food that has been contaminated by healthy typhoid carriers poses the greatest danger.

Prevention. There are four major public-health factors in preventing typhoid fever: sanitary control of domestic water supplies, pasteurization of milk, identification and treatment of typhoid carriers, and the practice of proper methods of nursing care for those who are ill with this disease.

The individual's best prospect of avoiding typhoid fever consists of being vaccinated against this disease. (See chapter 3, "Immunizations," in this volume.) Vaccination is very de-

503

sirable for persons who have had contact with a patient suffering from the disease, for any person traveling in areas where typhoid fever occurs or in areas where there is a question as to the purity of the water, and for those living in an area where an epidemic of typhoid fever has developed.

B. *Paratyphoid Fever.* There are two varieties of paratyphoid fever, caused by germs much like those that cause typhoid fever: paratyphoid A and paratyphoid B. Fever of either type tends to run a shorter course and tends to be less severe than typhoid fever, but the patient should receive similar care, and the same precautions should be taken against the spread of infection to other people.

What to Do

Certain of the antibiotic drugs are effective in shortening the course of illness with typhoid fever or with paratyphoid fever, in making the illness less severe, and in preventing serious complications. Good nursing care, however, is still a very important part of the treatment, as it relates both to the comfort and recovery of the patient and to the prevention of spread to other individuals. The care of the typhoid fever patient may be summarized as follows:

1. Instructions for preventing the spread of contagious diseases as given in the early part of this chapter should be carefully followed in caring for a patient with typhoid fever.

2. The patient should be kept in bed consistently from the time of onset of his symptoms until he recovers. He should use a bedpan instead of getting up to go to the bathroom.

3. The patient should be under a physician's supervision throughout the course of the illness.

4. He should receive an adequate supply of fluid, even beyond what he may choose to drink. His diet should be adequate to maintain good nutrition and should consist chiefly of milk, cream, buttermilk, gruels, broths, pureed vegetables, thickened soups, poached and soft-boiled eggs, fruit juices, and simple desserts.

5. The patient's mouth and teeth should be kept very clean, liberal use being made of a dentifrice with a magnesia or soap base.

6. Should it be necessary to administer an enema to bring about a bowel movement, great care should be taken to avoid undue pressure in administering the enema fluid. The physician's recommendations should be strictly followed in this matter.

7. High fever may be reduced by tepid sponge baths or alcohol rubs.

8. As a means of preventing bed sores, the patient's back should be rubbed with alcohol at least three times a day. The use of a very mild talcum powder after the alcohol rub is also helpful. The patient's position in bed should be changed frequently during the day, but he must be assisted in making these changes so as to avoid undue exertion.

9. If signs of intestinal hemorrhage or intestinal perforation appear, a physician must be notified at once.

TYPHUS.

(See chapter 32, "Warm-climate Ailments," in this volume.)

UNDULANT FEVER (BRUCELLOSIS).

This fever usually has an acute onset, with fever lasting for several days but with no signs that point to any particular part of the body. This is followed by a chronic stage in which there are repeated relapses characterized by fever, weakness, and vague aches and pains.

Undulant fever is caused by a specific germ which occurs in the blood and in certain organs, particularly the spleen. There are three types of the germ: Brucella melitensis from goats, Brucella abortus from cattle, and Brucella suis from swine. The disease is spread chiefly by raw milk or by butter or cheese made from raw milk, by handling or otherwise coming in contact with the body or carcass of an infected animal, or by eating the partially cooked flesh of such an animal. The disease was first recognized among soldiers who served on the island of Malta, hence the original name of the disease was "Malta fever."

At the beginning of the illness the patient develops headache, loss of appetite, weakness, and an irregularly increasing fever. In most cases there is constipation and in many a mild bronchitis with coughing. There may be night sweats.

After ten to fifteen days, there follows a period of relative freedom from symptoms, only to be followed later by a relapse. There may be from two to ten such waves of fever during the usual course of the disease. The patient gradually becomes weaker and anemic. At times his joints become swollen and painful. The kidneys are almost always affected, and it is usual for albumin to be present in the urine as indicated by a laboratory test. Typically, the patient feels better in the mornings than in the evenings. The usual course of the disease is from two to four months. In some cases the disease continues on in mild proporitons for a period of years.

In one sense undulant fever is not a serious disease because it seldom ends fatally, but it can weaken and disable a person for a very long period of time. Prevention, therefore, is important. Prevention consists in using milk and milk products which have been pasteurized and in making sure that meat is thoroughly cooked.

What to Do

The certain diagnosis of undulant fever requires interpretation of laboratory tests. Once the diagnosis is established, the physician has his choice of several antibacterial drugs. Best results are usually obtained when these are used in combination. Nursing care may be summarized as follows:

1. Bed rest throughout the acute phase of the illness is advised.

2. Tepid sponge baths and alcohol rubs are usually effective for the control of high fever.

3. The patient should be encouraged to drink adequate water and fruit juice.

4. The patient should be given an easily digested and adequately nourishing diet.

5. Because of the tendency for the disease to become chronic, attention must be given to maintaining the patient's courage and optimism.

6. Complications, if and when they develop, should be treated as recommended by the physician.

VALLEY FEVER.

(See *Coccidioidomycosis* in this chapter.)

VARICELLA.

(See *Chicken Pox* in this chapter.)

VARIOLA.

(See *Smallpox* in this chapter.)

WHOOPING COUGH (PERTUSSIS).

This acute, highly communicable disease involves the nose, throat, and other respiratory passages. It is characterized by a spasmodic cough which usually ends with a loud forced inspiration—the whoop. At the time of the whoop the patient may gag and vomit. In mild cases of the disease neither the whoop nor vomiting may be present.

Whooping cough is caused by a specific germ, Bordetella pertussis. It occurs throughout the world and often in epidemics. Although 50 percent of the cases occur before two years of age, persons of all ages who have not previously had the disease are susceptible. One attack usually confers immunity for life. The disease is most contagious during its early phases, when the germs are spread by contaminated droplets of moisture coughed into the air.

Whooping cough is most dangerous when it attacks young children, and for these it ranks first among the infectious diseases as a cause of death. Untreated cases involving babies under six months of age may have a death rate as high as 25 percent. With good medical care, this death rate, even for infants, can be reduced to as low as 1 or 2 percent.

For older children and vigorous adults, the disease is not considered to be serious in spite of its being troublesome. It may easily be prevented by a program of active immunization. (See chapter 3, "Immunizations," in this volume.) All infants should without fail receive the advantage of this immunization beginning at age two or three months.

The first stage of whooping cough begins a week or two after exposure. During a period of about two weeks the symptoms are essentially the same as those of an ordinary cold with the one difference that the cough becomes persistent and is particularly troublesome at night. After about two weeks of what appears to be a common cold, the coughing becomes spasmodic and the typical whoop is heard. At first this may occur only once or twice a day, but later it accompanies each spell of coughing. The patient's face becomes red and even bluish, and the veins stand out on his head and neck as he struggles for breath. Eventually his efforts serve to dislodge the tough mucus which has been obstructing the passage of air. But by this time he has become nauseated and may vomit. The stage of the disease in which whooping occurs lasts from three to six weeks. Less troublesome coughing may persist after that for several more months.

What to Do

1. The drug Erythromycin is used extensively for preventing whooping cough in those who are susceptible and who have had contact with a person who has this illness. The drug is also useful for treating those who are already ill with whooping cough. Some physicians recommend the use of pertussis immune globulin to protect very young patients and others who are not robust, once they have been exposed to whooping cough. The immune globulin is supposed to confer a temporary immunity. To be effective it must be administered before the symptoms begin.

2. For very young infants who have developed whooping cough, hospitalization is recommended. For the school-age child, the patient should be kept at home for at least three weeks after the characteristic whoop is first noticed.

3. The patient with whooping cough need not be kept in bed if he has sufficient vitality to engage in mild activities about the house without feeling tired. If the weather is fair, it is even good for the patient to be out of doors in the sunshine at least a part of each day. Great care should be taken to avoid his becoming chilled.

4. For patients who have great difficulty in getting their breath at the time of the paroxysms of coughing, it is well to have a mechanical suction machine available so that the heavy mucus can be sucked out of the patient's throat at the time of the coughing spells. For young children this procedure may even be lifesaving.

5. Steam inhalations are often helpful.

6. Fomentations to the patient's chest and neck two times a day may do a great deal to maintain his vitality and to hasten recovery. (See volume 3, chapter 20, "Simple Home Treatments.")

7. The wearing of a broad, snug binder around the abdomen will help to reduce the danger of muscle stress from violent coughing.

8. When vomiting becomes troublesome, it is well to feed the patient frequent small meals of soft food or liquid. It should be made certain that the patient drinks an adequate amount of fluid, particularly if he loses fluid by vomiting.

9. Particularly in the cases of young children, it may be advisable for the physician to use antibiotic drugs to control the possibility of complications.

YELLOW FEVER.
(See chapter 32, "Warm-climate Ailments," in this volume.)

Tuberculosis

Tuberculosis is generally thought of as a disease of the lungs; but, from a pulmonary focus, it may attack almost any part of the body. It is caused by a germ commonly called the tubercle bacillus. Tuberculosis germs can ride into the body on specks of dust or in tiny droplets sprayed out by an infected individual during coughing or sneezing. They may live for several days in moist sputum; they are fairly resistant to freezing, but they are somewhat less resistant to drying. They die instantly in boiling water, and in a few minutes or hours in sunlight and fresh air. Pasteurization, or heating a liquid to a temperature of 145° F. (63° C.) and holding the temperature at that level for half an hour, or heating it to 160° F. (71° C.) and holding for half a minute, will kill any tuberculosis germs in the liquid. If the living germs gain entrance to the lungs and get a foothold there, they grow fairly rapidly, at least for a time. One variety, the bovine type, prefers to attack cattle; but it will also grow in the human body, where it seems to prefer the lymph nodes or the bones rather than the lungs.

Tuberculosis germs are passed from person to person in numerous ways. Careless people spit on the floor, in public places, or on walks or paths. Germs may be in their sputum. Mixed with the dust, some of these germs may be blown about and breathed in by the passerby or may be carried into his home on his shoes. Children play in such places, soil their hands and playthings, and later carry the germs to their mouths. Germs may be left on a spoon, drinking cup, whistle, or pencil, and the next person who happens to put one of these articles into his mouth takes some of the germs into his body. If a cow has tuberculosis, germs may get into her milk. Also, if a person with tuberculosis handles milk, he may contaminate it. But, as noted above, pasteurization or boiling kills the germs.

Far more important and dangerous is the direct contact of a person with another who has the disease. A tuberculous mother who kisses her baby on the mouth is almost sure to plant some of her germs in the body of her child. Unfortunately, other members of the household—grandmothers, uncles, aunts—may have tuberculosis without knowing it and may not be aware of how dangerous it is for them to kiss children. It should never be forgotten that any moisture from the lungs or the lips of a tuberculous person may contain the germs whether or not he knows he has the disease.

When tubercle bacilli get into the body, they may be coughed or

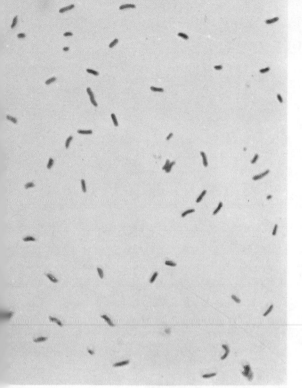

The tubercle bacillus multiplies
rapidly in a dark, moist place.

sneezed out before they do any damage. If swallowed, they may be killed by the acid in the stomach. If they get into the blood, they may be destroyed by the white blood cells. But if they elude these first defenses of the body, they will likely sooner or later find a lodging place, often in the lungs; and the discussion on the next few pages refers more directly to tuberculosis of the lungs than to other types.

The body, including the lungs, has special ways of fighting germ invaders of this type. Certain cells move to the spot where the germs have found lodgment. In a short time they build a wall or shell around them. This wall or shell with its contents is called a tubercle. Inside the tubercle, the bacilli continue to multiply and to destroy the small amount of lung tissue locked up with them. They may then perish without doing any further harm, or they may remain alive but quiescent inside the tubercle for a considerable length of time. A hard, gritty material—a calcium compound

—slowly replaces the destroyed lung substance if the normal resistance and repair processes of the body are in action, and the little shell finally becomes a stony prison for the germs.

If the tubercle bacillus were not a living thing, capable of multiplying, the above-described protective device would be perfect. But in the lung, where it is dark, warm, and moist, the germs tend to multiply rapidly. Then there is a race between the power of the cells to wall in the germs and the ability of the germs to multiply fast enough to escape. In most cases the cells win, but not always; and if they do, the first victory may not end the war. It takes a considerable period of time for the tubercles to become safe prisons. If at any time before this is accomplished the body's fighting power is decreased, some of the germs may escape and cause real trouble.

Two factors make the tubercle bacillus hard to kill and dangerous to keep around in the body. First, the surface of the germ has a waxy coating, which tends to protect it from the attacks of body cells whose business it is to fight germs. Second, the germ contains a special variety of protein called tuberculin. This protein, as is the case with all foreign proteins introduced into the body, stimulates the buildup of a specific sensitivity in the tissues. Thus it happens that if the germs shut up in the tubercle manage to escape—carrying their tuberculin with them, of course—they set up an allergic reaction in the sensitized tissues. Most of the tissue damage in a case of active pulmonary tuberculosis is the result of this type of allergic reaction.

Even though the focus in the lungs may be small, some of the germs may lodge in the lymph nodes, which abound in that part of the chest where the air passages and the large blood vessels enter or leave the lungs. Tubercles form in these nodes also, but they have a stronger tendency to calcify rather than to break down and let the germs escape than do tubercles in the lung tissue itself. If they should escape, however, they are already near tissue which they can easily attack and damage, since sensitivity has already been built up in this tissue by the presence of the germs in the body.

It is possible to test for this sensitivity, even though the person concerned has never had any symptoms of active tuberculosis. As can be understood from the foregoing discussions, sensitivity is being built up while the germs are being walled in; and it persists thereafter for a very long time—no doubt for life in many cases. The test is made by injecting a very small amount of tuberculin into the skin. If the body is sensitive to the germs, a spot of swelling and more or less redness will appear at the point of the injection within a day or two.

This does not mean that there is, or even that there ever has been, any active tuberculosis present, though, of course, there may be. It does mean that at some time in the past the body has been invaded by tuberculosis germs. Tests made on millions of apparently healthy individuals have provided evidence that a large proportion of the bodies of all people have been thus invaded, many of them during childhood. Obviously, then, many people from childhood onward are in danger of developing active, destructive tuberculosis if their general resistance falls low enough to allow a new infection to take root, or to allow living germs to escape from tubercles in which they have been lying dormant. Since, however, the tubercles tend to become safer and safer prisons, and the germs in them tend to die out with the passage of time, older people are less likely than younger poeple to be attacked by germs from broken-down tubercles.

So long as the body maintains its fighting power, all is likely to be well; but if its general resistance declines, the tide of battle may turn. This most often happens at about the time when young people are in their late teens or early twenties. It is then that they are

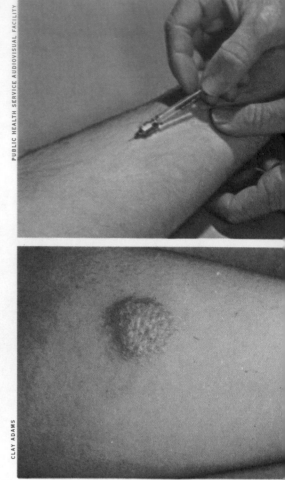

A positive tuberculin reaction indicates that tuberculosis germs have been present and that preventive treatment may be indicated.

most likely to use up energy in vigorous and exciting athletics or amusements. They often neglect to get enough rest and sleep, and they do not yet feel the need of paying attention to their eating habits. Too many girls become undernourished in their attempt to grow slender or to stay that way. The sex changes that have recently taken place may have upset the balance of their glandular activity and caused a drain on their nervous energy. It is therefore between the ages of fifteen and twenty-five that this disease has claimed its greatest number of victims. While a majority of tuberculosis deaths now occur at a later age, it is probable that the original active infection began during this critical period.

Only the tubercle bacillus can cause tuberculosis; but overwork, hard times, strain, dissipation, discouragement, and other burdens are great allies of the germ. They make it easier for it to get into the body and, once in, to secure a firm foothold. Surroundings are important too. Where, how, and with whom a child or other young person lives has much to do with deciding whether or not he will get tuberculosis. Most of us can overcome the few germs that invade our bodies through casual contact with other people. A child who lives daily with a person who has active tuberculosis is in constant danger unless every person in the household understands the danger and unless everything possible is done to prevent the germs from spreading from the infected person to others.

Whatever part of the body is attacked by tuberculosis germs, if an active disease results, there are generally a few outstanding symptoms and signs. The victim tires easily without sufficient reason and loses weight. He may have a poor appetite with indigestion. Cough is common if it is the lungs that are attacked. While these are the usual early symptoms and signs, they may not be the only ones. Sometimes blood spitting sounds the first alarm. This may be severe the first time or be so slight as merely to streak the sputum. There may be sharp pain in the chest due to pleurisy. Tuberculosis probably is the most common cause of that ailment, at least in young adults, though, of course, there are chest pains not caused by pleurisy. Any young or middle-aged adult who thinks he may have pleurisy should consult a physician and have him search for the cause of the pain. It may be tuberculosis, and the earlier its existence is discovered the better.

How does a physician determine whether or not a person has tuberculosis? First, he listens carefully to the person's description of his ailment. No symptom, however slight, is disregarded. All previous illnesses, especially those of childhood, have an important bearing on the question. What he hears enables him to judge whether or not there are grounds to suspect tuberculosis. Then he will make a careful physical examination. He will probably order a chest X ray taken and have the sputum examined.

An experienced physician may be able to make a diagnosis by physical examination, but many cases of early tuberculosis can be found only by means of X-ray studies. The X ray alone, however, may lead to a mistaken diagnosis, because a previously existing histoplasmosis or coccidioidomycosis may have produced findings which cannot be distinguished from those due to tuberculosis; and a chronic histoplasmosis may be the cause of lung cavities quite similar to those of advanced tuber-

An X ray of the chest reveals possible presence of tuberculosis.

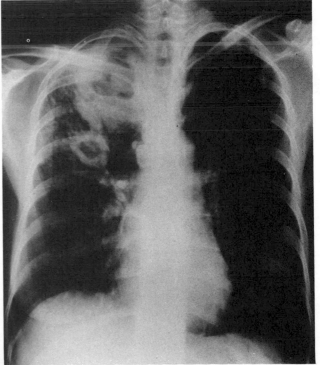

culosis. In cases of uncertainty from this point of view, both tuberculin, histoplasmin, and coccidioidin skin tests must be made to determine which disease is, or was, present.

Methods of Treatment

Tuberculosis can be cured if discovered before it has become too far advanced, and if the patient cooperates with the physician. The earlier the treatment is started the better are the chances for a cure. Delay is dangerous.

A. *Drug Therapy*. Fortunately, most patients with tuberculosis can now be treated quite successfully by medication—the result of many years of investigation and testing. Usually three drugs are used: streptomycin, para-aminosalicylic acid, and isoniazid. Each is used in amounts and in proportions one to the others in accord with the needs and relative responses of each patient. Such medication usually continues for a minimum of one year and frequently up to two years.

B. *Rest Cure*. In many cases, care in a sanatorium is indicated. In addition to medicines, rest has proved to be one of the most beneficial remedies. This means rest in the medical sense, not merely a change of scene or work. The degree and duration of rest is prescribed by the physician and depends upon evaluation of each patient. Rest gives the lungs their best chance to heal, and also it is an important part of the treatment of tuberculosis in any other part of the body.

Building up the body comes next in importance. This depends on good food and good digestion. A well-balanced diet, including milk, eggs, fruit, and vegetables, is best. Vitamins must be supplied in abundance.

While sunlight may be one of the most valuable remedies for bone or lymph node tuberculosis, it is easy for people with lung tuberculosis to get too much of it. Sunburn is especially harmful to people with pulmonary tuberculosis. Fresh air is important, but it is not necessary to lie out of doors in the broiling sun or in freezing weather in order to get it. Air that is clean, cool, and in slight motion is fresh air, so far as health is concerned. Cold weather does no harm, provided the patient is warmly covered; but a cold body is not comfortable, and comfort is one thing that the body needs in its fight against the tuberculosis germs.

C. *Phrenicectomy*. In recent years a number of ways have been found to give an infected lung extra rest in addition to that which it gets from its owner's lying in bed. Even in deep sleep, the lung is in constant motion, though to a much lesser degree than when a person is awake. Rest for a diseased lung may be increased by a slight operation on one of the phrenic nerves in the neck. This causes the corresponding half of the diaphragm, the large muscular partition between the chest and the abdomen, to stop working and ease the strain on the sick lung, since it cannot move as freely as before. Some time later, the nerve recovers and the normal action of the diaphragm is restored; but by that time the diseased condition of the lung is usually much improved.

D. *Pneumothorax*. Another device is to collapse a diseased lung by injecting air into the pleural sac between the chest wall and the lung. This is called pneumothorax. It is a safe procedure and causes but little pain. It may succeed in collapsing the lung so completely that it does little, if any, work; and, if necessary, the diseased lung can be kept collapsed for years. The other lung, if reasonably healthy, can do all the breathing work necessary for the body.

E. *Thoracoplasty*. The removal of portions of several ribs on the diseased side sometimes helps by permanently collapsing part of a lung. Surgical removal of that part of a lung that will not heal under ordinary treatments is proving to be increasingly successful; but of course neither of these rather serious surgical opera-

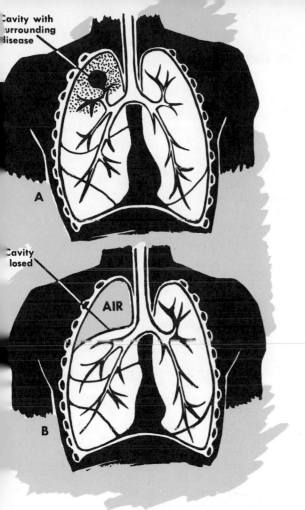

Cavity with surrounding disease

Cavity closed

AIR

A

B

Diseased lung (A). Collapsing it (B)
aids in recovery.

tions is advisable unless the other
lung is reasonably healthy.

Home Care

It is surprising how quickly most
tuberculosis patients improve after a
few weeks of bed rest. The fever goes
down, the cough stops, and the hollow
places begin to fill out. This improvement may deceive the patient
into thinking he can safely get up and
go about his business, but the experienced physician knows better. He
makes further examinations, including repeated X rays and sputum tests.
Frequently he finds that the fight in
the lung is not yet won. The enemy
has become quiet, but is only lying in
wait.

This is a dangerous time. To stop
fighting when the patient feels he is
about well would give the germs their
chance to break loose once more and
start a new battle in a fully sensitized
field. To win, the patient must keep
the enemy walled in until the organisms are destroyed or the germ
prisons are secure. He must stick
faithfully to the treatment program
until long after he feels well. Not until
his physician is sure that the tubercles
are tough and hard or that the bacilli
are no longer either alive or active will
he allow the patient to return to normal activity.

Sometimes sanatorium care cannot
be had. Then the rest treatment must
be carried out at home. With a physician to direct, it is often possible to
cure tuberculosis with the patient at
home; but it means that every household member, not only the sick one,
must strictly obey orders even though
it may be hard to do so.

A bright, sunny room with windows
on two sides is best for the sick person;
and he should be the only person living and sleeping in the room.

A. *Diet.* How to feed the tuberculosis patient is so important that the
physician should be consulted about a
diet plan. A general principle is that
the patient should not be overfed, but
he should eat enough to gain gradually up to his optimum weight. As a
rule, a good diet should include:

1. Milk—about one quart every day.
2. One or two eggs every day.
3. Plenty of vegetables (some fresh),
including one that grows above-
ground, like cabbage, and another that
grows beneath the ground, like
potatoes; but if any of these proves
hard to digest, change to another.
4. Leafy salads and raw fruits—one
or the other or both every day.
5. A tablespoonful of cod-liver oil
daily.
6. Easily digestible desserts.
7. Enough food to maintain or preferably gradually increase body
weight.

The patient should have his own set

of dishes, knife, fork, and spoon. These should be washed in very hot soapsuds, boiled five minutes after rinsing and kept apart from family dishes. His bed linen and washable clothes should also be kept apart from the family wash until they have been boiled in soapsuds.

B. *Precautionary Procedures. Getting rid of the sputum is very important.* All discharges from the patient's mouth or nose should be collected in paper cups which can be burned in an incinerator, stove, or furnace. In city apartments the cups may be enclosed in paper bags and arrangements made with the janitor to collect and burn the bags daily. Paper napkins or tissues used as handkerchiefs are useful to hold before the mouth when coughing.

Visits from friends and relatives are allowable, provided such visits cheer the patient and are not too long. Too many visits or too many visitors at one time tend to be exciting and tiring. The patient may join his friends in quiet talk, but should not discuss his illness or listen to the tales of woe of others. If the patient is coughing, the visitor should not stand or sit near him. *Children below the age of sixteen should not visit any tuberculosis sickroom* whether the patient coughs or not.

Every member of the household should be examined, not only once but as often as the physician considers advisable. Each child in the family should be given a tuberculin test. If it proves negative, the child is not infected. If it proves positive, the next step is to have the child's chest X-rayed. From the X-ray picture the physician can tell whether or not any measurable damage to the lungs has been done. Even if he sees no evidence of damage, he may still think a course of medical treatment would be additional insurance; and in any case he will want the child X-rayed and examined again from time to time to make sure that any possible beginning active infection is promptly discov-

ered. As long as a tuberculosis patient is in the home, and probably for a year longer, the physician will advise that any tuberculin-negative child there be retested at least as often as every six months.

Older people in the household may have chronic tuberculosis but not know it, even though they are troubled with coughing, or wheezing. They may mistakenly believe they have bronchitis, asthma, or heart trouble. Such people are especially dangerous to their associates because they usually take no care to protect others from possible infection. It is especially important that they be examined and, if found to be infected, put under careful medical supervision.

Miscellaneous Considerations

A. *Climate.* Years ago it was thought that certain climates are good for people with tuberculosis. Climate does help, but climate alone is no cure. Those who can afford to travel to a pleasant climate where they can have all else that is needed for the cure, and where they will not get homesick, may be wise in making the move. But if a person has to give up good home care, comfort, and friends for the sake of climate, it is a poor bargain.

A few people have claimed that exercise is good for a tuberculosis patient. This is a mistaken idea. Sitting up in a chair is usually the first exercise allowed, followed by going to meals and later by a little walking. Bit by bit other forms of light work or play may be allowed, but anything that causes fatigue is forbidden.

B. *Rules.* There are a few other miscellaneous rules worth remembering in the home treatment of a tuberculosis patient. The patient should avoid swallowing his sputum, for doing so may lead to intestinal tuberculosis. Sweeping and dusting of the patient's room should be done with damp mops and cloths only. Toothbrushes should be kept absolutely clean. The use of dental floss between the teeth, and a daily washing of the teeth with soap on a soft cloth, which can then be burned, is better treatment for the teeth and gums than the use of a toothbrush. Whoever takes care of the patient should form the habit of washing the hands frequently and well. This should always be done just before eating and before handling food or other objects that may be eaten or handled by others.

If all the rules given in foregoing paragraphs are obeyed, especially those concerning safe disposal of the patient's sputum, attendants need have no fear of contracting the disease. They should, however, lead a healthful life, take moderate outdoor exercise every day, and try to maintain a constant mental attitude of fearless service.

C. *Relapse*. A return of symptoms during the time when a patient is under treatment may occur. He should be instructed to be watchful for any sign or symptom of illness which he has experienced or has learned about. He should be warned not to blame some other disease, such as influenza or a cold, for signs or symptoms which may be caused by a relapse of tuberculosis. He should not ignore pink streaks in his sputum or imagine that they come from his gums or his throat. He should report any suspicious sign or symptom promptly to the physician and have a thorough reexamination.

Tuberculosis may become active again after its victims are apparently well, and due care should be taken to prevent this. Those who have completed a course of treatment often feel better than ever before, but this does not mean that they are necessarily entirely well. How well they really are depends not on how they feel but on the condition of their lungs, and these organs they cannot see.

People who have apparently fully recovered from tuberculosis need better care and more rest than do those who have never had the disease. They carry a handicap that cannot safely be ignored. Friends often do not understand that recovered patients are not safely well when they look so hale and strong; and the family must protect them from too much work, too much worry, too many visitors, too much entertainment, and too little rest.

D. *Testing Programs*. During recent decades many tuberculin testing campaigns have been carried on, in some cases among the general population but more commonly among groups of children and youth. These campaigns have discovered many tuberculin-positive individuals, most of whom had no other sign of infection by the tuberculosis germ. There has been considerable controversy as to whether or not children in this category should be treated. Experts in the field of tuberculosis seem increasingly to favor the idea that the positive tuberculin reaction indicates the presence of living tuberculosis germs in the body of the child concerned, and that a year's treatment, preferably with isoniazid, would decrease the likelihood that these germs would take hold and cause active disease. Such a program is especially needed for very young children living in home conditions conducive to the development of the disease.

E. *Preventive Measures*. Before going on to a discussion of tuberculosis in other parts of the body we should give attention to the prospects for preventing it by means similar to those used in preventing other germ diseases. Tuberculosis germs do not produce any true toxin, so there is no possibility of producing and using a specific antitoxin. One attack of the disease gives so little, if any, immunity against a later attack that we should not expect a vaccine made from the germs to be very effective. Since, however, a vaccine seems to offer the only hope of building up any useful amount of immunity at all, attempts have been made to produce one.

The most successful work along this

515

line was done by a French bacteriologist named Calmette. He made a vaccine from an attenuated culture of the living bacteria. The attenuated bacteria were named bacillus Calmette-Guérin after him and his associate Guérin. The vaccine is commonly called BCG. BCG has been rather widely used in several European countries, and it has seemed to have considerable preventive value. It is not recommended for general use, however, except in areas with a dense population and poor sanitary facilities. One objection to its use is that those who receive it become tuberculin-positive, so the tuberculin test is of no further use in detecting possible tuberculous infection in their cases.

What to Do

1. Remember that *rest and an easily digestible, nourishing diet* are the most important parts of the treatment for tuberculosis. Details of a recommended diet are noted above.

2. Do not waste time in trying out any advertised "cure."

3. Do not leave your home and family and go to some place with a "good climate" for tuberculosis without advice from a physician experienced in the treatment of this disease.

4. Consult such a physician and remain under his care. He will first make examinations and tests to make sure whether or not the suspected condition is really tuberculosis. If it is, he may advise you to go to a sanatorium for at least a few weeks or months. Follow this advice if you can. Sanatorium care is not only the best for the patient, but it provides an opportunity to learn how to plan and carry on a home program later suitable for the patient and protective for other members of the household.

5. Whether you are in a sanatorium or at home, your physician will probably prescribe remedies that have proved effective in fighting tuberculosis germs. The number of such remedies is growing, so no list will stay up-to-date very long. As this is being written, streptomycin sulfate, para-aminosalicylic acid (PAS), isonicotinic acid hydrazide (isoniazid, INH), pyrazinamide, viomycin, and cycloserine are worthy of mention. Combinations of the first three are generally used at the same time initially; and, as a rule, isoniazid is continued with or without PAS. One or another of the last three is occasionally used but only when the patient becomes sensitive, or the germs resistant, to the first three.

In pulmonary tuberculosis, the remedies may need to be taken for a year or two, and in some other types of the disease for an even longer period of time.

Nonpulmonary Tuberculosis

In addition to tuberculosis of the lungs, already discussed, certain other forms of the disease, or localities in which it may be found, merit discussion because they are more or less common. In all such cases the same general measures of treatment are suitable—that is, building up general health and resistance by such means as abundant rest, a proper diet, and fresh air. In some cases special types of treatment may be useful, and where this is true they will be mentioned.

A. *Bladder.* Tuberculosis of the bladder is usually a complication of tuberculosis of the kidney. A severe and persistent inflammation of the bladder is its chief manifestation, with markedly painful and frequent urination. So long as the kidney is actively infected, nothing can be done to cure the bladder disease. The infection can often be controlled by using antituberculosis drugs for a long time; but if this plan fails, the infected kidney may have to be surgically removed. This, of course, cannot be done unless the other kidney is free from infection.

B. *Bones and Joints.* Tuberculosis

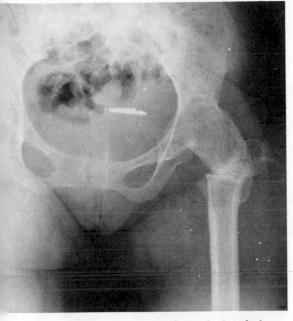

X ray showing tuberculosis of the joint, now comparatively rare.

of the bones and joints is growing less common at an even more rapid rate than is tuberculosis of the lungs. A large proportion of the cases have in times past been caused by the bovine variety of the germ, but increased tuberculin testing of dairy cattle and the pasteurization of milk have improved this situation.

Bone and joint tuberculosis usually occurs in children or youth. When the bones are affected, it is as a rule their end portions adjacent to the joints. In joint tuberculosis, the infection is nearly always present in the bone first, spreading to the joint later. (See *Arthritis, Tuberculous* in chapter 14 of this volume.)

If death comes from bone or joint tuberculosis, it is because of an extreme debility of the patient or because the germs break their way into a blood vessel and are disseminated throughout the body, giving rise to an acute general infection.

The treatment must be designed to fit each case. Proper treatment goes a long way toward preventing deformity and restoring or preserving function.

C. *Disseminated Tuberculosis.* If the germs of tuberculosis escape from one or more foci of infection anywhere in the body, there is a strong chance that they may find their way into the bloodstream and thus be scattered throughout the body. Wherever they go they are likely to lodge and start new tubercles, producing what is called disseminated tuberculosis, or, more commonly, miliary tuberculosis. This latter name is given to the condition because of the very large number of small tubercles that are formed. This condition tends to run a rapid course of from two to six weeks, with a fairly high fever, a rapid loss of weight and strength, profuse sweating, rapid pulse, headache, dizziness, dry tongue, distended abdomen, increasing anemia, and, until recently, an almost invariably fatal ending. The antituberculosis drugs have saved the lives of many victims of miliary tuberculosis, but this form of the disease is still serious.

D. *Epididymis.* The most common form of tuberculosis of the male sex organs is tuberculosis of the epididymis. At first this condition is usually onesided, but in nearly every case both sides are eventually involved. It causes swelling and tenderness, pain on ejaculation, a feeling of prostration after sexual intercourse, and eventually sterility and impotence. Tuberculosis of the epididymis rarely exists alone; it is associated with tuberculosis of the kidney, the bladder, the seminal vesicles, or foci of tuberculous infection elsewhere in the body.

E. *Intestines.* Tuberculosis germs can reach the intestine through the bloodstream or by means of the food. The most common way is by means of swallowed sputum that originated in an infected lung. The last few feet of the small intestine and the first few inches of the large intestine are most commonly attacked. Single tubercles, clumps of tubercles, and ulceration are common manifestations of intestinal tuberculosis; but in the caecum (first section of the large intestine) it is fairly common for a general thickening of the intestinal wall to take place, which may eventually result in partial or complete obstruction of the intestine.

Common symptoms are diarrhea or alternate constipation and diarrhea, abdominal pain, and tenderness. The stools often contain a little blood. If diarrhea is persistent, emaciation develops rapidly. If intestinal obstruction occurs, the symptoms will be similar to those of obstruction from other causes. In such cases surgery is needed, possibly also a valuable form of treatment for tuberculosis of the caecum without obstruction. As with other serious tuberculous infections, bed rest and an abundant, easily digestible diet are essential.

The acute inflammation usually responds well to modern treatment, and the use of antituberculosis drugs is making severe cases of intestinal tuberculosis increasingly rare, though scars resulting from the healing process may cause serious trouble.

F. *Kidneys.* Tuberculous infection of the kidneys occurs most commonly in young adults. As a rule, one kidney is first attacked; and the infection may become far advanced in this kidney before the other is affected. If symptoms respond promptly to the use of antituberculosis drugs, changing combinations of these should be used for two or more years. If the response is not prompt, surgical removal of the infected kidney should be considered. It should not be attempted, of course, if the other kidney is also infected. Examinations and tests made by a urologist are necessary to determine the true condition of both kidneys in such cases.

In a majority of cases the symptoms of tuberculosis of a kidney are wholly those of a bladder infection—especially painful and frequent urination. The urine is pale and slightly cloudy, and in advanced cases may contain albumin and pus. Tubercle bacilli are often found in it. Fever is rarely present; and the emaciation, weakness, loss of weight, and night sweats so characteristic of severe tuberculosis of other kinds are often slow in making their appearance.

G. *Larynx.* The larynx is occasionally infected in cases of tuberculosis of the lungs, as a rule by germs coughed up in the sputum. Inflammation and, later, ulceration take place; and the victim is troubled by hoarseness, cough, and pain on swallowing. These symptoms sometimes give the first indication that tuberculosis is present in the lungs. Accurate diagnosis of the condition requires careful examination, preferably by a throat specialist. The use of antituberculosis drugs usually brings prompt relief of the symptoms, but healing of the ulcers may take a long time.

H. *Lymph Nodes.* Most cases of tuberculosis of the lymph nodes begin in childhood, and at this time in life it is by far the most common type of tuberculosis. Besides the general forms of treatment advised for all types of tuberculosis, sun baths are of special value in cases of lymph-node tuberculosis. After tanning of the skin has occurred, frequent and long-continued exposures to sunlight are recommended.

If the nodes in the neck are affected, they show only as mildly painful swellings that may break down and discharge their pus and cheesy material through breaks in the skin. Surgical removal is often necessary, and it has a good chance of being a completely successful form of treatment. If not removed, the draining glands may eventually heal, but they leave much scarring behind. Attempts at surgical drainage without removal are unwise.

Nodes in the region of the air passages to the lungs are numerous, and they become infected with tuberculosis germs more often than do nodes in any other part of the body. Mild infections may produce no symptoms at all, but children with extensive involvement often run a low fever, have a poor appetite, become anemic, and lose weight and energy. Rest, a good diet, and sunbaths are of great benefit; but surgical removal of these nodes is not practical.

Tuberculous nodes in the region of the air passages to the lungs nearly always heal and attract deposits of calcium, which tend to persist throughout life. Chest X rays taken in later years show these small masses of calcium clearly and often provide the only proof that lymph-node tuberculosis in the chest ever existed. As mentioned earlier in this chapter, however, cases of active pulmonary tuberculosis may occasionally be caused by germs which may escape from tuberculous nodes in this region.

Nodes in the mesentery along the intestine are fairly often infected, but they usually produce no distinctive symptoms, and nearly all cases heal eventually. In severe cases in children there may be persistent diarrhea, weakness, fever, and loss of weight, with a distended abdomen tender to pressure.

I. *Meninges.* When tuberculosis germs attack the coverings of the brain and the spinal cord, particularly the delicate covering called the pia mater, a somewhat slowly progressive but always dangerous, tuberculous meningitis results. Nearly all cases occur in childhood or early youth. The patient becomes apathetic and drowsy. Sleep is disturbed. Headache of varying intensity is usually present, and its paroxysms may make the patient burst out with a sudden scream at times. Delirium tends to appear later in the course of the disease, and there may be other varying symptoms. When the case is fully developed, the forehead appears contracted, the facial expression blank, the eyeballs somewhat bloodshot and covered with thick mucus, and the pupils contracted. The abdomen is tense and retracted, the patient lies on his side with his limbs drawn up, localized paralyses appear, and the patient sinks into a complete coma which ends in death. At least this was the almost universal ending until recently.

Tuberculous meningitis is sometimes part of the picture in cases of miliary tuberculosis, and it is probably always secondary to a tuberculous focus elsewhere, usually primary in the lungs. Until recently, the best a physician could do was to give treatments that would relieve part of the sufferer's distress. The use of streptomycin in combination with other antituberculosis drugs has greatly reduced but has not eliminated fatalities. Some of those who live show signs of lifelong brain or nerve damage from the disease or from the drugs used to treat it.

J. *Oviducts.* Tuberculosis of the oviducts is the most common form of tuberculous infection of the female sex organs. It produces no characteristic symptoms different from those of infections or inflammations of these tubes caused by other kinds of germs. Since it is usually associated with tuberculosis of the intestine or the peritoneum, or is caused by germs that come by way of the bloodstream, any treatment that might be aimed at the oviducts themselves could hardly be expected to do much good.

K. *Peritoneum.* The peritoneum of tuberculous persons between the ages of twenty and forty is frequently infected with tuberculosis germs. In many cases no detectable symptoms are produced. In some, however, abdominal pain, tenderness, and distension are present, with irregular fever and progressive loss of weight. The abdominal distension is often from a collection of fluid. Diagnosis is difficult and requires careful study by a physician. Besides the ordinary types of treatment, sunbaths are of much value.

L. *Pleura.* The covering membrane of the lungs, the pleura, is nearly always affected when a tuberculous focus develops near the outer margin

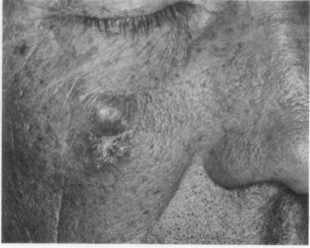

Lupus vulgaris, a common form of tuberculosis of the skin.

of a lung. Pleurisy results, and eventually fluid collects in the pleural cavity. A large proportion of all cases of pleurisy are tuberculous in origin.

M. *Skin.* The most common form of tuberculosis of the skin is lupus vulgaris. Any part of the skin surface may be attacked; but the face, particularly the nose, is by far the most common area. This disease most often attacks children, but it may persist until they are mature or even middle-aged. It is characterized by small, soft tubercles with an appearance similar to that of apple butter. These slowly increase in number and spread by the addition of new ones around the edges of those that are older. The tubercles tend to ulcerate and then to heal with scarring, leading to considerable deformity, disfigurement, and distress, but not to death.

There is no specific cure for lupus vulgaris. Antibacterial medication is helpful. X ray, radium, sunlight, other lights, cautery, and several other forms of treatment have been tried with fair success; but, as a rule, the treatment must be continued for a long time to do much good.

N. *Tonsils.* Tuberculosis of the tonsils is fairly common, but it is rarely present unless there is an already existing infection in the lungs. It does not often manifest itself by special signs or symptoms, though in severe cases the tonsils may become enlarged and ulcerated. In cases suspected of being tonsillar tuberculosis, a throat specialist should be consulted.

Venereal Infections

In one sense venereal infections do not differ from others. They are caused by specific disease organisms which can be seen and studied by means of a microscope and other facilities available in almost any clinical laboratory. But they differ in two important respects. First, they are usually transmitted by sexual intercourse, and more often than not by illicit activities of this kind. So long as prostitution continues, we shall have such infections to deal with. Also widespread promiscuity among teen-agers and college students has increased the problem to almost epidemic proportions in some areas. So the fight against venereal infections is at least as much a social problem as it is a medical problem. Second, with the most common of all venereal infections, gonorrhea, one attack does not immunize against future attacks; and there is no vaccine that can do this.

CHANCROID (SOFT CHANCRE).

Chancroid is a specific infection, transmitted as a rule by sexual contact. It may appear from one to ten days after exposure or contact. A small pimple appears first, nearly always somewhere on the genital organs. The pimple rapidly forms pus and ruptures, becoming a painful and pus-bathed ulcer, with considerable swelling in the surrounding tissues. The adjacent lymph nodes in the groin, usually on one side only, become swollen, tender, and often abscessed. The ulceration may become extensive and destructive if treatment is not begun early, but by use of the proper remedies most cases can be cured in a few days. Chancroids may be easily confused with syphilitic chancres, and for this reason a thorough examination by a physician is important, the treatment for the two conditions being entirely different.

What to Do

1. When a chancroid is suspected, immediately consult a physician, preferably a skin specialist, for a definite diagnosis. He will order such treatments as may be needed.

2. Avoid alcohol, stimulants, and unnecessary exercise. In severe cases hospitalization may be needed.

3. If abscessed nodes develop in the groin, the pus in them may have to be drawn out with a special needle.

4. Careful cleaning of the ulcers twice a day with mild soap and warm water is recommended.

5. Compresses wet with a

521

1 : 10,000 solution of potassium permanganate and kept applied to the ulcers two hours out of every three will hasten the healing.

6. Suitable sulfas and tetracycline antibiotics are effective medical remedies, but these must be prescribed by a physician.

GONORRHEA.

Gonorrhea is caused by a specific germ, the gonococcus. This germ is extremely active in invading mucous membranes, especially those of the eyes and the genital organs. As soon as infection takes place, the white cells of the blood attack the intruders by passing through the invaded membranes. The gonococci are mostly engulfed or swallowed by them, and may be seen inside of these cells, as well as outside of them, with the aid of a microscope. The mass of germs and white blood cells forms pus in abundance.

In men, gonorrheal infection causes inflammation, pain, burning, and a profuse discharge of rather thick, light-yellow pus from the urethra. In some parts of the world the great majority of males have this disease at least once in their lifetime. The male urethra, being much longer than that of the female, and having many glands and passages connected with it, is subject to a more severe early reaction to the germs of gonorrhea. Anterior urethritis, or disease in the terminal part of the urinary tract, easily becomes posterior urethritis also by backward extension of the infection. The germs may then gain access to the bladder, the prostate, the glands along the urethra, the seminal vesicle, the ductus deferens, and the epididymis; and they may cause inflammation in any or all of these organs or structures.

A condition which may follow gonorrhea, sometimes a long time after the acute infection has cleared up, is a narrowing or stricture of the urethra, which makes urination difficult and at times impossible, thus causing dangerous distention of the bladder. Stricture also develops in women, though much less often; but it does not develop in either sex until the disease becomes chronic. It tends to persist indefinitely, and must be treated by dilating or cutting the constriction. The treatment is painful and must be continued for many weeks and perhaps repeated later to prevent complications.

Stricture of the ductus deferens may also occur. If it does, sterility is the usual result. Epididymitis (see chapter 23 of this volume) may develop. It is a painful and sometimes serious complication.

Gonorrhea is less prevalent among women than among men, probably the chief reason being that a smaller proportion of women engage in illicit sexual relations. Many of the women who do become infected get the disease from their husbands who have contracted it before marriage and have not been entirely cured, or who have become infected through illicit sexual intercourse after marriage.

But, being internal, women's organs cannot be so readily treated as can those of men. Then, too, a married woman is not likely to begin treatment early, because, not suspecting that her husband has the disease, she does not apprehend any trouble until severe leucorrhea or pain compels her to seek medical aid. By that time the disease has become fully established.

Gonorrhea in a woman may begin with pain and burning on urination and a discharge of pus from the urethra, similar to the early symptoms in a man; but much more often the first noticeable sign is a profuse discharge of pus from the vagina, sometimes with fever and pain and tenderness in the lower part of the abdomen on one or both sides. Gonorrhea may be present and may persist in a woman, however, even though she has no noticeable symptoms; and sometimes it is difficult to determine definitely whether or not she has a gonorrheal infection.

The infection may travel up through

the uterus and the oviducts until it passes out through the open ends of these tubes into the abdominal cavity and causes peritonitis. If peritonitis is not caused, or if it quiets down without causing death or severe illness, the infection tends to become chronic in the oviducts and eventually to seal them shut in one or more places. Oviducts thus sealed shut will not allow ova to pass from the ovaries to the uterus, resulting in sterility. An oviduct sealed shut in two or more places forms one or more closed pus pockets. These pus pockets are dangerous foci of infection, and may lead to much pain, distress, and general ill health. Surgery finally becomes necessary in a considerable proportion of such cases to prevent complete invalidism.

In women, glands near the outlet of the vagina, especially the Bartholin's glands, may become infected and form painful and tender pus-filled pockets, requiring surgical drainage.

A very serious, though not very common, form of gonorrheal infection is called ophthalmia neonatorum, or sore eyes of the newborn. It is caused when germs get into the child's eyes during birth. So serious is infection of this kind that failure on the part of a physician to treat every newborn child so as to prevent this disease is considered a crime in many countries. The result of gonococcic infection in the eyes of an infant, if left untreated, is blindness in almost every case. The result of infection shows itself a few days after birth as a profuse discharge of pus from the eyes. It requires intensive and expert treatment if the little one's sight is to be saved.

Sometimes gonorrheal ophthalmia occurs in older children or adults. A person with genital gonorrhea may carry the germs to his eyes if he is not careful to disinfect his hands after urinating or changing dressings. If he tries to conceal his condition from other members of the household, they may unknowingly contaminate their hands by touching or handling objects

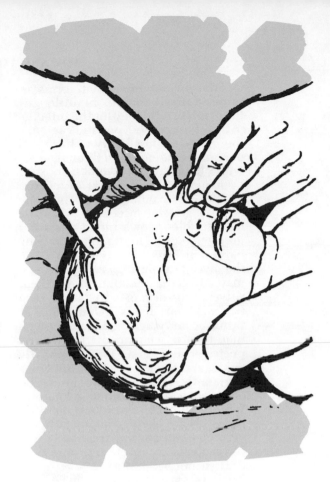

Treatment of the newborn against gonorrheal infection prevents possible blindness from such infection.

which he has carelessly contaminated, and then carry the germs to their eyes by rubbing them, though this rarely happens. Sometimes—also rarely—gonorrheal ophthalmia results from a blood-borne infection.

Gonorrhea sometimes occurs in little girls. It is characterized by a discharge of thick yellow pus from the vagina. The infection may come from diapers handled by the mother or a nurse who has the disease, from abnormal sex practices of older persons, occasionally from contaminated toilet seats, or from sleeping in the same bed with older persons who have gonorrhea. Not all vaginal discharges from little girls are due to gonorrhea, however, and it may require special laboratory procedures to determine

523

whether or not gonorrhea germs are present. Furthermore, in little girls there is less tendency for the infection to travel upward beyond the vagina, so the disease is less likely to have serious complications with them than it is with older girls and women.

Gonorrhea, while local in its early and usual manifestations, may become a general infection by getting into the blood. As a blood disease, it may gain access to the joints, causing painful arthritis; it may be carried to the eyes, causing ophthalmia; or it may result in infection of the heart valves, causing a usually fatal type of valvular heart disease. Gonorrheal arthritis occurs much more commonly in men than in women, as might be expected. The knee, the elbow, the ankle, and the hip are the joints most frequently attacked. The joints become hot and very tender and painful. When the acute symptoms subside, the joints are likely to be left stiff; and vigorous and painful treatment by a physician is necessary to restore them to their normal motion.

In its early stage, gonorrhea can usually be cured in a short time by proper treatment. For this reason, one who notices any smarting or burning or discharge from the urethra or the vagina a few days after sexual relations with a person not known to be free from the disease should immediately consult a physician for diagnosis, and for treatment if needed. It must be remembered that accurate diagnoses cannot be made without microscopic examinations and that it cannot be surely known that a cure has been accomplished until repeated microscopic examinations and cultures fail to find the germs. Relapses are not uncommon. Indulgence in alcohol and in sexual intercourse are the most potent causes of relapse.

What to Do

1. If any symptoms suspicious of gonorrhea are noticed, consult a physician without delay, preferably a urologist. It is perilous to postpone any needed treatment, to attempt self-treatment, or to depend on remedies sold without a physician's prescription.

2. Treatment of gonorrhea has been revolutionized by the use of certain sulfas, and especially of penicillin and certain other antibiotics. The use of these drugs can in most cases bring the infection under control within a very few days; but these remedies can be used safely and properly only under a physician's supervision.

3. Since exposure to infection with gonorrhea may carry with it the danger of exposure to infection with syphilis, anybody being treated for gonorrhea should also have a blood test for syphilis, and, if the first test proves to be negative, have it repeated one month later.

GRANULOMA INGUINALE (GRANULOMA VENEREUM).

Granuloma inguinale is a venereal infection, spread by sexual contact. It is believed to be caused by very small germs called Donovan bodies, which by microscopic examination can be seen packed inside the walls of certain rather large characteristic cells.

The first stage of this disease is a blister or small, flat pimple or nodule appearing on the external genital organs. Then a spreading ulcer develops, usually with new nodules forming around it as it extends. In severe cases there is much scarring and tissue destruction. More than one spot may be involved from the first, and the destructive ulceration may spread not only to the genital organs, but to the groins and thighs, or even farther. With proper treatment most cases are curable, but an occasional case is so resistant to treatment that it may progress until it comes to a fatal end.

What to Do

If granuloma inguinale is suspected, do not try self-treatment. Consult a physician at once. If he finds the condition actually present, he can use any one of several forms of antibiotics which are usually very effective in controlling this infection.

GENITAL HERPES SIMPLEX.

Genital herpes simplex is now the second most common venereal disease, being exceeded in frequency only by gonorrhea. It is caused by the herpes simplex virus type II which is a close relative of the herpes simplex virus type I that causes "cold sores" around the mouth and on the face.

There is no effective "cure" for the disease. Once the virus invades the tissues of a person's body, it remains for life, even though in latent state most of the time. The most severe symptoms occur when the virus is first acquired. These usually clear up spontaneously within three to six weeks. In the recurrent subsequent attacks which occur unpredictably, the symptoms are less severe and do not last as long.

For the specific manifestations that occur in the male and in the female, see the section on "Genital Herpes Simplex" in each of the chapters 23 and 24 of this volume. As noted there, the complications of this disease are more serious in the female than in the male.

What to Do

A person with this infection should report periodically to his physician for checkups.

LYMPHOGRANULOMA VENE-REUM (LYMPHOGRANULOMA INGUINALIS, CLIMATIC BUBO).

Venereal lymphogranuloma, which has at least a dozen other names, is an infectious virus disease, usually transmitted by sexual contact. A typical case begins as a papule or small ulcer somewhere on the external genital organs about two weeks after exposure. Next, the neighboring lymph nodes, usually in one or both groins in male patients but fairly often about the anus in females, become swollen and tender. The skin over these nodes turns purplish and then breaks down, forming persistent, tender ulcers into which more or less pus drains from the nodes beneath. During the period of swelling and ulceration there may be some fever and other general symptoms of an acute infection. The ulcers tend to heal, but very slowly and with much scarring. This scarring, especially in female patients, may cause a stricture of the anus or rectum, which is one of the most common and most troublesome of the late complications.

There is a rather simple test (the Frei test) by which the physician can know whether his patient has lymphogranuloma venereum. The test requires the injection of a small amount of test material into the patient's skin.

What to Do

1. As soon as venereal lymphogranuloma is suspected, consult a physician, preferably a skin specialist, to help find out the true nature of the disease. If needed, he can give or prescribe suitable sulfonamide and antibiotic remedies.

2. Choose foods that leave a small, or at least a smooth, residue after digestion.

3. Alternate hot and cold compresses over the swollen nodes in the groin will help to relieve pain and clear up the infection. (See volume 3, chapter 20, "Simple Home Treatments.")

SYPHILIS (LUES VENEREA, POX).

Syphilis is caused by a specific germ, *Treponema pallidum*. It is corkscrew-shaped and much larger than most bacteria. To contract syphilis, a person must get the germs from a living source, as a rule. They must enter the body through a break in the skin or mucous membrane, or be transmitted by a mother through the placenta to her unborn child. Syphilis contracted because of entrance of the germs into the body after birth is called acquired syphilis. Syphilis

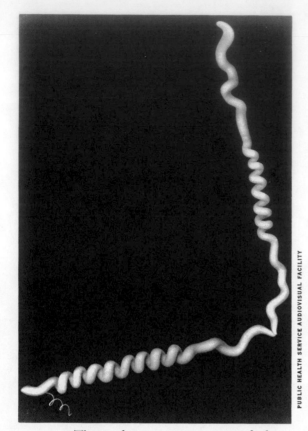

The corkscrew appearance of the syphilis germ (highly magnified).

transmitted before birth is called congenital syphilis.

Syphilis is usually contracted during sexual intercourse. Sometimes surgeons or dentists are infected through pricking or cutting their hands while operating on syphilitic patients. A few people are infected by using contaminated silverware, drinking glasses, or other utensils, but more by kissing people who have lesions of the disease in their mouths or on their lips. Even in such cases, the moist, living germs must enter through a break in the skin or penetrate a mucous membrane and get into the circulation before they can produce the disease. Drying kills syphilis germs very quickly. That is one reason why so few people get syphilis except by sexual intercourse.

The first sign of acquired syphilis is an ulcer called a chancre or Hunterian sore. The ulcer usually has well-defined edges and a small amount of slightly blood-tinged, watery discharge, but it is not painful. It may be easily seen, or entirely obscured by overlapping skin or mucous membrane. It appears from ten days to three or four weeks after exposure, and lasts from a few days to several weeks. It may disappear and soon be forgotten, but it usually leaves a scar. The chancre occurs most often on the mucous surfaces of the genital organs, but it may be on the skin. It may be in the mouth or on the lips. Women often contract syphilis without knowing it, because the chancre is likely to develop on the cervix or some other location within the vagina where it can be neither seen nor felt. This inability to detect early syphilis in a woman makes intercourse with prostitutes a frequent source of syphilitic infection.

From a few weeks to a few months after the appearance of the chancre, an eruption usually appears on the body. This may consist of only a few red, pimply blemishes, or it may be a profuse crop of various types of blotches. At this stage the germs are already widely distributed throughout the body. The infected person may have chills, fever, swollen lymph nodes, anemia, and pains in the bones and joints. The eruptive stage lasts for a few weeks, a few months, or, rarely, years. During this and a still later stage, very infectious lesions, known as mucous patches, are formed in the mouth and on other mucous surfaces of the body. From these, a considerable proportion of the new cases of syphilis are contracted.

The third stage of syphilis occurs generally from three to twenty years after the first lesion. Hard tumor masses called gummas appear in different parts of the body. These gummas may slough away and leave ulcers; they may form tumor masses in the abdomen, the lungs, the pelvis, or other parts of the body; and they may form in the bones and thus weaken

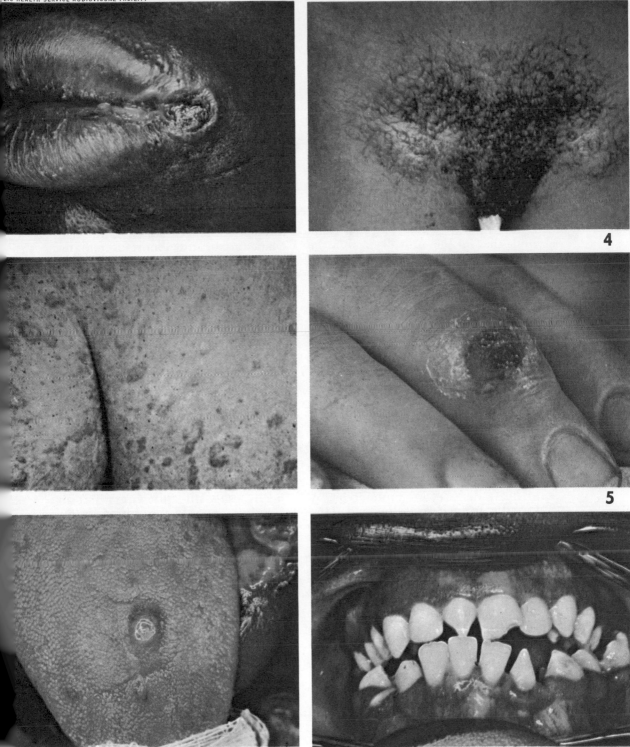

Manifestations, of syphilis as they appear on various parts of the body:
(1) chancre on the lip; (2) blotches on the skin; (3) chancre on the
tongue; (4) swollen lymph nodes of the groin; (5) chancre on finger; and
(6) notched, peg-shaped teeth (the latter a condition typical of syphilis
acquired prior to birth).

them, causing fractures. Large sores, difficult to heal, may develop on the skin and cover a large part of the body.

The most distressing features of syphilis come as late effects of the disease. A man, perhaps in the prime of life, begins to have abdominal pains which he cannot account for. These increase in severity, resembling a girdle-like constriction about his trunk. Excruciating pains shoot through his legs and body. He soon finds that he cannot walk well in the dark. He loses control of his legs. He cannot control the discharges from his bowels and bladder. He becomes a helpless invalid for the rest of his life because syphilis has wrecked his nervous system; yet he may live on for years in this pitiful state, for syphilis seldom kills quickly.

Tabes dorsalis, or locomotor ataxia, the terrible condition just described, is only one of many serious conditions or diseases caused by the germs of syphilis. Senile dementia or some cases of apoplexy, epilepsy, insanity, paralysis, and partial or complete blindness may have syphilis as their cause. Many of the rapidly fatal cases of heart disease are brought on by syphilis. In such cases, that part of the aorta near the heart is usually attacked first, and the aortic valve is so badly damaged that it cannot hold. The resultant excessive leakage throws such a heavy burden on the heart that it first enlarges greatly and finally fails completely.

Many inmates of mental institutions are there because of syphilis. The mental disease resulting from syphilis has various names, among which are general paresis, dementia paralytica, and general paralysis of the insane (GPI). While the victims of general paresis rarely suffer pain and often act as if they were "on top of the world," there is no cure for their condition; and they are a burden on public finances for the rest of their lives, which may drag on for many years.

The innocent children of syphilitic parents show some of the most pitiful effects of this disease. A large proportion of the babies born with syphilis die early, usually during their first year of life. A typical syphilitic baby has fissures about the angles of its mouth, a nasal discharge with "snuffles," a copper-brown-colored rash, and/or blisters on its buttocks and face. If it lives, it develops slowly, both physically and mentally, and is troubled with restlessness and disturbed sleep. Its bones grow in a characteristically abnormal manner, easily detectable by X ray. When the teeth come in, especially the permanent teeth, they are likely to be notched and peg-shaped. The eyes and ears may be diseased in various ways, with impairment or even loss of eyesight and hearing. Besides all this trouble, the unfortunate child has a strong chance of being an idiot or of being epileptic or neurotic in various ways; and he may later have any or all of the third-stage developments that characterize acquired syphilis.

Syphilis must be diagnosed and proper treatment begun early if grave aftereffects are to be avoided. Any ulcer or persistent sore on the genital organs, especially following illicit sex relations, should be immediately examined by a physician. No person should attempt to treat the sore himself; for improper treatment may so obscure the disease germ that the real condition cannot be reliably diagnosed, yet the disease will be permitted to go on and produce its terrible aftereffects.

When a doctor sees a sore which he suspects may be a chancre, he will probably make what is called a dark-field microscopic examination of scrapings or serum from the ulcer, or have such an examination made. This test offers about a fifty-fifty chance of discovering the germs if they are present. If they are found, treatment can begin at once. If not, a little later he will draw a specimen of blood for special tests which are much more likely than a dark-field examination to detect the true condition, though waiting for the results of such tests means unavoidable delay in starting treatment. These blood tests, of which there are several kinds, are applicable in all suspected cases of syphilis a few weeks after the initial infection—usually in time to make treatment fairly sure of success. Probably the best known of these blood tests is the Wassermann test.

Late syphilis is frequently detected by applying the Wassermann test or some equivalent test to fluid drawn from the spinal canal. When the disease has disappeared from all other tissues or fluids, the spinal fluid often gives evidence of its presence. The fluid must be drawn with great care by a physician and tested even more expertly than the blood is tested. While not all of the late ill effects of syphilis can be prevented if treatment is delayed until the central nervous system is invaded as shown by the spinal fluid test, modern treatment is so efficient that it can do a great deal of good if begun before actual symptoms of the third stage of syphilis have appeared. If begun during the first half of pregnancy, the treatment of an expectant mother who has syphilis may enable her to give birth to a baby who is free from the disease. If all such expectant mothers were thus treated, congenital syphilis could be practically wiped out, because a syphilitic child "catches" the disease from its mother and does not inherit it from its father.

Most people, at least most men, who have syphilis know they have been exposed; but many of them do not know they have the disease. An even larger number of women, especially married women, who have syphilis neither know they have it nor know that they have been exposed. The chancre is painless, and may develop in a place where it escapes notice. The skin eruptions and other signs and symptoms of the second stage may be so mild that they either go unnoticed or are mistaken for something of little importance. The interval between the second and third stages of the disease

may be very long. During this time the disease is called latent syphilis, and it shows no signs or symptoms of any kind; but a blood test taken during this period is likely to be positive. Treatment taken during this period will usually prevent the deplorable damage that comes with the third stage.

More than a few people scattered here and there have latent syphilis and do not know it, but its presence could usually be detected by a blood test, and its progression to the third stage could be checked. Knowledge of this fact has given rise to the almost universal practice of giving all expectant mothers blood tests fairly early in their pregnancy, so that if any of them happen to have latent syphilis its presence can be detected and they can be treated so as to prevent their passing the disease on to their unborn children. In many hospitals all patients admitted are given blood tests; and cases of latent syphilis are fairly often discovered in this way. In many communities blood-testing campaigns are carried on from time to time. Such practices, plus the vigorous case-finding programs of health departments, have greatly reduced the prevalence of syphilis; but much still remains to be done before the disease is stamped out.

What to Do

1. As soon as a suspicious sore or ulcer is discovered or there is any other reason to suspect a syphilitic infection, have a physician, preferably a urologist or a skin specialist, make such examinations and tests as are needed to determine the true condition.

2. Meanwhile, avoid sexual intercourse.

3. Remember that neither diet, hydrotherapy, nor any home treatment can cure syphilis; but there are remedies that can, and doctors can use them.

4. All effective remedies must be given or prescribed by a physician, but proper remedies correctly

given can come as near to curing syphilis in two weeks in our day as used to be possible in two years.

5. To help make medical treatments more effective, especially in cases of late syphilis, certain general health-building principles should receive attention. Some of these are:

A. Foods made largely from grains, fruits, nuts, and vegetables, together with milk and eggs in moderation, compose the best diet.

B. Alcohol, tobacco, stimulants, tea, coffee, and highly seasoned foods should be avoided.

C. The patient should drink water freely, especially between meals.

D. Plenty of sleep and a reasonable amount of outdoor exercise are important.

E. Frequent bathing is helpful. The practice of taking a hot bath for ten minutes before retiring, cooling the water to a little below body temperature at the end, and doing this at least two or three times a week, is recommended.

Allergy

It is not intended that this chapter will add significantly to our list of diseases. It is expected, rather, that it will improve the reader's understanding of the causes of some of the diseases described in other parts of the book.

In the broad sense, allergy is the body's response to the presence of some aggravating agent called an allergen. Individuals act differently in their responses to allergens; therefore some people are said to be more allergic than others.

It used to be assumed that all allergens were protein substances, and it was common to speak of "protein sensitivity," by which was meant that a given protein substance would cause certain tissues to react abnormally. It is now understood that some allergens are carbohydrates, and at least a few are chemically related to the fats. Regardless of their chemical nature, all allergens have one thing in common—they stimulate a sensitive individual to react by producing antibodies.

The mechanism by which tissues react unfavorably to the presence of an allergen is bound up with the body's intricate chemical processes, such as enzyme reactions, and is even related to the processes by which immunity is developed. Becoming immune to a certain germ whose products have served as an allergen is one form of allergic response. When the antibodies which a certain allergen produces are stationary within a group of the body's cells rather than being free in the bloodstream, then these cells in which the antibodies are located may be unfavorably affected when exposed to this specific allergen.

Kinds of Allergens

1. Some allergens enter the body by being inhaled. These include pollens; dusts; vapors, such as tobacco smoke; emanations from epithelium, such as dandruff, and strong odors, such as perfumes.

2. Certain foods provoke an allergic response in persons who may be sensitive. These include wheat, milk, chocolate, eggs, strawberries, nuts, pork, and fish.

3. Some persons become sensitive to drugs or biological agents. These, then, can serve as allergens.

4. Certain germs may function as allergens so that the symptoms produced when these germs invade a person's tissues are the indirect result of the allergic response and are not caused, primarily, by tissue injury through direct contact with the germs.

5. Some allergens cause the allergic response through a mere contact with the skin or the mucous membranes of a sensitive person. These include products from plants such as poison

oak and poison ivy, and certain dyes, metals, plastics, furs, leathers, rubber products, cosmetics, and chemicals such as insecticides.

6. Even physical agents such as heat, cold, light, and pressure occasionally awaken an allergic response. Many a sufferer from hay fever has noticed that he begins to sneeze when he steps into bright sunlight.

Preventing the Allergic Response

In general, the allergic response may be prevented or its symptoms modified in four ways.

A. *Avoiding the Allergen.* The simplest way to prevent the allergic response is to prevent the allergens to which a person is sensitive from entering his body. Sufferers from hay fever can often prevent their attacks by staying indoors during the time of year when the plants bloom that produce the pollens to which they are sensitive. If these plants are limited to a certain locality, the sufferers can avoid symptoms by staying away from this locality. Allergy to a drug can be avoided by not using the drug. Allergy to some specific food may be handled by excluding this food from the diet. Persons sensitive to a particular dust may benefit by wearing a filtering mask. Airconditioning systems with good filters often bring relief to victims of hay fever and asthma.

B. *Desensitization.* Just as it is possible to make a person immune to snake venom by injecting gradually increasing doses of this venom into his tissues, so it is possible to build up a person's tolerance to most allergens by a carefully controlled program of administering gradually increasing doses of this allergen. Physicians can obtain preparations of the usual allergens from medical supply houses and can inject these into a sensitive patient, beginning with very small doses and building up gradually week by week, until the patient's tolerance has improved to the point where he will no longer develop symptoms when exposed to the allergen. This method has proved quite successful in bringing relief to many patients suffering from hay fever and from the types of asthma which result in large part from allergy. It may be necessary to administer doses of these preparations at regular intervals the year round in order to maintain the individual's tolerance to the offending substance.

C. *The Use of Antihistamines.* In many cases of allergy, histamine is one of the chemicals which the body's tissues liberate in response to the presence of an allergen. An antihistamine drug, which counteracts histamine, may relieve the allergic response in such cases. There are many varieties of antihistamine drugs, and it happens that one kind will benefit some allergic persons and another kind, others. It may be necessary to use the trial-and-error method to determine which form of antihistamine will bring the greatest benefit in a particular case. Some hay fever sufferers derive such benefit from the use of antihistamines that they prefer using them to obtaining relief by the more time-consuming method desensitization.

Some hazard is involved in the use of antihistamine drugs, because in some cases these have the side effect of making a person stuporous. It is dangerous, therefore, for the person taking such drugs to drive a car lest his reactions have been slowed to the extent that his driving is unsafe.

D. *The Use of Hormones.* In cases of extremely serious allergic reactions, the appropriate use of steroid preparations derived from the cortex of the adrenal gland may provide some benefit. These powerful medicinal agents should be used only under the direct supervision of a physician.

HAY FEVER.

The symptoms of this illness depend typically upon an allergic response to an offending protein substance breathed in by way of the inspired air. The symptoms of this illness are de-

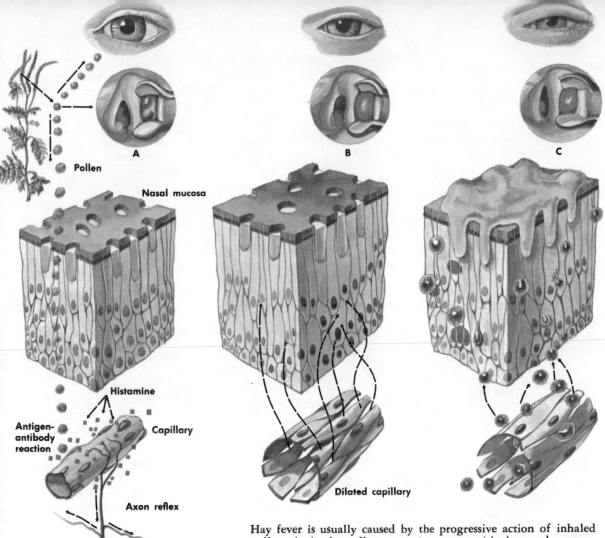

A   **B**   **C**

Pollen

Nasal mucosa

Histamine

Antigen-
antibody
reaction

Capillary

Axon reflex

Dilated capillary

Hay fever is usually caused by the progressive action of inhaled pollen: A. As the pollen comes in contact with the nasal mucosa, the antigen-antibody reaction ensues, with a release of histamine. B. Capillaries and venules dilate, eyes and nasal passages become red, followed by (C) swelling and exudation of serum.

scribed in chapter 16, "Diseases of the Ear, Nose, and Throat," in this volume.

ASTHMA.

At least half the cases of asthma seem to be caused or aggravated by allergy. Asthma as a disease is discussed in chapter 17, "Diseases of the Respiratory Organs," in this volume. Emergency treatment for an acute attack is described in volume 3, chapter 18, "Handling Emergencies."

HIVES (URTICARIA).

This skin manifestation is usually the result of an allergic response to some offending allergen. The condition is discussed in chapter 12, "Skin Diseases," in this volume.

ANGIONEUROTIC EDEMA.

This peculiar manifestation of the allergic response involves the skin in much the same manner as in hives except that here we have one or more large swollen skin areas. In some forms of the disease, this area of swelling may involve the lining of the larynx in such a way as to interfere with breathing and even endanger the victim's life. In other cases it is the face, hands, feet, and genitalia that become swollen. What to do for this condition is discussed in chapter 12, "Skin Diseases," in this volume.

SERUM SICKNESS.

Serum sickness is an allergic reaction triggered by the injection of a serum of animal origin (usually horse serum). Certain antitoxins, valuable in the treatment of specific infections, are contained in animal serum. This allergic reaction typically occurs in persons who have had a previous injection of this same kind of serum and have had time to become sensitive to it. It is because of the possibility of serum sickness that physicians prefer to use toxoid preparations, when available, rather than the antiserums.

Symptoms of serum sickness may develop as long as fourteen days after the injection. However, they may occur much more promptly in previously sensitized persons. The illness begins with a skin eruption which may appear like hives. There is fever, enlargement of the lymph nodes, pain in the joints, nausea, and abdominal pain.

Emergency treatment for serum sickness requires the use of carefully graduated small injections of a 1:1,000 solution of epinephrine. Usually the beginning injection consists of .5 ml. of this dilute solution. It is followed a few minutes later by an injection of 1 ml. Depending upon the patient's condition, the injection may need to be repeated two or three times at intervals of a few minutes.

DRUG ALLERGY.

An allergic reaction may occur in sensitive individuals after the taking of certain drugs. There are said to be more than one hundred drugs which at one time or another have provoked an allergic response in sensitive persons. Certain drugs are more common offenders than others, the notable ones among the modern drugs being some of the sulfonamides and penicillin.

The development of a skin rash is the usual manifestation of a drug allergy. Fever and symptoms of shock may occur in the more extreme cases. Discontinuance of the offending drug is the obvious method of treatment, the symptoms usually disappearing within a very few days after the drug is discontinued. This problem is also discussed in chapter 12, "Skin Diseases," under the heading of *Drug Rash*, in this volume.

Warm-Climate Ailments

Certain diseases—quite a large group—occur usually only in warm-climate areas. These are commonly called tropical diseases, the subject of the present chapter.

The prevalence of disease is greater, on the average, in warm climates than in temperate zones; for, in addition to the tropical diseases, the illnesses which occur in other parts of the world are present there too. This factor, plus several others, contributes to the higher incidence of disease in warm climates.

Hot weather is debilitating. Warmth favors the growth of germs. Insect and animal germ carriers abound, and many of them breed the year round. Sanitary facilities are often inadequate. Good personal health habits, sanitation, and the fight against germs and potential disease-carrying insects are important anywhere; but they are particularly important in regions with warm climates, even more so than elsewhere.

Two features of sanitation in warm climates need special emphasis, one having to do with water and the other with food. Many warm-climate areas have modern water systems, but even with them the danger of contamination is not always eliminated. For safety in places without fully adequate water sanitation, all drinking water should be boiled. After it is

boiled, it should be kept in a tightly covered container, and preferably drawn out by means of a faucet. The container and the faucet should frequently be cleaned, rinsed with clean water, and thoroughly scalded.

Only such fruits and vegetables should be eaten raw as can be thoroughly cleansed with a detergent solution and disinfected by chlorination or scalding, unless it is known beyond question that they have not come in contact with the soil or with contaminated hands or insects—points about which one can rarely be sure. Solutions of chloride of lime, or of such ordinary household bleaching agents as Clorox or Purex, may be used as disinfectants. Government or mission doctors or local public-health officials should be consulted as to the kind and strength of solution preferred in the locality concerned, and the recommended period of time for immersion in it.

The fruits and vegetables should first be cleansed in a detergent solution. In the case of lettuce, each leaf should be cleansed individually. Then after being rinsed with cooled, boiled water, they should be soaked in a solution of two tablespoons of Clorox to one gallon of boiled water for thirty minutes, then rinsed again with cooled, boiled water, and finally kept where they will not be exposed to in-

535

sects or handling until immediately before serving. It is recommended that the housewife handle such foods herself or else supervise their handling so carefully that they are sure not to become recontaminated after being disinfected; and it is better to limit the choice to such fruits and vegetables as have a firm peel or rind that can be removed after disinfection is complete.

Now we will consider the various warm-climate ailments.

AFRICAN SLEEPING SICKNESS (TRYPANOSOMIASIS).

There are several varieties of trypanosomes that may live in the human body, but African sleeping sickness is the most serious disease which they may cause. At times this disease has almost depopulated large areas in Africa.

The parasites causing African sleeping sickness are spindle-shaped, actively wriggling organisms of microscopic size, but much larger than a red blood cell. They can often be found in the blood, the cerebrospinal fluid, and certain tissues of the body, but they are most numerous in enlarged lymph nodes. They are transmitted by the bites of tsetse flies, which become infective within from eighteen to thirty-four days after taking an infective meal. Many species of wild or domestic animals can harbor the parasites, some species being made ill by them and some not. These animals form the usual reservoirs from which the organisms are transmitted to man, though it is quite possible for the organisms to be passed from man to man in the same way.

The fly bite produces some irritation, and within two days is marked by a red nodule surrounded by a white zone. In a typical case fever develops within two or three weeks, but its onset may be much longer delayed. It may continue in an irregular way for months or years, or it may be relapsing in character with considerable periods of quiescence. Headache,

neuralgic pains, insomnia, and loss of ability to concentrate are common, and the pulse is likely to be rapid. Pink or reddish patches may appear from time to time on the trunk and thighs and persist for a few days. The lymph nodes in any or all parts of the body may become enlarged, but those that are most commonly and noticeably so are on the sides of the neck below and behind the ears. This last is an important diagnostic sign.

Sometimes the disease runs an acute course. The brain becomes severely involved early; and the victim dies following convulsions, epileptiform seizures, and coma. In the usual case it progresses slowly. The victim becomes gradually more and more emaciated and mentally and physically feeble, but subject to tremors, especially of the tongue, fingers, and forearms.

Apparently, when the parasites have gained a firm foothold in the central nervous system, the peculiar lethargy that gives the common name to the disease comes on and increases gradually in severity until the victim becomes completely helpless. Prior to this stage the disease sometimes terminates of itself, and in other cases it has a fair chance of being cured. But when it really develops into sleeping sickness, the end is almost certainly fatal.

The best chance for a cure comes when specific treatment begins before central nervous system symptoms develop. When what seem to be possible early signs and symptoms of the disease are observed, therefore, trained medical aid should be sought without delay. Neither diet, home remedies, nor the best of personal hygiene can be trusted to overcome the infection.

The fight against African sleeping sickness, however, resolves itself largely into a fight against the tsetse fly. Government authorities in practically all areas known to be infested by these insects have much information about their habits and habitat, and frequently have campaigns under way to keep them under control. A person going to such regions should take care to become acquainted with these authorities and their plans for tsetse-fly control and cooperate with them in every possible way.

What to Do

1. Consult a physician as soon as the first suspicious signs or symptoms of trypanosomiasis are observed. If he finds evidence that the organisms are present in the body, he can give injections of suramin sodium (Antrypol) for the gambiense type of the disease, or tryparsamide or Melarsen for the rhodesiense type.

2. Have the physician search for and try to clear up any additional infections that may be present and be complicating the case.

3. Unless the lethargic stage of the disease has already set in, try to keep the victim's general health built up by means of plenty of rest, cleanliness, and a liberal diet.

4. In any case, after apparent cure, keep the victim under a physician's supervision for at least two years, if possible. There may be a relapse.

5. As preventive measures:

A. Try to avoid the bites of tsetse flies.

B. Try to prevent infected persons from being bitten by them.

C. Promote all practical measures for the fly's extermination.

D. If possible, move to some area not infested by them.

E. If compelled to live in an infested area, consult a physician about the advisability of periodic injections of Naphuride, et cetera.

AMERICAN TRYPANOSOMIASIS.

(See *Chagas' Disease* in this chapter.)

ANCYLOSTOMIASIS.

(See *Hookworm Infection* in chapter 21.)

BARTONELLOSIS (OROYA FEVER).

Bartonellosis is limited to that part of South America between latitudes 2 degrees north and 13 degrees south, and occurs chiefly in certain valleys on the western slopes of the Andes. It is caused by a very small germ that attacks the red blood cells and delicate structures within many of the body's organs. The disease is transmitted by the bites of infected sand flies.

The disease begins with lassitude and an irregular fever that seldom rises very high. Headache commonly occurs, along with pain and tenderness of the bones and joints. The liver and spleen are likely to be swollen and tender. A severe anemia develops rapidly. Between 20 and 40 percent of the untreated victims die.

A milder and more chronic form of the infection is characterized by nodules under the skin and a skin eruption. The nodules and some of the eruptive spots tend to ulcerate and bleed easily. This mild form of the disease is called verruga peruana, and it is seldom fatal.

What to Do

1. Do not attempt home treatments. They will not cure.

2. Consult a physician if possible. He can give or prescribe penicillin, chloramphenicol, streptomycin, or tetracycline antibiotics, all of which have proved reasonably effective. He may also prescribe symptomatic remedies or treatments and give attention to the anemia that may be present.

BLACKWATER FEVER.

Blackwater fever is a serious complication of malaria. It occurs almost exclusively in falciparum malaria, which is by far the most serious type of the disease. It is called blackwater fever because dark-colored urine is a prominent sign of this complication. It is characterized by severe blood damage, and large amounts of albumin and hemoglobin are lost through the kidneys. It is the decomposed hemoglobin that gives the dark color to the urine.

The onset of blackwater fever is usually sudden, with a chill, prostration, fever, and pain in the regions of the kidneys and bladder. Nausea and vomiting are often troublesome and persistent. The skin takes on a yellow tint. The urine, which becomes progressively darker in color, may be passed in increasingly scanty amounts, and in some cases urination becomes completely suppressed. It is of little use to list more symptoms here, however, because in the course of a severe attack of blackwater fever a great variety of alarming and dangerous symptoms may develop; and cases differ widely. The disease does not develop except in people who have, or have had, malaria; and the characteristic symptoms and signs already listed are enough to make the diagnosis easy. At least a quarter of the victims of this disease die of it. A first attack predisposes to another and more severe attack. Very few individuals survive a third attack. For additional information on malaria, see under *Malaria* later in this chapter.

What to Do

1. Keep the victim in bed, lying down.

2. A physician should attend the victim, because blood transfusions and various other supportive therapy that can be given only by a physician may be needed to save life. There is no specific remedy.

3. If the victim's stomach will retain food, give him a bland, liquid or soft diet, avoiding any foods hard for him to digest.

4. Urge him to drink water freely if he can retain it.

5. Fomentations applied to the upper abdomen every three hours may help control the nausea. (See volume 3, chapter 20, "Simple Home Treatments.")

6. Avoid moving the victim while he is ill, but when he becomes better he should go to a nonmalarial region and stay there.

BLINDING DISEASE.
(See *Filariasis: C. Onchocerciasis* in this chapter.)

BREAKBONE FEVER.
(See *Dengue* in this chapter.)

BLOOD FLUKES.
(See *Fluke Infestations: A. Blood Flukes* in this chapter.)

CALABAR SWELLING.
(See *Filariasis: B. Loiasis* in this chapter.)

CHAGAS' DISEASE (AMERICAN TRYPANOSOMIASIS).
Chagas' disease is caused by Trypanosoma cruzi, a blood-dwelling parasite found chiefly in the south central and southeastern parts of the United States, in Mexico, and in Central and South America. The organism resembles that which causes African sleeping sickness. It is transmitted by assassin bugs, or kissing bugs, which usually attack the face and are night biters. The organisms are not directly transmitted by the bites, however, but are excreted in the bug's feces which are passed at the time of the bite, and then rubbed or scratched into the itching bite wound. Armadillos, opossums, and several species of rodents are known to be or suspected of being animal reservoirs of infection, so that transmission may be either from animal to man or from man to man via the bugs.

The disease is much more severe in children than in adults. A continuously high fever is a common feature. Edema of one side of the face and inflammation of the corresponding eye is a characteristic sign. Additional signs and symptoms may be swelling of local lymph nodes, enlarged liver and spleen, nervous and mental disturbances, convulsions, rapid pulse, and enlargement and irregular beat-

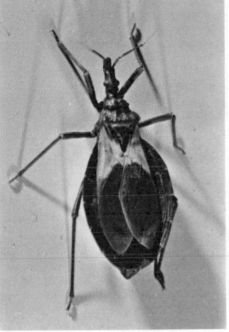

PUBLIC HEALTH SERVICE AUDIOVISUAL FACILITY

Kissing bug, vector of the parasite involved in Chagas' disease.

ing of the heart. The acute symptoms do not persist very long, but they fairly often bring death to young children. A chronic infection may show very few outward signs. Enlargement of the thyroid, baldness, mental dullness, and nervous disorders are fairly often noticeable; but heart damage is the most prominent feature in adults.

What to Do

1. Try to make the victim as comfortable as possible and conserve his strength. No specific remedy has yet been discovered.

2. Prevention is obviously important. There are three points to pay attention to: (1) Avoid sleeping in houses that afford harborage for the bugs. Cracks in the plaster are the usual hideouts for kissing bugs. (2) Sleep under a good bed net. (3) Try to exterminate the animals that may carry the infective organisms. No practical method of direct extermination of the bugs has yet been devised.

CHOLERA.

Cholera is caused by specific germs taken into the body by way of the mouth. If this fact is understood, a person can live in a community where cholera is raging, yet avoid contracting the disease. The bowel discharges of people sick with cholera are teeming with cholera germs. If these bowel discharges are thrown out without having first been boiled or otherwise thoroughly disinfected, or if they are used as fertilizer, the wells, ponds, and streams in the vicinity become contaminated. Flies, ants, cockroaches, and mice are all carriers of cholera germs. They feed on the bowel discharges, along with other filth, and carry the germs on their feet and in the discharges from their intestines. In this way they contaminate any foodstuffs to which they gain access. It is contaminated food and water, therefore, that must be guarded against if cholera is to be avoided. There are no other important sources of infection.

Whenever there is any known or suspected danger of contracting cholera, everybody concerned should make it an inflexible rule to boil all water before drinking it. Milk should also be boiled. All dishes and cooking utensils should be thoroughly scalded with boiling hot water every time *before* they are used. As described in the opening paragraphs of this chapter, vegetables and fruits to be eaten raw should first be washed and disinfected. The hands should always be thoroughly washed with soap and warm water before handling food. These precautions apply at all seasons and everywhere in what is known to be "cholera country," even though no cases are known to exist in the immediate vicinity at the time.

When cholera is actually present in a community, additional care needs to be taken. No cold cooked foods should be eaten. Any item of food to be peeled and eaten raw should be treated as described for raw vegetables and then peeled with a sterilized knife shortly before being served. Take additional care to keep all foodstuffs where they cannot come in contact with flies, cockroaches, or other insects, or with rats. Take a course of cholera vaccine, even though you have previously taken such a course. The vaccine has considerable preventive value if taken often enough.

The incubation period of cholera varies from a few hours to four or five days. The onset is usually sudden, with severe cramps in the back or limbs. It may begin with diarrhea and colicky pains. Shortly after the onset the stools become thin and contain small, white, curdlike masses. These are the "rice-water" stools. Generally there is severe vomiting also at the onset. So much fluid is lost in the vomitus, and especially in the stools, that the victim suffers extreme thirst, his urine diminishes, his skin dries, and his face has a pinched appearance. His skin feels cold, and his lips, face, and fingernails become bluish. What has just been described is a severe case; but in every epidemic there are many cases that run a comparatively light course and, except for the diarrhea, exhibit few symptoms.

The chief principles in treatment are to relieve the distressing symptoms and to compensate for the extremely rapid loss of body fluids with the sodium and potassium salts which they contain. It is especially important to give enough fluid to maintain kidney activity, for cessation of kidney function brings grave consequences. If the body can be supplied with sufficient fluid and essential minerals for a few days, its defense forces have a good chance to overcome the cholera germs, and recovery is quite likely; but about half of the untreated cases end fatally within from three to five days.

What to Do

1. Have a physician in attendance as early as possible. The prompt giving of large amounts of salt solution by vein and of other special preparations either by vein or by mouth often improves the patient's condition dramatically. The physician may also give streptomycin or soluble sulfas, plus plasma or other remedies.

2. Read carefully "Home Care for Contagious Diseases" in the first part of chapter 28 in this volume and follow the instruction as far as possible.

3. Keep the patient in bed.

4. Until a physician is in attendance, give the patient all the water he can hold without vomiting.

5. Do not allow the patient to become chilled. If necessary, apply a hot-water bottle to his feet and another to his spine.

6. Apply hot fomentations to the abdomen every three hours. (See volume 3, chapter 20, "Simple Home Treatments.")

7. Give no solid food during the acute stage. Strained vegetable broths and strained cereal gruels may be given in as large amounts as the patient can take.

8. Protect others from infection:

A. Boil or otherwise disinfect all bowel discharges from the cholera patient.

B. Do not handle contaminated clothing or bedding until it has been disinfected.

C. Protect all foods and beverages from flies and other insects.

D. Urge every exposed person to take a course of cholera vaccine.

DENGUE (BREAKBONE FEVER).

This epidemic virus disease is usually transmitted by the Aedes aegypti mosquito, but sometimes by other species. It is as yet uncommon in most parts of the United States, but airplane travel to and from foreign countries bids fair to bring about an increase.

The symptoms appear about four to ten days after the bite of the mosquito. The onset is abrupt, the fever rising rapidly, and in severe cases as high as 106° F. (41.2° C.). The face becomes

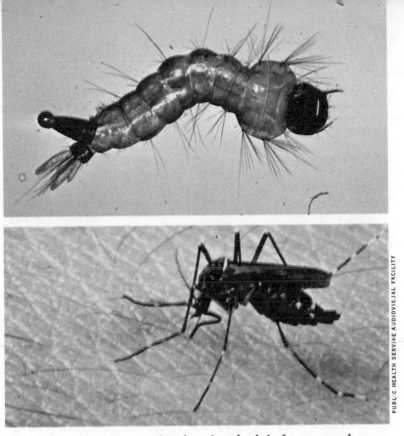

The Aedes aegypti mosquito, larval and adult forms, usual transmitter of dengue (breakbone fever).

congested, and there may be marked soreness in the eyeballs. The throat is sore, and there are pains in the head, lower back, and joints. The victim is usually nervous and depressed, and sleep is often disturbed. Prostration may be great. In spite of the fever, the pulse tends to be relatively slow and the blood pressure low.

About the third or fourth day the temperature drops to normal, and the victim feels much better physically and recovers from his mental depression. In typical cases after one to three days the temperature again rises, and the pains and mental depression reappear. The second wave of illness is shorter than the first. During this period an eruption appears on the hands and feet and then spreads to the arms, legs, and body. The rash may resemble that of measles or scarlet fever, or may be like neither. It soon fades. Convalescence is usually slow, but the disease is self-limited, and the acute symptoms do not last long.

Dengue can be prevented by the destruction of mosquitoes or by protecting people from their bites. Good nursing is the most important part of the treatment. There is no known specific remedy. Deaths from the disease are almost unknown, although it causes a great deal of distress to those who have it.

What to Do

1. Keep the victim in bed, and give him plenty of water to drink.

2. If his fever goes as high as 104° F. (40° C.), reduce it by means of cool enemas, tepid sponges, or alcohol sponges.

3. Hot fomentations over painful areas may give relief. (See volume 3, chapter 20, "Simple Home Treatments.")

4. An ice bag to the head may help to relieve headache.

5. A physician may order remedies for the relief of pain.

6. Convalescence may be has-

541

tened by giving cold mitten frictions daily after the acute symptoms are past. (See volume 3, chapter 20.)

DRACUNCULOSIS (DRACONTIASIS, GUINEA WORM).

Embryo Guinea worms, barely large enough to be visible to the unaided eye, are discharged into water in large numbers by the mature female parasites. This most frequently happens when infected persons are wading or immersed in water. An embryo must enter the body of a member of some suitable species of copepod (tiny, water-dwelling crustacean) for a period of preliminary development. The usual way by which the partly developed embryo enters the human body is by way of drinking water containing the infected copepods. In the tissues it grows to maturity, at which time the female is a smooth, slender, white worm about a yard long, lying in an irregularly coiled position in the connective tissues beneath the skin. It is believed that the development in the tissues takes from several months to a year.

As maturity approaches, the worm migrates to those parts of the body most frequently in contact with water, usually the legs and feet. At maturity the head end of the worm approaches the skin surface and excretes an irritating and toxic substance which causes a blister to form. When this blister ruptures, a slightly raw area with a small opening in its center is seen. Whenever cool or cold water comes in contact with this area, the worm discharges a milky cloud of coiled embryos through this opening, out of which the worm's head may protrude slightly, especially when most of the embryos have been discharged.

Previous to the time when the Guinea worm approaches the skin surface and prepares to discharge embryos, it causes few or no symptoms in the infected person. The most marked symptoms are associated with the blister formation. They usually consist of itching, vomiting, diarrhea, dizziness,

and difficulty in breathing. Secondary infection of the ulcerated area is very common, and may cause troublesome sores and extensive abscess formation.

If the worm should be killed, broken, or lacerated while lying in the tissues, especially if this should happen while its body still contains numerous embryos, the affected body part becomes extremely painful, inflamed, and swollen; and abscesses, sloughing of the tissues, arthritis, tendon contractions, stiffening of neighboring joints, and various other dangerous or distressing symptoms are likely to develop. When the worm's body has become empty of embryos, it becomes less tanacious, and causes less trouble if it should happen to be broken or lacerated in the process of extraction.

What to Do

1. When a typical blister is discovered, the opening of the blister and the discharge of the embryos can be hastened by continuous wet dressings or frequent douchings of the area with cool water.

2. When the discharge of embryos seems to be complete or nearly so, and the worm's head has protruded sufficiently, tie a silk thread to it and, by winding it around a small stick, apply very slow and gentle traction to it and try to pull the worm out of its sheath, taking care not to break the worm and leave part of it in the tissues. Extraction may take as long as two weeks.

3. A physician may be able to loosen the worm and hasten its extraction by means of injections of an olive-oil emulsion of phenothiazine, or he may be able to remove the worm surgically. He may also give or prescribe antibiotics to help control secondary infections.

4. There are three useful preventive measures:

A. Promote all practicable measures to free domestic water

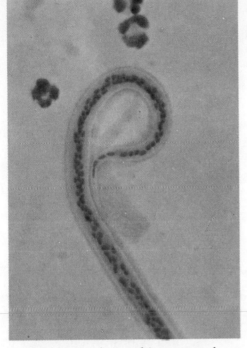

Wuchereria bancrofti, a parasite responsible for elephantiasis.

supplies from the copepods which harbor the embryo parasites.

B. Promote all practicable measures to keep infected people from contaminating water supplies.

C. Boil all drinking water that is not known to be safe.

DUMDUM FEVER.
(See *Leishmaniasis: B. Kala Azar* in this chapter.)

ELEPHANTIASIS.
(See *Filariasis: A. Elephantiasis* in this chapter.)

ESPUNDIA.
(See *Leishmaniasis: A. Espundia* in this chapter.)

FILARIASIS.
Four of the six well-known species of filarial parasites produce definite disease in humans. Two of them—Loa loa and Onchocerca volvulus—are discussed separately below. The other two—Wuchereria bancrofti and Wuchereria malayi—are responsible for elephantiasis. (See A. Elephantiasis in this section.)

All of them are small, extremely slender worms, most of the adults varying between one and three inches (2.5 and 7.5 cm.) in length, though adult females of one species sometimes reach a length of 20 inches (50 cm.). There are few tropical or subtropical countries in which filarial worms are not found, and in some places more than half of the population harbor them.

The mature Wuchereria worms may live in the body for many years, and throughout their adult lives the females may continue to discharge large numbers of embryos, called microfilariae. A perculiarity often found is that the embryos abound in the circulating blood during the night, being most abundant between midnight and morning, but are scarce in the daytime. Sometimes, however, this periodicity is reversed; and there seem to be some localities where there is no definite periodicity.

The night-swarming microfilariae are taken into the bodies of mosquitoes which bite infected persons. In the mosquitoes' bodies the embryos undergo partial development. When the mosquito host infected with the partly developed forms bites a person, some of these parasites escape into the victim's skin. Within this victim's body they gradually grow to maturity and begin the production of new multitudes of microfilariae. Microfilariae that swarm in the daytime depend on bloodsucking flies for their transmission in much the same way that the night-swarming ones do on mosquitoes.

There are three obvious parts of the program of preventing infections with filariae: (1) guarding healthy people against the bites of infected insects, (2) keeping infected people from being bitten by insects, and (3) extermination of the insects themselves. Success in carrying out this program has proved so difficult in some localities that it is advisable not to stay in them if it is possible to live elsewhere. The program has been

543

somewhat facilitated recently by the discovery that administration of diethylcarbamazine (Hetrazan) will cause a marked reduction of microfilariae in the blood, hence reducing the danger of transmission by blood-sucking insects.

Oddly, the presence of millions of microfilariae in the blood causes no distress. It is the adult worms that cause symptoms and diseases, many of them brought on by irritation or obstruction of the lymph vessels by the parasites, and others resulting from local damage or irritation in other tissues or structures.

When the lymph vessels become so irritated that inflammation sets in, the condition is called lymphangitis, a name which is also used to denote lymph-vessel inflammation from other causes. This condition often brings about the death of the worms that caused it. Filarial lymphangitis, therefore, though a distressing condition while it lasts, has a chance of put-

Enormous swelling of the legs commonly characterizes elephantiasis.

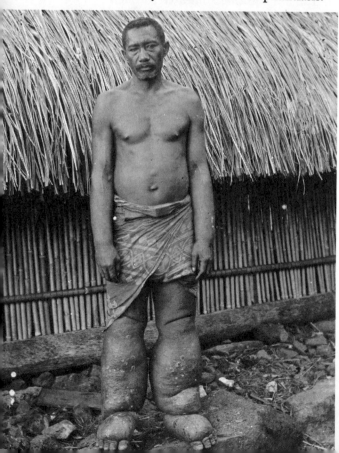

ting an end to the infection, which is not true of most other conditions caused by these parasites.

The commonest and most extensive site of lymph-vessel obstruction and consequent dilation or varicosity is in the abdomen. It may involve the thoracic duct, which is the largest lymph channel and empties lymph into the bloodstream in one of the large veins at the base of the neck, and which in connection with this function carries fat in an emulsified form from the digestive organs to the blood. The emulsified fat is what gives the milky appearance to the contents of the lymph vessels of the abdomen during the digestion and absorption of fats, and these milky-appearing contents are called chyle. When the thoracic duct is obstructed so that it cannot carry the chyle to the bloodstream in the normal way, it travels by other channels, sometimes seeping through the damaged walls of lymph vessels. This may result in chylous ascites (a collection of chyle in the abdominal cavity), chylous diarrhea, and chyluria (a mixture of chyle with the urine). Other complications that sometimes develop include inflammation of the lymph nodes (lymphadenitis), of the testis (orchitis), of the spermatic cord (funiculitis), and of the epididymis (epididymitis). Enlargement of the scrotum due to the accumulation of fluid (hydrocele) may also occur.

Elephantiasis is a late complication of filariasis. Afflicted individuals usually have a history of long residence in a filarial area, where they have been exposed to the bites of infected mosquitoes. Loiasis and onchocerciasis are filarial diseases transmitted by flies rather than by mosquitoes. Each of these disease entities calls for a more extended discussion, which will appear in its order on the following pages.

A. *Elephantiasis.* Elephantiasis is the name given to a firm, somewhat rubbery, slowly developing swelling of various parts of the body. The legs are most often affected. Other parts of the body often affected are the feet, the arms, the scrotum, the breasts, and the vulva. The enlargement is caused by chronic obstruction of lymph drainage. Examination of the tissues by operation shows that the deeper layers of the skin, together with the underlying connective tissues, are enormously thickened and changed into a blubbery mass which oozes lymph freely when punctured or cut.

The chief drawbacks in elephantiasis are the awkwardness and repulsive appearance caused by the swellings. These are, in some cases, so extensive as to make it impossible for the victim to work or even to move about much without help. There is no known cure for elephantiasis. There would be more hope of finding one sometime if the lymph-vessel obstruction were always caused by living worms which could move about; but in many cases it is caused by the dead and calcified bodies of these parasites which perpetuate the obstruction to lymph flow, no matter what medication or local treatment is used. These facts make preventive measures all the more important.

It is chiefly during the period when the microfilariae are developing into mature worms in the lymphatics that the acute symptoms preceding the appearance of elephantiasis occur. These may be fever, inflammation of the lymph vessels, enlargement of the lymph nodes, abscess formation, tissue destruction, scarring, and most of the other inflammatory or irritative conditions named in the next to the last paragraph of the above general discussion on *Filariasis*. It is during this period that courses of treatment with diethylcarbamazine (Hetrazan) do the most good.

What to Do

1. If the development of elephantiasis is discovered early enough, while many of the causative parasites are still living in the tissues, it is wise to have a physician give a series of treatments with diethylcarbamazine (Hetrazan). The series may extend over a period as long as two years. The treatments will kill most of the filariae in circulation at the time and make the final outcome less serious.

2. In the early stages of the swelling of a limb, it will be found that elevation of the limb, the wearing of elastic bandages, and alternate hot and cold applications two or three times daily will prove helpful. (See volume 3, chapter 20, "Simple Home Treatments.")

3. Surgical removal of the thickened subcutaneous tissue has, in some cases, restored a leg to a more normal appearance and to a degree of usefulness.

B. *Loiasis (Calabar Swelling).* The mature form of Loa loa does not live in the lymph vessels, but migrates about in the body, chiefly in the connective tissues. The immature ones are transmitted by the bites of tabanid flies.

While the migration may cause itching, pricking, or creeping sensations, and temporary swellings or puffiness, Calabar swellings, in various parts of the body, it is strange that more distress does not result, since there is good evidence that the parasite can travel through the tissues as fast as half an inch (1.25 cm.) a minute. In a few parts of the body considerable pain and swelling are caused by its presence. One of these is beneath the conjunctiva covering the eyeball; and, rather oddly, this seems to be one of its favorite haunts. The death of the worm in the tissues may result in an abscess.

What to Do

1. Cold compresses may reduce discomfort in the swellings.

2. A physician may be able to remove the parasite if it is detected migrating near the surface of the body. He may also use diethylcarbamazine (Hetrazan) in some stages or forms of the infection.

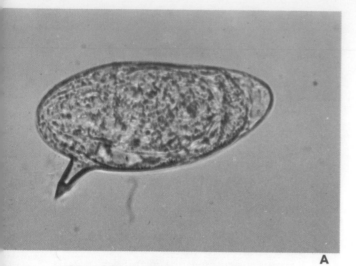

A

One of the parasites responsible for bilharziasis: A. egg; B. young; and C. adult form.

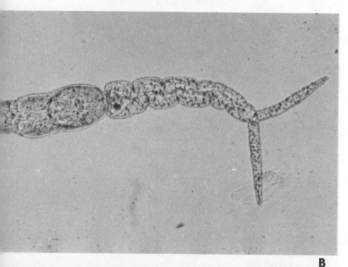

B

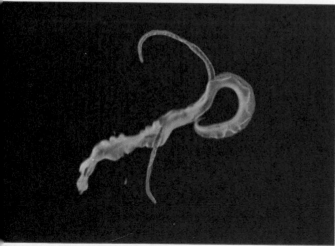

C

C. Onchocerciasis (Blinding Disease). Onchocerciasis is caused by a filarial parasite called Onchocerca volvulvus, the immature parasite being transmitted by bites of the black fly or buffalo gnat. As a rule, the presence of the mature parasites in the tissues causes itching, and later local inflammation, with the formation of slowly growing nodules surrounding the parasites beneath the skin. These nodules are firm to the touch and swarm with microfilariae, which do not circulate in the blood. They sometimes cause pain, but usually only itching. They occur chiefly on those parts of the body where bone tissue closely underlies the skin. In the course of time, various structures in the eyes may be attacked, and blindness be the result. This is not likely to occur, however, until the infection has persisted for several years.

What to Do

There is no very effective remedy, but a physician can give a series of treatments with diethylcarbamazine (Hetrazan), which is the best remedy now known. Tumors near the skin surface may be surgically excised. This should be done, if possible, especially in the case of any tumors that may be near the eyes.

FLUKE INFESTATION (TREMATODIASIS).

Several kinds of flukes (trematodes) are parasitic in man and animals, infestation resulting from the ingestion of uncooked or insufficiently cooked fish, crustaceans, and vegetation which are the intermediate hosts of the trematodes. Four common human infestations are discussed in the following paragraphs.

A. Blood Flukes (Schistosomiasis, Bilharziasis). Schistosomiasis occurs in many tropical or subtropical regions. It may be caused by any one of three somewhat similar parasites, the adult forms of which look like small, slender worms. If body discharges containing the eggs of these parasites find their way into water, the eggs hatch and the tiny young parasites swim about until they find a suitable snail to harbor them. In the snail's body they undergo further development, and then they once more escape into the water, where they await an opportunity to come in contact with, and penetrate the skin of, some human or other warm-blooded animal. Their penetration in considerable numbers may set up an irritation that is sometimes called "swimmer's itch." They might, of course, enter their victim's body if he should happen to drink water containing them.

Having entered the body, the parasites travel by way of the blood or lymph channels, seeming to prefer the small veins of the bladder, the liver, or the mesentery of the intestines as a place in which to congregate. In these veins the eggs are laid. The eggs produce a lytic enzyme which enables many of them to work through the walls of these veins into the lumen of the bladder or the intestine, from which they are expelled in the urine or the feces. They can sometimes be found in these discharges.

Depending on the type of parasite, the infection may give rise to bladder irritation and inflammation with blood in the urine; to irritation or ulceration and swelling of the intestines, chiefly the sigmoid and the rectum, with occasional diarrhea and mucus and blood in the stools; or to involvement chiefly of the small intestine with enlargement of the liver and the spleen and a collection of fluid in the abdominal cavity in the later stages.

Those cases characterized by blood in the urine may not have much pain, but they tend to be extremely chronic and to lead to general debility and the formation of bladder stones. Diagnosis is easy, because the urine contains multitudes of the characteristically shaped eggs of the parasite Schistosoma haematobium.

The intestinal form is characterized by more noticeable illness with frequent dysenterylike symptoms, growths resembling hemorrhoids, spells of fever, abdominal pain, loss of appetite, chills, cough, and enlargement of the liver and spleen. The hemorrhoidlike growths sometimes demand surgery. The dysenteric stools abound with the eggs of the parasites. In the late stages of the disease blood vessels may become clogged with eggs, and collections of eggs in other parts of the body may cause firm swellings, pneumonia, or large abdominal tumors.

Infections that chiefly affect the liver and spleen lead to great enlargement of these organs, irregular fever, loss of weight, pallor, vomiting, diarrhea, and fluid distension of the abdomen; but the course of the disease may extend to twenty years or more. Surgical removal of the spleen is sometimes beneficial. Eggs are found in the stools, but are seldom abundant.

The intestines, liver, and spleen are the chief points of attack of Schistosoma mansoni and Schistosoma japonicum, the latter organism being spread largely as a result of the wet cultivation of rice as practiced so largely in Japan and other Oriental lands.

What to Do

1. If any form of schistosomiasis is suspected, have a physician determine the true nature of the case. If this condition is found, he may give injections of some suitable antimony compound, which is likely to be effective *if the case is treated early*.

2. If the case is advanced, he may use the same remedy, but may need to do major surgery as well. Other treatment must by symptomatic only.

3. The general health needs to be conserved by means of abundant rest and a well-balanced, easily digestible diet.

4. As preventive measures:

547

A. Avoid bathing or wading in, or otherwise coming in contact with, the water of rivers, canals, ponds, or rice fields in regions in which the parasites may be found.

B. Boil all questionable drinking water.

C. Make sure of sanitary disposal of human excreta.

B. *Liver Flukes (Clonorchiasis)*. In some parts of the tropical or subtropical world, particularly where raw fish forms a part of the diet, as many as half of the population may be infested with liver flukes; but only a few of the victims may be made noticeably ill thereby. In light infestations, mild indigestion may be the only symptom. In severe cases, an enlarged liver, edema, and recurring attacks of jaundice are typical. Mild cases of "liver trouble," with diarrhea, if patients come from fluke-infested regions, should lead to a suspicion of clonorchiasis. The finding of the flukes' eggs in the patient's stools provides evidence of the presence of the infestation.

Adult liver flukes are oblong and flat, averaging about half an inch in length and about a quarter as broad. In the human victim they abound in the small bile ducts of the liver. The eggs pass out with the bile into the intestine. They do not hatch unless they find their way into water, and usually not until they are swallowed by some fresh-water snail, in whose body the first stage of development occurs. The next stage takes place in the body of some fish that has eaten the snail. Carp seem to be especially susceptible. Humans or lower animals become infested by eating raw or insufficiently cooked fish. Once started, the infestation may persist for several years, even though no new parasites enter the victim's body.

The presence of a few flukes may produce no symptoms, and even heavy infestations are not likely to be directly fatal, though they may seriously reduce the victim's resistance to other diseases.

What to Do

1. Gentian violet in enteric-coated tablets may do some good. The adult dose is 1 grain (60 mg.) three times a day, and treatment should continue for two weeks. Sodium antimony tartrate and chloroquine have proved to be of some value, but they must be given or prescribed by a physician.

2. Have the victim move to some noninfested region, if possible, and try to build up his general health by means of a nourishing and well-balanced diet, *not including raw fish*.

3. There are two useful preventive measures:

A. Avoid eating raw or insufficiently cooked fish.

B. Make sure of the sanitary disposal of bowel discharges.

C. *Liver Rot (Fascioliasis)*. Most commonly a disease of sheep, fascioliasis may also affect mankind. It is caused by Fasciola hepatica, a comparatively large liver fluke. The eggs of this fluke pass out of the body in the feces, pass their first stage of development in the bodies of snails, and then attach themselves in the form of cysts to certain water plants, usually watercress, or other green vegetation. If the cysts happen to be swallowed by sheep or by humans, they become active, penetrate the wall of the intestine, grow to maturity in the bile ducts, and produce more or less liver damage.

Fascioliasis may cause vomiting, joint pains, abdominal pain, jaundice, itching, diarrhea, and an irregular fever; but it is seldom fatal. Diagnosis is made by finding the eggs in the stools.

What to Do

1. If the disease is suspected, have a physician arrange for a stool examination to detect the presence of the eggs. Meanwhile, keep the victim in bed.

548

2. If the disease is found, the physician can give injections of emetine hydrochloride, the most effective remedy now known.

3. Preventive measures include:

A. Avoid eating uncooked plants to which the cysts might be attached.

B. Avoid eating sheep liver that is insufficiently cooked.

D. *Lung Flukes (Paragonimiasis, Endemic Hemoptysis).* Lung flukes are found in many parts of the Far East. The mature forms may reach a length of a bit less than an inch (about 2 cm.), and they are about half as wide as they are long. They may infect several species of domestic and wild animals as well as humans, and they may be found in several different parts of the body, but their characteristic habitat is the human lung. The victim's sputum contains numerous eggs. These must find their way into water, or at least into the body of a fresh-water snail, in order to begin their development. The second stage of development takes place in the body of a fresh-water crab or crayfish, and results in the formation of a small, quiescent mass called a cyst. When a living cyst is swallowed, it begins its development into the mature form in the intestine. Later it penetrates the intestinal wall and the diaphragm and migrates to the lung.

A typical case of the disease comes on gradually, and it does not make its victim feel noticeably ill. There is a chronic cough and vague distress in the chest and an abundant, sticky, reddish-brown sputum, which, on microscopic examination, is found to contain many red blood cells and the eggs of the parasite. The victim occasionally spits blood, and he may become very anemic. Observation of the typical sputum and finding the characteristic eggs in it make detection of the disease easy; but its cure is difficult or impossible because no means of expelling the parasites from the lungs has yet been discovered. Further-

more, other parts of the body may be invaded, especially the abdominal organs, the spinal cord, and the brain; and the parasites cannot be expelled from these places either. Even a moderate infection may persist for several years; and heavy infections may prove fatal, especially if the brain becomes involved.

Obviously, prevention is of prime importance. This should not be difficult to ensure if people would simply refrain from eating the raw or insufficiently cooked flesh of fresh-water crabs or crayfish.

What to Do

1. Do not try any cough remedy or other home treatment.

2. Consult a physician as soon as possible. He may use emetine hydrochloride, chloroquine, or some other remedy with benefit if the disease is still in its early stage. Later, they may be useless.

3. As further preventive measures:

A. Burn the infected person's sputum or treat it with a very strong disinfectant.

B. Boil all water used for domestic purposes unless it is known to be free from the immature parasites that cause the disease.

GNATHOSTOMIASIS.

This infection is caused by a parasitic worm transmitted in a way much like that of the liver fluke. (See *Fluke Infestations* above.) It comes from eating raw fish. Usually only one or a very few of the worms are found in a single host, but they migrate through the body all the time until they die. Occasionally uncomfortable or even dangerous complications arise when the parasite is migrating in deep tissues or internal organs, but the usual result is only a painless swelling surrounding the parasite.

What to Do

1. There is no useful home treatment, and no known remedy.

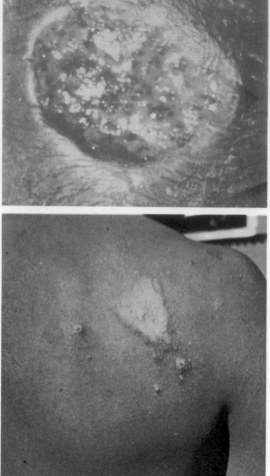

In one form of leishmaniasis the parasites causing it abound beneath the skin and give rise to sores.

PUBLIC HEALTH SERVICE AUDIOVISUAL FACILITY

2. If a migrating worm is detected near the body surface, have it removed surgically. It may be the only one in the body.

GUINEA WORM.
(See *Dracunculosis* in this chapter.)

HANSEN'S DISEASE.
(See *Leprosy* in this chapter.)

HOOKWORM INFECTION.
(See chapter 21 of this volume.)

KALA AZAR.
(See *Leishmaniasis:* B. *Kala Azar* in the next item.)

LEISHMANIASIS.

The various forms of leishmaniasis are all caused by minute parasites, called Leishman-Donovan bodies, which may be found by a microscopic study of the blood cells of an infected person, but which multiply in certain other body cells, especially the cells which line the blood vessels. These parasites, much smaller than red blood cells, are transmitted, at least mainly, by various species of Phlebotomus, or sand flies. In some regions leishmaniasis is common among infants and rare among adults. In other regions the opposite is true. In one common form the spleen and liver are chiefly involved, causing a disease called kala azar. In another form the parasites abound in and beneath the skin in one or more circumscribed areas, giving rise to slowly developing ulcers, to which the common name oriental sores has been given. Espundia is a name that has been applied to an American form of leishmaniasis, in which both skin and mucous membranes are attacked.

Three preventive measures have some value, and would have more if they were easier to carry out. First, if possible, avoid living in places where leishmaniasis abounds. Second, since the parasites may infect rodents and several domestic animals, especially dogs, try to exterminate rodents and destroy all domestic animals known to be infected. (The infection can be detected by a study of the blood cells.) Third, use all practical means to guard against insect bites, especially sand-fly bites. (See *Sand-fly Fever* in this chapter.)

A. *Espundia (American Leishmaniasis. Mucocutaneous Leishmaniasis).* Espundia occurs chiefly in forest workers in various parts of Central and South America. The disease is similar to oriental sore (see paragraph C in this listing) except that in some cases the mucous membranes of the nose, mouth, and throat are affected. Such an extension of the infection is very dangerous, since there is likely to be more or less destruction of the deep tissues of these parts of the body, bringing about disfigurement in some cases, and more or less impairment of the normal function of these parts in all cases. Death may result from secondary bacterial infection.

What to Do

1. Follow the treatment outline given for oriental sore (see paragraph C in this listing) insofar as it is applicable.

2. A physician should give the specific remedies and supervise other treatments, partly because of the great danger of secondary infection.

B. *Kala Azar (Dumdum Fever, Internal Leishmaniasis, Tropical Splenomegaly)*. Typical kala azar in adults is marked by a slowly developing, chronic, irregular but not very high fever; emaciation; anemia; and, most outstanding signs of all, an enlarged liver and a greatly enlarged and hardened spleen. The parasites abound in the spleen and the liver, and may be found in the bone marrow and the blood. In some cases the onset is more abrupt; and comparatively high fever, periodic chills, and sweats are common, giving rise to a suspicion of malaria or undulant fever. In some regions painless enlargement of the lymph nodes is common. In women a cessation of menstruation usually develops early in the course of the disease.

Some victims are plagued with rheumatic pains. Late in the disease dropsy of the legs and fluid in the abdomen are common. In many cases the skin takes on a dusky color, which fact explains the native name for the disease—kala azar, meaning literally "the black disease." In infants kala azar is marked by pallor, malarialike fever, diarrhea, and nosebleed, with enlargement of the spleen later.

Peculiarly, the kala azar victim, in spite of being feverish, weak, and emaciated, does not feel seriously ill.

He is likely to keep a good appetite, a clean tongue, and a desire to work, with little or no sense of malaise or apathy. Probably not more than 5 percent of untreated kala azar victims recover, but death is usually from some other infection that takes hold of the weakened victim rather than from kala azar itself. With suitable treatment, especially if begun early, 95 or more percent of kala azar victims can be saved.

What to Do

1. If the victim is not too much troubled with abdominal distress, give him a liberal and well-balanced diet, abundant in protein, vitamins, and iron-containing foods.

2. At the time of writing ethylstibamine (Neostibosan), a compound containing antimony, is the remedy of choice. It is administered intravenously.

3. The physician should also treat the anemia that is almost sure to be present.

C. *Oriental Sore (Aleppo Boil, Cutaneous Leishmaniasis, Delhi Boil)*. A typical oriental sore begins after a long incubation period as a small, itchy, slightly raised spot on the skin. It slowly enlarges and becomes scaly. When the scaly crust is removed, a moist and bleeding ulcer is revealed. The ulcer, having a scanty discharge, becomes crusted again from time to time, and slowly increases in size, often reaching a diameter of more than an inch (2.5 cm.).

Within two months to a year or more, slow healing begins, usually in the center. When healing is complete, a somewhat depressed and contracted scar is left. When scarring is extensive, it may cause much disfigurement or deformity. Oriental sores, however, are not fatal; and one attack usually protects the victim against further infection of the same sort.

As a rule the sores are neither pain-

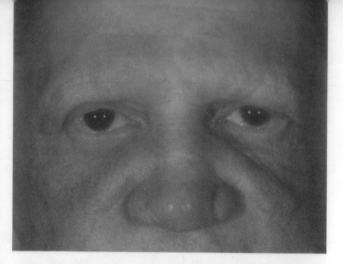

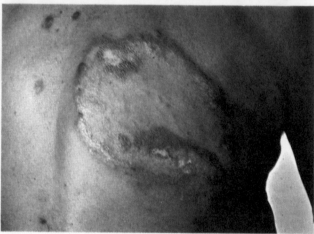

PUBLIC HEALTH SERVICE AUDIOVISUAL FACILITY

In the lepromatous variety of leprosy, loss of eyebrows constitutes an early symptom, and in the tuberculoid, spots on the skin.

ful nor dangerous, but secondary infection may make them so. Treatment is aimed as much toward prevention or control of this secondary infection as it is toward influencing the original infection that caused the sore. While we have been speaking of the sore in the singular, however, a person may have several or many of them at the same time.

What to Do

1. Apply hot fomentations to the affected area or areas once a day (see volume 3, chapter 20), and follow with antiseptic dressings or ointments, using saturated boric acid solution, 5 percent boric acid

ointment, or 5 percent ammoniated mercury ointment.

2. Have a physician give injections of suitable antimony compounds, which are the most effective specific remedies.

3. The physician may recommend still other remedies that his experience has proved to be effective, and he may use suitable sulfas or antibiotics in case of secondary infection, which is very common.

LEPROSY (HANSEN'S DISEASE).

Leprosy, sometimes called Hansen's disease, is a chronic infectious disease caused by a germ which greatly resembles the germ of tuberculosis. It has been found in tears, in sputum, and in nasal, urethral, and vaginal secretions; it abounds in scrapings from the diseased and thickened skin; and it has been detected after death in the liver, the spleen, and other internal organs.

The germs are believed to gain entrance to the body through the membrane lining the nose or through breaks in the skin. Biting insects may possibly introduce the germs into the skin, and there may be other modes of infection. Leprosy is apparently mildly contagious in some of its stages, but not in others; but, on account of its seriousness, it should for safety be handled as a contagious disease. Some cases have apparently been contracted through long contact with an infected person. It does not seem to be hereditary, but there are a few known cases in which infection apparently took place through the placenta.

Leprosy has a gradual onset. From two to three years, and occasionally a much longer period, may elapse from the time of the first exposure until it begins to show definite signs or symptoms; and then it runs a slow and lengthy course. Any unnatural patch on the surface of the skin, if void of sensibility to temperature, pain, or touch, should be a warning of the possible onset of this disease. Other early symptoms are nosebleed, headache, and fever. Certain areas of the body may lose sensitiveness, since it is the skin and the nerve trunks that are chiefly attacked by the disease.

Two fairly well defined varieties of leprosy exist: the lepromatous, in which the patient manifests no resistance to the disease, and the tuberculoid, in which there is considerable biological resistance. The lepromatous variety is characterized by the formation of nodules and a diffuse infiltration of the skin. The nodules, frequently most abundant on the face, soon alter the appearance of the victim. They cause the beard and the eyebrows to drop out, and the cheeks, brows, and ears to have an irregular swollen appearance. The tendency of these nodules is to break down and ulcerate, sometimes destroying the ears, and at other times the nose; sometimes laying bare the bones of the skull; sometimes attacking the eyes; and sometimes making large openings through the cheek into the mouth. At times the mastication of food is almost impossible and swallowing is difficult. When the larynx is involved, the voice becomes hoarse and is sometimes entirely lost. The respiration is greatly hindered, the gums tend to ulcerate, and the teeth to fall out. The senses of smell and taste are usually lost. These nodules may also appear on the extremities, from which the flesh may drop off, leaving the bones exposed. The lymph nodes show generalized involvement and enlargement.

In a considerable proportion of cases the nerve trunks are primarily involved. These tend to become much swollen and hardened. There is irritation and pain at first, which may be followed by loss of sensation in spots. More often the nerves are paralyzed, with foot drop or inability to move the forearm or to walk. The waste of muscles supplied by these nerves and the absorption of other tissues, even to the dissolving of bones, is not at all uncommon.

The tuberculoid variety is less severe and more superficial. It progresses slowly, if at all. It is often confined to discolored and insensitive spots on the skin. Even in this variety, the damage to nerves may be considerable. The nerve damage is less responsive to treatment than in the lepromatous variety.

With modern treatment there is hope for all types of cases, but the treatment must be long-continued, and improvement is slow. Unless properly treated, leprosy is never really checked; but there are times when it seems to subside somewhat. The disease leaves victims in such a weakened condition that they often die from an attack by some other disease. Only a few live until they succumb to the wasting effects of the leprosy itself.

What to Do

1. If leprosy is suspected, have a physician make the necessary examinations and tests to determine the true nature of the condition.

2. If leprosy is found, the physician can prescribe and supervise the use of one of the sulfone drugs, which are quite effective in the long run.

3. A nutritious diet, a hygienic environment, and a good mental attitude help the patient to recover. Individuals with mild infections do much better when they keep active than when at bed rest.

4. While danger of contagion is not great, all persons not infected should avoid body contact with a leper, handling objects that he has handled, wearing clothing that he has worn, or eating food that he has touched or that has been exposed to flies or other insects that could have been in contact with him. Care should also be taken not to come in contact with food or any other substance or object that could have become contaminated by any of his body discharges, especially those of his nose.

LEPTOSPIROSIS (SPIROCHETAL JAUNDICE, WEIL'S DISEASE).

Leptospirosis is caused by any one of a family of parasites, the most important member of which is Leptospira icterohaemorrhagiae, which abounds in the liver of the victim and which can be found in his blood early in the course of his disease, and in his urine later. The other members of this family are associated with animals other than rats, and they cause less severe infections.

The usual method of infection is contact of the broken skin with, or accidental swallowing of, food or water contaminated by the urine of rats, which harbor the causative organisms without apparent harm to themselves. The incubation period is from five to thirteen days. In the typical case the onset is fairly sudden, with chills, nausea, vomiting, headache, and muscle and abdominal pains. Within a few hours fever rises, the headache becomes worse, and extreme thirst and severe aching of the limbs develop. The blood vessels of the eyeballs become markedly dilated, which is a characteristic sign.

The fever remains irregularly high for a few days, falls for a short time, then shows a secondary rise for a few more days. Jaundice appears in about half of the cases some time after the onset. In cases with jaundice the liver is enlarged and tender and the output of urine is decreased. Simple herpes (fever blisters) and rashes of various types are common. A hemorrhagic rash is a serious danger sign. In most of the regions where the disease is common between 10 and 20 percent of the victims who develop jaundice die.

Cases of leptospirosis with jaundice, also called Weil's disease, may vary widely in their symptoms and may easily be mistaken for any one of several other diseases. For that reason, whenever this disease is suspected it is important to have a physician study the case to find out just what is wrong.

What to Do

1. If Weil's disease is present, keep the victim at rest in bed.

2. If his stomach can retain food, give him a liquid diet and urge him to take all the fluid he can.

3. For itching apply 1 percent phenol in calamine lotion or 1 percent menthol in petrolatum.

4. It is important to watch for and deal with the complications that may arise and to have the physician give or order suitable antibiotics, which are the most effective known remedies.

5. Important measures to prevent the spread of the disease are:

A. Sterilize the victim's body discharges. (For approved methods see chapter 28 of this volume under sub-heading "Home Care for Contagious Diseases.")

B. Do what is possible to exterminate rats.

C. Avoid swimming in, or other contact with, water that may be contaminated with the parasites, especially by means of rat urine.

LIVER FLUKE.

(See *Fluke Infestations: B. Liver Fluke* in this chapter.)

LIVER ROT.

(See *Fluke Infestations: C. Liver Rot* in this chapter.)

LUNG FLUKE.

(See *Fluke Infestations: D. Lung Fluke* in this chapter.)

MADUROMYCOSIS (MADURA FOOT, MYCETOMA).

Mycetoma is caused by one of a family of fungi similar to the organism that causes actinomycosis. (See chapter 28 in this volume.) While other parts of the body are occasionally attacked, the infection usually begins on the sole of the foot, with slow formation of a firm, rounded, somewhat discolored, painless swelling. After a few weeks the swelling softens and ruptures, persistently discharging a viscid, syrupy- or oily-appearing, occasionally blood-streaked, pus, containing granules of fish-egg size, grayish, yellowish, reddish, or black in color. As time goes on, more and more swellings form and break down, the entire foot enlarges to two to four times its normal size, the discharging openings persist, and the leg muscles shrink from disuse. All the tissues of the foot, including the bones, become involved; and bits of diseased bone are discharged in the pus at times. Pain is not often a problem, even in advanced cases.

If the disease is not checked in its early stages, the crippled victim may suffer with it for ten or twenty years. He finally dies from general debility or from some other infection that attacks him in his weakened condition.

What to Do

1. **Consult a physician for suitable remedies, which may be sulfonamides or antibiotics. The medication may have to be continued over a long period of time.**

2. **If medication is begun too late to bring about a cure, amputation of the diseased foot may be necessary.**

MALARIA (AGUE, CHILLS AND FEVER).

The signs and symptoms of ordinary malaria are too well known to need any extended description. The attacks of "chills and fever" for a few hours, followed by drenching sweats, every day or, more often, every alternate or every third day, make the typical case of the disease easily recognizable. It is also quite generally known that malaria is caused by one or more of four types of parasites that are introduced into the blood by the bite of an anopheles mosquito that has previously bitten a person with malaria, that the blood is the place where these parasites live and do most of their damage, and that a chronic case results in general debility, anemia, and an enlarged spleen.

Four types of malaria affect humans:

Vivax and tertian malaria are caused by the parasites Plasmodium vivax and Plasmodium ovale. These are the common types of malaria, the mildest, and the most likely to recur. Once the infection becomes established, the paroxysms of fever typically occur every second day for the vivax and every third day for the tertian. They may occur daily, however, in cases where there is a double brood of parasites, one brood segmenting on days two, four, and six and the other on days one, three, five, et cetera.

A third type, quartan malaria, is caused by the Plasmodium malariae. This type is slightly more severe than vivax malaria. The paroxysms of fever occur every three days. When there is a double infection, the paroxysms occur on days one and two and again on days four and five, et cetera.

The fourth, falciparum malaria, is caused by the Plasmodium falciparum. This is the most serious type of malaria, the type in which the often fatal complications of cerebral malaria or blackwater fever occur. The paroxysms occur at irregular intervals. When recognized early and treated promptly, however, this type responds well to therapy.

It is wise for persons living in a malarial region to learn as much as possible about the disease so as to be able to detect its presence early. In such a region any illness accompanied by fever, whether characterized by intermittent attacks or not, also any tendency to increasing weakness or fatigability or any obscure malady the nature of which is not understood, should arouse suspicion of malaria and prompt the individual to seek professional help for diagnosis and prompt treatment. To be successful, the early treatment of an acute attack may need to be very intensive.

Drugs for Prevention: In areas where malaria is widespread, it is advisable for preventive drugs to be taken continuously. Two of these are

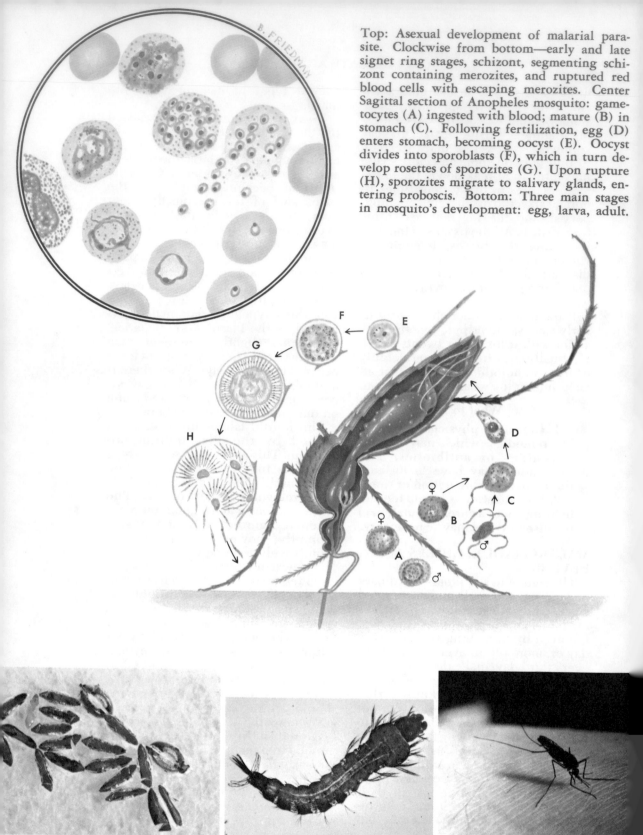

Top: Asexual development of malarial parasite. Clockwise from bottom—early and late signet ring stages, schizont, segmenting schizont containing merozites, and ruptured red blood cells with escaping merozites. Center Sagittal section of Anopheles mosquito: gametocytes (A) ingested with blood; mature (B) in stomach (C). Following fertilization, egg (D) enters stomach, becoming oocyst (E). Oocyst divides into sporoblasts (F), which in turn develop rosettes of sporozites (G). Upon rupture (H), sporozites migrate to salivary glands, entering proboscis. Bottom: Three main stages in mosquito's development: egg, larva, adult.

CHAS. PFIZER & CO., INC., PUBLIC HEALTH SERVICE AUDIOVISUAL FACILIT chloroquine and amodiaquine. One or the other (not both) should be used. Recommended dosages are as follows:

1. Chloroquine (Aralen)—0.5 gram (2 tablets) taken once a week on the same day each week.

2. Amodiaquine (Camoquin)—0.4 to 0.6 gram (2 or 3 tablets) taken once a week.

What to Do

1. During attacks of chills, keep the victim warm and in bed.

2. If fever rises as high as 104° F. (40° C.), try to reduce it by means of cool enemas, cool sponges, or alcohol sponges.

3. If there is tenderness in the region of the spleen, apply fomentations three times a day. (See volume 3, chapter 20, "Simple Home Treatments.")

4. During acute attacks the diet should be liquid.

5. The victim should avoid overexertion, even on fever-free days.

6. Most of the effective drug remedies require the supervision of a physician for best results.

7. In case of emergency, if no physician is available at the time, and if no instructions have been given as to the use of the above-named or other remedies, the old-time remedy quinine sulfate may be used for a course of treatments, though it is best not to rely on it permanently. The dose for an adult should be 10 grains (0.65 gm.) three times a day for seven days. The course of treatment may be repeated at the first sign of a relapse, but a real cure of malaria may not be possible with quinine sulfate.

8. Do all possible to prevent the victim from being bitten by mosquitoes, as a means of preventing the transmission of the disease to others.

9. Preventive measures include:

A. Killing of adult mosquitoes by the use of insecticides.

B. Killing larval mosquitoes by means of oiling or poisoning ponds or other standing water, draining swamps or ponds, or planting suitable small fish in them.

C. Avoiding mosquito bites by screening doors and windows, using bed nets, or wearing suitable clothing and using mosquito repellents, such as dimethyl phthalate, when going outside at night.

NOCARDIOSIS.

Nocardiosis is a condition caused by one or more subtypes of fungus closely related to that which causes actinomycosis. When introduced into the skin, these organisms cause damage similar to that of actinomycosis or maduromycosis (See chapter 28, "Infectious Diseases," in this volume; also *Maduromycosis* above.) When inhaled, they may cause severe lung disease, the early symptoms of which may resemble those of tuberculosis. Cough and the raising of pussy sputum are the chief symptoms, but the infection can cause large areas of consolidation, also cavities, in the lungs; and the disease may spread to the ribs and burrow through the chest wall.

Any part of the body may be attacked, but involvement of the brain and its coverings is the most serious development. Recovery is usual if the treatment is thorough and begun early enough. Delay may be fatal.

What to Do

1. Since nocardiosis may simulate any one of several other conditions, any suspicion of its presence should lead to a thorough study by a physician to determine what is really wrong.

2. No home remedy is of any use, but long-continued treatment with suitable sulfonamides and antibiotics will usually bring about a cure.

ORIENTAL SORE.

(See *Leishmaniasis: C. Oriental Sore* in this chapter.)

OROYA FEVER.
(See *Bartonellosis* in this chapter.)

PHLEBOTOMUS FEVER.
(See *Sand-fly Fever* in this chapter.)

PINTA (AZUL, CARATE, MAL DEL PINTO).
Pinta is a spirochetal infection of the skin caused by Treponema carateum. The skin of the hands, wrists, feet, and ankles is most commonly attacked. The means of spread are not definitely known, though actual contact with an open sore and indirect contact through flies are suspected. While the causative organism is much like that which causes syphilis, pinta is not a venereal disease.

The first stage consists of one or more papules. The second stage is marked by a spreading eruption of flat, reddish spots called pintids. In the third stage there are spots of various colors; but these spots eventually lose their color and become whitish, thickened, and hardened. If such spots are on the palms or soles, they tend to crack and cause inconvenience or discomfort. The disease is not otherwise dangerous, or even distressing, except for the unpleasing appearance of the skin.

What to Do

1. Consult a physician. He can give injections of penicillin, an effective remedy.

2. Preventive measures similar to those for yaws are recommended. (See *Yaws* in this chapter.)

PLAGUE.
Plague is caused by a specific organism called Pasteurella pestis. There are two distinct forms of the disease. The bubonic is characterized by swellings of the lymph nodes. The swollen nodes are called buboes. The pneumonic form affects the lungs and produces a type of pneumonia so serious that death occurs in two or three days in untreated cases.

A. *Bubonic*. This form of plague is

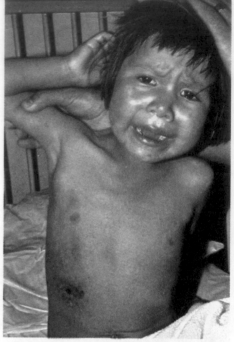

In bubonic plague, buboes usually appear in armpits the second day.

primarily a disease of rats, and it is usually transmitted to man by the bites of rat fleas. Wild rodents have occasionally been found infected, and they must be considered as a possible source of the disease. This is particularly true in the western part of the United States. Limited experience indicates that the plague organism becomes somewhat less virulent when it infects wild rodents, so that cases of plague from this source are comparatively mild.

The incubation period of bubonic plague is from two to ten days. A typical case of the disease begins suddenly with a high fever, great weakness, chills, severe headache, and pains in the back and limbs. There may be vomiting and diarrhea. In most cases buboes begin to appear in the groins, under the arms, and in the neck during the second day. The fever may go as high as 104° F. (40° C.) the first day. There is intense thirst. The disease causes great prostration; and if the case is fatal, death commonly comes between the third and sixth day.

The disease may become septicemic and involve all parts of the body. It is especially dangerous when the brain is involved. In the more hopeful cases the fever goes down gradually and the victim recovers after a long convalescence. The prospect for recovery in plague cases, however, is much brighter since the discovery of the value of the sulfas and the antibiotics.

What to Do

It is especially important that all plague victims be isolated in a contagious-disease hospital, if at all possible. The advice given below is applicable only in cases where hospitalization is impossible.

1. A physician should begin treatment as soon as possible. Streptomycin, tetracycline antibiotics, and chloramphenicol have proved quite effective in treating victims of plague.

2. Keep the victim in bed.

3. If the fever rises as high as 104° F. (40° C.), reduce it by means of cool sponges and cool enemas.

4. Apply ice bags to the painful buboes. If doing so does not give relief, try fomentations three times a day. (See volume 3, chapter 20.)

5. I pus forms in a bubo, it should be opened and drained by a physician.

6. Keep an ice bag over the heart, also on the head if the victim is delirious.

7. Apply hot fomentations to the lower back three times a day.

8. Try to keep the victim's kidneys active by urging him to take all the liquid he can.

9. His diet should consist of milk, soups, and broths.

10. To help protect others from contracting the disease, destroy rats and fleas and try to secure plague vaccinatoin for all individuals who are in danger of infection.

B. *Pneumonic*. The pneumonic form of plague is one of the most contagious diseases known. It is not spread by rats, but it travels from man to man through the air. The invisible droplets thrown out of the mouth and nose in coughing, sneezing, or forcible talking contain the plague bacilli. Inhalation of germs carried by dust is also a possible source of infection.

The incubation period of the pneumonic form of plague is short. It may be only a few hours and is rarely as long as five days. The symptoms at the onset are much like those of ordinary pneumonia. (See chapter 17 of this volume.) It starts with a chill and headache, the fever rises rapidly, the pulse becomes rapid, and the victim soon begins to cough and has difficulty in getting his breath. The sputum consists of mucus at first, but soon becomes bloody. In fatal cases, which used to be the great majority of all cases, the victim becomes delirious and dies within a few hours to three days. If treatment is to save life, it must be begun promptly.

What to Do

The patient should be hospitalized if possible. If he must be cared for at home, follow these directions:

1. The same remedies recommended for bubonic plague should be used, but they are quite ineffective unless given within fifteen hours of the onset of the attack.

2. Read carefully the subsection "Home Care for Contagious Diseases" in chapter 28 of this volume and follow the instructions given. The attendant, for his own protection, should wear a face mask made of several layers of gauze; and nobody should attend a victim of this disease unless already vaccinated against plague. If possible, the attendant should also wear sterilized coveralls, goggles, and rubber gloves. Nobody but the attendant and the physician should come anywhere near the victim.

RAT-BITE FEVER (SODOKU).

Rat-bite fever is common in Japan, but it also occurs in many other parts of the world. It is caused by a tiny spiral organism found sometimes in the blood but more easily found in tissue fluids from the area of the bite and from adjacent lymph nodes.

As a rule the bite heals; but a few days later the spot becomes inflamed, swollen, hardened, painful, and dark-colored. The nearby lymph nodes swell and become tender. The acute stage of the disease begins with chills and a rising fever, headache, nausea, weakness, muscle and joint pains, and a rapid pulse. A dusky-red rash appears on the body and limbs. One or more relapses at intervals of several days are common. Of the victims who do not receive proper treatment, about one in ten dies; but nearly all recover when given modern remedies.

Rat-bite fever victims need expert medical attention for two reasons: (1) The disease may closely resemble malaria or relapsing fever, and it is important to find out early what is wrong. (2) The only really effective remedies must be given or ordered by a doctor.

What to Do

1. Have a physician study the case to make sure what is wrong. If it proves to be rat-bite fever, the physician can give or prescribe suitable antibiotics. All other treatment of value can be symptomatic only, and the physician can advise what it should be.

2. As preventive measures:

A. Have rat bites cauterized without delay.

B. Exterminate rats.

SAND-FLY FEVER (PHLEBOTO-MUS FEVER, PAPPATACI FEVER).

Sand-fly fever is caused by a virus transmitted by the bites of infected sand flies. These flies are also responsible for the transmission of several other diseases. They choose dark,

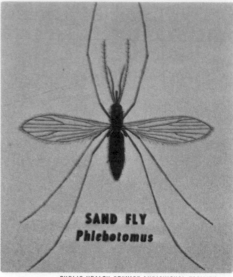

SAND FLY
Phlebotomus

PUBLIC HEALTH SERVICE AUDIOVISUAL FACILITY

damp places, especially those with cracks or crannies, in which to lay their eggs; and they hide in weeds or shrubbery during daylight. They are weak fliers, seldom rising to a height of more than ten feet (3 meters) above the ground. They are too small to be kept out by ordinary screens or nets, but they may be repelled by camphor or strong-smelling oils or ointments. Small as they are, however, their bites are decidedly irritating.

Sand-fly fever is, in its typical form, much like dengue—distressing, but not at all deadly. It may resemble a case of influenza without upper respiratory symptoms. Its onset is sudden, with fever, severe headache, dizziness, general aching, and pain behind the eyes. As a rule the fever is fairly high, and it persists for three or four days, but the pulse is slow. Marked debility, both physical and mental, persists for a week or two after the temperature falls to normal. Since atypical forms of disease may resemble malaria or typhus, which are often found in the same parts of the world, careful study of all suspicious cases by a physician is important.

What to Do

1. Since no known curative remedy is availalble, only symptomatic treatment is useful.

2. Apply mild tincture of iodine to sand-fly bites.

3. Home remedies do not seem to be effective in relieving the headache of sand-fly fever. A physician may use remedies that bring relief.

4. Prevention of sand-fly bites is obviously important. The following measures are recommended:

A. Spray known or suspected breeding or hiding places, both indoors and out.

B. Clear away brush or high weeds or grass from the vicinity of the dwelling.

C. Use very fine-mesh bed nets.

D. Avoid exposure out of doors after dark.

E. Wear close-woven clothing and apply dimethyl phthalate or some other good insect repellent to exposed skin areas when it is necessary to be out at night. It may be necessary to do this indoors as well if provision cannot be made to keep sand flies out of the house.

SPIROCHETAL JAUNDICE.

(See *Leptospirosis* in this chapter.)

SPOROTRICHOSIS.

Sporotrichosis is a persistent fungous infection, due to Sporotrichum schenckii. It begins as a firm, elastic, movable nodule underneath the skin. As the nodule enlarges, it becomes attached to the skin, which develops inflammation and then breaks down, forming an ulcer. Other nodules form along the lymph vessels draining the originally infected area. The lymph vessels may become inflamed and thickened, feeling like cords beneath the skin. Nodules may form in scattered locations almost anywhere in the body, including bones, joints, muscles, and various organs. The lungs seem most likely of all organs to be damaged. If left without proper treatment, the infection may persist several years, but the general health is not often much affected by it.

What to Do

1. Do not attempt self-treatment. No local treatment will do any good, and symptomatic treatment is not often needed.

2. Consult a physician. If he finds sporotrichosis present, he will probably prescribe heavy doses of potassium iodide. He may order Amphotericin B, which has proved useful in cases with bone and joint involvement.

SPRUE (PSILOSIS, TROPICAL DIARRHEA).

Sprue in now believed to be at least partly caused by a dietary deficiency, but there is increasing evidence that at least in some cases there is an allergic factor also. It is a serious malady that often attacks people who go to certain tropical or subtropical regions from temperate zones, but it is not at all common among those who are native to such regions. The cause is not strictly associated with the climate, however, because individuals living in high, cool areas are attacked as well as those who live in the warm or hot lowlands. An increasing number of cases of what has been called nontropical sprue have been recognized in parts of the world not formerly believed to be conducive to this disease, but in these cases the factor of food allergy seems to be prominent.

Sprue is rarely found among young adults. Occasionally it develops years later in a person who may have lived in a sprue region for many months or years without showing any signs of the disease while living there. Body changes that come along with advancing years apparently have something to do with preparing the way for sprue, but just what these changes are or how they operate is not fully understood.

Cases vary widely, but the typical one usually begins with nothing more than a mild morning looseness of the bowels, which may persist for some time before any other signs or symptoms develop. Later, at least dur-

561

ing active periods of the disease, there are four outstanding symptoms: sore mouth, indigestion with bloating, diarrhea, and weight loss. The severely affected individual has a dark or muddy complexion, is emaciated, anemic, weak, irritable, unreasonable, and is troubled with loss of memory and inability to concentrate. Most of the time his tongue is comparatively smooth, congested, more or less eroded beneath and at the edges, and fissured in the center. It and the lining of his mouth are so tender and irritable that almost intolerable pain and burning are caused by putting anything more harsh than the blandest of foods into his mouth.

In chronic sprue cases the stools are characteristic, being copious, pasty, pale gray in color, fermenting, spongy, and extremely foul-smelling. If chemically examined, they will be found to contain much fat, particularly fatty acids. There are often two or more bowel movements early in the day, with no abnormal bowel movements or looseness during the afternoon or evening.

By spells some or all of the signs and symptoms of sprue may decrease in severity, or even entirely disappear, only to return later in a more aggravated form if suitable treatment has not been perseveringly given. There are many cases that have only a few of the characteristic symptoms, however; and the nature of the malady may be entirely overlooked if the victim does not have the benefit of expert medical study and laboratory tests.

Early cases of sprue, properly treated, nearly always end in recovery. The outlook is bad for people past fifty, or for long-standing cases, for careless victims, and for people who cannot or will not carefully follow a suitable diet.

Nontropical sprue is characterized by poor absorption of fats, proteins, and vitamins A, B12, D, and K. Softening of the bones may develop. It bears a close relationship to celiac disease of children.

What to Do

1. If sprue is suspected, have a physician make needed examinations and tests. If he finds sprue present, he will arrange for the treatment, but home nursing care is still important.

2. The victim needs to be carefully protected from chilling. He needs a warm room and warm clothing, and he must avoid bad weather and cold baths.

3. He should have daily sunbaths, if possible.

4. If sunbaths are not possible, try to arrange for ultraviolet-light treatments.

5. Diet is of prime importance. The following general principles are recommended as a guide:

A. Make the diet high-protein and high-vitamin, but low-fat.

B. Include in the diet 2 ounces (60 c.c.) of brewer's yeast or 1 ounce (30 c.c.) of rice polishings daily.

C. No detailed diet lists are given here because cases vary widely in the kinds of food that can be handled by the irritated digestive organs without distress—a point of prime importance to consider in feeding victims of sprue. Even though the victim is emaciated, he must not be given more food than his digestive organs can handle satisfactorily. Milk agrees with most sprue victims, however, and it is usually the mainstay of sprue diets, at least in the early weeks of treatment.

6. The victim should be kept under the care or supervision of a physician to arrange for the following remedies and to watch the effects carefully:

A. Vitamin B12, folic acid, vitamin D, some calcium compound, and vitamin K.

B. A suitable mouthwash, the nature of which must depend on the special condition of the individual victim's mouth.

C. Suitable means of controlling

diarrhea, also constipation in the later stages of some cases.

D. Blood transfusions or other measures to combat anemia, which may be extreme and possibly of a pernicious type.

7. When the victim is able to travel, he should leave the sprue area and, preferably, never return.

TROPICAL ULCER (NAGA SORE).

Tropical ulcers occur in many parts of the tropics, but especially those with much wet weather. Actual cause of the ulcers remains uncertain, but it is probable that a poorly balanced diet, especially one short in vitamin A, is an important causative factor.

The condition begins as a blister or a small inflamed spot. This develops into a rapidly spreading ulcer, which may reach a diameter of as much as 4 inches (10 cm.). Fever, pain, a general toxic condition, and marked disability may be present.

What to Do

1. Bed rest and a nutritious diet are important.

2. Keep the ulcer cleansed by washing from time to time with a 5 percent solution of magnesium sulfate, or apply locally a 1:1,000 solution of acriflavine.

3. After cleansing, dust thickly with sulfathiazole powder, and keep the powder in place with a gauze dressing.

4. A physician can give suitable antibiotics, which are the most effective remedies.

5. Cod-liver oil ointment dressings may be used when healing is well-advanced.

6. In severe cases surgical skin grafting may be necessary.

TYPHUS FEVER.

Several diseases that used to be considered unrelated to each other, or only slightly related, are now grouped together under the general name "typhus fevers," largely because of the similarity of the organisms causing them and the fact that these organisms are usually transmitted by the bites of lice, fleas, ticks, or mites.

A. *Epidemic Typhus (Jail Fever, Louse Typhus, Ship Fever).* The germs of typhus fever are very small and are related to those of Rocky Mountain spotted fever. Germs of this type are called rickettsiae. Louse-borne typhus is transmitted from person to person by the body louse, called Pediculus corporis, or Pediculus humanus. Spread of the lice from the body or clothing of one person to those of others is favored by close contact and lack of personal cleanliness, especially in cold weather when warm clothing is worn. Extermination of body lice is the secret of success in preventing typhus fever. Dusting powders developed especially for this purpose during and following World War II proved very effective.

Shortly before the appearance of typical symptoms, the typhus victim may seem to have a common cold. The real onset of the disease is sudden, with chills, high fever, headache, general pains, prostration, nausea, vomiting, constipation or diarrhea, with possible delirium or stupor developing early. About the fifth day small pink spots appear on the skin of the neck, chest, abdomen, and limbs. They change to red, then to purple, and finally to a brownish color. In nearly all cases there is marked bronchitis with cough and sputum. The pulse is rapid, but the blood pressure is low.

It is somewhat difficult to distinguish typhus in its early stages from Rocky Mountain spotted fever and several other diseases, though the location and circumstances involved make the distinction easier. This problem need not bother the victim nor his family, however, because the home care and nursing for all of these conditions are similar.

Typhus is not a serious disease among young persons, but among the elderly it may be deadly. The mortality has run from 4 percent to as high as

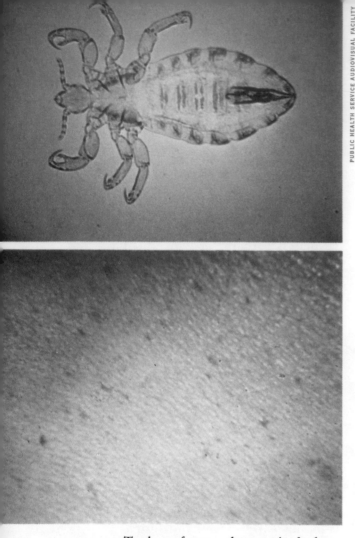

Typhus fever, characterized by pink spots on the skin, is caused by organisms transmitted by body lice.

70 percent, depending on age and locality; but the availability of modern remedies makes the prospect much brighter.

What to Do

1. For the safety of the attendant and others, be sure that no living lice are left on the victim's body. His body should be repeatedly dusted with an efficient lousicide, and his clothing should be sterilized, preferably by heat.

2. Since dried louse feces may contain living typhus germs, attendants while working with victims of the disease should wear masks, goggles, and gloves, as well as protective gowns.

3. A physician should be in charge of the case, since chloromycetin, the tetracycline antibiotics, and all other effective remedies must be ordered or given by a physician.

4. In nursing the victim, follow (2 to 6) and (8) under *Typhoid Fever.* (See chapter 28, "Infectious Diseases," in this volume.)

5. Before attending a typhus victim, or before going into a region where typhus cases may exist, it is advisable to be vaccinated against the disease.

B. *Flea Typhus and Tick Typhus.* During recent years a mild type of typhus fever, sometimes called endemic typhus, flea typhus, or murine typhus, has become increasingly prevalent, a rising incidence usually accompanying an increase in the rat population. Most of the cases are spread by rat fleas instead of by lice. While the disease is seldom fatal, the control problem is difficult. It is virtually impossible to exterminate the fleas that carry it. They do not stay on the body or in the clothing, or even always in the house of the victim; and there is no way of fumigating the outdoors. Rat extermination, however, is a valuable control measure.

Tick-borne typhus fevers occur in many tropical countries. The infected ticks are most commonly found on dogs, but they will occasionally bite humans. In removing the ticks from dogs in such regions, it is wise to use forceps or a piece of paper rather than the bare fingers.

What to Do

Secure the services of a physician, if possible. The same remedies that have proved useful in cases of epidemic typhus (see above) should be used in cases of flea typhus or tick typhus.

C. *Scrub Typhus (Japanese Flood Fever, Kedani Fever, Mite Fever,*

Tsutsugamushi). The riskettsial organisms that cause scrub typhus are transmitted by numerous species of mites. They can pick up or transmit the organisms only in their larval or blood-sucking stage, but they can carry them in their bodies until maturity and pass them on to the next generation of mites through the eggs. It is possible that rodents may act as reservoirs of infection.

In a typical case, a painless papule first appears, usually on some part of the body ordinarily covered by clothing. It enlarges and becomes dark in the center, eventually forming an ulcer that is less than half an inch (1.2 cm.) in diameter and that leaves a scar when it heals. The lymph nodes in its vicinity swell and become tender.

As the disease develops, there is a gradually rising fever, which eventually becomes high; but the pulse rate is much slower than might be expected. In many cases, but not all, a body rash appears about the fifth day, spreads widely, and lasts from one to ten days. The spleen is enlarged and tender. At the height of the disease severe headache behind the eyes, loss of appetite, nausea, vomiting, muscular twitching, difficult breathing, cough, deep prostration, and delirium may be present. Without specific treatment up to 20 percent of the victims die, the mortality differing widely in different localities.

What to Do

1. Follow the instructions as to what should be done in a case of epidemic typhus (see above), except for louse-extermination measures.

2. Keep the victim from returning to regular work until long after convalescence seems complete, for undetected heart damage may be present.

3. As preventive measures:

A. As far as possible, avoid mite-infested localities.

B. Try to clear away or burn vegetation infested by mites.

C. Wear clothing that will keep the mites from gaining access to the skin (close-woven fabrics, long legs, leggings, long sleeves, tight collars, tight wristbands, et cetera, being desirable).

D. Apply a thin layer of dimethyl or dibutyl phthalate or other proved insect repellent to those parts of the clothing which mites must pass in order to reach the skin.

YAWS (FRAMBESIA, PIAN).

In many ways the effects of yaws resemble those of syphilis, and most of the remedies used in treating the one disease are also effective in treating the other. (See chapter 30, "Venereal Infections," in this volume.) Yaws, however, cannot be classed as venereal disease; but it is highly contagious. It is caused by a spirochete which looks much like the spirochete of syphilis. The organism must enter through some break in the skin or mucous membrane in order to cause the disease.

The first sore, or "mother yaw," may appear almost anywhere on the body, commonly on the legs or feet. It is not characteristic in appearance at first; but it usually becomes covered by a yellowish crust, and it is not painful unless it is firmly pressed. It may persist for several months. Its persistence, its painlessness, and the fact that the victim lives in a yaws area are the outstanding features that justify a suspicion that the condition is really yaws.

The appearance of the "mother yaw" may not be accompanied by any noticeable illness of the victim; but mild fever, headache, digestive upsets, and pain in the bones and joints may occur. The lymph nodes near the sore are enlarged. The Wassermann reaction usually becomes positive within a month of the time the sore first appears, and it remains strongly so thereafter. In doubtful cases, this reaction is a valuable diagnostic aid.

The second stage of yaws begins within six weeks to three months after

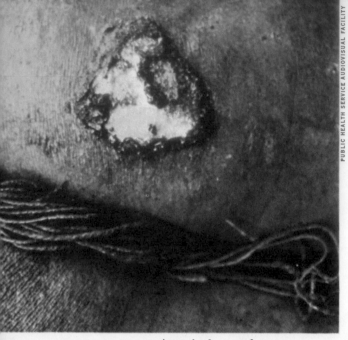

A typical case of yaws.

the first. Tiny, flat pimples appear and grow to various-sized, considerably elevated, raspberrylike, itchy, but practically painless, yellow-crusted sores or ulcers. If a crust is removed, serum oozes out and another crust soon forms. A laboratory examination of the serum or crust shows it to be swarming with the causative organisms. It often happens that a large ulcer has several small ones grouped around it. Within a few weeks the sore dries and the crust falls off, leaving a pale spot which later darkens. The sores may be the only signs of the second stage, but fever and the other distressing symptoms that sometimes occur during the first stage are somewhat more likely to accompany the second.

The third stage of yaws is much like the third stage of syphilis. It is chiefly characterized by more or less destructive and persistent ulcers, more common about the nose than elsewhere, which may cause much disfigurement and deformity; and it is this prospect more than anything else that makes the early treatment of yaws important for the victim. The bones, especially the tibia, are often attacked; but the brain, the heart, and the internal or-

gans are not often affected. Even though the victim's general resistance may run low, making him unusually susceptible to other infections, death from yaws itself is extremely rare.

What to Do

1. Have a physician give injections of penicillin or dichlorophenarsine hydrochloride (Clorarsen), or prescribe one or more of the tetracycline antibiotics.

2. Take care to support the victim's general health by means of fresh air, cleanliness, and good food.

3. Both victims and contacts need education in personal hygiene.

4. As preventive measures:

A. Isolate yaws victims until their open sores have healed.

B. Apply antiseptic ointments or dusting powders to such sores, and keep them covered with dressings so that flies cannot get to them.

C. Carefully dress and treat wounds in healthy persons who may come in contact with yaws victims, and keep flies away from these wounds.

D. Thoroughly disinfect, or burn if it is impossible to disinfect otherwise, houses or huts in which persons with open yaws sores have recently lived.

YELLOW FEVER (YELLOW JACK).

Yellow fever is a frequently fatal, epidemic, virus disease, transmitted by the bite of the Aedes aegypti mosquito or one of several closely related species. In the past there have been widespread epidemics in the eastern and southern parts of the United States, and the disease is more or less prevalent in many other parts of the world, chiefly in tropical areas. Increase of airplane travel from country to country is increasing the danger of spread of yellow fever. Furthermore, since the discovery of animal reservoirs of infection in the jungle, hope of real eradication of yellow fever from the world is less than it used to be.

566

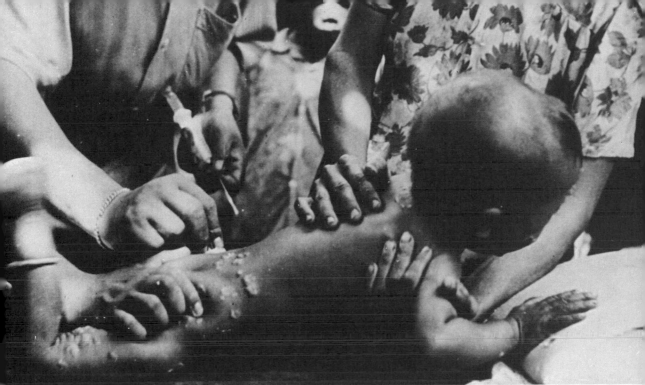

A yaws patient receiving an injection, an important early treatment.

About three to six days after a person is bitten by an infected mosquito, the illness begins. The onset is abrupt, with a rapid rise in temperature to 103° F. (39.4° C.) or more. A person may feel perfectly well, and then within a few hours he may become critically ill. The face is flushed and swollen, and the eyes are bloodshot. All the typical symptoms of an acute infection are present. There are severe pains in the head, both front and back, and extending down the spine and to the legs. The pulse is rapid in the early course of the disease.

Vomiting, first of mucus and then of bile, comes on early. The kidneys are affected, and a large amount of albumin can be found in the urine by the third or fourth day. The fever remains high for a few days, being a little higher in the evenings than in the mornings, but then it begins to decline steadily. A characteristic finding is a marked slowing of the pulse while a considerable amount of fever is still present.

With the decline in temperature, improvement in the acute symptoms occurs; but the victim may become increasingly toxic along with the appearance of the most characteristic features of yellow fever—jaundice and hemorrhages. The whites of the eyes first become yellow, and the jaundice can soon be observed over the whole body. The gums swell up and bleed. Then hemorrhages from the bowels and the stomach appear, characterized by bloody stools and vomitus appearing like coffee grounds. Frequently there are hemorrhages under the skin showing up as black-and-blue spots. Liver damage may be very marked.

Severe yellow fever is frequently fatal. If the victim survives for as long as nine days, he will probably get well. The first evidence of probable survival is a fall of the temperature to near normal. Up until this happens, however, even a moderately severe attack must be considered dangerous, because a sudden turn for the worse often occurs.

Prevention of the spread of yellow fever to others is equally as important as the treatment of people who al-

567

ready have it. Since the causative virus circulates in the blood during the first three days of the illness, the victim should be kept within screens during this period so that no mosquito can bite him, either by day or by night. The mosquito that spreads yellow fever flies and bites freely by daylight as well as by night.

A considerable degree of protection against infection is given by an effective live-virus vaccine, and people going to yellow fever regions should be thus protected.

Everybody in the neighborhood of the sick person should take as much care as possible to avoid being bitten by mosquitoes, since the disease is not transmitted in any other way than by mosquito bites. All possible measures should be taken to destroy mosquitoes and to keep them from breeding. Yellow-fever mosquitoes prefer to breed near houses, and they do not fly as far as do malaria mosquitoes. For safety, no standing water should be allowed anywhere near the house. Yellow-fever mosquitoes can breed in a very small amount of water. The eggs may be deposited in a roof gutter, an old tin can, or any hole or depression in a tree or in the ground or elsewhere that can catch and hold a little rainwater for a few days.

Experience has shown that the thorough and repeated use of a mosquito-killing spray in houses in a neighborhood in which there is a case of yellow fever is a very valuable procedure—even more valuable than careful screening of the houses. After feeding on an infected person, or any other person for that matter, the mosquito tends to find some dark corner in the house and remain quiet for a few days. If killed during this period, it will never transmit the infection; and spraying in dark corners, under beds, and under and around other furniture is quite likely to find and kill such hiding disease carriers.

What to Do

1. The victim should be under a physician's care, preferably in a hospital; but the damage that may be done by moving a very ill patient should not be ignored. If the moving must be for a considerable distance or if it cannot be done without putting the patient under strain, it may be better to do without hospital care.

2. There is no specific remedy, but the physician may prescribe suitable symptomatic remedies or treatments. Good nursing is important.

3. Keep the patient at absolute rest in bed.

4. Put him on a high-protein, high-carbohydrate liquid diet for three days.

5. Give the patient all the weak lemonade he will drink; or give him all the water he can be persuaded to take.

6. If vomiting is severe, so that water cannot be retained in the stomach, give an enema every two hours of about half a pint (225 c.c.) of tepid water to which half a teaspoonful of baking soda has been added. Give these enemas slowly so that they will not disturb or irritate the patient and so that he can retain and absorb the solution. (It may be that the physician will want to give the patient fluid by vein.)

7. Beginning with the fourth day the patient can have milk, vegetable broths, and eggnogs.

8. Give fomentations to the spine with hot foot bath and cold compress to the head twice a day unless the patient is too ill to be disturbed at all. (See volume 3, chapter 20, "Simple Home Treatments.")

9. If the fever rises above 103° F. (39.4° C.), reduce it somewhat by means of very gently given tepid sponges or alcohol sponges.

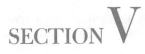

SECTION V

Illustrated Study
of Cells

Microscopic Views of
Normal and Abnormal Tissues

In diagnosing an illness the doctor frequently calls for laboratory tests, which could include microscopic examination of blood cells or of tissue samples obtained from organs suspected of being diseased. Because many systemic diseases produce unique effects on the blood and on the tissues, such tests give clues to possible infection or to incipient stages of abnormalities such as cancer or degenerative diseases.

Normal cells and abnormal cells often look so near alike that it takes a trained eye to detect malformation or disease. A physician skilled in recognizing specific changes produced by disease is called a pathologist, and the method of removing a small portion of tissue for special study, a biopsy examination.

The following magnifications show what a doctor sees when he looks through a microscope at normal and abnormal cells and tissues. They are not medical drawings but illustrations showing actual tissue mounted on glass slides by a special technique known as microtomy.

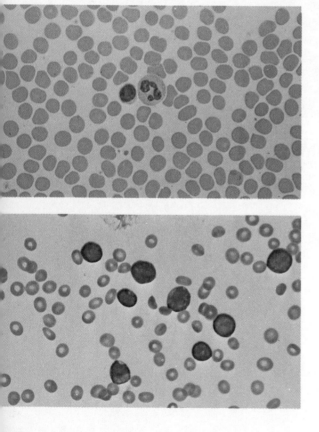

A microscopic view of a normal blood preparation in which occasional white blood cells are seen among numerous red blood cells. Seen here, a lymphocyte (dark cell) and a neutrophilic granulocyte.

A microscopic view of a blood preparation in a case of lymphocytic leukemia. In this disease lymphocytes increase tremendously.

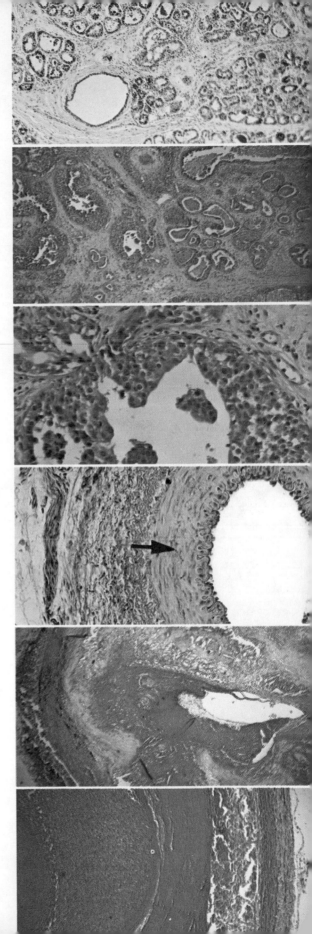

A microscopic view showing gland tissue of the normal breast during pregnancy.

A microscopic view of a small area of breast tissue showing clusters of cells of a malignant tumor (carcinoma).

A microscopic view of a small portion of a carcinoma of the breast (a malignant tumor). The tumor cells manifest a tendency to invade the adjacent tissue.

A microscopic view of a normal small artery showing its scalloped lining and the surrounding narrow layer of smooth muscle. During life, the pressure of blood within the artery smooths out the scallops of the lining. The pointer indicates the layer of smooth muscle that forms most of the artery's wall.

A microscopic view of a coronary artery in which the passageway for blood has been almost occluded by arteriosclerosis.

A microscopic view of a section of the wall of a vein which contains a thrombus—material consisting mostly of clotted blood.

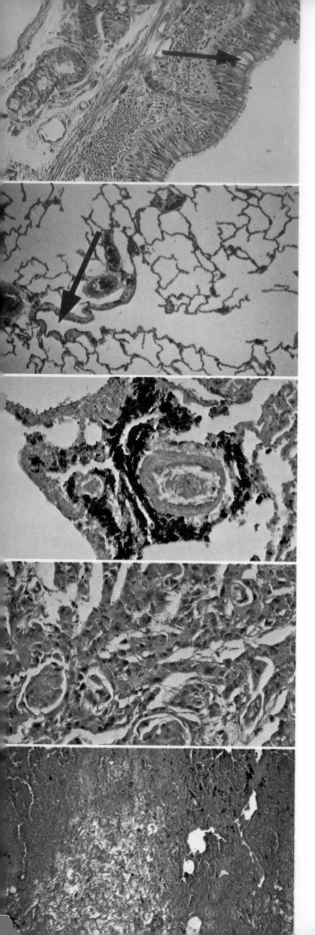

A microscopic view of a portion of the wall of the normal trachea. The epithelium lining the trachea is equipped with tiny villi—fingerlike structures which, by their waving action, sweep out foreign material which has been carried in by the inhaled air. The arrow indicates two goblet cells which produce mucus. In the deeper areas are glands which also produce mucus.

A microscopic view of normal lung tissue. The arrow points to a bronchiole, which represents the final branching of the system of tubes which bring air into the lung.

A microscopic view of a small area of lung tissue indicating how carbon which is inhaled remains in the lung tissue. Inasmuch as carbon is insoluble and inert, these deposits remain for the duration of life.

A high-power microscopic view of an area of lung which has been invaded by a bronchiogenic carcinoma—the highly malignant tumor which is so commonly caused by the use of cigarettes.

Microscopic view of an area of lung which has become involved in bronchopneumonia. Notice that the air sacs have become filled with defense cells and tissue debris.

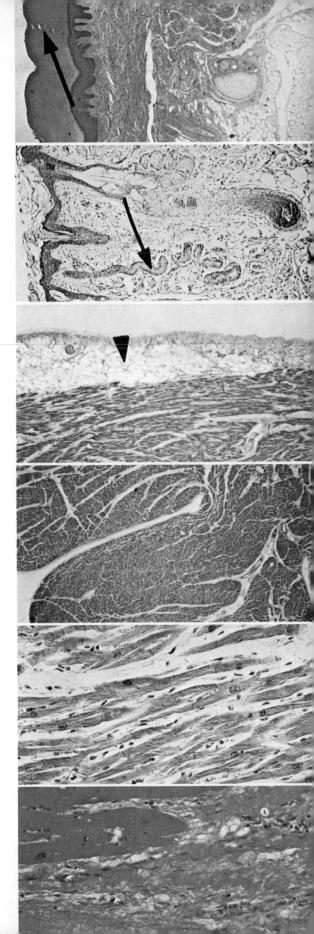

A microscopic view of normal skin from the palm of the hand. The two heavy bands at the left constitute the epidermis, the intermediate zone of tissue arranged as a "feltwork" is the dermis, and the looser tissue at the right is the subcutaneous area. The arrow indicates the duct of a sweat gland spiraling to the surface.

A microscopic view of normal thin skin such as occurs on the arm. The arrow points to the duct of a sweat gland. To the extreme right is the root of a hair. Left of the hair root and continuing to the free surface is a portion of a hair follicle with its associated sebaceous gland.

A microscopic view of a portion of the wall of a normal heart showing its external surface. The arrow indicates a delicate layer of fat just beneath the heart's outer wall.

A microscopic view of a small portion of the wall of the normal heart showing its lining membrane as it extends between two folds of muscle tissue.

A microscopic view of the muscle contained in the wall of a normal heart.

A microscopic view of a portion of the heart wall in which healing has occurred following a typical "heart attack" caused by the occlusion of a branch of a coronary artery. The lighter areas consist of scar tissue; the darker structures are remaining heart muscle fibers.

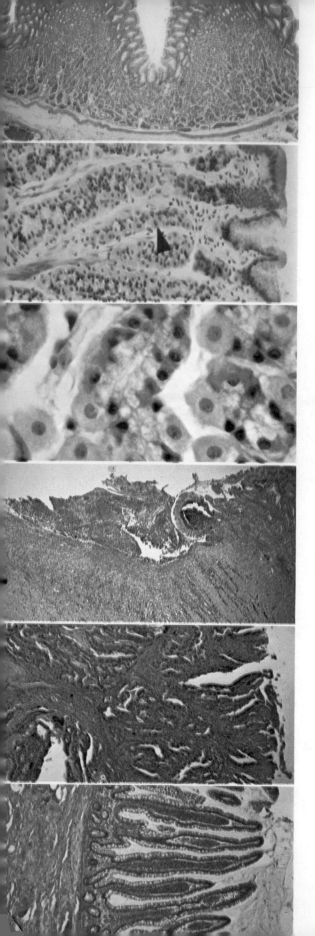

A low-power microscopic view of the normal glandular membrane of the stomach.

A microscopic view of the glandular membrane which lines the stomach and produces gastric juice. Arrow points to a "parietal cell" which produces hydrochloric acid.

A high magnification of some of the gland cells in the lining of the stomach. The large, conspicuous cells are the "parietal cells" which produce hydrochloric acid.

A low-power microscopic view of the lining membrane of the stomach showing an area in which an ulcer has developed.

A microscopic view of a portion of the glandular lining of the stomach which has become involved by a malignant tumor.

A microscopic view of the elaborate membrane lining the normal small intestine. The fingerlike extensions are called villi.

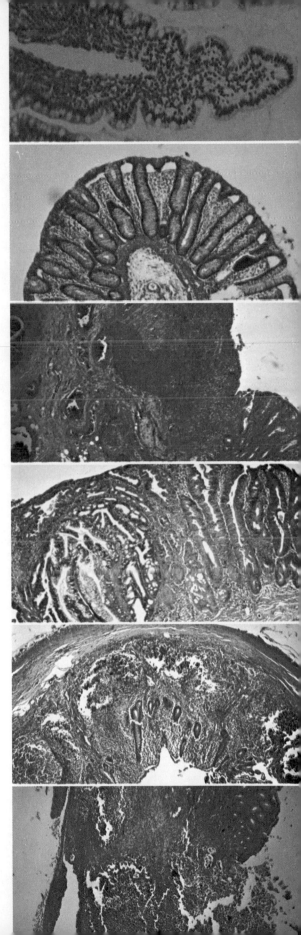

A high magnification of the villi which occur in the lining of the small intestine. Many of the cells covering a villus secrete mucus. At the center of each villus is a lacteal vessel which carries away the fatty component of the food as it is absorbed.

A low-power microscopic view of a fold of the mucosa lining the normal large intestine. Many tube-shaped glands are present.

A low-power microscopic view of the large intestine in a case of ulcerative colitis. Notice that a portion of the glandular lining has been destroyed.

A microscopic view of a beginning carcinoma in the large intestine. As yet the malignant tumor has not invaded the adjacent deeper tissues and is therefore called a "carcinoma in situ."

A low-power microscopic view of a sector of the wall of a normal appendix.

A microscopic view of a portion of the wall of the appendix in a case of acute appendicitis. The tissue is inflamed and fragile.

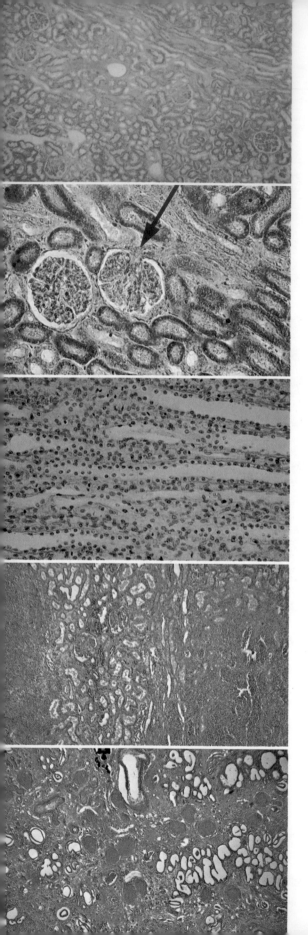

A low-power microscopic view of the cortical region of a normal kidney showing both glomeruli and tubules.

A high magnification of the cortical region of normal kidney tissue. The arrow points to that part of a glomerulus at which the tiny blood vessels enter and leave.

A microscopic view of the medullary region of a normal kidney showing the minute parallel tubules.

A microscopic view of kidney tissue in active pyelonephritis.

A microscopic view of kidney tissue in chronic glomerulonephritis.

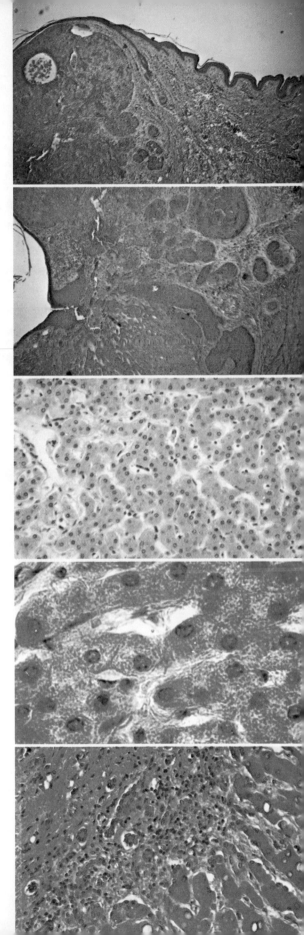

A microscopic view of thin skin in which there is a beginning basal cell carcinoma (skin cancer) at the left.

A microscopic view of a portion of a basal cell carcinoma of the skin showing how the cell groups of this tumor tend to invade the deeper dermal tissues.

A microscopic view of normal liver tissue. During life the cords of liver cells are bathed by the blood which routinely passes through the liver.

A high-power microscopic view of normal liver tissue showing the individual cells.

A microscopic view of liver tissue in cirrhosis. In this disease, large areas of normal tissue are replaced by dense scarlike tissue.

Photos and Illustrations

Credits for illustrations used in volume 2 of *Your and Your Health:*

Pages 4, 6, 7, 11, 12, 15, 18, 20, 26, 27, 28, 31, 35, 36, 38, 39, 42, 44, 52, 54, 57, 59, 60, 62, 65, 68, 70, 75, 88, 91, 96, 118, 121, 130, 137, 142, 145, 223, 225, 226, 232, 265, 370, 401, 443, 465, 466, 472—James Converse

Pages 80, 174—Ralph Sweet

Pages 84, 90, 100, 240, 280, 284, 291, 292, 302, 306, 318, 332, 375, 379, 533—Lester Quade

Pages 109, 245, 258, 260, 513—Howard Larkin

Pages 200, 251, 259, 376, 523—Margery Gardephe

Pages 212, 491—Joe Maniscalco

Pages 243, 270, 381, 419, 448, 451—Kelly Solis-Novarro

Page 249—Lucille Innes

Pages 324, 373, 377, 412, 448—Robert Eldridge

Page 328—Dolores Sither

Special acknowledgment is due Ciba Pharmaceutical Company for the Frank H. Netter, M.D., illustrations taken from "The Ciba Collection of Medical Illustrations"; to Lederle Laboratories for the Paul Peck illustrations taken from their "Selective Atlas of Normal Anatomy"; to the Upjohn Company, Chas. Pfizer & Co., Inc., Eli Lilly, Sandoz Pharmaceuticals, Spirt & Co., American Cancer Society, Veterans Administration, and the National Institute of Health of Atlanta, Georgia, and Bethesda, Maryland for their contributions to this volume.

General Index

GENERAL INDEX

GENERAL INDEX

GENERAL INDEX

GENERAL INDEX